W9-AAZ-476

JOHNS HOPKINS
SYMPTOMS & REMEDIES

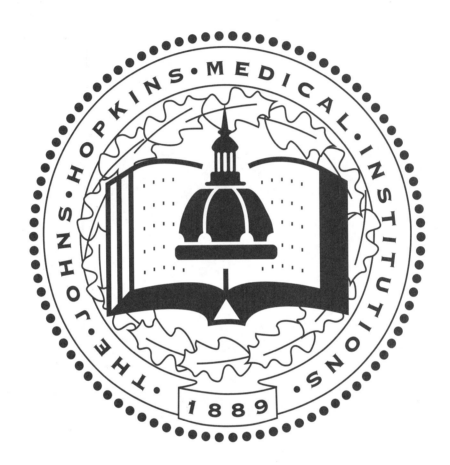

JOHNS HOPKINS

Symptoms AND Remedies

Revised and Updated New Edition

THE COMPLETE HOME
MEDICAL REFERENCE

Medical Editor
Simeon Margolis, M.D., Ph.D.

Prepared by the Editors of
The Johns Hopkins Medical Letter
HEALTH AFTER 50

REBUS • NEW YORK
DISTRIBUTED BY RANDOM HOUSE

THE JOHNS HOPKINS MEDICAL LETTER
HEALTH AFTER 50

JOHNS HOPKINS SYMPTOMS AND REMEDIES *is published in association with* THE JOHNS HOPKINS MEDICAL LETTER HEALTH AFTER 50. *This monthly eight-page newsletter provides practical, timely information for anyone concerned with taking control of his or her own health care. The newsletter is written in clear, nontechnical, easy-to-understand language and comes from the century-old tradition of Johns Hopkins excellence. For information on how to subscribe to this newsletter, please write to Medletter Associates, Inc., Department 1106, 632 Broadway, New York, New York 10012.*

This book is not intended as a substitute for the advice of a physician. Readers who suspect they may have specific medical problems should consult a physician about any suggestions made in this book.

Revised and Updated New Edition
Copyright © 1999 Medletter Associates, Inc.

All rights reserved.
No part of this book may be reproduced or transmitted in any form or by any means, electronic, mechanical, photocopying, recording, or otherwise, without the prior written permission of the publisher.

For information about permission to reproduce selections from this book,
write to Permissions, Medletter Associates, Inc., 632 Broadway, New York, New York 10012.

Johns Hopkins was ranked America's best overall medical center in a survey conducted by *U.S. News & World Report*, published July 27, 1998.

Library of Congress Cataloging-in-Publication Data

Johns Hopkins symptoms and remedies: the complete home medical reference / medical editor, Simeon Margolis; prepared by the editors of the Johns Hopkins medical letter health after 50.—Rev. and updated new ed.
p. cm.
Includes index.
ISBN 0-929661-52-4 (HARDCOVER)
1. Medicine, Popular—Handbooks, manuals, etc. 2. Symptomatology—Handbooks, manuals, etc.
I. Margolis, Simeon, 1931- . II. Johns Hopkins Medical Institutions. III. Johns Hopkins medical letter health after 50. IV. Title: Symptoms and remedies.
  [DNLM: 1. Medicine—handbooks. 2. Self Medication—methods—handbooks.]
RC81.J66 1999
616.02'4—dc21
DNLM/DLC
for Library of Congress   99-19107
                              CIP

Printed in the United States of America
10 9 8 7 6 5 4 3 2 1
Distributed by Random House, Inc.

**Johns Hopkins Medical Books
are published under the auspices of
The Johns Hopkins Medical Letter
HEALTH AFTER 50.**

RODNEY FRIEDMAN
Editor and Publisher

EVAN HANSEN
Executive Editor

PATRICE BENNEWARD
Senior Writer

NATASHA RAYMOND
Managing Editor

TINA PAVANE, R.N.
Medical Researcher

TOM R. DAMRAUER, M.L.S.
Chief of Information Resources

ELLEN TULCHINSKY, M.L.S.
Librarian

LESLIE MALTESE–McGILL
Copy Editor

———————

HELEN MULLEN
Circulation Director

BARBARA MAXWELL O'NEILL
Associate Publisher

DAVID ALEXANDER
Circulation Manager

JERRY LOO
Product Manager

DEBORAH BOYER
Promotions Manager

LISA NATOLI
Special Sales

Johns Hopkins Symptoms and Remedies

EVAN HANSEN
Editorial Director

EDWARD PETONIAK
Executive Editor

JEREMY D. BIRCH
Managing Editor

TIMOTHY JEFFS
Art Director

YOHEVED GERTZ
Designer

JOHN P. LYNCH
Assistant Editor

CARNEY W. MIMMS III
Production Database Designer

JOHN VASILIADIS
Production Database Programmer

ROBERT DUCKWALL
Medical Illustrator

KIMBERLY GRIEGER
DONALD HOMOLKA
Copy Editors

The Johns Hopkins Medical Institutions
Baltimore, Maryland 21205

MEDICAL EDITOR

SIMEON MARGOLIS, M.D., PH.D.
Professor, Medicine & Biological Chemistry

EDITORIAL BOARD OF ADVISORS

MARTIN D. ABELOFF, M.D.
Professor, Oncology
Director, Oncology Center

BARBARA DE LATEUR, M.D.
Professor & Director
Physical Medicine & Rehabilitation

JOHN A. FLYNN, M.D.
Assistant Professor, Medicine
Clinical Director, Division of General Internal Medicine

LINDA P. FRIED, M.D., M.P.H.
Professor, Medicine & Epidemiology
Director, Center on Aging & Health

H. FRANKLIN HERLONG, M.D.
Associate Dean, School of Medicine
Associate Professor, Medicine

KEITH D. LILLEMOE, M.D.
Professor & Vice-Chairman, Surgery

PETER RABINS, M.D.
Professor, Psychiatry
Director, Division of Geriatric & Neuropsychiatry

ANDREW P. SCHACHAT, M.D.
Professor, Ophthalmology
Director, Retinal Vascular Center

EDWARD E. WALLACH, M.D.
Professor, Gynecology & Obstetrics

PATRICK C. WALSH, M.D.
Professor & Chairman, Urology

JAMES WEISS, M.D.
Professor, Medicine
Cardiology Division

OFFICE OF COMMUNICATIONS &
PUBLIC AFFAIRS

ELAINE FREEMAN
Executive Director

JOANN RODGERS
Deputy Director

KRISTIN BRUNNWORTH
Editorial Assistant

How to use this book

This book is divided into two distinct sections: The first is a collection of charts, each of which covers a specific symptom and indicates one or more of the disorders commonly associated with it. You can then look up any one of these potential diagnoses in the second half of the book, which provides a comprehensive explanation of each disorder, what to do about it, whether or not you can treat it yourself (and how), and when to call a doctor.

Suppose, for example, that you are suffering from eye pain. When you look this up in the symptoms charts, you find 17 possible diagnoses listed. However, you see that only eight of these also involve the associated symptom "with eye discharge or excessive tearing," which, in your case, is applicable. After reading the distinguishing features of each of these eight disorders, you determine that perhaps only three of them produce a profile of symptoms that resembles your own. You may then refer to the Disorders section to read more about these ailments—and to help you determine what to do next. (This book is not, however, intended as a substitute for the advice and expertise of a physician. Readers should always consult a doctor about any suggestions made in these pages.) The Disorder section can also serve as a valuable resource when you already know the diagnosis and simply want more information.

SYMPTOMS

In this section of the book, you will find charts covering a wide range of common symptoms. These charts are designed to help you narrow down the number of disorders that may be associated with a given symptom. You can then find further information on any potential diagnosis in the Disorder section. Please bear in mind, however, that these charts are not intended to establish a definitive diagnosis—only your doctor can do that after performing a physical examination and conducting the appropriate tests. Indeed, some of the less common disorders that can cause a specific symptom may not be covered in this book, and some symptoms (such as dry skin, for example) may develop even when no underlying disease is involved.

THE EDITORS

Abdominal pain

Associated Symptoms	Possible Diagnosis	Distinguishing Features
	Amyloidosis *Accumulation of amyloid, a waxy substance, in tissues and organs*	Symptoms vary greatly depending on the body parts affected and may include fatigue and weakness; weight loss; heart palpitations; shortness of breath; swelling of the legs; difficulty swallowing due to swelling of the tongue; diarrhea; abdominal pain; raised spots on the armpits, groin, face, and neck; numbness or tingling of the hands or feet; dizziness on standing; joint pains.
	Appendicitis, acute	Pain near the navel, spreading to the lower right abdomen; nausea and vomiting; constipation; possibly diarrhea; low-grade fever; loss of appetite.
	Cirrhosis *Chronic damage to the cells of the liver*	No symptoms in early stages; loss of weight and appetite; nausea; swollen legs, ankles and abdomen; itching; jaundice; black stools; vomiting blood; fatigue; impotence; memory loss; confusion.
	Colitis, ulcerative *Inflammation of the lining of the colon*	Pain on the left side of the abdomen that lessens after bowel movements; bloody diarrhea; pain in the rectal area; possibly, fever, rapid heartbeat, nausea and vomiting, loss of appetite, dehydration with severe attacks.
	Colon Polyps	Rectal bleeding; blood in the stool; abdominal pain; change in bowel habits.
	Crohn's disease *Inflammation of the lining of the small intestine*	Episodes of abdominal pain or cramps in lower abdomen; nausea; diarrhea; loss of weight and appetite; possibly, fever; rectal bleeding or blood in stools; fatigue; anal fissures; joint pains; inflammation of the eyes.
	Diarrhea, acute	Loose, watery stools; increased frequency of bowel movements; abdominal cramping and pain. In infants, possibly drowsiness, slack skin, dry, sticky mouth and tongue, or persistent crying.
	Diverticular disorders *Swellings in the wall of the colon*	Usually no symptoms unless diverticulae become inflamed. Tenderness or pain in the lower left abdomen relieved by passing stools or gas; constipation or diarrhea; blood in the stool; severe, spasmodic abdominal pain that becomes constant; possibly, fever and nausea.
	Dysentery, bacillary	Watery diarrhea that may contain mucus or blood; rectal pain upon defecation; abdominal pain; rapid dehydration and weight loss; nausea and vomiting.
	Food poisoning	Symptoms vary greatly depending on the type and extent of poisoning and may include nausea, vomiting, diarrhea, bloody stools, abdominal pain, and collapse.

Abdominal pain *continued*

Associated Symptoms	Possible Diagnosis	Distinguishing Features
	Gallbladder disorders	Moderate to severe pain in the upper right side of the abdomen, chest, upper back, or right shoulder. Pain often follows the ingestion of high-fat foods and is episodic, lasting 20 minutes to several hours. Nausea and vomiting; low-grade fever; belching; heartburn; gas; possibly, jaundice, pale stools, and itchy skin.
	Hepatitis, acute viral	Fever; fatigue; loss of appetite; aching muscles and joints; abdominal pain or discomfort; jaundice; dark urine and pale stools.
	Hepatitis, chronic	Fatigue; nausea; vomiting; loss of appetite; jaundice; dark urine; clay-colored stools; depression; pain or discomfort in the upper right abdomen; abdominal swelling; fever; in women, cessation of menstruation, acne, and the appearance of male pattern facial hair.
	Intestinal obstruction	Abdominal pain and cramps; nausea; vomiting; weakness; gas; bloating; possible diarrhea; progressive constipation culminating in inability to pass stools or gas.
	Irritable bowel syndrome	Cramps in the middle or to one side of the lower abdomen that are usually relieved with bowel movements; nausea; bloating; gas; alternating diarrhea and constipation.
	Leukemias	Symptoms vary depending on the type of leukemia and may include: loss of appetite and weight; increased bruising and bleeding; bone pain, especially in the legs; abdominal pain and distention; nausea; heart palpitations; severe fatigue; pallor; breathing difficulty; fever; night sweats; headache; enlarged lymph nodes; joint pains (due to gout).
	Liver tumors	Pain or discomfort in the upper right portion of the abdomen; abdominal swelling; loss of weight and appetite; nausea and vomiting; fever; excessive perspiration; jaundice; pallor; severe fatigue.
	Malabsorption, digestive *A failure of the small intestine to absorb nutrients in the diet*	Diarrhea; weight loss; yellowish, foul-smelling stools; abdominal cramps, gas, and bloating; weakness and lethargy.
	Myelofibrosis *An increase of fibrous scar tissue within the bone marrow*	Weakness and fatigue; abdominal fullness; a tendency to bleed easily; bone pain; pallor; shortness of breath during physical exertion; increased susceptibility to bruising and infections; weight loss.

Abdominal pain *continued*

Associated Symptoms	Possible Diagnosis	Distinguishing Features
	Ovarian cysts	In many cases, no symptoms. Painless swelling in the lower abdomen; possibly, pain during intercourse; brown vaginal discharge; lack of or heavier than usual menstrual periods; vomiting; unusual hair growth on face or body.
	Pancreatitis *Inflammation of the pancreas*	Sudden, extreme abdominal pain; nausea and vomiting; weakness; fever; clammy skin; abdominal bloating and tenderness.
	Peritonitis *Inflammation of the abdominal membrane*	Sudden abdominal pain, rigidity, and swelling; chills and fever; weakness; rapid heartbeat; nausea and vomiting; extreme thirst; low urine output.
	Rheumatoid arthritis, juvenile	Fever; rash; abdominal pain; weight loss; swelling, stiffness, and pain in the affected joints; enlarged lymph glands; fatigue; pallor; red, painful eyes.
	Stomach cancer	Discomfort in the upper abdomen; black, tarry stools; vomiting of blood; loss of appetite and weight; vomiting after meals.
	Systemic lupus erythematosus *Inflammation of connective tissues throughout the body*	Red, blotchy, butterfly-shaped rash on the cheeks and bridge of the nose; fatigue; fever; loss of appetite and weight; nausea; joint and abdominal pain; headaches; blurred vision; increased sensitivity to sun exposure; depression; psychosis; mental confusion.
	Tapeworm infestation	Often asymptomatic. Unexplained weight loss; presence of white eggs or ribbon-like segments of worm in the stool, bedding, or clothing; symptoms of pernicious anemia.
	Testicular torsion *Twisting of the spermatic cord*	Severe pain and swelling on one side of the scrotum; skin on the scrotum may appear red or purple; lightheadedness or fainting; possibly, abdominal pain, nausea and vomiting.
with back pain	Bladder infection *Cystitis*	Burning during urination; frequent and urgent urination with only small amounts of urine passed; blood in the urine; lower abdominal pain; low-grade fever; pain during sexual intercourse and, in men, during ejaculation.
	Endometriosis *The migration of the uterine lining to other reproductive or abdominal organs*	Pain in the lower abdomen, vagina, and lower back beginning just prior to menses and intensifying after blood flow has ceased; heavy bleeding during periods; pain during intercourse; diarrhea; constipation; pain during bowel movements; bleeding from the rectum; bloody urine during menses; nausea and vomiting prior to menses; infertility.

Abdominal pain *continued*

Associated Symptoms	Possible Diagnosis	Distinguishing Features
with back pain *continued*	Kidney cancer	Blood in the urine; abdominal and lower back pain; low-grade fever; loss of weight and appetite.
	Kidney infection *Pyelonephritis*	Sudden fever and shaking chills; severe fatigue; burning and frequent urination; cloudy or bloody urine; pain in the abdomen, back, or flanks, sometimes severe; nausea and vomiting.
	Pancreatic cancer	Often, no symptoms until far advanced. Upper abdominal pain which spreads to the back; loss of weight and appetite; jaundice; nausea, vomiting, and indigestion; diarrhea; fatigue; depression.
	Pelvic inflammatory disease	Initially, lower pelvic pain; pain during intercourse; irregular menstrual bleeding; vaginal discharge with abnormal color or odor; low-grade fever; chills; frequent urination; fatigue; loss of appetite; later, severe abdominal pain and high fever.
	Prostate cancer	Difficulty urinating; frequent urination with decreased urine output; pain in the pelvic area and lower back; painful ejaculation or bowel movements; impotence.
	Prostatitis *Inflammation of the prostate gland*	Burning during urination; urgent and frequent urination; fever and chills; discharge from the penis; lower abdominal and back pain; blood in the urine.
	Renal calculi *Kidney stones*	Intermittent spasms of pain in the back and flanks, radiating through the lower abdomen towards the groin; nausea and vomiting; blood in the urine; urge to urinate but only small amounts of urine are passed.
	Renal failure, acute *Severe kidney failure*	Asymptomatic in early stages. Possibly, mental confusion; shortness of breath; abdominal pain; decreased sex drive; fatigue; muscle and bone pain; numbness in the legs and feet; headache; impaired mental acuity; bad breath.
with chest pain	Aortic aneurysm *A sac-like ballooning at a weak spot in the wall of the aorta, the body's primary artery*	Usually asymptomatic; occasionally, severe abdominal and back pain; chest pain; swallowing difficulty; dizziness and fainting; hoarseness; cough.
	Congestive heart failure	Shortness of breath; fatigue; need to sleep on several pillows; weakness; cough; heart palpitations; swelling in the legs, ankles, and abdomen; frequent urination at night; indigestion; nausea and vomiting; loss of appetite.

Abdominal pain *continued*

Associated Symptoms	Possible Diagnosis	Distinguishing Features
with chest pain *continued*	Peptic ulcer	Intermittent, burning or gnawing pain in the upper abdomen or lower chest; indigestion; loss of appetite and weight. Pain may be relieved by eating or antacids. Possible nausea and vomiting. Black, tarry stools, vomiting blood.
	Pleurisy *Inflammation of the membranes lining the lungs and chest cavity*	Sudden chest pain worse on inspiration that may also radiate into the shoulder or abdomen; rapid breathing; coughing; sneezing; possibly, fever.
	Pneumothorax *Accumulation of air between the two membranes lining the lungs and the chest cavity*	Chest pain that may radiate into the abdomen or shoulder; shortness of breath; dry cough.
	Uterine cancer	Heavy bleeding during menses; bleeding between menses or after intercourse; postmenopausal bleeding; abnormal vaginal discharge usually watery and blood-streaked; weight loss.

Abdominal swelling

Associated Symptoms	Possible Diagnosis	Distinguishing Features
with swollen legs/ ankles (edema)	Cirrhosis *Chronic damage to the cells of the liver*	No symptoms in early stages; loss of weight and appetite; nausea; swollen legs, ankles and abdomen; itching; jaundice; black stools; vomiting blood; fatigue; impotence; memory loss; confusion.
	Congestive heart failure	Shortness of breath; fatigue; need to sleep on several pillows; weakness; cough; heart palpitations; swelling in the legs, ankles, and abdomen; frequent urination at night; indigestion; nausea and vomiting; loss of appetite.
	Glomerulonephritis, acute *Sudden or intense inflammation of the glomeruli, tiny structures that filter blood in the kidneys*	Blood in the urine; passing only small amounts of urine; swelling of the ankles or the tissues around the eyes; shortness of breath; possibly, fatigue, nausea and vomiting, loss of appetite, headaches, back pain, fever, impaired vision.
	Glomerulonephritis, chronic *Persistent inflammation of the glomeruli, tiny structures that filter blood in the kidneys*	Blood in the urine; passing only small amounts of urine; swelling of the legs or ankles; shortness of breath; possibly, fatigue, nausea and vomiting, loss of appetite, itching, headaches, impaired vision.
	Nephrotic syndrome *Damage to the filtering units of the kidneys*	Swelling in the ankles and around the eyes; weight gain, due to fluid retention throughout the body; shortness of breath; passing only small amounts of urine that has an unusually foamy appearance; fatigue; diarrhea; loss of appetite.
	Pericarditis *Inflammation of the membrane surrounding the heart*	Sharp chest pain that may spread to the neck and shoulders; pain may be relieved by sitting up and leaning forward; swollen legs and abdomen; breathing difficulty; chills; fever; fatigue.
	Renal failure, acute *Severe kidney failure*	Initially, decreased urine output, weight gain and swelling due to edema, loss of appetite, nausea and vomiting, fatigue. If untreated, confusion, seizures, and drowsiness.
	Renal failure, chronic *Persistent, mild kidney failure*	Asymptomatic in early stages. Possibly, mental confusion; shortness of breath; abdominal pain; decreased sex drive; fatigue; muscle and bone pain; numbness in the legs and feet; headache; impaired mental acuity; bad breath.
without swollen legs/ankles	Appendicitis, acute	Pain near the navel, spreading to the lower right abdomen; nausea and vomiting; constipation; possibly diarrhea; low-grade fever; loss of appetite.

Abdominal swelling *continued*

Associated Symptoms	Possible Diagnosis	Distinguishing Features
without swollen legs/ankles *continued*	Colitis, ulcerative *Inflammation of the lining of the colon*	Pain on the left side of the abdomen that lessens after bowel movements; bloody diarrhea; pain in the rectal area; possibly, fever, rapid heartbeat, nausea and vomiting, loss of appetite, dehydration with severe attacks.
	Constipation, chronic	Infrequent and possibly painful bowel movements; straining during bowel movements; hard, dry stool; abdominal swelling; continued sensation of fullness after evacuating bowels.
	Diverticular disorders *Swellings in the wall of the colon*	Usually no symptoms unless diverticulae become inflamed. Tenderness or pain in the lower left abdomen relieved by passing stools or gas; constipation or diarrhea; blood in the stool; severe, spasmodic abdominal pain that becomes constant; possibly, fever and nausea.
	Gallbladder disorders	Moderate to severe pain in the upper right side of the abdomen, chest, upper back, or right shoulder. Pain often follows the ingestion of high-fat foods and is episodic, lasting 20 minutes to several hours. Nausea and vomiting; low-grade fever; belching; heartburn; gas; possibly, jaundice, pale stools, and itchy skin.
	Hepatitis, chronic	Fatigue; nausea; vomiting; loss of appetite; jaundice; dark urine; clay-colored stools; depression; pain or discomfort in the upper right abdomen; abdominal swelling; fever; in women, cessation of menstruation, acne, and the appearance of male pattern facial hair.
	Intestinal obstruction	Abdominal pain and cramps; nausea; vomiting; weakness; gas; bloating; possible diarrhea; progressive constipation culminating in inability to pass stools or gas.
	Irritable bowel syndrome	Cramps in the middle or to one side of the lower abdomen that are usually relieved with bowel movements; nausea; bloating; gas; alternating diarrhea and constipation.
	Kidney cancer	Blood in the urine; abdominal and lower back pain; low-grade fever; loss of weight and appetite.
	Lactose intolerance *Difficulty digesting milk and dairy products*	Abdominal cramps; diarrhea; nausea; bloating; flatulence.

Abdominal swelling *continued*

Associated Symptoms	Possible Diagnosis	Distinguishing Features
without swollen legs/ankles *continued*	Leukemias	Symptoms vary depending on the type of leukemia and may include: loss of appetite and weight; increased bruising and bleeding; bone pain, especially in the legs; abdominal pain and distention; nausea; heart palpitations; severe fatigue; pallor; breathing difficulty; fever; night sweats; headache; enlarged lymph nodes; joint pains (due to gout).
	Liver tumors	Pain or discomfort in the upper right portion of the abdomen; abdominal swelling; loss of weight and appetite; nausea and vomiting; fever; excessive perspiration; jaundice; pallor; severe fatigue.
	Megacolon, toxic *Distention of the colon*	Severe constipation; abdominal bloating; loss of weight and appetite; possible diarrhea; in newborns, failure to pass a stool within 48 hours after birth; in children, slow growth from infancy to age five.
	Mesenteric ischemia *A blood clot blocking blood flow to the intestine*	Severe abdominal cramping, usually around the navel, that is exacerbated by eating and alleviated by fasting. Possibly, bloody stools.
	Ovarian cancer	Often asymptomatic until widespread. Possibly, abdominal swelling or discomfort, nausea, and vomiting. In advanced stages, excessive hair growth, unexplained weight loss, abnormal menstrual bleeding or post-menopausal bleeding; urinary frequency.
	Ovarian cysts	In many cases, no symptoms. Painless swelling in the lower abdomen; possibly, pain during intercourse; brown vaginal discharge; lack of or heavier than usual menstrual periods; vomiting; unusual hair growth on face or body.
	Peritonitis *Inflammation of the abdominal membrane*	Sudden abdominal pain, rigidity, and swelling; chills and fever; weakness; rapid heartbeat; nausea and vomiting; extreme thirst; low urine output.

Agitation

Associated Symptoms	Possible Diagnosis	Distinguishing Features
	Alzheimer's disease	Symptoms vary greatly in different individuals. Initially, minor forgetfulness gradually developing into severe, short-term memory loss, disorientation, an inability to concentrate, and sudden mood and personality changes. In later stages, severe confusion, possible hallucinations or paranoid delusions, loss of social and sexual inhibitions, impaired judgment, anxiety, depression, agitation and combativeness, wandering and getting lost, inability to write, urinary and fecal incontinence.
	Bipolar disorder *Manic-depressive illness*	Symptoms vary depending on phase of the disorder; mania: inflated self-esteem, elation, euphoria, grandiosity, increased activity, and a decreased need for sleep; depression: persistent feelings of sadness, apathy, or hopelessness; diminished interest in activities; loss of appetite and weight or unusual increase in appetite and weight; insomnia or drowsiness; difficulty concentrating; agitation in older patients.
	Depression	Persistent feelings of sadness, apathy, or hopelessness; diminished interest in activities; loss of or unusual increase in appetite and weight; insomnia or drowsiness; difficulty concentrating; agitation.
	Hypoglycemia *Low blood sugar*	Anxiety; hunger; trembling; headache; palpitations; perspiration; confusion; irritability; loss of coordination; possibly, double vision, seizures, or coma.
	Rabies	Low-grade fever; headache; loss of appetite; difficulty swallowing; tingling at site of animal bite; intense thirst exacerbated by the inability to drink without violent, painful throat spasms; paralysis of facial muscles; drooling. Agitation and violent behavior, confusion, convulsions, coma.
	Renal failure, chronic *Persistent, mild kidney failure*	Asymptomatic in early stages. Possibly, mental confusion; shortness of breath; abdominal pain; decreased sex drive; fatigue; muscle and bone pain; numbness in the legs and feet; headache; impaired mental acuity; bad breath.
	Schizophrenia	Delusions; hallucinations; rambling, nonsensical, or minimal speech; extremely disorganized behavior; inappropriate emotional responses or emotional detachment; lack of willful movement.
	Septic shock *Severe drop in blood pressure due to the presence of microorganisms or their toxins in the bloodstream*	Nausea and vomiting; prostration; diarrhea; sudden high fever; chills; rapid breathing; mental confusion or agitation; decreased urine output; severe fatigue; rapid heartbeat.

Ankle pain

Associated Symptoms	Possible Diagnosis	Distinguishing Features
	Ankylosing spondylitis *Inflammation of the joints between the spine and the pelvis*	Initially, pain and stiffness in the lower back and hips that becomes worse after resting; neck or chest pain; possible pain in the hip, knee, and ankle joints; pain in the heel of the foot; eye pain; blurred vision.
	Bone cancer	Pain, tenderness, and swelling in the affected bones and joints, often intensifying at night; a noticeable tumor or mass; increased susceptibility to bone fractures.
	Bursitis *Inflammation of the bursas, the lubricant-filled sacs in and around the joints*	Pain and swelling around a joint, usually the elbow, knee, or shoulder; painful movement in the affected joint; possibly, fever.
	Dislocations/subluxations	Deformity of the affected joint; joint pain and tenderness; difficulty moving a joint; swelling and stiffness within 30 minutes after joint injury.
	Gout	Most commonly affects the joints of the big toe. Affected joints are red, swollen, hot, and severely painful. In late stages, joint deformity. Kidney stones.
	Infectious arthritis	Pain, swelling, stiffness, and redness, usually in one joint. Fever. Severity varies from a mild ache to severe, debilitating pain and eventual joint deformity.
	Osteoarthritis *Degeneration of the cartilage that lines the joints*	Pain, swelling, and stiffness in one or more joints; enlargement and distortion of affected joints.
	Osteomalacia and Rickets *Softening and weakening of the bones, usually due to poor calcification*	Bone pain, especially in the neck, legs, hips and ribs. Muscle weakness, numbness, or spasms in the hands, feet, and throat; increased susceptibility to bone fractures.
	Peripheral vascular disease *Narrowing of blood vessels in the legs or arms*	Muscle pain on one or both legs that occurs with exercise and subsides with rest; possible pain in the fingers, arms, buttocks, lower back, or the arch of the foot; impotence. Severe symptoms include: muscle pain at rest that intensifies at night; discolored or blue toes; open sores; cold or numb feet; heightened sensitivity to cold; weak or absent pulse in the affected limb; scaly or hairless skin over the affected area.
	Rheumatoid arthritis	Fatigue and weakness; joint pain, stiffness, and inflammation, especially in the hands, feet, and arms; joint deformity; dry mouth; dry, painful eyes. Morning stiffness.

Ankle pain *continued*

Associated Symptoms	Possible Diagnosis	Distinguishing Features
	Rheumatoid arthritis, juvenile	Fever; rash; abdominal pain; weight loss; swelling, stiffness, and pain in the affected joints; enlarged lymph glands; fatigue; pallor; red, painful eyes.
	Sprains and strains	Swelling, pain or tenderness in the affected joints; impaired joint function.
	Tendinitis *Inflammation of a tendon*	Pain over a tendon anywhere in the body; if involved tendon is near or part of a joint, restricted movement of the joint.

Ankles swollen Edema

Associated Symptoms	Possible Diagnosis	Distinguishing Features
with shortness of breath	Amyloidosis *Accumulation of amyloid, a waxy substance, in tissues and organs*	Symptoms vary greatly depending on the body parts affected and may include fatigue and weakness; weight loss; heart palpitations; shortness of breath; swelling of the legs; difficulty swallowing due to swelling of the tongue; diarrhea; abdominal pain; raised spots on the armpits, groin, face, and neck; numbness or tingling of the hands or feet; dizziness on standing; joint pains.
	Chronic obstructive pulmonary disease	Shortness of breath; wheezing; persistent, mucus-producing cough, especially in the morning; possibly, chest pain, swollen legs and ankles.
	Congestive heart failure	Shortness of breath; fatigue; need to sleep on several pillows; weakness; cough; heart palpitations; swelling in the legs, ankles, and abdomen; frequent urination at night; indigestion; nausea and vomiting; loss of appetite.
	Glomerulonephritis, acute *Sudden or intense inflammation of the glomeruli, tiny structures that filter blood in the kidneys*	Blood in the urine; passing only small amounts of urine; swelling of the ankles or the tissues around the eyes; shortness of breath; possibly, fatigue, nausea and vomiting, loss of appetite, headaches, back pain, fever, impaired vision.
	Glomerulonephritis, chronic *Persistent inflammation of the glomeruli, tiny structures that filter blood in the kidneys*	Blood in the urine; passing only small amounts of urine; swelling of the legs or ankles; shortness of breath; possibly, fatigue, nausea and vomiting, loss of appetite, itching, headaches, impaired vision.
	Nephrotic syndrome *Damage to the filtering units of the kidneys*	Swelling in the ankles and around the eyes; weight gain, due to fluid retention throughout the body; shortness of breath; passing only small amounts of urine that has an unusually foamy appearance; fatigue; diarrhea; loss of appetite.
	Pericarditis *Inflammation of the membrane surrounding the heart*	Sharp chest pain that may spread to the neck and shoulders; pain may be relieved by sitting up and leaning forward; swollen legs and abdomen; breathing difficulty; chills; fever; fatigue.
	Renal failure, acute *Severe kidney failure*	Initially, decreased urine output, weight gain and swelling due to edema, loss of appetite, nausea and vomiting, fatigue. If untreated, confusion, seizures, and drowsiness.
	Renal failure, chronic *Persistent, mild kidney failure*	Asymptomatic in early stages. Possibly, mental confusion; shortness of breath; abdominal pain; decreased sex drive; fatigue; muscle and bone pain; numbness in the legs and feet; headache; impaired mental acuity; bad breath.

Ankles swollen Edema *continued*

Associated Symptoms	Possible Diagnosis	Distinguishing Features
with shortness of breath *continued*	Systemic lupus erythematosus *Inflammation of connective tissues throughout the body*	Red, blotchy, butterfly-shaped rash on the cheeks and bridge of the nose; fatigue; fever; loss of appetite and weight; nausea; joint and abdominal pain; headaches; blurred vision; increased sensitivity to sun exposure; depression; psychosis; mental confusion.
without shortness of breath	Cirrhosis *Chronic damage to the cells of the liver*	No symptoms in early stages; loss of weight and appetite; nausea; swollen legs, ankles and abdomen; itching; jaundice; black stools; vomiting blood; fatigue; impotence; memory loss; confusion.
	Dislocations/subluxations	Deformity of the affected joint; joint pain and tenderness; difficulty moving a joint; swelling and stiffness within 30 minutes after joint injury.
	Gout	Most commonly affects the joints of the big toe. Affected joints are red, swollen, hot, and severely painful. In late stages, joint deformity. Kidney stones.
	Sprains and strains	Swelling, pain or tenderness in the affected joints; impaired joint function.
	Thrombophlebitis *Inflammation associated with a blood clot*	Redness, swelling, pain, and tenderness in the affected area; most often occurs in the leg; swelling of the leg; prominent superficial veins around affected area; possibly, fever.
	Varicose veins	Blue or purplish, knotted veins, usually in the legs; itching or discomfort in the affected area; swollen feet and ankles. Possible scaly skin, muscle cramps, or skin ulcers.

Anxiety

Associated Symptoms	Possible Diagnosis	Distinguishing Features
	Anxiety states	Sudden attacks of unreasonable fear and panic; rapid heartbeat or palpitations; perspiration; dry mouth; irritability; muscle tension; trembling; shortness of breath; restlessness; poor concentration; insomnia; fatigue; weakness.
	Bipolar disorder *Manic-depressive illness*	Symptoms vary depending on phase of the disorder; mania: inflated self-esteem, elation, euphoria, grandiosity, increased activity, and a decreased need for sleep; depression: persistent feelings of sadness, apathy, or hopelessness; diminished interest in activities; loss of appetite and weight or unusual increase in appetite and weight; insomnia or drowsiness; difficulty concentrating; agitation in older patients.
	Chronic obstructive pulmonary disease	Shortness of breath; wheezing; persistent, mucus-producing cough, especially in the morning; possibly, chest pain, swollen legs and ankles.
	Congestive heart failure	Shortness of breath; fatigue; need to sleep on several pillows; weakness; cough; heart palpitations; swelling in the legs, ankles, and abdomen; frequent urination at night; indigestion; nausea and vomiting; loss of appetite.
	Depression	Persistent feelings of sadness, apathy, or hopelessness; diminished interest in activities; loss of or unusual increase in appetite and weight; insomnia or drowsiness; difficulty concentrating; agitation.
	Hyperthyroidism *Overactivity of the thyroid gland*	Protruding eyes; weight loss despite increased appetite; intolerance to heat; excessive perspiration; nervousness or restlessness; possibly, swelling in the neck (goiter); palpitations; tremor; diarrhea.
	Hypoglycemia *Low blood sugar*	Anxiety; hunger; trembling; headache; palpitations; perspiration; confusion; irritability; loss of coordination; possibly, double vision, seizures, or coma.
	Myocardial infarction *Heart attack*	Sudden chest pain or pressure that may spread to the arm, shoulder and jaw; excessive perspiration; shortness of breath. Possible nausea and vomiting.
	Pheochromocytoma *Tumor in central part of the adrenal, the glands above the kidneys*	Headaches, sometimes severe; rapid heartbeat or heart palpitations; excessive perspiration; faintness, especially when standing up; chest pain; abdominal pain; constipation; weight loss; nervousness, irritability, or anxiety; mental confusion or psychosis.

Anxiety *continued*

Associated Symptoms	Possible Diagnosis	Distinguishing Features
	Pulmonary edema *An accumulation of fluid in the lungs*	Severe shortness of breath; rapid breathing; pallor; excessive perspiration; bluish nails and lips; cough with frothy sputum; wheezing; anxiety and restlessness.
	Pulmonary embolism *A blood clot traveling from legs or heart that lodges in an artery supplying the lungs*	Sudden shortness of breath and severe breathing difficulty; chest pain worse on inspiration; rapid heartbeat; cough, possibly with bloody sputum; wheezing; excessive perspiration.
	Rabies	Low-grade fever; headache; loss of appetite; difficulty swallowing; tingling at site of animal bite; intense thirst exacerbated by the inability to drink without violent, painful throat spasms; paralysis of facial muscles; drooling. Agitation and violent behavior, confusion, convulsions, coma.

Appetite loss Anorexia

Associated Symptoms	Possible Diagnosis	Distinguishing Features
	Bipolar disorder *Manic-depressive illness*	Symptoms vary depending on phase of the disorder; mania: inflated self-esteem, elation, euphoria, grandiosity, increased activity, and a decreased need for sleep; depression: persistent feelings of sadness, apathy, or hopelessness; diminished interest in activities; loss of appetite and weight or unusual increase in appetite and weight; insomnia or drowsiness; difficulty concentrating; agitation in older patients.
	Depression	Persistent feelings of sadness, apathy, or hopelessness; diminished interest in activities; loss of or unusual increase in appetite and weight; insomnia or drowsiness; difficulty concentrating; agitation.
	Hepatitis, chronic	Fatigue; nausea; vomiting; loss of appetite; jaundice; dark urine; clay-colored stools; depression; pain or discomfort in the upper right abdomen; abdominal swelling; fever; in women, cessation of menstruation, acne, and the appearance of male pattern facial hair.
	Lymphoma, Hodgkin's *Cancer of the lymph nodes and lymphoid tissue*	Painless swelling of the lymph nodes usually in the neck or armpits; loss of appetite; night sweats.
	Lymphoma, non-Hodgkin's *Cancer of the lymph nodes and lymphoid tissue*	Painless swelling of lymph nodes in the neck or groin; possible abdominal pain, vomiting of blood, headache.
	Mumps	Pain in the ear, below the ear, and in the jaw; swollen glands in the neck; headache; pain on swallowing and chewing; sore muscles; joint pain; loss of appetite. Testicular swelling and tenderness in adults.
	Renal failure, acute *Severe kidney failure*	Initially, decreased urine output, weight gain and swelling due to edema, loss of appetite, nausea and vomiting, fatigue. If untreated, confusion, seizures, and drowsiness.
	Tuberculosis	Often, asymptomatic. Possibly, low-grade fever; excessive perspiration; cough producing sputum or blood; weight loss; chronic fatigue; chest pain; shortness of breath; night sweats.
with abdominal pain	Appendicitis, acute	Pain near the navel, spreading to the lower right abdomen; nausea and vomiting; constipation; possibly diarrhea; low-grade fever; loss of appetite.

Appetite loss Anorexia *continued*

Associated Symptoms	Possible Diagnosis	Distinguishing Features
with abdominal pain *continued*	Colorectal cancer *A growth of malignant cells in the colon or rectum*	Change in bowel habits; diarrhea; constipation; narrow stools; bloody or dark stools; lower abdominal pain; bloating; cramps; gas; loss of weight and appetite; fatigue and heart palpitations due to anemia.
	Crohn's disease *Inflammation of the lining of the small intestine*	Episodes of abdominal pain or cramps in lower abdomen; nausea; diarrhea; loss of weight and appetite; possibly, fever; rectal bleeding or blood in stools; fatigue; anal fissures; joint pains; inflammation of the eyes.
	Hepatitis, acute viral	Fever; fatigue; loss of appetite; aching muscles and joints; abdominal pain or discomfort; jaundice; dark urine and pale stools.
	Kidney cancer	Blood in the urine; abdominal and lower back pain; low-grade fever; loss of weight and appetite.
	Leukemias	Symptoms vary depending on the type of leukemia and may include: loss of appetite and weight; increased bruising and bleeding; bone pain, especially in the legs; abdominal pain and distention; nausea; heart palpitations; severe fatigue; pallor; breathing difficulty; fever; night sweats; headache; enlarged lymph nodes; joint pains (due to gout).
	Liver tumors	Pain or discomfort in the upper right portion of the abdomen; abdominal swelling; loss of weight and appetite; nausea and vomiting; fever; excessive perspiration; jaundice; pallor; severe fatigue.
	Megacolon, toxic *Distention of the colon*	Severe constipation; abdominal bloating; loss of weight and appetite; possible diarrhea; in newborns, failure to pass a stool within 48 hours after birth; in children, slow growth from infancy to age five.
	Mesenteric ischemia *A blood clot blocking blood flow to the intestine*	Severe abdominal cramping, usually around the navel, that is exacerbated by eating and alleviated by fasting. Possibly, bloody stools.
	Pancreatic cancer	Often, no symptoms until far advanced. Upper abdominal pain which spreads to the back; loss of weight and appetite; jaundice; nausea, vomiting, and indigestion; diarrhea; fatigue; depression.
	Pelvic inflammatory disease	Initially, lower pelvic pain; pain during intercourse; irregular menstrual bleeding; vaginal discharge with abnormal color or odor; low-grade fever; chills; frequent urination; fatigue; loss of appetite; later, severe abdominal pain and high fever.

Appetite loss Anorexia *continued*

Associated Symptoms	Possible Diagnosis	Distinguishing Features
with abdominal pain *continued*	Stomach cancer	Discomfort in the upper abdomen; black, tarry stools; vomiting of blood; loss of appetite and weight; vomiting after meals.
	Tapeworm infestation	Often asymptomatic. Unexplained weight loss; presence of white eggs or ribbon-like segments of worm in the stool, bedding, or clothing; symptoms of pernicious anemia.
with headache	Anemia, folic acid deficiency	Fatigue and weakness; pallor; shortness of breath, heart palpitations, or noticeably rapid heartbeat on exertion; sore, red, and glazed looking tongue; loss of weight and appetite; nausea and diarrhea; abdominal distention.
	Anemia, pernicious	Fatigue; inability to concentrate; sore, red tongue; weakness; dizziness; pallor; shortness of breath on exertion; palpitations; numbness and tingling in extremities; incoordination; headache; loss of weight and appetite; possibly, jaundice.
	Hydrocephalus *Overaccumulation of cerebrospinal fluid, the liquid surrounding the brain*	In infants, an enlarged head, rigidity of the legs, irritability, projectile vomiting, drowsiness, seizures, and lethargy. In older persons, headache, vomiting, loss of coordination, deterioration of mental faculties, speech difficulty, and loss of appetite.
	Influenza *Flu*	Chills, muscle aches, and loss of appetite followed by a cough, sore throat, nasal congestion, and fever; possible chest pain.
	Mononucleosis, infectious	Headache; high fever; swollen glands in the neck, groin, and armpits; severe sore throat; swallowing difficulty.
	Rabies	Low-grade fever; headache; loss of appetite; difficulty swallowing; tingling at site of animal bite; intense thirst exacerbated by the inability to drink without violent, painful throat spasms; paralysis of facial muscles; drooling. Agitation and violent behavior, confusion, convulsions, coma.
with rash/spots	AIDS *Acquired immunodeficiency syndrome*	Recurrent infections affecting the skin and respiratory system; cough; shortness of breath; loss of appetite; weight loss; fatigue; diarrhea; fever; dementia; malignant skin lesions; swollen lymph glands throughout the body; purplish skin nodules; memory loss; confusion; personality changes.
	Measles	Cough; fever; watery nasal discharge; loss of appetite; red, watering eyes; sore throat; body aches; red, slightly itchy rash that gradually spreads all over the body.

Appetite loss Anorexia *continued*

Associated Symptoms	Possible Diagnosis	Distinguishing Features
with rash/spots *continued*	Rocky Mountain spotted fever	Within a week after exposure, high fever, loss of appetite, headache, muscle aches, nausea and vomiting; dry cough; sensitivity to light. Within six days, the appearance of small pink spots on wrists and ankles, eventually spreading over the entire body, where they then grow, darken in color, and bleed.
	Sarcoidosis *Accumulation of inflammatory cells in the lymph nodes and other tissues throughout the body*	Often no symptoms. Swollen lymph nodes in the neck or armpits; muscle aches; fever; breathing difficulty; possibly, purple rash on the face; reddish or brownish skin spots on the forearms, face, or legs; numbness; joint pain or stiffness; a painful, red eye; blurred vision; loss of appetite and weight.
	Syphilis	Initially, painless, ulcerated, red sore on the genitals, mouth, or rectum; swollen glands in the neck, armpit, or groin; rash with small, red, scaly bumps; fever; headache. If left untreated, damage to heart valves leading to congestive heart failure; mental deterioration; loss of balance; seizures; dementia; personality changes.
	Systemic lupus erythematosus *Inflammation of connective tissues throughout the body*	Red, blotchy, butterfly-shaped rash on the cheeks and bridge of the nose; fatigue; fever; loss of appetite and weight; nausea; joint and abdominal pain; headaches; blurred vision; increased sensitivity to sun exposure; depression; psychosis; mental confusion.
	Typhoid fever	Headache; fever, loss of appetite; abdominal pain and tenderness; extreme weakness; constipation followed by diarrhea; drowsiness, stupor, or coma; raised, pink skin eruptions on the chest and abdomen; joint aches; sore throat.
with swollen legs/ ankles (edema)	Cirrhosis *Chronic damage to the cells of the liver*	No symptoms in early stages; loss of weight and appetite; nausea; swollen legs, ankles and abdomen; itching; jaundice; black stools; vomiting blood; fatigue; impotence; memory loss; confusion.
	Glomerulonephritis, acute *Sudden or intense inflammation of the glomeruli, tiny structures that filter blood in the kidneys*	Blood in the urine; passing only small amounts of urine; swelling of the ankles or the tissues around the eyes; shortness of breath; possibly, fatigue, nausea and vomiting, loss of appetite, headaches, back pain, fever, impaired vision.
	Glomerulonephritis, chronic *Persistent inflammation of the glomeruli, tiny structures that filter blood in the kidneys*	Blood in the urine; passing only small amounts of urine; swelling of the legs or ankles; shortness of breath; possibly, fatigue, nausea and vomiting, loss of appetite, itching, headaches, impaired vision.

Appetite loss Anorexia *continued*

Associated Symptoms	Possible Diagnosis	Distinguishing Features
with swollen legs/ ankles (edema) *continued*	Nephrotic syndrome *Damage to the filtering units of the kidneys*	Swelling in the ankles and around the eyes; weight gain, due to fluid retention throughout the body; shortness of breath; passing only small amounts of urine that has an unusually foamy appearance; fatigue; diarrhea; loss of appetite.
	Renal failure, chronic *Persistent, mild kidney failure*	Asymptomatic in early stages. Possibly, mental confusion; shortness of breath; abdominal pain; decreased sex drive; fatigue; muscle and bone pain; numbness in the legs and feet; headache; impaired mental acuity; bad breath.

Arm pain

Associated Symptoms	Possible Diagnosis	Distinguishing Features
	Bone cancer	Pain, tenderness, and swelling in the affected bones and joints, often intensifying at night; a noticeable tumor or mass; increased susceptibility to bone fractures.
	Bursitis *Inflammation of the bursas, the lubricant-filled sacs in and around the joints*	Pain and swelling around a joint, usually the elbow, knee, or shoulder; painful movement in the affected joint; possibly, fever.
	Carpal tunnel syndrome	Numbness, tingling, and pain in the hand and wrist, often intensifying at night; weakness of the fingers and hand.
	Dislocations/subluxations	Deformity of the affected joint; joint pain and tenderness; difficulty moving a joint; swelling and stiffness within 30 minutes after joint injury.
	Hypoparathyroidism *Underactivity of the parathyroid glands*	Numbness and tingling and painful, cramp-like spasms of the face, hands, arms, and feet; cataracts; possible seizures.
	Infectious arthritis	Pain, swelling, stiffness, and redness, usually in one joint. Fever. Severity varies from a mild ache to severe, debilitating pain and eventual joint deformity.
	Intervertebral disk, herniated	Severe lower back or neck pain that is exacerbated by movement or lifting heavy objects, sneezing, coughing, straining at stool. Pain, tingling, or numbness in a leg or an arm, usually on one side.
	Myocardial infarction *Heart attack*	Sudden chest pain or pressure that may spread to the arm, shoulder and jaw; excessive perspiration; shortness of breath. Possible nausea and vomiting.
	Osteoarthritis *Degeneration of the cartilage that lines the joints*	Pain, swelling, and stiffness in one or more joints; enlargement and distortion of affected joints.
	Osteomalacia and Rickets *Softening and weakening of the bones, usually due to poor calcification*	Bone pain, especially in the neck, legs, hips and ribs. Muscle weakness, numbness, or spasms in the hands, feet, and throat; increased susceptibility to bone fractures.
	Osteomyelitis *Infection of bone and bone marrow*	Fever; severe pain in the affected bone; inflammation and swelling of the skin over the affected area; deformity. In children, arrested growth of the affected bone.

Arm pain *continued*

Associated Symptoms	Possible Diagnosis	Distinguishing Features
	Peripheral vascular disease *Narrowing of blood vessels in the legs or arms*	Muscle pain on one or both legs that occurs with exercise and subsides with rest; possible pain in the fingers, arms, buttocks, lower back, or the arch of the foot; impotence. Severe symptoms include: muscle pain at rest that intensifies at night; discolored or blue toes; cold or numb feet; open sores; heightened sensitivity to cold; weak or absent pulse in the affected limb; scaly or hairless skin over the affected area.
	Rheumatoid arthritis	Fatigue and weakness; joint pain, stiffness, and inflammation, especially in the hands, feet, and arms; joint deformity; dry mouth; dry, painful eyes. Morning stiffness.
	Rotator cuff injury	Pain in the shoulder; difficulty raising and lowering the arm; recurring dull ache in the shoulder; pain after sleeping on the shoulder; shoulder weakness.
	Sprains and strains	Swelling, pain or tenderness in the affected joints; impaired joint function.
	Tendinitis *Inflammation of a tendon*	Pain over a tendon anywhere in the body; if involved tendon is near or part of a joint, restricted movement of the joint.

Back pain

Associated Symptoms	Possible Diagnosis	Distinguishing Features
with abdominal pain/discomfort	Aortic aneurysm *A sac-like ballooning at a weak spot in the wall of the aorta, the body's primary artery*	Usually asymptomatic; occasionally, severe abdominal and back pain; chest pain; swallowing difficulty; dizziness and fainting; hoarseness; cough.
	Bladder stones	Interruption of urine stream; inability to urinate except in certain positions; frequent and urgent urination with only small amounts of urine passed; blood in the urine; pain in the genitals, lower back, or abdomen; low-grade fever.
	Cervical cancer	Initially, asymptomatic. In later stages, unexpected vaginal bleeding or discharge between periods, after intercourse, or after menopause. If untreated, pelvic pain.
	Cervical disorders, non-malignant	Vaginal discharge; vaginal burning and itching; vaginal bleeding after intercourse, between periods, or after bowel movements.
	Disseminated intravascular coagulation *Bleeding disorder marked by excessive and inappropriate blood coagulation*	Abnormal bleeding possibly at several sites at once; vomiting blood; bloody or black stools; abnormal vaginal bleeding; blood in the urine; severe abdominal or back pain; possibly, convulsions, or coma.
	Endometriosis *The migration of the uterine lining to other reproductive or abdominal organs*	Pain in the lower abdomen, vagina, and lower back beginning just prior to menses and intensifying after blood flow has ceased; heavy bleeding during periods; pain during intercourse; diarrhea; constipation; pain during bowel movements; bleeding from the rectum; bloody urine during menses; nausea and vomiting prior to menses; infertility.
	Fibroids, uterine *Benign growths of the muscular wall of the uterus*	Heavier or prolonged bleeding during menses; abdominal discomfort; lower back pain; pressure on the bladder and frequent urination; constipation. Possible, sharp, sudden, lower abdominal pain.
	Gallbladder disorders	Moderate to severe pain in the upper right side of the abdomen, chest, upper back, or right shoulder. Pain often follows the ingestion of high-fat foods and is episodic, lasting 20 minutes to several hours. Nausea and vomiting; low-grade fever; belching; heartburn; gas; possibly, jaundice, pale stools, and itchy skin.
	Kidney cancer	Blood in the urine; abdominal and lower back pain; low-grade fever; loss of weight and appetite.

Back pain *continued*

Associated Symptoms	Possible Diagnosis	Distinguishing Features
with abdominal pain/discomfort *continued*	Kidney cysts	Pain or tenderness in the lower back or abdomen; blood in the urine. In infants, symmetrical, protruding masses visible in the flanks.
	Kidney infection *Pyelonephritis*	Sudden fever and shaking chills; severe fatigue; burning and frequent urination; cloudy or bloody urine; pain in the abdomen, back, or flanks, sometimes severe; nausea and vomiting.
	Pancreatitis *Inflammation of the pancreas*	Sudden, extreme abdominal pain; nausea and vomiting; weakness; fever; clammy skin; abdominal bloating and tenderness.
	Prostate cancer	Difficulty urinating; frequent urination with decreased urine output; pain in the pelvic area and lower back; painful ejaculation or bowel movements; impotence.
	Renal calculi *Kidney stones*	Intermittent spasms of pain in the back and flanks, radiating through the lower abdomen towards the groin; nausea and vomiting; blood in the urine; urge to urinate but only small amounts of urine are passed.
	Testicular cancer	Firm, usually painless mass, usually in one testicle. In later stages, a dull ache in the groin or lower abdomen may occur. Possibly, male breast development. In advanced cases, swollen lymph glands; abdominal or back pain; weight loss; breathing difficulty.
	Uterine prolapse	Often asymptomatic. Possibly, difficulty passing urine or stools, pain during intercourse, backache that intensifies when lifting, sensation of heaviness or dragging within the pelvis, painful or heavy menstrual periods, or bleeding between periods. In severe cases, uterus visibly protrudes outside of vagina.
without abdominal pain/discomfort	Ankylosing spondylitis *Inflammation of the joints between the spine and the pelvis*	Initially, pain and stiffness in the lower back and hips that becomes worse after resting; neck or chest pain; possible pain in the hip, knee, and ankle joints; pain in the heel of the foot; eye pain; blurred vision.
	Fibromyalgia	Muscle aches, pains, and stiffness; specific points on the body that feel sore when pressed; fatigue; headaches; feeling unrefreshed upon awakening in the morning.
	Hyperparathyroidism *Overactivity of the parathyroid glands*	Increased susceptibility to bone fractures; depression; indigestion; increased thirst and urine output; fatigue, lethargy; somnolence; muscle weakness; nausea and vomiting; loss of appetite; weight loss.

Back pain *continued*

Associated Symptoms	Possible Diagnosis	Distinguishing Features
without abdominal pain/discomfort *continued*	Intervertebral disk, herniated	Severe lower back or neck pain that is exacerbated by movement or lifting heavy objects, sneezing, coughing, straining at stool. Pain, tingling, or numbness in a leg or an arm, usually on one side.
	Multiple myeloma *Production of malignant plasma cells in the bone marrow*	Bone pain, especially progressive, constant back pain that intensifies with movement; unexplained bone fractures; fatigue; pallor; shortness of breath; increased bleeding, such as bleeding gums or nosebleeds; easily bruised skin; increased susceptibility to infection; headache; vision disturbances; loss of height.
	Obesity	Symptoms such as chest pain or shortness of breath from heart disease, knee or hip pain, or abdominal pain from gallstones all result from the complications of obesity.
	Osteoarthritis *Degeneration of the cartilage that lines the joints*	Pain, swelling, and stiffness in one or more joints; enlargement and distortion of affected joints.
	Osteomalacia and Rickets *Softening and weakening of the bones, usually due to poor calcification*	Bone pain, especially in the neck, legs, hips and ribs. Muscle weakness, numbness, or spasms in the hands, feet, and throat; increased susceptibility to bone fractures.
	Osteomyelitis *Infection of bone and bone marrow*	Fever; severe pain in the affected bone; inflammation and swelling of the skin over the affected area; deformity. In children, arrested growth of the affected bone.
	Osteoporosis *Loss of bone mass due to calcium depletion*	Backache; easily fractured bones, especially in the wrists, hips, and spine; gradual loss of height; stooped or hunched posture.
	Paget's disease *A weakening, thickening, and deformity of the bones*	Often asymptomatic. Possibly, bone pain or deformity, especially bowing of the legs, bent spine, and facial deformity; unexplained bone fractures; joint pain or stiffness; hearing loss; headaches; ringing in ears.
	Pelvic inflammatory disease	Initially, lower pelvic pain; pain during intercourse; irregular menstrual bleeding; vaginal discharge with abnormal color or odor; low-grade fever; chills; frequent urination; fatigue; loss of appetite; later, severe abdominal pain and high fever.
	Spinal cord trauma	Severe pain and swelling in the affected area; loss of sensation, muscle weakness, or paralysis below the site of the injury; urinary or fecal incontinence or retention; impotence; breathing difficulty; shock.

Back pain *continued*

Associated Symptoms	Possible Diagnosis	Distinguishing Features
without abdominal pain/discomfort *continued*	Spinal stenosis *Narrowing of the spinal canal due to bony overgrowth*	Numbness, pain, and weakness in the legs and back that is exacerbated by walking and alleviated by sitting.
	Spinal tumor	Progressive numbness, tingling, and muscle weakness; fecal or urinary incontinence; persistent back pain.
	Sprains and strains	Swelling, pain or tenderness in the affected joints; impaired joint function.

Bad breath Halitosis

Associated Symptoms	Possible Diagnosis	Distinguishing Features
with mouth pain	Gingivitis	Red-purple gums that are swollen, shiny, and bleed easily; bad breath.
	Impacted teeth	Gum pain; unpleasant taste in mouth, especially when biting down; red, swollen gums around the affected tooth; headache or jaw ache; possibly, bad breath.
	Periodontitis *Inflammation of the tissues supporting the teeth*	Red, swollen, painful gums that bleed easily; loose teeth; bad breath; possible pus discharge.
	Sinusitis *Inflammation of the mucous membranes lining the sinuses*	Throbbing pain above or below one or both eyes that intensifies when bending the head forward or coughing; nasal congestion; loss of sense of smell; often, pus-like nasal discharge; possible dental pain in the upper jaw; fever.
	Sjögren's syndrome	Dry, itching, burning eyes; sensation of a foreign body under the eyelids; dry mouth; difficulty swallowing; vaginal dryness; dry skin; frequent dental cavities; joint pain; swelling of glands (parotids) in front of the ears; Raynaud's phenomenon.
	Tongue disorders	Symptoms vary depending on the specific disorder and include: dark or bright red, black, or dark brown tongue; sore, swollen, or smooth tongue; hair-like growths on the tongue; adjacent areas of the mouth may be inflamed; ulcers or raised, white patches on the tongue; excessive salivation; swallowing difficulty; bad breath.
	Tooth abscess	Persistent tooth pain; pain when biting or chewing; difficulty swallowing; swollen glands in the neck; earache; fever; possibly, foul taste in the mouth or bad breath.
	Tooth decay	Tooth pain, especially after eating sweet or sour foods; tooth sensitivity to hot and cold; bad breath; unpleasant taste in the mouth.
	Trench mouth	Grayish film on the gums; red, swollen, painful, bleeding gums; bad breath; bad taste in the mouth; pain on swallowing or speaking; excessive salivation.
without mouth pain	Bronchiectasis *Lung condition that stretches and distorts the walls of the bronchial tubes*	Cough that produces dark green sputum; bad breath; possibly, shortness of breath; loss of appetite and weight; clubbed fingers.

Bad breath Halitosis *continued*

Associated Symptoms	Possible Diagnosis	Distinguishing Features
without mouth pain *continued*	Diverticular disorders *Swellings in the wall of the colon*	Usually no symptoms unless diverticulae become inflamed. Tenderness or pain in the lower left abdomen relieved by passing stools or gas; constipation or diarrhea; blood in the stool; severe, spasmodic abdominal pain that becomes constant; possibly, fever and nausea.
	Esophageal cancer	Swallowing difficulty and pain; weight loss; drooling; possibly, vomiting or coughing up of bloody mucus, regurgitation of food; chest pain; repeated respiratory infections.
	Intestinal obstruction	Abdominal pain and cramps; nausea; vomiting; weakness; gas; bloating; possible diarrhea; progressive constipation culminating in inability to pass stools or gas.
	Lung abscess	Cough producing foul-smelling sputum; bad breath; fever; chills; weight loss; possible chest pain.
	Pharyngitis *Inflammation of the pharynx, the part of the throat between the mouth and the esophagus*	Sore or red throat; speaking and swallowing difficulties; sensitive, swollen glands in the neck; fever; headache; possible earache.
	Renal failure, chronic *Persistent, mild kidney failure*	Asymptomatic in early stages. Possibly, mental confusion; shortness of breath; abdominal pain; decreased sex drive; fatigue; muscle and bone pain; numbness in the legs and feet; headache; impaired mental acuity; bad breath.

Behavior abnormalities/changes

Associated Symptoms	Possible Diagnosis	Distinguishing Features
	Adrenal insufficiency *Inadequate production of steroid hormones by the adrenal gland*	Loss of weight and appetite; fatigue; weakness; darkening of the skin; abdominal pain; diarrhea; indigestion; nausea and vomiting; constipation; lack of sex drive; dizziness when rising from sitting or lying position.
	AIDS *Acquired immunodeficiency syndrome*	Recurrent infections affecting the skin and respiratory system; cough; shortness of breath; loss of appetite; weight loss; fatigue; diarrhea; fever; dementia; malignant skin lesions; swollen lymph glands throughout the body; purplish skin nodules; memory loss; confusion; personality changes.
	Alzheimer's disease	Symptoms vary greatly in different individuals. Initially, minor forgetfulness gradually developing into severe, short-term memory loss, disorientation, an inability to concentrate, and sudden mood and personality changes. In later stages, severe confusion, possible hallucinations or paranoid delusions, loss of social and sexual inhibitions, impaired judgment, anxiety, depression, agitation and combativeness, wandering and getting lost, inability to write, urinary and fecal incontinence.
	Anemia, pernicious	Fatigue; inability to concentrate; sore, red tongue; weakness; dizziness; pallor; shortness of breath on exertion; palpitations; numbness and tingling in extremities; incoordination; headache; loss of weight and appetite; possibly, jaundice.
	Anxiety states	Sudden attacks of unreasonable fear and panic; rapid heartbeat or palpitations; perspiration; dry mouth; irritability; muscle tension; trembling; shortness of breath; restlessness; poor concentration; insomnia; fatigue; weakness.
	Bipolar disorder *Manic-depressive illness*	Symptoms vary depending on phase of the disorder; mania: inflated self-esteem, elation, euphoria, grandiosity, increased activity, and a decreased need for sleep; depression: persistent feelings of sadness, apathy, or hopelessness; diminished interest in activities; loss of appetite and weight or unusual increase in appetite and weight; insomnia or drowsiness; difficulty concentrating; agitation in older patients.
	Brain tumors	Headaches that become more severe when reclining; nausea and vomiting; memory loss; double vision; muscle weakness; numbness, tingling, or partial paralysis; vision loss; speech disturbances; seizures; drowsiness.

Behavior abnormalities/changes *continued*

Associated Symptoms	Possible Diagnosis	Distinguishing Features
	Cushing's syndrome	Red, oval-shaped face; humped upper back and obese trunk; acne; purple stretch marks on the abdomen, thighs, and breasts; thin and easily bruised skin; easily fractured bones; depression or euphoria; insomnia; fatigue; muscle weakness; hirsutism (in women).
	Depression	Persistent feelings of sadness, apathy, or hopelessness; diminished interest in activities; loss of or unusual increase in appetite and weight; insomnia or drowsiness; difficulty concentrating; agitation.
	Hydrocephalus *Overaccumulation of cerebrospinal fluid, the liquid surrounding the brain*	In infants, an enlarged head, rigidity of the legs, irritability, projectile vomiting, drowsiness, seizures, and lethargy. In older persons, headache, vomiting, loss of coordination, deterioration of mental faculties, speech difficulty, and loss of appetite.
	Hyperparathyroidism *Overactivity of the parathyroid glands*	Increased susceptibility to bone fractures; depression; indigestion; increased thirst and urine output; fatigue, lethargy; somnolence; muscle weakness; nausea and vomiting; loss of appetite; weight loss.
	Hypoglycemia *Low blood sugar*	Anxiety; hunger; trembling; headache; palpitations; perspiration; confusion; irritability; loss of coordination; possibly, double vision, seizures, or coma.
	Hypopituitarism *Underactivity of the pituitary gland*	Intolerance to cold; chronic headaches; decreased sex drive; fatigue; dizziness; fine wrinkles around the eyes and mouth; dry skin; extreme thirst and excessive urination; loss of appetite; vaginal dryness; absence of milk production in new mothers; in men, reduced muscular strength, shrinking of the testes, and loss of body hair; growth retardation in children and adolescents.
	Renal failure, acute *Severe kidney failure*	Initially, decreased urine output, weight gain and swelling due to edema, loss of appetite, nausea and vomiting, fatigue. If untreated, confusion, seizures, and drowsiness.
	Schizophrenia	Delusions; hallucinations; rambling, nonsensical, or minimal speech; extremely disorganized behavior; inappropriate emotional responses or emotional detachment; lack of willful movement.
	Stroke	Symptoms vary with the location of brain injury. Sudden onset of weakness, paralysis, or loss of sensation, usually on one side of the body; a sudden heaviness in a limb; speech abnormalities; headache; vision disturbances; dizziness; confusion; coma; urinary and fecal incontinence.

Behavior abnormalities/changes *continued*

Associated Symptoms	Possible Diagnosis	Distinguishing Features
	Syphilis	Initially, painless, ulcerated, red sore on the genitals, mouth, or rectum; swollen glands in the neck, armpit, or groin; rash with small, red, scaly bumps; fever; headache. If left untreated, damage to heart valves leading to congestive heart failure; mental deterioration; loss of balance; seizures; dementia; personality changes.
	Systemic lupus erythematosus *Inflammation of connective tissues throughout the body*	Red, blotchy, butterfly-shaped rash on the cheeks and bridge of the nose; fatigue; fever; loss of appetite and weight; nausea; joint and abdominal pain; headaches; blurred vision; increased sensitivity to sun exposure; depression; psychosis; mental confusion.
	Wilson's disease *An accumulation of copper in the liver, brain, and other tissues*	Anemia; fluid accumulation in the abdomen; vomiting blood; progressive intellectual impairment; tremor; weakness; walking difficulty; rigidity of limbs; personality changes; speech difficulties; dementia.

Belching/burping

Associated Symptoms	Possible Diagnosis	Distinguishing Features
	Colorectal cancer *A growth of malignant cells in the colon or rectum*	Change in bowel habits; diarrhea; constipation; narrow stools; bloody or dark stools; lower abdominal pain; bloating; cramps; gas; loss of weight and appetite; fatigue and heart palpitations due to anemia.
	Esophageal cancer	Swallowing difficulty and pain; weight loss; drooling; possibly, vomiting or coughing up of bloody mucus, regurgitation of food; chest pain; repeated respiratory infections.
	Esophageal stricture *Narrowing of the esophagus, the passageway from the mouth to the stomach*	Sudden or gradual decrease in the ability to swallow solid food or liquids; chest pain after eating; regurgitation of food and liquids; increased salivation; weight loss. Aspiration into lungs can cause cough, wheezing, shortness of breath.
	Gallbladder disorders	Moderate to severe pain in the upper right side of the abdomen, chest, upper back, or right shoulder. Pain often follows the ingestion of high-fat foods and is episodic, lasting 20 minutes to several hours. Nausea and vomiting; low-grade fever; belching; heartburn; gas; possibly, jaundice, pale stools, and itchy skin.
	Gastroesophageal reflux *Heartburn*	Burning sensation in the middle of the chest; pain and difficulty swallowing; slight regurgitation of stomach's contents into the mouth, especially when reclining or bending forward; mild abdominal pain.
	Peptic ulcer	Intermittent, burning or gnawing pain in the upper abdomen or lower chest; indigestion; loss of appetite and weight. Pain may be relieved by eating or antacids. Possible nausea and vomiting. Black, tarry stools, vomiting blood.

Bleeding gums

Associated Symptoms	Possible Diagnosis	Distinguishing Features
	Anemia, aplastic	Fatigue and weakness; shortness of breath; heart palpitations; pallor; bleeding gums; nosebleeds; tendency to bruise easily; small red dots under the skin (petechiae). Increased susceptibility to infection.
	Cirrhosis *Chronic damage to the cells of the liver*	No symptoms in early stages; loss of weight and appetite; nausea; swollen legs, ankles and abdomen; itching; jaundice; black stools; vomiting blood; fatigue; impotence; memory loss; confusion.
	Gingivitis	Red-purple gums that are swollen, shiny, and bleed easily; bad breath.
	Hemophilia	Profuse bleeding from minor injuries and tooth extractions; internal bleeding that may cause blood in the urine; bleeding into joints; symptoms of stroke due to intracerebral bleeding; possibly, extensive bruising.
	Leukemias	Symptoms vary depending on the type of leukemia and may include: loss of appetite and weight; increased bruising and bleeding; bone pain, especially in the legs; abdominal pain and distention; nausea; heart palpitations; severe fatigue; pallor; breathing difficulty; fever; night sweats; headache; enlarged lymph nodes; joint pains (due to gout).
	Multiple myeloma *Production of malignant plasma cells in the bone marrow*	Bone pain, especially progressive, constant back pain that intensifies with movement; unexplained bone fractures; fatigue; pallor; shortness of breath; increased bleeding, such as bleeding gums or nosebleeds; easily bruised skin; increased susceptibility to infection; headache; vision disturbances; loss of height.
	Periodontitis *Inflammation of the tissues supporting the teeth*	Red, swollen, painful gums that bleed easily; loose teeth; bad breath; possible pus discharge.
	Platelet function disorders	Minor bleeding in the mouth or just beneath the surface of the skin, often appearing as clusters of small, pinpoint-sized red specks; frequent nosebleeds; easy bruising; prolonged menstrual periods; fatigue; pallor; dark-colored stools.
	Trench mouth	Grayish film on the gums; red, swollen, painful, bleeding gums; bad breath; bad taste in the mouth; pain on swallowing or speaking; excessive salivation.
	Von Willebrand's disease *Chronic bleeding disorder*	Frequent nosebleeds; excessive bleeding from cuts; bleeding gums; easy bruising; abnormal or excessive menstrual bleeding; blood in the stool.

Blemishes/skin discolorations

Associated Symptoms	Possible Diagnosis	Distinguishing Features
	Acne	Blackheads, whiteheads, pimples, pustules, or cysts usually on the face, chest, back, shoulders, and neck. May result in pockmarks and scarring.
	Adrenal insufficiency *Inadequate production of steroid hormones by the adrenal gland*	Loss of weight and appetite; fatigue; weakness; darkening of the skin; abdominal pain; diarrhea; indigestion; nausea and vomiting; constipation; lack of sex drive; dizziness when rising from sitting or lying position.
	AIDS *Acquired immunodeficiency syndrome*	Recurrent infections affecting the skin and respiratory system; cough; shortness of breath; loss of appetite; weight loss; fatigue; diarrhea; fever; dementia; malignant skin lesions; swollen lymph glands throughout the body; purplish skin nodules; memory loss; confusion; personality changes.
	Dermatomyositis *Inflammation of the muscles and skin*	Red rash on the neck, upper torso, and upper arms and legs; purple discoloration and swelling of the eyelids; areas of thickened skin; muscle weakness and stiffness, usually in the shoulders and pelvis; cold hands and feet; speaking or swallowing difficulty; weight loss.
	Hemochromatosis *An excess accumulation of iron in the liver, pancreas, heart, testes, skin, and other organs*	A bronze or slate-grey tone to skin that is normally fair; chronic abdominal pain; heart palpitations; joint pain; drowsiness. In men, a decrease in the size of the testes, loss of sexual desire, and impotence.
	Hepatitis, chronic	Fatigue; nausea; vomiting; loss of appetite; jaundice; dark urine; clay-colored stools; depression; pain or discomfort in the upper right abdomen; abdominal swelling; fever; in women, cessation of menstruation, acne, and the appearance of male pattern facial hair.
	Oral herpes *Cold sores*	Initially, a tingling sensation or discomfort around the mouth, followed by small, raw, open sores on outside edge of lips; scabbing of sores.
	Polycythemia vera *An overproduction of red and white blood cells and platelets*	Headache; ringing in the ears; blurred vision; flushed skin; itching; dizziness; fatigue; night sweats; frequent nose bleeds and bruises.
	Rosacea *Redness, swelling, and blemishes around the nose, cheeks, and forehead*	Facial flushing; stinging, burning, or feeling of skin pulled tight across face; bumps, blemishes, and swelling of nose and cheeks; severe swelling or enlargement of the nose.

Blemishes/skin discolorations *continued*

Associated Symptoms	Possible Diagnosis	Distinguishing Features
	Scleroderma	Shiny, tight, and hardened skin, especially on the fingers, arms, and face; hands or feet may successively turn blue, white, and red upon exposure to cold (Raynaud's phenomenon); swallowing difficulty; bloating after eating; weight loss; shortness of breath on exertion; high blood pressure; symptoms of renal failure. Possibly, heartburn, muscle aches and weakness, joint pain, fever, or fatigue.
	Vitiligo *Loss of skin pigmentation*	White or abnormally pale patches of skin, usually on the face, hands, armpits, and groin.

Blood in the urine

Associated Symptoms	Possible Diagnosis	Distinguishing Features
with urinary difficulty or incontinence	Appendicitis, acute	Pain near the navel, spreading to the lower right abdomen; nausea and vomiting; constipation; possibly diarrhea; low-grade fever; loss of appetite.
	Bladder cancer	Blood in the urine; painful and frequent urination; pelvic pain; feeling of pressure in the back; persistent fever.
	Bladder infection *Cystitis*	Burning during urination; frequent and urgent urination with only small amounts of urine passed; blood in the urine; lower abdominal pain; low-grade fever; pain during sexual intercourse and, in men, during ejaculation.
	Bladder stones	Interruption of urine stream; inability to urinate except in certain positions; frequent and urgent urination with only small amounts of urine passed; blood in the urine; pain in the genitals, lower back, or abdomen; low-grade fever.
	Glomerulonephritis, acute *Sudden or intense inflammation of the glomeruli, tiny structures that filter blood in the kidneys*	Blood in the urine; passing only small amounts of urine; swelling of the ankles or the tissues around the eyes; shortness of breath; possibly, fatigue, nausea and vomiting, loss of appetite, headaches, back pain, fever, impaired vision.
	Glomerulonephritis, chronic *Persistent inflammation of the glomeruli, tiny structures that filter blood in the kidneys*	Blood in the urine; passing only small amounts of urine; swelling of the legs or ankles; shortness of breath; possibly, fatigue, nausea and vomiting, loss of appetite, itching, headaches, impaired vision.
	Kidney cysts	Pain or tenderness in the lower back or abdomen; blood in the urine. In infants, symmetrical, protruding masses visible in the flanks.
	Kidney infection *Pyelonephritis*	Sudden fever and shaking chills; severe fatigue; burning and frequent urination; cloudy or bloody urine; pain in the abdomen, back, or flanks, sometimes severe; nausea and vomiting.
	Penile cancer	Sore, ulcer, or wart-like lump on the penis, usually near the head, possibly painful; bleeding or unusual discharge from the penis. Possibly, pain during urination, or enlarged lymph nodes in the groin.
	Prostatic hyperplasia, benign *Prostate enlargement*	Slow or delayed urination; dribbling urine; the need to urinate several times during the night; possibly, pain during urination; blood in the urine.

Blood in the urine *continued*

Associated Symptoms	Possible Diagnosis	Distinguishing Features
with urinary difficulty or incontinence *continued*	Prostatitis *Inflammation of the prostate gland*	Burning during urination; urgent and frequent urination; fever and chills; discharge from the penis; lower abdominal and back pain; blood in the urine.
	Renal calculi *Kidney stones*	Intermittent spasms of pain in the back and flanks, radiating through the lower abdomen towards the groin; nausea and vomiting; blood in the urine; urge to urinate but only small amounts of urine are passed.
	Urethritis *Infection of the urethra, the passageway that drains urine from the bladder*	Frequent and painful urination; blood in the urine; yellow, pus-filled discharge; possible difficulty passing urine; urinary urgency; pain during intercourse; in men, painful ejaculation.
without urinary difficulty or incontinence	Disseminated intravascular coagulation *Bleeding disorder marked by excessive and inappropriate blood coagulation*	Abnormal bleeding possibly at several sites at once; vomiting blood; bloody or black stools; abnormal vaginal bleeding; blood in the urine; severe abdominal or back pain; possibly, convulsions, or coma.
	Endometriosis *The migration of the uterine lining to other reproductive or abdominal organs*	Pain in the lower abdomen, vagina, and lower back beginning just prior to menses and intensifying after blood flow has ceased; heavy bleeding during periods; pain during intercourse; diarrhea; constipation; pain during bowel movements; bleeding from the rectum; bloody urine during menses; nausea and vomiting prior to menses; infertility.
	Hemophilia	Profuse bleeding from minor injuries and tooth extractions; internal bleeding that may cause blood in the urine; bleeding into joints; symptoms of stroke due to intracerebral bleeding; possibly, extensive bruising.
	Kidney cancer	Blood in the urine; abdominal and lower back pain; low-grade fever; loss of weight and appetite.
	Renal vein thrombosis *Blood clot in the vein leaving the kidney*	Severe lower back and flank pain, swelling of legs and face from edema.
	Systemic lupus erythematosus *Inflammation of connective tissues throughout the body*	Red, blotchy, butterfly-shaped rash on the cheeks and bridge of the nose; fatigue; fever; loss of appetite and weight; nausea; joint and abdominal pain; headaches; blurred vision; increased sensitivity to sun exposure; depression; psychosis; mental confusion.

Bloody sputum

Associated Symptoms	Possible Diagnosis	Distinguishing Features
with fever	Bronchitis, acute	Shortness of breath; persistent cough producing yellow or green sputum; possibly, chest pain; wheezing; fever.
	Legionnaire's disease	Dry cough progressing to one with blood-streaked sputum; high fever; chills; breathing difficulty; chest pain; headache; muscle aches; diarrhea; nausea; vomiting; mental confusion and disorientation.
	Lung abscess	Cough producing foul-smelling sputum; bad breath; fever; chills; weight loss; possible chest pain.
	Pneumonia	High fever; shortness of breath; cough with sputum; chest pain; fatigue.
	Systemic lupus erythematosus *Inflammation of connective tissues throughout the body*	Red, blotchy, butterfly-shaped rash on the cheeks and bridge of the nose; fatigue; fever; loss of appetite and weight; nausea; joint and abdominal pain; headaches; blurred vision; increased sensitivity to sun exposure; depression; psychosis; mental confusion.
	Tuberculosis	Often, asymptomatic. Possibly, low-grade fever; excessive perspiration; cough producing sputum or blood; weight loss; chronic fatigue; chest pain; shortness of breath; night sweats.
without fever	Aortic aneurysm *A sac-like ballooning at a weak spot in the wall of the aorta, the body's primary artery*	Usually asymptomatic; occasionally, severe abdominal and back pain; chest pain; swallowing difficulty; dizziness and fainting; hoarseness; cough.
	Bronchiectasis *Lung condition that stretches and distorts the walls of the bronchial tubes*	Cough that produces dark green sputum; bad breath; possibly, shortness of breath; loss of appetite and weight; clubbed fingers.
	Chronic obstructive pulmonary disease	Shortness of breath; wheezing; persistent, mucus-producing cough, especially in the morning; possibly, chest pain, swollen legs and ankles.
	Congestive heart failure	Shortness of breath; fatigue; need to sleep on several pillows; weakness; cough; heart palpitations; swelling in the legs, ankles, and abdomen; frequent urination at night; indigestion; nausea and vomiting; loss of appetite.
	Esophageal cancer	Swallowing difficulty and pain; weight loss; drooling; possibly, vomiting or coughing up of bloody mucus, regurgitation of food; chest pain; repeated respiratory infections.

Bloody sputum *continued*

Associated Symptoms	Possible Diagnosis	Distinguishing Features
without fever *continued*	Lung cancer	Persistent cough; wheezing; shortness of breath; chest pain; fatigue; weight loss.
	Pulmonary edema *An accumulation of fluid in the lungs*	Severe shortness of breath; rapid breathing; pallor; excessive perspiration; bluish nails and lips; cough with frothy sputum; wheezing; anxiety and restlessness.
	Pulmonary embolism *A blood clot traveling from legs or heart that lodges in an artery supplying the lungs*	Sudden shortness of breath and severe breathing difficulty; chest pain worse on inspiration; rapid heart-beat; cough, possibly with bloody sputum; wheezing; excessive perspiration.

Bluish skin/lips Cyanosis

Associated Symptoms	Possible Diagnosis	Distinguishing Features
	Anaphylaxis	Itching and hives; swelling of the eyes, lips, and tongue; weakness or faintness; tightening in the chest or throat; wheezing; shortness of breath; profuse sweating; palpitations; sudden, intense distress; feelings of impending doom; stomach cramps; nausea, vomiting, or diarrhea; bluish tinge (cyanosis) to the skin, lips, and nail beds due to oxygen insufficiency.
	Chronic obstructive pulmonary disease	Shortness of breath; wheezing; persistent, mucus-producing cough, especially in the morning; possibly, chest pain, swollen legs and ankles.
	Congestive heart failure	Shortness of breath; fatigue; need to sleep on several pillows; weakness; cough; heart palpitations; swelling in the legs, ankles, and abdomen; frequent urination at night; indigestion; nausea and vomiting; loss of appetite.
	Hypothermia *Low body temperature (below 94°)*	Shivering; pallor; puffy face; fatigue and confusion; slow, shallow breathing; muscle stiffness; normally warm areas of the body are cold; loss of consciousness.
	Pneumonia	High fever; shortness of breath; cough with sputum; chest pain; fatigue.
	Pneumothorax *Accumulation of air between the two membranes lining the lungs and the chest cavity*	Chest pain that may radiate into the abdomen or shoulder; shortness of breath; dry cough.
	Pulmonary edema *An accumulation of fluid in the lungs*	Severe shortness of breath; rapid breathing; pallor; excessive perspiration; bluish nails and lips; cough with frothy sputum; wheezing; anxiety and restlessness.

Blurred or double vision

Associated Symptoms	Possible Diagnosis	Distinguishing Features
with eye pain	Conjunctivitis *Pinkeye*	Itching and redness in the affected eye; discharge from the eye, clear or pus-filled; excessive tearing; aversion to bright lights; possibly, swollen eyelids.
	Corneal ulcers and infections	Severe eye pain; blurred vision; increased tear production; aversion to light.
	Eye cancers	Often initially asymptomatic. In later stages, gradual blurring and loss of vision, bulging eyes. Possibly, crossed eyes, change in eye color, or a tumor visible through the pupil. Painful red eye.
	Glaucoma	Often initially asymptomatic. In later stages, the symptoms of closed angle glaucoma include: the appearance of halos and rainbows around lights; dilated pupil in the affected eye; severe headache and eye pain; possibly, nausea and vomiting. Open angle glaucoma symptoms include: blurred vision and a gradual loss of peripheral vision.
	Hyphema *Blood within the eye*	Visible bleeding within the front portion of the eye in and around the iris; impaired vision.
	Optic neuritis	Sudden, partial loss of vision, usually in the central portion of the field of vision; blurred vision; pain in affected eye.
	Uveitis and iritis *Inflammation of the uvea,* *a group of structures in the* *eye including the iris*	Moderate to severe eye pain; aversion to light; redness in the eye; excessive tearing; blurred vision; spots in the field of vision.
without eye pain	Cataracts	Painless, increasingly blurred vision; appearance of halos around lights; changes in color perception; increased sensitivity to light and glare.
	Macular degeneration	Gradual loss of vision in the central portion of the field of vision, interfering with reading or any close work requiring keen near-vision; blurred vision.
	Retinal detachment	Possibly, bright flashes of light in the peripheral vision, blurred vision, shadows or blindness in part of the field of vision.
	Retinal vessel occlusion *Blockage of the retinal* *arteries and veins*	Sudden blurring or loss of vision in all or a portion of the field of vision in one eye, bleeding in the eye.

Blurred or double vision *continued*

Associated Symptoms	Possible Diagnosis	Distinguishing Features
with headache	Brain hemorrhage	Sudden loss of consciousness; sudden, severe headache; mental confusion; stiff neck; nausea and vomiting; paralysis on one side of the face or body; weakness and dizziness; loss of speech; blurred or double vision; dilated pupils.
	Concussion	Brief loss of consciousness following a blow to the head. Occasionally causes nausea and vomiting.
	Headache, migraine	Throbbing pain in the temple which spreads to the side of the head; nausea; vomiting. Pain may be preceded by blurred or impaired vision with bright spots and zig-zag patterns.
	Hyperprolactinemia *Overproduction of the hormone prolactin by the pituitary gland*	Symptoms may vary depending on gender; in women: cessation of menstrual periods, decreased menstrual flow, excess facial hair; in men: erectile dysfunction, infertility, decreased libido, enlarged breasts; in men and women: abnormal production of breast milk, headaches, decreased vision.
	Sarcoidosis *Accumulation of inflammatory cells in the lymph nodes and other tissues throughout the body*	Often no symptoms. Swollen lymph nodes in the neck or armpits; muscle aches; fever; breathing difficulty; possibly, purple rash on the face; reddish or brownish skin spots on the forearms, face, or legs; numbness; joint pain or stiffness; a painful, red eye; blurred vision; loss of appetite and weight.
	Systemic lupus erythematosus *Inflammation of connective tissues throughout the body*	Red, blotchy, butterfly-shaped rash on the cheeks and bridge of the nose; fatigue; fever; loss of appetite and weight; nausea; joint and abdominal pain; headaches; blurred vision; increased sensitivity to sun exposure; depression; psychosis; mental confusion.
with speech difficulty	Botulism	Difficulty swallowing and speaking; nausea; vomiting; blurred or double vision.
	Brain tumors	Headaches that become more severe when reclining; nausea and vomiting; memory loss; double vision; muscle weakness; numbness, tingling, or partial paralysis; vision loss; speech disturbances; seizures; drowsiness.
	Encephalitis *Inflammation of the brain*	Initially, headache and fever followed by confusion, hallucinations, and paralysis on one side of the body; memory loss; difficulty with speech and eye movements; drowsiness; possible coma or epileptic seizures; loss of hearing; sensitivity to light; stiff neck.

Blurred or double vision *continued*

Associated Symptoms	Possible Diagnosis	Distinguishing Features
with speech difficulty *continued*	Multiple sclerosis *Gradual degeneration of the protective sheaths surrounding the nerves within the brain and spinal cord*	Symptoms may appear suddenly and then disappear; persistent symptoms may take years to develop and include numbness or tingling in any part of the body, weakness in the extremities, an unsteady walk, slurred speech, urinary incontinence, fatigue, depression, temporary loss of vision, double or blurred vision, mental confusion, and memory loss.
	Myasthenia gravis *Nerve degeneration causing gradual loss of voluntary muscle control*	Drooping eyelids; double or blurred vision; muscle weakness especially in the face, throat, and neck; chewing and swallowing difficulties; possible breathing difficulty. Slurred, nasal-sounding speech.

Bone pain

Associated Symptoms	Possible Diagnosis	Distinguishing Features
	Bone cancer	Pain, tenderness, and swelling in the affected bones and joints, often intensifying at night; a noticeable tumor or mass; increased susceptibility to bone fractures.
	Infectious arthritis	Pain, swelling, stiffness, and redness, usually in one joint. Fever. Severity varies from a mild ache to severe, debilitating pain and eventual joint deformity.
	Multiple myeloma *Production of malignant plasma cells in the bone marrow*	Bone pain, especially progressive, constant back pain that intensifies with movement; unexplained bone fractures; fatigue; pallor; shortness of breath; increased bleeding, such as bleeding gums or nosebleeds; easily bruised skin; increased susceptibility to infection; headache; vision disturbances; loss of height.
	Myelofibrosis *An increase of fibrous scar tissue within the bone marrow*	Weakness and fatigue; abdominal fullness; a tendency to bleed easily; bone pain; pallor; shortness of breath during physical exertion; increased susceptibility to bruising and infections; weight loss.
	Osteomalacia and Rickets *Softening and weakening of the bones, usually due to poor calcification*	Bone pain, especially in the neck, legs, hips and ribs. Muscle weakness, numbness, or spasms in the hands, feet, and throat; increased susceptibility to bone fractures.
	Osteomyelitis *Infection of bone and bone marrow*	Fever; severe pain in the affected bone; inflammation and swelling of the skin over the affected area; deformity. In children, arrested growth of the affected bone.
	Osteoporosis *Loss of bone mass due to calcium depletion*	Backache; easily fractured bones, especially in the wrists, hips, and spine; gradual loss of height; stooped or hunched posture.
	Paget's disease *A weakening, thickening, and deformity of the bones*	Often asymptomatic. Possibly, bone pain or deformity, especially bowing of the legs, bent spine, and facial deformity; unexplained bone fractures; joint pain or stiffness; hearing loss; headaches; ringing in ears.

Bones, frequent or easy breakage

Associated Symptoms	Possible Diagnosis	Distinguishing Features
	Bone cancer	Pain, tenderness, and swelling in the affected bones and joints, often intensifying at night; a noticeable tumor or mass; increased susceptibility to bone fractures.
	Cushing's syndrome	Red, oval-shaped face; humped upper back and obese trunk; acne; purple stretch marks on the abdomen, thighs, and breasts; thin and easily bruised skin; easily fractured bones; depression or euphoria; insomnia; fatigue; muscle weakness; hirsutism (in women).
	Hyperparathyroidism *Overactivity of the parathyroid glands*	Increased susceptibility to bone fractures; depression; indigestion; increased thirst and urine output; fatigue, lethargy; somnolence; muscle weakness; nausea and vomiting; loss of appetite; weight loss.
	Multiple myeloma *Production of malignant plasma cells in the bone marrow*	Bone pain, especially progressive, constant back pain that intensifies with movement; unexplained bone fractures; fatigue; pallor; shortness of breath; increased bleeding, such as bleeding gums or nosebleeds; easily bruised skin; increased susceptibility to infection; headache; vision disturbances; loss of height.
	Osteomalacia and Rickets *Softening and weakening of the bones, usually due to poor calcification*	Bone pain, especially in the neck, legs, hips and ribs. Muscle weakness, numbness, or spasms in the hands, feet, and throat; increased susceptibility to bone fractures.
	Osteoporosis *Loss of bone mass due to calcium depletion*	Backache; easily fractured bones, especially in the wrists, hips, and spine; gradual loss of height; stooped or hunched posture.
	Paget's disease *A weakening, thickening, and deformity of the bones*	Often asymptomatic. Possibly, bone pain or deformity, especially bowing of the legs, bent spine, and facial deformity; unexplained bone fractures; joint pain or stiffness; hearing loss; headaches; ringing in ears.
	Rheumatoid arthritis	Fatigue and weakness; joint pain, stiffness, and inflammation, especially in the hands, feet, and arms; joint deformity; dry mouth; dry, painful eyes. Morning stiffness.

Breathing difficulty

Associated Symptoms	Possible Diagnosis	Distinguishing Features
with chest pain	Asthma	Shortness of breath; wheezing; cough; tightness in the chest; possibly, excessive perspiration or rapid heartbeat.
	Cardiomyopathy *Disease of the heart muscle causing a reduction in the force of heart contractions*	Fatigue; chest pain and palpitations; shortness of breath; swelling of the legs; wheezing; cough.
	Chronic obstructive pulmonary disease	Shortness of breath; wheezing; persistent, mucus-producing cough, especially in the morning; possibly, chest pain, swollen legs and ankles.
	Empyema *Collection of pus in any body cavity, usually between the membranes covering the lungs*	Chest pain exacerbated by deep inhalation; shortness of breath; dry cough; fever and chills; exhaustion; weight loss; night sweats; abdominal pain and jaundice.
	Esophageal rupture *A tear in the esophagus, the passageway from the mouth to the stomach*	Chest pain; rapid, shallow breathing; excessive perspiration; fever.
	Legionnaire's disease	Dry cough progressing to one with blood-streaked sputum; high fever; chills; breathing difficulty; chest pain; headache; muscle aches; diarrhea; nausea; vomiting; mental confusion and disorientation.
	Lung cancer	Persistent cough; wheezing; shortness of breath; chest pain; fatigue; weight loss.
	Myocardial infarction *Heart attack*	Sudden chest pain or pressure that may spread to the arm, shoulder and jaw; excessive perspiration; shortness of breath. Possible nausea and vomiting.
	Pericarditis *Inflammation of the membrane surrounding the heart*	Sharp chest pain that may spread to the neck and shoulders; pain may be relieved by sitting up and leaning forward; swollen legs and abdomen; breathing difficulty; chills; fever; fatigue.
	Pleurisy *Inflammation of the membranes lining the lungs and chest cavity*	Sudden chest pain worse on inspiration that may also radiate into the shoulder or abdomen; rapid breathing; coughing; sneezing; possibly, fever.
	Pneumonia	High fever; shortness of breath; cough with sputum; chest pain; fatigue.
	Pneumothorax *Accumulation of air between the two membranes lining the lungs and the chest cavity*	Chest pain that may radiate into the abdomen or shoulder; shortness of breath; dry cough.

Breathing difficulty *continued*

Associated Symptoms	Possible Diagnosis	Distinguishing Features
with chest pain *continued*	Pulmonary embolism *A blood clot traveling from legs or heart that lodges in an artery supplying the lungs*	Sudden shortness of breath and severe breathing difficulty; chest pain worse on inspiration; rapid heartbeat; cough, possibly with bloody sputum; wheezing; excessive perspiration.
	Tuberculosis	Often, asymptomatic. Possibly, low-grade fever; excessive perspiration; cough producing sputum or blood; weight loss; chronic fatigue; chest pain; shortness of breath; night sweats.
without chest pain	Amyloidosis *Accumulation of amyloid, a waxy substance, in tissues and organs*	Symptoms vary greatly depending on the body parts affected and may include fatigue and weakness; weight loss; heart palpitations; shortness of breath; swelling of the legs; difficulty swallowing due to swelling of the tongue; diarrhea; abdominal pain; raised spots on the armpits, groin, face, and neck; numbness or tingling of the hands or feet; dizziness on standing; joint pains.
	Amyotrophic lateral sclerosis *Progressive degeneration of nerve cells of the central nervous system*	Progressive loss of strength and coordination in the limbs; muscle twitching and cramps that begin in the hands and spread to the arms, shoulders, and legs; stiff, clumsy gait; swallowing, breathing, or speaking difficulty; weight loss; drooling; involuntary laughing or crying.
	Anaphylaxis	Itching and hives; swelling of the eyes, lips, and tongue; weakness or faintness; tightening in the chest or throat; wheezing; shortness of breath; profuse sweating; palpitations; sudden, intense distress; feelings of impending doom; stomach cramps; nausea, vomiting, or diarrhea; bluish tinge (cyanosis) to the skin, lips, and nail beds due to oxygen insufficiency.
	Botulism	Difficulty swallowing and speaking; nausea; vomiting; blurred or double vision.
	Congestive heart failure	Shortness of breath; fatigue; need to sleep on several pillows; weakness; cough; heart palpitations; swelling in the legs, ankles, and abdomen; frequent urination at night; indigestion; nausea and vomiting; loss of appetite.
	Croup *Inflammation of the air passages in children*	Barking cough; hoarseness; wheezing; possibly, breathing difficulty; chest discomfort.
	Epiglottitis *Inflammation of the epiglottis, the flap of tissue lying behind the tongue*	Sore throat; sudden fever; breathing difficulty which may become severe within hours of onset; pain or difficulty swallowing; muffled speech; hoarseness; drooling.

Breathing difficulty *continued*

Associated Symptoms	Possible Diagnosis	Distinguishing Features
without chest pain *continued*	Goiter *A swelling of the thyroid gland*	A swelling in the neck that can vary from a small lump to a huge growth. Possible breathing or swallowing difficulties. Can be associated with symptoms of hyper- or hypothyroidism.
	Jaw dislocation or fracture	Inability to close the jaw normally; painful, swollen, or numb jaw; misalignment of teeth; speaking difficulty; possible breathing difficulty.
	Leukemias	Symptoms vary depending on the type of leukemia and may include: loss of appetite and weight; increased bruising and bleeding; bone pain, especially in the legs; abdominal pain and distention; nausea; heart palpitations; severe fatigue; pallor; breathing difficulty; fever; night sweats; headache; enlarged lymph nodes; joint pains (due to gout).
	Liver tumors	Pain or discomfort in the upper right portion of the abdomen; abdominal swelling; loss of weight and appetite; nausea and vomiting; fever; excessive perspiration; jaundice; pallor; severe fatigue.
	Myasthenia gravis *Nerve degeneration causing gradual loss of voluntary muscle control*	Drooping eyelids; double or blurred vision; muscle weakness especially in the face, throat, and neck; chewing and swallowing difficulties; possible breathing difficulty. Slurred, nasal-sounding speech.
	Nephrotic syndrome *Damage to the filtering units of the kidneys*	Swelling in the ankles and around the eyes; weight gain, due to fluid retention throughout the body; shortness of breath; passing only small amounts of urine that has an unusually foamy appearance; fatigue; diarrhea; loss of appetite.
	Obesity	Symptoms such as chest pain or shortness of breath from heart disease, knee or hip pain, or abdominal pain from gallstones all result from the complications of obesity.
	Peripheral neuropathies *Degeneration of the nerves that supply the extremities*	Tingling or numbness commonly beginning in the hands and feet and gradually spreading toward the center of the body; sensitive skin; muscle weakness; possibly, pain in the hands and feet; lack of coordination; shooting pains exacerbated by touch or changes in temperature; breathing difficulty; urinary or fecal incontinence.
	Poliomyelitis *Polio*	Low fever; sore throat; headache; nausea and vomiting. In severe cases, paralysis without loss of sensation; stiff neck and back; twitching; swallowing and breathing difficulty; drooling.

Breathing difficulty *continued*

Associated Symptoms	Possible Diagnosis	Distinguishing Features
without chest pain *continued*	Pulmonary edema *An accumulation of fluid in the lungs*	Severe shortness of breath; rapid breathing; pallor; excessive perspiration; bluish nails and lips; cough with frothy sputum; wheezing; anxiety and restlessness.
	Renal failure, acute *Severe kidney failure*	Initially, decreased urine output, weight gain and swelling due to edema, loss of appetite, nausea and vomiting, fatigue. If untreated, confusion, seizures, and drowsiness.
	Sarcoidosis *Accumulation of inflammatory cells in the lymph nodes and other tissues throughout the body*	Often no symptoms. Swollen lymph nodes in the neck or armpits; muscle aches; fever; breathing difficulty; possibly, purple rash on the face; reddish or brownish skin spots on the forearms, face, or legs; numbness; joint pain or stiffness; a painful, red eye; blurred vision; loss of appetite and weight.
	Thyroid cancer	Painless lump in the front of the neck; possibly, swallowing or breathing difficulty; hoarseness or loss of voice; enlarged lymph nodes in the neck.
	Thyroid nodules	Usually painless lump in the front of the neck; possibly, breathing or swallowing difficulty.

Bruising, easy or frequent

Associated Symptoms	Possible Diagnosis	Distinguishing Features
	Anemia, aplastic	Fatigue and weakness; shortness of breath; heart palpitations; pallor; bleeding gums; nosebleeds; tendency to bruise easily; small red dots under the skin (petechiae). Increased susceptibility to infection.
	Anemia, iron deficiency	Fatigue and weakness; pallor; shortness of breath and heart palpitations on exertion; irritability or inability to concentrate; sore tongue or tiny cracks at the corners of the mouth; black, tarry or bloody stools; unusual craving for dirt, paint, or ice.
	Cirrhosis *Chronic damage to the cells of the liver*	No symptoms in early stages; loss of weight and appetite; nausea; swollen legs, ankles and abdomen; itching; jaundice; black stools; vomiting blood; fatigue; impotence; memory loss; confusion.
	Cushing's syndrome	Red, oval-shaped face; humped upper back and obese trunk; acne; purple stretch marks on the abdomen, thighs, and breasts; thin and easily bruised skin; easily fractured bones; depression or euphoria; insomnia; fatigue; muscle weakness; hirsutism (in women).
	Hemophilia	Profuse bleeding from minor injuries and tooth extractions; internal bleeding that may cause blood in the urine; bleeding into joints; symptoms of stroke due to intracerebral bleeding; possibly, extensive bruising.
	Hepatitis, acute viral	Fever; fatigue; loss of appetite; aching muscles and joints; abdominal pain or discomfort; jaundice; dark urine and pale stools.
	Hepatitis, chronic	Fatigue; nausea; vomiting; loss of appetite; jaundice; dark urine; clay-colored stools; depression; pain or discomfort in the upper right abdomen; abdominal swelling; fever; in women, cessation of menstruation, acne, and the appearance of male pattern facial hair.
	Leukemias	Symptoms vary depending on the type of leukemia and may include: loss of appetite and weight; increased bruising and bleeding; bone pain, especially in the legs; abdominal pain and distention; nausea; heart palpitations; severe fatigue; pallor; breathing difficulty; fever; night sweats; headache; enlarged lymph nodes; joint pains (due to gout).
	Liver tumors	Pain or discomfort in the upper right portion of the abdomen; abdominal swelling; loss of weight and appetite; nausea and vomiting; fever; excessive perspiration; jaundice; pallor; severe fatigue.

Bruising, easy or frequent *continued*

Associated Symptoms	Possible Diagnosis	Distinguishing Features
	Lymphoma, Hodgkin's *Cancer of the lymph nodes and lymphoid tissue*	Painless swelling of the lymph nodes usually in the neck or armpits; loss of appetite; night sweats.
	Lymphoma, non-Hodgkin's *Cancer of the lymph nodes and lymphoid tissue*	Painless swelling of lymph nodes in the neck or groin; possible abdominal pain, vomiting of blood, headache.
	Multiple myeloma *Production of malignant plasma cells in the bone marrow*	Bone pain, especially progressive, constant back pain that intensifies with movement; unexplained bone fractures; fatigue; pallor; shortness of breath; increased bleeding, such as bleeding gums or nosebleeds; easily bruised skin; increased susceptibility to infection; headache; vision disturbances; loss of height.
	Myelofibrosis *An increase of fibrous scar tissue within the bone marrow*	Weakness and fatigue; abdominal fullness; a tendency to bleed easily; bone pain; pallor; shortness of breath during physical exertion; increased susceptibility to bruising and infections; weight loss.
	Platelet function disorders	Minor bleeding in the mouth or just beneath the surface of the skin, often appearing as clusters of small, pinpoint-sized red specks; frequent nosebleeds; easy bruising; prolonged menstrual periods; fatigue; pallor; dark-colored stools.
	Polycythemia vera *An overproduction of red and white blood cells and platelets*	Headache; ringing in the ears; blurred vision; flushed skin; itching; dizziness; fatigue; night sweats; frequent nose bleeds and bruises.
	Systemic lupus erythematosus *Inflammation of connective tissues throughout the body*	Red, blotchy, butterfly-shaped rash on the cheeks and bridge of the nose; fatigue; fever; loss of appetite and weight; nausea; joint and abdominal pain; headaches; blurred vision; increased sensitivity to sun exposure; depression; psychosis; mental confusion.
	Typhoid fever	Headache; fever, loss of appetite; abdominal pain and tenderness; extreme weakness; constipation followed by diarrhea; drowsiness, stupor, or coma; raised, pink skin eruptions on the chest and abdomen; joint aches; sore throat.
	Von Willebrand's disease *Chronic bleeding disorder*	Frequent nosebleeds; excessive bleeding from cuts; bleeding gums; easy bruising; abnormal or excessive menstrual bleeding; blood in the stool.
	Wilson's disease *An accumulation of copper in the liver, brain, and other tissues*	Anemia; fluid accumulation in the abdomen; vomiting blood; progressive intellectual impairment; tremor; weakness; walking difficulty; rigidity of limbs; personality changes; speech difficulties; dementia.

Bumps on the skin

Associated Symptoms	Possible Diagnosis	Distinguishing Features
	Acne	Blackheads, whiteheads, pimples, pustules, or cysts usually on the face, chest, back, shoulders, and neck. May result in pockmarks and scarring.
	Herpes zoster *Shingles*	A sensitive band of skin on one side of the body that becomes severely painful and develops slightly raised red spots that blister, dry and crust over. Pain may persist for months or years after skin has healed.
	Lyme disease	A small red bump, surrounded by a concentric bulls-eye-like red rash with a pale center. Over the following month: fever and chills; extreme fatigue; headaches. Symptoms may progress over several months or years and may include: palpitations; joint or muscle pain; and chronic joint inflammation, especially in the knees.
	Rosacea *Redness, swelling, and blemishes around the nose, cheeks, and forehead*	Facial flushing; stinging, burning, or feeling of skin pulled tight across face; bumps, blemishes, and swelling of nose and cheeks; severe swelling or enlargement of the nose.
	Sarcoidosis *Accumulation of inflammatory cells in the lymph nodes and other tissues throughout the body*	Often no symptoms. Swollen lymph nodes in the neck or armpits; muscle aches; fever; breathing difficulty; possibly, purple rash on the face; reddish or brownish skin spots on the forearms, face, or legs; numbness; joint pain or stiffness; a painful, red eye; blurred vision; loss of appetite and weight.
	Syphilis	Initially, painless, ulcerated, red sore on the genitals, mouth, or rectum; swollen glands in the neck, armpit, or groin; rash with small, red, scaly bumps; fever; headache. If left untreated, damage to heart valves leading to congestive heart failure; mental deterioration; loss of balance; seizures; dementia; personality changes.

Chest pain

Associated Symptoms	Possible Diagnosis	Distinguishing Features
with shortness of breath	Asthma	Shortness of breath; wheezing; cough; tightness in the chest; possibly, excessive perspiration or rapid heartbeat.
	Bronchitis, acute	Shortness of breath; persistent cough producing yellow or green sputum; possibly, chest pain; wheezing; fever.
	Cardiomyopathy *Disease of the heart muscle causing a reduction in the force of heart contractions*	Fatigue; chest pain and palpitations; shortness of breath; swelling of the legs; wheezing; cough.
	Chronic obstructive pulmonary disease	Shortness of breath; wheezing; persistent, mucus-producing cough, especially in the morning; possibly, chest pain, swollen legs and ankles.
	Coronary artery disease *Blockage in the arteries supplying blood to the heart muscle*	Initially, asymptomatic. In later stages, dull chest pain that may spread to the neck or the arms usually exacerbated by physical exertion and alleviated with rest; heart palpitations; shortness of breath.
	Empyema *Collection of pus in any body cavity, usually between the membranes covering the lungs*	Chest pain exacerbated by deep inhalation; shortness of breath; dry cough; fever and chills; exhaustion; weight loss; night sweats; abdominal pain and jaundice.
	Esophageal rupture *A tear in the esophagus, the passageway from the mouth to the stomach*	Chest pain; rapid, shallow breathing; excessive perspiration; fever.
	Esophageal stricture *Narrowing of the esophagus, the passageway from the mouth to the stomach*	Sudden or gradual decrease in the ability to swallow solid food or liquids; chest pain after eating; regurgitation of food and liquids; increased salivation; weight loss. Aspiration into lungs can cause cough, wheezing, shortness of breath.
	Legionnaire's disease	Dry cough progressing to one with blood-streaked sputum; high fever; chills; breathing difficulty; chest pain; headache; muscle aches; diarrhea; nausea; vomiting; mental confusion and disorientation.
	Lung cancer	Persistent cough; wheezing; shortness of breath; chest pain; fatigue; weight loss.
	Myocardial infarction *Heart attack*	Sudden chest pain or pressure that may spread to the arm, shoulder and jaw; excessive perspiration; shortness of breath. Possible nausea and vomiting.

Chest pain *continued*

Associated Symptoms	Possible Diagnosis	Distinguishing Features
with shortness of breath *continued*	Pericarditis *Inflammation of the membrane surrounding the heart*	Sharp chest pain that may spread to the neck and shoulders; pain may be relieved by sitting up and leaning forward; swollen legs and abdomen; breathing difficulty; chills; fever; fatigue.
	Pleurisy *Inflammation of the membranes lining the lungs and chest cavity*	Sudden chest pain worse on inspiration that may also radiate into the shoulder or abdomen; rapid breathing; coughing; sneezing; possibly, fever.
	Pneumonia	High fever; shortness of breath; cough with sputum; chest pain; fatigue.
	Pneumothorax *Accumulation of air between the two membranes lining the lungs and the chest cavity*	Chest pain that may radiate into the abdomen or shoulder; shortness of breath; dry cough.
	Pulmonary embolism *A blood clot traveling from legs or heart that lodges in an artery supplying the lungs*	Sudden shortness of breath and severe breathing difficulty; chest pain worse on inspiration; rapid heartbeat; cough, possibly with bloody sputum; wheezing; excessive perspiration.
	Valvular heart disease	Depends on which heart valve is affected. Often asymptomatic. Possibly, fatigue and weakness; dizziness; chest pain; shortness of breath; heart palpitations; fainting; edema; stroke from embolism to the brain.
without shortness of breath	Ankylosing spondylitis *Inflammation of the joints between the spine and the pelvis*	Initially, pain and stiffness in the lower back and hips that becomes worse after resting; neck or chest pain; possible pain in the hip, knee, and ankle joints; pain in the heel of the foot; eye pain; blurred vision.
	Aortic aneurysm *A sac-like ballooning at a weak spot in the wall of the aorta, the body's primary artery*	Usually asymptomatic; occasionally, severe abdominal and back pain; chest pain; swallowing difficulty; dizziness and fainting; hoarseness; cough.
	Costochondritis *Inflammation of the cartilage of the rib cage*	Pain in the chest, sometimes severe, aggravated by motion of the rib cage; possible swelling around the rib cage.
	Gastroesophageal reflux *Heartburn*	Burning sensation in the middle of the chest; pain and difficulty swallowing; slight regurgitation of stomach's contents into the mouth, especially when reclining or bending forward; mild abdominal pain.
	Influenza *Flu*	Chills, muscle aches, and loss of appetite followed by a cough, sore throat, nasal congestion, and fever; possible chest pain.

Chest pain *continued*

Associated Symptoms	Possible Diagnosis	Distinguishing Features
without shortness of breath *continued*	Lung abscess	Cough producing foul-smelling sputum; bad breath; fever; chills; weight loss; possible chest pain.
	Pancreatitis *Inflammation of the pancreas*	Sudden, extreme abdominal pain; nausea and vomiting; weakness; fever; clammy skin; abdominal bloating and tenderness.
	Peptic ulcer	Intermittent, burning or gnawing pain in the upper abdomen or lower chest; indigestion; loss of appetite and weight. Pain may be relieved by eating or antacids. Possible nausea and vomiting. Black, tarry stools, vomiting blood.
	Pheochromocytoma *Tumor in central part of the adrenal, the glands above the kidneys*	Headaches, sometimes severe; rapid heartbeat or heart palpitations; excessive perspiration; faintness, especially when standing up; chest pain; abdominal pain; constipation; weight loss; nervousness, irritability, or anxiety; mental confusion or psychosis.
	Tuberculosis	Often, asymptomatic. Possibly, low-grade fever; excessive perspiration; cough producing sputum or blood; weight loss; chronic fatigue; chest pain; shortness of breath; night sweats.

Chewing difficulty

Associated Symptoms	Possible Diagnosis	Distinguishing Features
	Amyotrophic lateral sclerosis *Progressive degeneration of nerve cells of the central nervous system*	Progressive loss of strength and coordination in the limbs; muscle twitching and cramps that begin in the hands and spread to the arms, shoulders, and legs; stiff, clumsy gait; swallowing, breathing, or speaking difficulty; weight loss; drooling; involuntary laughing or crying.
	Dry mouth	Dry or burning sensation in the mouth; difficulty chewing, swallowing, and speaking; possibly, cracked lips, changes in the tongue's surface, mouth ulcers, changes in taste perception, or tooth decay.
	Jaw dislocation or fracture	Inability to close the jaw normally; painful, swollen, or numb jaw; misalignment of teeth; speaking difficulty; possible breathing difficulty.
	Mumps	Pain in the ear, below the ear, and in the jaw; swollen glands in the neck; headache; pain on swallowing and chewing; sore muscles; joint pain; loss of appetite. Testicular swelling and tenderness in adults.
	Myasthenia gravis *Nerve degeneration causing gradual loss of voluntary muscle control*	Drooping eyelids; double or blurred vision; muscle weakness especially in the face, throat, and neck; chewing and swallowing difficulties; possible breathing difficulty. Slurred, nasal-sounding speech.
	Oral cancers	Sore in the mouth that bleeds and does not heal; lump in the cheek; white or red patch on the gums; swallowing and chewing difficulties; numbness of the tongue; swelling of the jaw.
	Osteoarthritis *Degeneration of the cartilage that lines the joints*	Pain, swelling, and stiffness in one or more joints; enlargement and distortion of affected joints.
	Osteomyelitis *Infection of bone and bone marrow*	Fever; severe pain in the affected bone; inflammation and swelling of the skin over the affected area; deformity. In children, arrested growth of the affected bone.
	Peritonsillar abscess *A collection of pus between the tonsils and surrounding tissue due to infection*	Sore throat; severe pain when swallowing; fever; headache; impaired speech; drooling; swollen glands in the neck.
	Rheumatoid arthritis	Fatigue and weakness; joint pain, stiffness, and inflammation, especially in the hands, feet, and arms; joint deformity; dry mouth; dry, painful eyes. Morning stiffness.

Chewing difficulty *continued*

Associated Symptoms	Possible Diagnosis	Distinguishing Features
	Temporomandibular joint syndrome	Pain in the joints connecting the jaw to the skull; headache; tender jaw muscles; dull facial pain; clicking noise when opening or closing the mouth; pain when yawning and chewing. Jaw may temporarily lock in position.
	Tetanus	Often, lockjaw; stiffness and, later, muscle spasms in the neck and face; drooling; abdominal and back pain; extreme perspiration; swallowing difficulty; possible convulsions; fever.
	Tooth abscess	Persistent tooth pain; pain when biting or chewing; difficulty swallowing; swollen glands in the neck; earache; fever; possibly, foul taste in the mouth or bad breath.

Chills

Associated Symptoms	Possible Diagnosis	Distinguishing Features
with cough	AIDS *Acquired immunodeficiency syndrome*	Recurrent infections affecting the skin and respiratory system; cough; shortness of breath; loss of appetite; weight loss; fatigue; diarrhea; fever; dementia; malignant skin lesions; swollen lymph glands throughout the body; purplish skin nodules; memory loss; confusion; personality changes.
	Common cold	Nasal congestion; watery eyes; sneezing; sore throat; cough; muscle aches; mild headache; listlessness; possibly, low-grade fever.
	Empyema *Collection of pus in any body cavity, usually between the membranes covering the lungs*	Chest pain exacerbated by deep inhalation; shortness of breath; dry cough; fever and chills; exhaustion; weight loss; night sweats; abdominal pain and jaundice.
	Influenza *Flu*	Chills, muscle aches, and loss of appetite followed by a cough, sore throat, nasal congestion, and fever; possible chest pain.
	Legionnaire's disease	Dry cough progressing to one with blood-streaked sputum; high fever; chills; breathing difficulty; chest pain; headache; muscle aches; diarrhea; nausea; vomiting; mental confusion and disorientation.
	Lung abscess	Cough producing foul-smelling sputum; bad breath; fever; chills; weight loss; possible chest pain.
	Pneumonia	High fever; shortness of breath; cough with sputum; chest pain; fatigue.
	Rocky Mountain spotted fever	Within a week after exposure, high fever, loss of appetite, headache, muscle aches, nausea and vomiting; dry cough; sensitivity to light. Within six days, the appearance of small pink spots on wrists and ankles, eventually spreading over the entire body, where they then grow, darken in color, and bleed.
without cough	Anemia, hemolytic	Fatigue and weakness; shortness of breath on exertion; pallor; heart palpitations; jaundice and dark urine.
	Appendicitis, acute	Pain near the navel, spreading to the lower right abdomen; nausea and vomiting; constipation; possibly diarrhea; low-grade fever; loss of appetite.
	Ear infection, middle *Inflammation of the middle ear*	Earache; deafness; ringing in the ear; possibly, a discharge of pus from the ear; fever; dizziness.

Chills *continued*

Associated Symptoms	Possible Diagnosis	Distinguishing Features
without cough *continued*	Hypothermia *Low body temperature (below 94°)*	Shivering; pallor; puffy face; fatigue and confusion; slow, shallow breathing; muscle stiffness; normally warm areas of the body are cold; loss of consciousness.
	Kidney infection *Pyelonephritis*	Sudden fever and shaking chills; severe fatigue; burning and frequent urination; cloudy or bloody urine; pain in the abdomen, back, or flanks, sometimes severe; nausea and vomiting.
	Laryngitis	Hoarseness that often progresses to loss of the voice; throat pain; dry cough; possible fever.
	Lyme disease	A small red bump, surrounded by a concentric bulls-eye-like red rash with a pale center. Over the following month: fever and chills; extreme fatigue; headaches. Symptoms may progress over several months or years and may include: palpitations; joint or muscle pain; and chronic joint inflammation, especially in the knees.
	Lymphoma, Hodgkin's *Cancer of the lymph nodes and lymphoid tissue*	Painless swelling of the lymph nodes usually in the neck or armpits; loss of appetite; night sweats.
	Malaria	Initially, severe chills and shivering. In later stages, extremely high fever followed by a period of profuse perspiration as fever subsides; headache, sometimes severe; vomiting.
	Pelvic inflammatory disease	Initially, lower pelvic pain; pain during intercourse; irregular menstrual bleeding; vaginal discharge with abnormal color or odor; low-grade fever; chills; frequent urination; fatigue; loss of appetite; later, severe abdominal pain and high fever.
	Pericarditis *Inflammation of the membrane surrounding the heart*	Sharp chest pain that may spread to the neck and shoulders; pain may be relieved by sitting up and leaning forward; swollen legs and abdomen; breathing difficulty; chills; fever; fatigue.
	Peritonitis *Inflammation of the abdominal membrane*	Sudden abdominal pain, rigidity, and swelling; chills and fever; weakness; rapid heartbeat; nausea and vomiting; extreme thirst; low urine output.
	Prostatitis *Inflammation of the prostate gland*	Burning during urination; urgent and frequent urination; fever and chills; discharge from the penis; lower abdominal and back pain; blood in the urine.

Chills *continued*

Associated Symptoms	Possible Diagnosis	Distinguishing Features
without cough *continued*	Septic shock *Severe drop in blood pressure due to the presence of microorganisms or their toxins in the bloodstream*	Nausea and vomiting; prostration; diarrhea; sudden high fever; chills; rapid breathing; mental confusion or agitation; decreased urine output; severe fatigue; rapid heartbeat.
	Sinusitis *Inflammation of the mucous membranes lining the sinuses*	Throbbing pain above or below one or both eyes that intensifies when bending the head forward or coughing; nasal congestion; loss of sense of smell; often, pus-like nasal discharge; possible dental pain in the upper jaw; fever.
	Typhoid fever	Headache; fever, loss of appetite; abdominal pain and tenderness; extreme weakness; constipation followed by diarrhea; drowsiness, stupor, or coma; raised, pink skin eruptions on the chest and abdomen; joint aches; sore throat.

Confusion

Associated Symptoms	Possible Diagnosis	Distinguishing Features
	AIDS *Acquired immunodeficiency syndrome*	Recurrent infections affecting the skin and respiratory system; cough; shortness of breath; loss of appetite; weight loss; fatigue; diarrhea; fever; dementia; malignant skin lesions; swollen lymph glands throughout the body; purplish skin nodules; memory loss; confusion; personality changes.
	Alzheimer's disease	Symptoms vary greatly in different individuals. Initially, minor forgetfulness gradually developing into severe, short-term memory loss, disorientation, an inability to concentrate, and sudden mood and personality changes. In later stages, severe confusion, possible hallucinations or paranoid delusions, loss of social and sexual inhibitions, impaired judgment, anxiety, depression, agitation and combativeness, wandering and getting lost, inability to write, urinary and fecal incontinence.
	Bipolar disorder *Manic-depressive illness*	Symptoms vary depending on phase of the disorder; mania: inflated self-esteem, elation, euphoria, grandiosity, increased activity, and a decreased need for sleep; depression: persistent feelings of sadness, apathy, or hopelessness; diminished interest in activities; loss of appetite and weight or unusual increase in appetite and weight; insomnia or drowsiness; difficulty concentrating; agitation in older patients.
	Cirrhosis *Chronic damage to the cells of the liver*	No symptoms in early stages; loss of weight and appetite; nausea; swollen legs, ankles and abdomen; itching; jaundice; black stools; vomiting blood; fatigue; impotence; memory loss; confusion.
	Depression	Persistent feelings of sadness, apathy, or hopelessness; diminished interest in activities; loss of or unusual increase in appetite and weight; insomnia or drowsiness; difficulty concentrating; agitation.
	Diabetes mellitus *Insufficiency of or resistance to insulin*	Fatigue; excessive thirst; frequent urination; weight loss despite increased appetite; blurred vision; numbness and tingling of feet and hands; impotence.
	Hyperparathyroidism *Overactivity of the parathyroid glands*	Increased susceptibility to bone fractures; depression; indigestion; increased thirst and urine output; fatigue, lethargy; somnolence; muscle weakness; nausea and vomiting; loss of appetite; weight loss.
	Hypothermia *Low body temperature (below 94°)*	Shivering; pallor; puffy face; fatigue and confusion; slow, shallow breathing; muscle stiffness; normally warm areas of the body are cold; loss of consciousness.

Confusion *continued*

Associated Symptoms	Possible Diagnosis	Distinguishing Features
	Hypothyroidism *Underactivity of the thyroid gland*	Unexplained weight gain; fatigue; muscle weakness; cramps; dry skin; hair loss; deepening of the voice; intolerance for cold; constipation; chest pain; insomnia; puffiness around eyes; loss of sex drive; depression; menstrual abnormalities; possible swelling in the neck.
	Multiple sclerosis *Gradual degeneration of the protective sheaths surrounding the nerves within the brain and spinal cord*	Symptoms may appear suddenly and then disappear; persistent symptoms may take years to develop and include numbness or tingling in any part of the body, weakness in the extremities, an unsteady walk, slurred speech, urinary incontinence, fatigue, depression, temporary loss of vision, double or blurred vision, mental confusion, and memory loss.
	Renal failure, acute *Severe kidney failure*	Initially, decreased urine output, weight gain and swelling due to edema, loss of appetite, nausea and vomiting, fatigue. If untreated, confusion, seizures, and drowsiness.
	Reye's syndrome *Childhood disease marked by brain and liver damage*	Following recovery from an upper respiratory infection, nausea and vomiting; memory loss; confusion or delirium; possible seizures; drowsiness; lethargy.
	Schizophrenia	Delusions; hallucinations; rambling, nonsensical, or minimal speech; extremely disorganized behavior; inappropriate emotional responses or emotional detachment; lack of willful movement.
	Seizures	Involuntary twitching or jerking; muscle rigidity; loss of consciousness; confusion; drooling; hallucinations.
	Septic shock *Severe drop in blood pressure due to the presence of microorganisms or their toxins in the bloodstream*	Nausea and vomiting; prostration; diarrhea; sudden high fever; chills; rapid breathing; mental confusion or agitation; decreased urine output; severe fatigue; rapid heartbeat.
with headache	Brain abscess	Headaches; drowsiness; nausea and vomiting; fever; seizures; possible partial paralysis; confusion; speaking difficulty.
	Brain hemorrhage	Sudden loss of consciousness; sudden, severe headache; mental confusion; stiff neck; nausea and vomiting; paralysis on one side of the face or body; weakness and dizziness; loss of speech; blurred or double vision; dilated pupils.
	Brain tumors	Headaches that become more severe when reclining; nausea and vomiting; memory loss; double vision; muscle weakness; numbness, tingling, or partial paralysis; vision loss; speech disturbances; seizures; drowsiness.

Confusion *continued*

Associated Symptoms	Possible Diagnosis	Distinguishing Features
with headache *continued*	Chronic fatigue syndrome	Severe fatigue made worse by exercise; recurrent flu-like symptoms; persistent sore throat; low-grade fever; muscle and joint aches; headache; painful, swollen lymph nodes; depression and mental confusion; memory loss; sleep difficulties.
	Concussion	Brief loss of consciousness following a blow to the head. Occasionally causes nausea and vomiting.
	Encephalitis *Inflammation of the brain*	Initially, headache and fever followed by confusion, hallucinations, and paralysis on one side of the body; memory loss; difficulty with speech and eye movements; drowsiness; possible coma or epileptic seizures; loss of hearing; sensitivity to light; stiff neck.
	Heatstroke	Sudden dizziness; weakness; headache; hot, dry, red skin which later turns grey; high body temperature; muscle cramps; confusion; seizures; loss of consciousness.
	Hydrocephalus *Overaccumulation of cerebrospinal fluid, the liquid surrounding the brain*	In infants, an enlarged head, rigidity of the legs, irritability, projectile vomiting, drowsiness, seizures, and lethargy. In older persons, headache, vomiting, loss of coordination, deterioration of mental faculties, speech difficulty, and loss of appetite.
	Hypertension	Usually asymptomatic except in severe cases. Possibly, headache, easy fatigability, palpitations, chest pain, blurred vision, dizziness, nose bleeds, and confusion.
	Hypoglycemia *Low blood sugar*	Anxiety; hunger; trembling; headache; palpitations; perspiration; confusion; irritability; loss of coordination; possibly, double vision, seizures, or coma.
	Legionnaire's disease	Dry cough progressing to one with blood-streaked sputum; high fever; chills; breathing difficulty; chest pain; headache; muscle aches; diarrhea; nausea; vomiting; mental confusion and disorientation.
	Meningitis *Inflammation of the membranes covering the brain and spinal cord*	Severe headache; nausea and vomiting; sensitivity to light; stiffness in the neck; possible red skin rash; fever; mental confusion; drowsiness; loss of consciousness; seizures.
	Pheochromocytoma *Tumor in central part of the adrenal, the glands above the kidneys*	Headaches, sometimes severe; rapid heartbeat or heart palpitations; excessive perspiration; faintness, especially when standing up; chest pain; abdominal pain; constipation; weight loss; nervousness, irritability, or anxiety; mental confusion or psychosis.

Confusion *continued*

Associated Symptoms	Possible Diagnosis	Distinguishing Features
with headache *continued*	Rabies	Low-grade fever; headache; loss of appetite; difficulty swallowing; tingling at site of animal bite; intense thirst exacerbated by the inability to drink without violent, painful throat spasms; paralysis of facial muscles; drooling. Agitation and violent behavior, confusion, convulsions, coma.
	Renal failure, acute *Severe kidney failure*	Initially, decreased urine output, weight gain and swelling due to edema, loss of appetite, nausea and vomiting, fatigue. If untreated, confusion, seizures, and drowsiness.
	Stroke	Symptoms vary with the location of brain injury. Sudden onset of weakness, paralysis, or loss of sensation, usually on one side of the body; a sudden heaviness in a limb; speech abnormalities; headache; vision disturbances; dizziness; confusion; coma; urinary and fecal incontinence.
	Systemic lupus erythematosus *Inflammation of connective tissues throughout the body*	Red, blotchy, butterfly-shaped rash on the cheeks and bridge of the nose; fatigue; fever; loss of appetite and weight; nausea; joint and abdominal pain; headaches; blurred vision; increased sensitivity to sun exposure; depression; psychosis; mental confusion.
	Toxic shock syndrome	Lethargy; conjunctivitis; confusion; sudden high fever accompanied by nausea, watery diarrhea, sore throat, and headache. Red rash on the palms and soles of the feet, which, after a week or two, begins to peel.
	Transient ischemic attack *Temporary blockage in an artery supplying the brain*	Weakness or numbness in a limb; slurred speech; short-lived, temporary partial blindness; numbness and tingling; speech difficulties; confusion; dizziness.
	Typhoid fever	Headache; fever, loss of appetite; abdominal pain and tenderness; extreme weakness; constipation followed by diarrhea; drowsiness, stupor, or coma; raised, pink skin eruptions on the chest and abdomen; joint aches; sore throat.

Constipation

Associated Symptoms	Possible Diagnosis	Distinguishing Features
	Adrenal insufficiency *Inadequate production of steroid hormones by the adrenal gland*	Loss of weight and appetite; fatigue; weakness; darkening of the skin; abdominal pain; diarrhea; indigestion; nausea and vomiting; constipation; lack of sex drive; dizziness when rising from sitting or lying position.
	Anal fissures	Rectal pain or burning during and immediately after bowel movements; blood in the stool or on toilet paper; rectal itching.
	Appendicitis, acute	Pain near the navel, spreading to the lower right abdomen; nausea and vomiting; constipation; possibly diarrhea; low-grade fever; loss of appetite.
	Colorectal cancer *A growth of malignant cells in the colon or rectum*	Change in bowel habits; diarrhea; constipation; narrow stools; bloody or dark stools; lower abdominal pain; bloating; cramps; gas; loss of weight and appetite; fatigue and heart palpitations due to anemia.
	Constipation, chronic	Infrequent and possibly painful bowel movements; straining during bowel movements; hard, dry stool; abdominal swelling; continued sensation of fullness after evacuating bowels.
	Diverticular disorders *Swellings in the wall of the colon*	Usually no symptoms unless diverticulae become inflamed. Tenderness or pain in the lower left abdomen relieved by passing stools or gas; constipation or diarrhea; blood in the stool; severe, spasmodic abdominal pain that becomes constant; possibly, fever and nausea.
	Endometriosis *The migration of the uterine lining to other reproductive or abdominal organs*	Pain in the lower abdomen, vagina, and lower back beginning just prior to menses and intensifying after blood flow has ceased; heavy bleeding during periods; pain during intercourse; diarrhea; constipation; pain during bowel movements; bleeding from the rectum; bloody urine during menses; nausea and vomiting prior to menses; infertility.
	Fibroids, uterine *Benign growths of the muscular wall of the uterus*	Heavier or prolonged bleeding during menses; abdominal discomfort; lower back pain; pressure on the bladder and frequent urination; constipation. Possible, sharp, sudden, lower abdominal pain.
	Hemorrhoids	Pain during defecation; anal itching; mucus discharge from the anus. Bright, red blood on toilet paper, stool, or in toilet bowl after a bowel movement.
	Hyperparathyroidism *Overactivity of the parathyroid glands*	Increased susceptibility to bone fractures; depression; indigestion; increased thirst and urine output; fatigue, lethargy; somnolence; muscle weakness; nausea and vomiting; loss of appetite; weight loss.

Constipation *continued*

Associated Symptoms	Possible Diagnosis	Distinguishing Features
	Hypothyroidism *Underactivity of the thyroid gland*	Unexplained weight gain; fatigue; muscle weakness; cramps; dry skin; hair loss; deepening of the voice; intolerance for cold; constipation; chest pain; insomnia; puffiness around eyes; loss of sex drive; depression; menstrual abnormalities; possible swelling in the neck.
	Intestinal obstruction	Abdominal pain and cramps; nausea; vomiting; weakness; gas; bloating; possible diarrhea; progressive constipation culminating in inability to pass stools or gas.
	Irritable bowel syndrome	Cramps in the middle or to one side of the lower abdomen that are usually relieved with bowel movements; nausea; bloating; gas; alternating diarrhea and constipation.
	Megacolon, toxic *Distention of the colon*	Severe constipation; abdominal bloating; loss of weight and appetite; possible diarrhea; in newborns, failure to pass a stool within 48 hours after birth; in children, slow growth from infancy to age five.
	Mesenteric ischemia *A blood clot blocking blood flow to the intestine*	Severe abdominal cramping, usually around the navel, that is exacerbated by eating and alleviated by fasting. Possibly, bloody stools.
	Multiple sclerosis *Gradual degeneration of the protective sheaths surrounding the nerves within the brain and spinal cord*	Symptoms may appear suddenly and then disappear; persistent symptoms may take years to develop and include numbness or tingling in any part of the body, weakness in the extremities, an unsteady walk, slurred speech, urinary incontinence, fatigue, depression, temporary loss of vision, double or blurred vision, mental confusion, and memory loss.
	Pheochromocytoma *Tumor in central part of the adrenal, the glands above the kidneys*	Headaches, sometimes severe; rapid heartbeat or heart palpitations; excessive perspiration; faintness, especially when standing up; chest pain; abdominal pain; constipation; weight loss; nervousness, irritability, or anxiety; mental confusion or psychosis.
	Proctitis *Inflammation of the rectum*	Soreness in the rectal area; mucus discharge from the anus; constipation; painful bowel movements; possibly, rectal bleeding.
	Typhoid fever	Headache; fever, loss of appetite; abdominal pain and tenderness; extreme weakness; constipation followed by diarrhea; drowsiness, stupor, or coma; raised, pink skin eruptions on the chest and abdomen; joint aches; sore throat.

Cough, dry

Associated Symptoms	Possible Diagnosis	Distinguishing Features
with fever	Chlamydia *Contagious, infectious disease caused by chlamydia, a group of microorganisms*	Usually asymptomatic; possibly, pain or burning during urination, watery discharge from the penis or vagina, swelling of the testicles, breathing difficulty, cough, high fever, inflammation of the inner lining of the eyelids and the membrane covering the whites of the eyes.
	Common cold	Nasal congestion; watery eyes; sneezing; sore throat; cough; muscle aches; mild headache; listlessness; possibly, low-grade fever.
	Congestive heart failure	Shortness of breath; fatigue; need to sleep on several pillows; weakness; cough; heart palpitations; swelling in the legs, ankles, and abdomen; frequent urination at night; indigestion; nausea and vomiting; loss of appetite.
	Croup *Inflammation of the air passages in children*	Barking cough; hoarseness; wheezing; possibly, breathing difficulty; chest discomfort.
	Empyema *Collection of pus in any body cavity, usually between the membranes covering the lungs*	Chest pain exacerbated by deep inhalation; shortness of breath; dry cough; fever and chills; exhaustion; weight loss; night sweats; abdominal pain and jaundice.
	Laryngitis	Hoarseness that often progresses to loss of the voice; throat pain; dry cough; possible fever.
	Legionnaire's disease	Dry cough progressing to one with blood-streaked sputum; high fever; chills; breathing difficulty; chest pain; headache; muscle aches; diarrhea; nausea; vomiting; mental confusion and disorientation.
	Lung cancer	Persistent cough; wheezing; shortness of breath; chest pain; fatigue; weight loss.
	Measles	Cough; fever; watery nasal discharge; loss of appetite; red, watering eyes; sore throat; body aches; red, slightly itchy rash that gradually spreads all over the body.
	Pleurisy *Inflammation of the membranes lining the lungs and chest cavity*	Sudden chest pain worse on inspiration that may also radiate into the shoulder or abdomen; rapid breathing; coughing; sneezing; possibly, fever.
	Pneumonia	High fever; shortness of breath; cough with sputum; chest pain; fatigue.

Cough, dry *continued*

Associated Symptoms	Possible Diagnosis	Distinguishing Features
with fever *continued*	Rocky Mountain spotted fever	Within a week after exposure, high fever, loss of appetite, headache, muscle aches, nausea and vomiting; dry cough; sensitivity to light. Within six days, the appearance of small pink spots on wrists and ankles, eventually spreading over the entire body, where they then grow, darken in color, and bleed.
	Sarcoidosis *Accumulation of inflammatory cells in the lymph nodes and other tissues throughout the body*	Often no symptoms. Swollen lymph nodes in the neck or armpits; muscle aches; fever; breathing difficulty; possibly, purple rash on the face; reddish or brownish skin spots on the forearms, face, or legs; numbness; joint pain or stiffness; a painful, red eye; blurred vision; loss of appetite and weight.
	Systemic lupus erythematosus *Inflammation of connective tissues throughout the body*	Red, blotchy, butterfly-shaped rash on the cheeks and bridge of the nose; fatigue; fever; loss of appetite and weight; nausea; joint and abdominal pain; headaches; blurred vision; increased sensitivity to sun exposure; depression; psychosis; mental confusion.
	Tuberculosis	Often, asymptomatic. Possibly, low-grade fever; excessive perspiration; cough producing sputum or blood; weight loss; chronic fatigue; chest pain; shortness of breath; night sweats.
	Whooping cough	Initially, mild cough, sneezing, nasal congestion, and irritated eyes. Within approximately two weeks, cough becomes severe and persistent, and is accompanied by characteristic high-pitched "whooping" sound during inhalation; loss of appetite; listlessness; vomiting or choking spells. Most common among young children.
without fever	Anaphylaxis	Itching and hives; swelling of the eyes, lips, and tongue; weakness or faintness; tightening in the chest or throat; wheezing; shortness of breath; profuse sweating; palpitations; sudden, intense distress; feelings of impending doom; stomach cramps; nausea, vomiting, or diarrhea; bluish tinge (cyanosis) to the skin, lips, and nail beds due to oxygen insufficiency.
	Aortic aneurysm *A sac-like ballooning at a weak spot in the wall of the aorta, the body's primary artery*	Usually asymptomatic; occasionally, severe abdominal and back pain; chest pain; swallowing difficulty; dizziness and fainting; hoarseness; cough.
	Asthma	Shortness of breath; wheezing; cough; tightness in the chest; possibly, excessive perspiration or rapid heartbeat.

Cough, dry *continued*

Associated Symptoms	Possible Diagnosis	Distinguishing Features
without fever *continued*	Cardiomyopathy *Disease of the heart muscle causing a reduction in the force of heart contractions*	Fatigue; chest pain and palpitations; shortness of breath; swelling of the legs; wheezing; cough.
	Esophageal stricture *Narrowing of the esophagus, the passageway from the mouth to the stomach*	Sudden or gradual decrease in the ability to swallow solid food or liquids; chest pain after eating; regurgitation of food and liquids; increased salivation; weight loss. Aspiration into lungs can cause cough, wheezing, shortness of breath.
	Pneumothorax *Accumulation of air between the two membranes lining the lungs and the chest cavity*	Chest pain that may radiate into the abdomen or shoulder; shortness of breath; dry cough.

Cough, wet

Associated Symptoms	Possible Diagnosis	Distinguishing Features
	Allergic rhinitis *Hay fever*	Nasal congestion; frequent sneezing; itchy eyes, nose, and throat.
	Asthma	Shortness of breath; wheezing; cough; tightness in the chest; possibly, excessive perspiration or rapid heartbeat.
	Bronchiectasis *Lung condition that stretches and distorts the walls of the bronchial tubes*	Cough that produces dark green sputum; bad breath; possibly, shortness of breath; loss of appetite and weight; clubbed fingers.
	Chronic obstructive pulmonary disease	Shortness of breath; wheezing; persistent, mucus-producing cough, especially in the morning; possibly, chest pain, swollen legs and ankles.
	Congestive heart failure	Shortness of breath; fatigue; need to sleep on several pillows; weakness; cough; heart palpitations; swelling in the legs, ankles, and abdomen; frequent urination at night; indigestion; nausea and vomiting; loss of appetite.
	Esophageal cancer	Swallowing difficulty and pain; weight loss; drooling; possibly, vomiting or coughing up of bloody mucus, regurgitation of food; chest pain; repeated respiratory infections.
	Lung cancer	Persistent cough; wheezing; shortness of breath; chest pain; fatigue; weight loss.
	Pulmonary edema *An accumulation of fluid in the lungs*	Severe shortness of breath; rapid breathing; pallor; excessive perspiration; bluish nails and lips; cough with frothy sputum; wheezing; anxiety and restlessness.
	Pulmonary embolism *A blood clot traveling from legs or heart that lodges in an artery supplying the lungs*	Sudden shortness of breath and severe breathing difficulty; chest pain worse on inspiration; rapid heartbeat; cough, possibly with bloody sputum; wheezing; excessive perspiration.
with fever	AIDS *Acquired immunodeficiency syndrome*	Recurrent infections affecting the skin and respiratory system; cough; shortness of breath; loss of appetite; weight loss; fatigue; diarrhea; fever; dementia; malignant skin lesions; swollen lymph glands throughout the body; purplish skin nodules; memory loss; confusion; personality changes.
	Bronchitis, acute	Shortness of breath; persistent cough producing yellow or green sputum; possibly, chest pain; wheezing; fever.
	Common cold	Nasal congestion; watery eyes; sneezing; sore throat; cough; muscle aches; mild headache; listlessness; possibly, low-grade fever.

Cough, wet *continued*

Associated Symptoms	Possible Diagnosis	Distinguishing Features
with fever *continued*	Influenza *Flu*	Chills, muscle aches, and loss of appetite followed by a cough, sore throat, nasal congestion, and fever; possible chest pain.
	Legionnaire's disease	Dry cough progressing to one with blood-streaked sputum; high fever; chills; breathing difficulty; chest pain; headache; muscle aches; diarrhea; nausea; vomiting; mental confusion and disorientation.
	Lung abscess	Cough producing foul-smelling sputum; bad breath; fever; chills; weight loss; possible chest pain.
	Measles	Cough; fever; watery nasal discharge; loss of appetite; red, watering eyes; sore throat; body aches; red, slightly itchy rash that gradually spreads all over the body.
	Pneumonia	High fever; shortness of breath; cough with sputum; chest pain; fatigue.
	Tuberculosis	Often, asymptomatic. Possibly, low-grade fever; excessive perspiration; cough producing sputum or blood; weight loss; chronic fatigue; chest pain; shortness of breath; night sweats.
	Whooping cough	Initially, mild cough, sneezing, nasal congestion, and irritated eyes. Within approximately two weeks, cough becomes severe and persistent, and is accompanied by characteristic high-pitched "whooping" sound during inhalation; loss of appetite; listlessness; vomiting or choking spells. Most common among young children.

Depression

Associated Symptoms	Possible Diagnosis	Distinguishing Features
	Alzheimer's disease	Symptoms vary greatly in different individuals. Initially, minor forgetfulness gradually developing into severe, short-term memory loss, disorientation, an inability to concentrate, and sudden mood and personality changes. In later stages, severe confusion, possible hallucinations or paranoid delusions, loss of social and sexual inhibitions, impaired judgment, anxiety, depression, agitation and combativeness, wandering and getting lost, inability to write, urinary and fecal incontinence.
	Bipolar disorder *Manic-depressive illness*	Symptoms vary depending on phase of the disorder; mania: inflated self-esteem, elation, euphoria, grandiosity, increased activity, and a decreased need for sleep; depression: persistent feelings of sadness, apathy, or hopelessness; diminished interest in activities; loss of appetite and weight or unusual increase in appetite and weight; insomnia or drowsiness; difficulty concentrating; agitation in older patients.
	Congestive heart failure	Shortness of breath; fatigue; need to sleep on several pillows; weakness; cough; heart palpitations; swelling in the legs, ankles, and abdomen; frequent urination at night; indigestion; nausea and vomiting; loss of appetite.
	Depression	Persistent feelings of sadness, apathy, or hopelessness; diminished interest in activities; loss of or unusual increase in appetite and weight; insomnia or drowsiness; difficulty concentrating; agitation.
	Diabetes mellitus *Insufficiency of or resistance to insulin*	Fatigue; excessive thirst; frequent urination; weight loss despite increased appetite; blurred vision; numbness and tingling of feet and hands; impotence.
	Encephalitis *Inflammation of the brain*	Initially, headache and fever followed by confusion, hallucinations, and paralysis on one side of the body; memory loss; difficulty with speech and eye movements; drowsiness; possible coma or epileptic seizures; loss of hearing; sensitivity to light; stiff neck.
	Hepatitis, acute viral	Fever; fatigue; loss of appetite; aching muscles and joints; abdominal pain or discomfort; jaundice; dark urine and pale stools.
	Hepatitis, chronic	Fatigue; nausea; vomiting; loss of appetite; jaundice; dark urine; clay-colored stools; depression; pain or discomfort in the upper right abdomen; abdominal swelling; fever; in women, cessation of menstruation, acne, and the appearance of male pattern facial hair.

Depression *continued*

Associated Symptoms	Possible Diagnosis	Distinguishing Features
	Hyperthyroidism *Overactivity of the thyroid gland*	Protruding eyes; weight loss despite increased appetite; intolerance to heat; excessive perspiration; nervousness or restlessness; possibly, swelling in the neck (goiter); palpitations; tremor; diarrhea.
	Hypothyroidism *Underactivity of the thyroid gland*	Unexplained weight gain; fatigue; muscle weakness; cramps; dry skin; hair loss; deepening of the voice; intolerance for cold; constipation; chest pain; insomnia; puffiness around eyes; loss of sex drive; depression; menstrual abnormalities; possible swelling in the neck.
	Multiple sclerosis *Gradual degeneration of the protective sheaths surrounding the nerves within the brain and spinal cord*	Symptoms may appear suddenly and then disappear; persistent symptoms may take years to develop and include numbness or tingling in any part of the body, weakness in the extremities, an unsteady walk, slurred speech, urinary incontinence, fatigue, depression, temporary loss of vision, double or blurred vision, mental confusion, and memory loss.
	Pancreatic cancer	Often, no symptoms until far advanced. Upper abdominal pain which spreads to the back; loss of weight and appetite; jaundice; nausea, vomiting, and indigestion; diarrhea; fatigue; depression.
	Parkinson's disease *Degeneration of the basal ganglia, a cluster of nerve cells in the brain*	Tremors in the hands; stiffness and weakness; impaired voluntary movement; shuffling gait; stooped posture; unblinking, fixed expression; possibly, slow, hesitant speech; difficulty swallowing; drooling; depression. Tremors occur at rest (not with voluntary movements) and disappear during sleep.
	Schizophrenia	Delusions; hallucinations; rambling, nonsensical, or minimal speech; extremely disorganized behavior; inappropriate emotional responses or emotional detachment; lack of willful movement.

Diarrhea

Associated Symptoms	Possible Diagnosis	Distinguishing Features
may or may not occur with nausea/vomiting	AIDS *Acquired immunodeficiency syndrome*	Recurrent infections affecting the skin and respiratory system; cough; shortness of breath; loss of appetite; weight loss; fatigue; diarrhea; fever; dementia; malignant skin lesions; swollen lymph glands throughout the body; purplish skin nodules; memory loss; confusion; personality changes.
	Amebiasis *Parasitic infection*	Usually asymptomatic; possibly, diarrhea; loose stools may contain mucus and blood; abdominal cramps; fatigue; weight loss; gas and flatulence. In severe cases, large amount of bloody stools daily; fever, nausea and vomiting, and abdominal tenderness.
	Amyloidosis *Accumulation of amyloid, a waxy substance, in tissues and organs*	Symptoms vary greatly depending on the body parts affected and may include fatigue and weakness; weight loss; heart palpitations; shortness of breath; swelling of the legs; difficulty swallowing due to swelling of the tongue; diarrhea; abdominal pain; raised spots on the armpits, groin, face, and neck; numbness or tingling of the hands or feet; dizziness on standing; joint pains.
	Anemia, folic acid deficiency	Fatigue and weakness; pallor; shortness of breath, heart palpitations, or noticeably rapid heartbeat on exertion; sore, red, and glazed looking tongue; loss of weight and appetite; nausea and diarrhea; abdominal distention.
	Carcinoid tumors and carcinoid syndrome	May be asymptomatic; flushing or redness of the face and neck; gas and profuse diarrhea; abdominal cramping; watery, swollen eyes; shortness of breath or wheezing.
	Colitis, ulcerative *Inflammation of the lining of the colon*	Pain on the left side of the abdomen that lessens after bowel movements; bloody diarrhea; pain in the rectal area; possibly, fever, rapid heartbeat, nausea and vomiting, loss of appetite, dehydration with severe attacks.
	Diverticular disorders *Swellings in the wall of the colon*	Usually no symptoms unless diverticulae become inflamed. Tenderness or pain in the lower left abdomen relieved by passing stools or gas; constipation or diarrhea; blood in the stool; severe, spasmodic abdominal pain that becomes constant; possibly, fever and nausea.
	Food poisoning	Symptoms vary greatly depending on the type and extent of poisoning and may include nausea, vomiting, diarrhea, bloody stools, abdominal pain, and collapse.
	Pancreatic cancer	Often, no symptoms until far advanced. Upper abdominal pain which spreads to the back; loss of weight and appetite; jaundice; nausea, vomiting, and indigestion; diarrhea; fatigue; depression.

Diarrhea *continued*

Associated Symptoms	Possible Diagnosis	Distinguishing Features
with nausea/vomiting	Adrenal insufficiency *Inadequate production of steroid hormones by the adrenal gland*	Loss of weight and appetite; fatigue; weakness; darkening of the skin; abdominal pain; diarrhea; indigestion; nausea and vomiting; constipation; lack of sex drive; dizziness when rising from sitting or lying position.
	Appendicitis, acute	Pain near the navel, spreading to the lower right abdomen; nausea and vomiting; constipation; possibly diarrhea; low-grade fever; loss of appetite.
	Crohn's disease *Inflammation of the lining of the small intestine*	Episodes of abdominal pain or cramps in lower abdomen; nausea; diarrhea; loss of weight and appetite; possibly, fever; rectal bleeding or blood in stools; fatigue; anal fissures; joint pains; inflammation of the eyes.
	Dysentery, bacillary	Watery diarrhea that may contain mucus or blood; rectal pain upon defecation; abdominal pain; rapid dehydration and weight loss; nausea and vomiting.
	Endometriosis *The migration of the uterine lining to other reproductive or abdominal organs*	Pain in the lower abdomen, vagina, and lower back beginning just prior to menses and intensifying after blood flow has ceased; heavy bleeding during periods; pain during intercourse; diarrhea; constipation; pain during bowel movements; bleeding from the rectum; bloody urine during menses; nausea and vomiting prior to menses; infertility.
	Intestinal obstruction	Abdominal pain and cramps; nausea; vomiting; weakness; gas; bloating; possible diarrhea; progressive constipation culminating in inability to pass stools or gas.
	Irritable bowel syndrome	Cramps in the middle or to one side of the lower abdomen that are usually relieved with bowel movements; nausea; bloating; gas; alternating diarrhea and constipation.
	Lactose intolerance *Difficulty digesting milk and dairy products*	Abdominal cramps; diarrhea; nausea; bloating; flatulence.
	Legionnaire's disease	Dry cough progressing to one with blood-streaked sputum; high fever; chills; breathing difficulty; chest pain; headache; muscle aches; diarrhea; nausea; vomiting; mental confusion and disorientation.
	Toxic shock syndrome	Lethargy; conjunctivitis; confusion; sudden high fever accompanied by nausea, watery diarrhea, sore throat, and headache. Red rash on the palms and soles of the feet, which, after a week or two, begins to peel.

Diarrhea *continued*

Associated Symptoms	Possible Diagnosis	Distinguishing Features
with nausea/vomiting *continued*	Trichinosis *Parasitic infestation*	Initially, crampy abdominal pain, diarrhea, vomiting, and fever, followed within one to two weeks by swelling around the eyes, muscle aches and tenderness, fever, and weakness. Possibly, coughing up of bloody phlegm; delirium; coma; heart failure symptoms.
without nausea/ vomiting	Colorectal cancer *A growth of malignant cells in the colon or rectum*	Change in bowel habits; diarrhea; constipation; narrow stools; bloody or dark stools; lower abdominal pain; bloating; cramps; gas; loss of weight and appetite; fatigue and heart palpitations due to anemia.
	Diarrhea, acute	Loose, watery stools; increased frequency of bowel movements; abdominal cramping and pain. In infants, possibly drowsiness, slack skin, dry, sticky mouth and tongue, or persistent crying.
	Malabsorption, digestive *A failure of the small intestine to absorb nutrients in the diet*	Diarrhea; weight loss; yellowish, foul-smelling stools; abdominal cramps, gas, and bloating; weakness and lethargy.
	Megacolon, toxic *Distention of the colon*	Severe constipation; abdominal bloating; loss of weight and appetite; possible diarrhea; in newborns, failure to pass a stool within 48 hours after birth; in children, slow growth from infancy to age five.
	Tapeworm infestation	Often asymptomatic. Unexplained weight loss; presence of white eggs or ribbon-like segments of worm in the stool, bedding, or clothing; symptoms of pernicious anemia.
	Typhoid fever	Headache; fever, loss of appetite; abdominal pain and tenderness; extreme weakness; constipation followed by diarrhea; drowsiness, stupor, or coma; raised, pink skin eruptions on the chest and abdomen; joint aches; sore throat.

Dizziness

Associated Symptoms	Possible Diagnosis	Distinguishing Features
	Acoustic neuroma *A benign tumor in the cells covering the auditory nerve*	Gradual hearing loss; ringing in the ear; headache; numbness in the face; unsteady walk. In later stages, swallowing and speaking difficulties; possibly, slight paralysis.
	Amyloidosis *Accumulation of amyloid, a waxy substance, in tissues and organs*	Symptoms vary greatly depending on the body parts affected and may include fatigue and weakness; weight loss; heart palpitations; shortness of breath; swelling of the legs; difficulty swallowing due to swelling of the tongue; diarrhea; abdominal pain; raised spots on the armpits, groin, face, and neck; numbness or tingling of the hands or feet; dizziness on standing; joint pains.
	Anemia, aplastic	Fatigue and weakness; shortness of breath; heart palpitations; pallor; bleeding gums; nosebleeds; tendency to bruise easily; small red dots under the skin (petechiae). Increased susceptibility to infection.
	Anemia, folic acid deficiency	Fatigue and weakness; pallor; shortness of breath, heart palpitations, or noticeably rapid heartbeat on exertion; sore, red, and glazed looking tongue; loss of weight and appetite; nausea and diarrhea; abdominal distention.
	Anemia, hemolytic	Fatigue and weakness; shortness of breath on exertion; pallor; heart palpitations; jaundice and dark urine.
	Anemia, iron deficiency	Fatigue and weakness; pallor; shortness of breath and heart palpitations on exertion; irritability or inability to concentrate; sore tongue or tiny cracks at the corners of the mouth; black, tarry or bloody stools; unusual craving for dirt, paint, or ice.
	Anemia, pernicious	Fatigue; inability to concentrate; sore, red tongue; weakness; dizziness; pallor; shortness of breath on exertion; palpitations; numbness and tingling in extremities; incoordination; headache; loss of weight and appetite; possibly, jaundice.
	Cardiac arrhythmias *Irregularities in the heartbeat*	Frequently, asymptomatic; possibly; heart palpitations; light-headedness; shortness of breath; sudden weakness; loss of consciousness.
	Cardiomyopathy *Disease of the heart muscle causing a reduction in the force of heart contractions*	Fatigue; chest pain and palpitations; shortness of breath; swelling of the legs; wheezing; cough.
	Cervical acceleration/ deceleration injuries *Whiplash*	Pain and stiffness in the neck that usually intensifies 24 hours after a head injury or neck sprain.

Dizziness *continued*

Associated Symptoms	Possible Diagnosis	Distinguishing Features
	Cholesteatoma *Infected cyst in the eardrum or middle ear*	Hearing loss; discharge of pus from ear; headaches and earaches; weakness of facial muscles; dizziness.
	Concussion	Brief loss of consciousness following a blow to the head. Occasionally causes nausea and vomiting.
	Ear infection, middle *Inflammation of the middle ear*	Earache; deafness; ringing in the ear; possibly, a discharge of pus from the ear; fever; dizziness.
	Hypertension	Usually asymptomatic except in severe cases. Possibly, headache, easy fatigability, palpitations, chest pain, blurred vision, dizziness, nose bleeds, and confusion.
	Hypoglycemia *Low blood sugar*	Anxiety; hunger; trembling; headache; palpitations; perspiration; confusion; irritability; loss of coordination; possibly, double vision, seizures, or coma.
	Otosclerosis *An overgrowth of bone in the middle ear*	Progressive hearing loss; ringing in the ears; dizziness. Hearing is more distinct when background noise is present.
	Paget's disease *A weakening, thickening, and deformity of the bones*	Often asymptomatic. Possibly, bone pain or deformity, especially bowing of the legs, bent spine, and facial deformity; unexplained bone fractures; joint pain or stiffness; hearing loss; headaches; ringing in ears.
	Polycythemia vera *An overproduction of red and white blood cells and platelets*	Headache; ringing in the ears; blurred vision; flushed skin; itching; dizziness; fatigue; night sweats; frequent nose bleeds and bruises.
	Toxic shock syndrome	Lethargy; conjunctivitis; confusion; sudden high fever accompanied by nausea, watery diarrhea, sore throat, and headache. Red rash on the palms and soles of the feet, which, after a week or two, begins to peel.
	Transient ischemic attack *Temporary blockage in an artery supplying the brain*	Weakness or numbness in a limb; slurred speech; short-lived, temporary partial blindness; numbness and tingling; speech difficulties; confusion; dizziness.
with nausea/vomiting	Adrenal insufficiency *Inadequate production of steroid hormones by the adrenal gland*	Loss of weight and appetite; fatigue; weakness; darkening of the skin; abdominal pain; diarrhea; indigestion; nausea and vomiting; constipation; lack of sex drive; dizziness when rising from sitting or lying position.
	Benign paroxysmal positional vertigo	Sudden sensation of spinning that occurs after changing the position of the head; loss of balance; nausea and vomiting.

Dizziness *continued*

Associated Symptoms	Possible Diagnosis	Distinguishing Features
with nausea/vomiting *continued*	Brain tumors	Headaches that become more severe when reclining; nausea and vomiting; memory loss; double vision; muscle weakness; numbness, tingling, or partial paralysis; vision loss; speech disturbances; seizures; drowsiness.
	Headache, migraine	Throbbing pain in the temple which spreads to the side of the head; nausea; vomiting. Pain may be preceded by blurred or impaired vision with bright spots and zig-zag patterns.
	Hypopituitarism *Underactivity of the pituitary gland*	Intolerance to cold; chronic headaches; decreased sex drive; fatigue; dizziness; fine wrinkles around the eyes and mouth; dry skin; extreme thirst and excessive urination; loss of appetite; vaginal dryness; absence of milk production in new mothers; in men, reduced muscular strength, shrinking of the testes, and loss of body hair; growth retardation in children and adolescents.
	Labyrinthitis *Inflammation of the semicircular canals of the inner ear*	Severe dizziness, loss of balance, jerky movements of the eyes; nausea and vomiting; ringing in the ears. In later stages, possible hearing loss.
	Ménière's disease *Dysfunction of structures in the inner ear*	Sudden attack of severe vertigo; nausea and vomiting; impaired sense of balance; ringing in the ears; hearing loss in the affected ear. Jerky movements of the eyes.

Drooling

Associated Symptoms	Possible Diagnosis	Distinguishing Features
with twitching, convulsions, or tremors	Amyotrophic lateral sclerosis *Progressive degeneration of nerve cells of the central nervous system*	Progressive loss of strength and coordination in the limbs; muscle twitching and cramps that begin in the hands and spread to the arms, shoulders, and legs; stiff, clumsy gait; swallowing, breathing, or speaking difficulty; weight loss; drooling; involuntary laughing or crying.
	Parkinson's disease *Degeneration of the basal ganglia, a cluster of nerve cells in the brain*	Tremors in the hands; stiffness and weakness; impaired voluntary movement; shuffling gait; stooped posture; unblinking, fixed expression; possibly, slow, hesitant speech; difficulty swallowing; drooling; depression. Tremors occur at rest (not with voluntary movements) and disappear during sleep.
	Poliomyelitis *Polio*	Low fever; sore throat; headache; nausea and vomiting. In severe cases, paralysis without loss of sensation; stiff neck and back; twitching; swallowing and breathing difficulty; drooling.
	Rabies	Low-grade fever; headache; loss of appetite; difficulty swallowing; tingling at site of animal bite; intense thirst exacerbated by the inability to drink without violent, painful throat spasms; paralysis of facial muscles; drooling. Agitation and violent behavior, confusion, convulsions, coma.
	Seizures	Involuntary twitching or jerking; muscle rigidity; loss of consciousness; confusion; drooling; hallucinations.
	Tetanus	Often, lockjaw; stiffness and, later, muscle spasms in the neck and face; drooling; abdominal and back pain; extreme perspiration; swallowing difficulty; possible convulsions; fever.
without twitching, convulsions, or tremors	Bell's palsy *Paralysis of muscles on one side of the face*	Drooping muscles and weakness on one side of the face resulting in a distorted smile or an expressionless look; drooping brow, tearing and an inability to close the affected eyelid; drooling; possibly, ear pain on the affected side of the face; possibly, changes in taste perception; increased sensitivity to noise.
	Esophageal cancer	Swallowing difficulty and pain; weight loss; drooling; possibly, vomiting or coughing up of bloody mucus, regurgitation of food; chest pain; repeated respiratory infections.
	Myasthenia gravis *Nerve degeneration causing gradual loss of voluntary muscle control*	Drooping eyelids; double or blurred vision; muscle weakness especially in the face, throat, and neck; chewing and swallowing difficulties; possible breathing difficulty. Slurred, nasal-sounding speech.

Drooling *continued*

Associated Symptoms	Possible Diagnosis	Distinguishing Features
without twitching, convulsions, or tremors *continued*	Peritonsillar abscess *A collection of pus between the tonsils and surrounding tissue due to infection*	Sore throat; severe pain when swallowing; fever; headache; impaired speech; drooling; swollen glands in the neck.
	Salivary gland disorders	Swollen, painful glands behind the ear or under the tongue; soft, painful, swollen glands in the neck; bitter taste in the mouth; fever; dry mouth; increased number of dental cavities; difficulty swallowing.
	Tongue disorders	Symptoms vary depending on the specific disorder and include: dark or bright red, black, or dark brown tongue; sore, swollen, or smooth tongue; hair-like growths on the tongue; adjacent areas of the mouth may be inflamed; ulcers or raised, white patches on the tongue; excessive salivation; swallowing difficulty; bad breath.

Drowsiness

Associated Symptoms	Possible Diagnosis	Distinguishing Features
	Bipolar disorder *Manic-depressive illness*	Symptoms vary depending on phase of the disorder; mania: inflated self-esteem, elation, euphoria, grandiosity, increased activity, and a decreased need for sleep; depression: persistent feelings of sadness, apathy, or hopelessness; diminished interest in activities; loss of appetite and weight or unusual increase in appetite and weight; insomnia or drowsiness; difficulty concentrating; agitation in older patients.
	Brain abscess	Headaches; drowsiness; nausea; vomiting; fever; seizures; possible partial paralysis; confusion; speaking difficulty.
	Depression	Persistent feelings of sadness, apathy, or hopelessness; diminished interest in activities; loss of or unusual increase in appetite and weight; insomnia or drowsiness; difficulty concentrating; agitation.
	Encephalitis *Inflammation of the brain*	Initially, headache and fever followed by confusion, hallucinations, and paralysis on one side of the body; memory loss; difficulty with speech and eye movements; drowsiness; possible coma or epileptic seizures; loss of hearing; sensitivity to light; stiff neck.
	Hemochromatosis *An excess accumulation of iron in the liver, pancreas, heart, testes, skin, and other organs*	A bronze or slate-grey tone to skin that is normally fair; chronic abdominal pain; heart palpitations; joint pain; drowsiness. In men, a decrease in the size of the testes, loss of sexual desire, and impotence.
	Hydrocephalus *Overaccumulation of cerebrospinal fluid, the liquid surrounding the brain*	In infants, an enlarged head, rigidity of the legs, irritability, projectile vomiting, drowsiness, seizures, and lethargy. In older persons, headache, vomiting, loss of coordination, deterioration of mental faculties, speech difficulty, and loss of appetite.
	Insomnia	Difficulty falling asleep or staying asleep; daytime fatigue; irritability.
	Renal failure, acute *Severe kidney failure*	Initially, decreased urine output, weight gain and swelling due to edema, loss of appetite, nausea and vomiting, fatigue. If untreated, confusion, seizures, and drowsiness.
	Sleep apnea *Recurrent episodes of breathing cessation during sleep*	Loud snoring; morning fatigue and headache; sleep disturbances; daytime sleepiness; difficulty concentrating; memory loss. Most common among overweight men.
	Typhoid fever	Headache; fever, loss of appetite; abdominal pain and tenderness; extreme weakness; constipation followed by diarrhea; drowsiness, stupor, or coma; raised, pink skin eruptions on the torso; joint aches; sore throat.

Ear, ringing or buzzing Tinnitus

Associated Symptoms	Possible Diagnosis	Distinguishing Features
with dizziness	Anemia, aplastic	Fatigue and weakness; shortness of breath; heart palpitations; pallor; bleeding gums; nosebleeds; tendency to bruise easily; small red dots under the skin (petechiae). Increased susceptibility to infection.
	Anemia, folic acid deficiency	Fatigue and weakness; pallor; shortness of breath, heart palpitations, or noticeably rapid heartbeat on exertion; sore, red, and glazed looking tongue; loss of weight and appetite; nausea and diarrhea; abdominal distention.
	Anemia, hemolytic	Fatigue and weakness; shortness of breath on exertion; pallor; heart palpitations; jaundice and dark urine.
	Anemia, iron deficiency	Fatigue and weakness; pallor; shortness of breath and heart palpitations on exertion; irritability or inability to concentrate; sore tongue or tiny cracks at the corners of the mouth; black, tarry or bloody stools; unusual craving for dirt, paint, or ice.
	Concussion	Brief loss of consciousness following a blow to the head. Occasionally causes nausea and vomiting.
	Ear infection, middle *Inflammation of the middle ear*	Earache; deafness; ringing in the ear; possibly, a discharge of pus from the ear; fever; dizziness.
	Hypertension	Usually asymptomatic except in severe cases. Possibly, headache, easy fatigability, palpitations, chest pain, blurred vision, dizziness, nose bleeds, and confusion.
	Labyrinthitis *Inflammation of the semicircular canals of the inner ear*	Severe dizziness, loss of balance, jerky movements of the eyes; nausea and vomiting; ringing in the ears. In later stages, possible hearing loss.
	Ménière's disease *Dysfunction of structures in the inner ear*	Sudden attack of severe vertigo; nausea and vomiting; impaired sense of balance; ringing in the ears; hearing loss in the affected ear. Jerky movements of the eyes.
	Otosclerosis *An overgrowth of bone in the middle ear*	Progressive hearing loss; ringing in the ears; dizziness. Hearing is more distinct when background noise is present.
	Paget's disease *A weakening, thickening, and deformity of the bones*	Often asymptomatic. Possibly, bone pain or deformity, especially bowing of the legs, bent spine, and facial deformity; unexplained bone fractures; joint pain or stiffness; hearing loss; headaches; ringing in ears.
	Polycythemia vera *An overproduction of red and white blood cells and platelets*	Headache; ringing in the ears; blurred vision; flushed skin; itching; dizziness; fatigue; night sweats; frequent nose bleeds and bruises.

Ear, ringing or buzzing Tinnitus *continued*

Associated Symptoms	Possible Diagnosis	Distinguishing Features
without dizziness	Acoustic neuroma *A benign tumor in the cells covering the auditory nerve*	Gradual hearing loss; ringing in the ear; headache; numbness in the face; unsteady walk. In later stages, swallowing and speaking difficulties; possibly, slight paralysis.
	Ear drum, perforated	Earache or sudden pain in the ear; partial hearing loss; slight bleeding or discharge from the ear; ringing or buzzing in the affected ear.
	Presbycusis *Loss of hearing due to age*	Progressive inability to hear well in the presence of background noise; difficulty understanding speech.
	Tinnitus *Ringing in one or both ears*	Ringing, buzzing, humming, or hissing sound in the ear, which may be continuous or episodic; possible hearing loss.

Earache

Associated Symptoms	Possible Diagnosis	Distinguishing Features
with hearing loss	Acoustic neuroma *A benign tumor in the cells covering the auditory nerve*	Gradual hearing loss; ringing in the ear; headache; numbness in the face; unsteady walk. In later stages, swallowing and speaking difficulties; possibly, slight paralysis.
	Cholesteatoma *Infected cyst in the eardrum or middle ear*	Hearing loss; discharge of pus from ear; headaches and earaches; weakness of facial muscles; dizziness.
	Ear drum, perforated	Earache or sudden pain in the ear; partial hearing loss; slight bleeding or discharge from the ear; ringing or buzzing in the affected ear.
	Ear infection, middle *Inflammation of the middle ear*	Earache; deafness; ringing in the ear; possibly, a discharge of pus from the ear; fever; dizziness.
	Ear infection, outer	Redness and itching of the ear canal; discharge from the ear; ear pain; possibly, temporary loss of hearing.
without hearing loss	Laryngitis	Hoarseness that often progresses to loss of the voice; throat pain; dry cough; possible fever.
	Neuralgia *Pain due to nerve damage or irritation*	Symptoms vary depending on the area affected and include: recurring episodes of sharp pain on one side of the lips, gums, cheek, or chin; radiating pain around the eyes; a burning pain along the path of a nerve encircling the torso. Pain may last from a few seconds to several minutes and always affects the same location. Attacks may occur several times a day for weeks with asymptomatic periods of weeks or months in between and may be triggered by touching or blowing on the affected area. Mouth pain may be exacerbated by talking, eating, or swallowing.
	Pharyngitis *Inflammation of the pharynx, the part of the throat between the mouth and the esophagus*	Sore or red throat; speaking and swallowing difficulties; sensitive, swollen glands in the neck; fever; headache; possible earache.
	Sinusitis *Inflammation of the mucous membranes lining the sinuses*	Throbbing pain above or below one or both eyes that intensifies when bending the head forward or coughing; nasal congestion; loss of sense of smell; often, pus-like nasal discharge; possible dental pain in the upper jaw; fever.
	Temporomandibular joint syndrome	Pain in the joints connecting the jaw to the skull; headache; tender jaw muscles; dull facial pain; clicking noise when opening or closing the mouth; pain when yawning and chewing. Jaw may temporarily lock in position.

Earache *continued*

Associated Symptoms	Possible Diagnosis	Distinguishing Features
without hearing loss *continued*	Tonsillitis	Sore, inflamed throat; swallowing difficulty; headache; swollen glands in the neck; fever; loss of voice. In children, nausea, vomiting, and abdominal pain.
	Tooth abscess	Persistent tooth pain; pain when biting or chewing; difficulty swallowing; swollen glands in the neck; earache; fever; possibly, foul taste in the mouth or bad breath.
	Tooth decay	Tooth pain, especially after eating sweet or sour foods; tooth sensitivity to hot and cold; bad breath; unpleasant taste in the mouth.

Ejaculation, painful

Associated Symptoms	Possible Diagnosis	Distinguishing Features
	Bladder cancer	Blood in the urine; painful and frequent urination; pelvic pain; feeling of pressure in the back; persistent fever.
	Bladder infection *Cystitis*	Burning during urination; frequent and urgent urination with only small amounts of urine passed; blood in the urine; lower abdominal pain; low-grade fever; pain during sexual intercourse and, in men, during ejaculation.
	Candidiasis *Fungal infection of the mouth, genitals, or mucous membranes*	Thick, white discharge from the vagina; itching and irritation in the vaginal area; pain while urinating or during intercourse; in men, inflammation of the head of the penis; possibly, yellow raised patches in the mouth.
	Chlamydia *Contagious, infectious disease caused by chlamydia, a group of microorganisms*	Usually asymptomatic; possibly, pain or burning during urination, watery discharge from the penis or vagina, swelling of the testicles, breathing difficulty, cough, high fever, inflammation of the inner lining of the eyelids and the membrane covering the whites of the eyes.
	Epididymitis *Inflammation of the coiled sperm conduit that rests on each testicle*	Severe pain and swelling at the back of a testicle; possibly, redness and swelling of the scrotum; burning on urination.
	Neurogenic bladder *Inability to control passage of urine due to damage to nerves to the bladder*	Inability to control urine flow which may involuntarily release in large volumes or in a continuous dribbling. Bed-wetting during sleep; feeling the need to urinate though no urine is passed; pain or burning during urination.
	Orchitis *Inflammation of a testicle*	Swelling and severe pain in the affected testicle; possible bloody discharge in the semen; pain during intercourse; fever.
	Prostate cancer	Difficulty urinating; frequent urination with decreased urine output; pain in the pelvic area and lower back; painful ejaculation or bowel movements; impotence.
	Prostatitis *Inflammation of the prostate gland*	Burning during urination; urgent and frequent urination; fever and chills; discharge from the penis; lower abdominal and back pain; blood in the urine.
	Testicular torsion *Twisting of the spermatic cord*	Severe pain and swelling on one side of the scrotum; skin on the scrotum may appear red or purple; light-headedness or fainting; possibly, abdominal pain, nausea and vomiting.

Ejaculation, painful *continued*

Associated Symptoms	Possible Diagnosis	Distinguishing Features
	Urethritis *Infection of the urethra, the passageway that drains urine from the bladder*	Frequent and painful urination; blood in the urine; yellow, pus-filled discharge; possible difficulty passing urine; urinary urgency; pain during intercourse; in men, painful ejaculation.
	Varicocele *Varicose veins in the scrotum*	Visibly enlarged, twisted veins in the scrotum; swelling around the testicles, usually on the left side, that may subside when reclining; sensation of heaviness or dragging in the groin; possibly, scrotal pain or discomfort.

Elbow pain

Associated Symptoms	Possible Diagnosis	Distinguishing Features
	Bone cancer	Pain, tenderness, and swelling in the affected bones and joints, often intensifying at night; a noticeable tumor or mass; increased susceptibility to bone fractures.
	Bursitis *Inflammation of the bursas, the lubricant-filled sacs in and around the joints*	Pain and swelling around a joint, usually the elbow, knee, or shoulder; painful movement in the affected joint; possibly, fever.
	Dislocations/subluxations	Deformity of the affected joint; joint pain and tenderness; difficulty moving a joint; swelling and stiffness within 30 minutes after joint injury.
	Infectious arthritis	Pain, swelling, stiffness, and redness, usually in one joint. Fever. Severity varies from a mild ache to severe, debilitating pain and eventual joint deformity.
	Osteoarthritis *Degeneration of the cartilage that lines the joints*	Pain, swelling, and stiffness in one or more joints; enlargement and distortion of affected joints.
	Osteomyelitis *Infection of bone and bone marrow*	Fever; severe pain in the affected bone; inflammation and swelling of the skin over the affected area; deformity. In children, arrested growth of the affected bone.
	Rheumatoid arthritis	Fatigue and weakness; joint pain, stiffness, and inflammation, especially in the hands, feet, and arms; joint deformity; dry mouth; dry, painful eyes. Morning stiffness.
	Rheumatoid arthritis, juvenile	Fever; rash; abdominal pain; weight loss; swelling, stiffness, and pain in the affected joints; enlarged lymph glands; fatigue; pallor; red, painful eyes.
	Sprains and strains	Swelling, pain or tenderness in the affected joints; impaired joint function.
	Tendinitis *Inflammation of a tendon*	Pain over a tendon anywhere in the body; if involved tendon is near or part of a joint, restricted movement of the joint.

Erectile dysfunction Impotence

Associated Symptoms	Possible Diagnosis	Distinguishing Features
	Acromegaly *Overproduction of growth hormone by the pituitary gland*	In adults (acromegaly): Gradual thickening of the bones of the face, jaw, and the extremities in adults; oily skin; severe headache; excessive hair growth; excessive perspiration; joint pains. In children (in which the disease is called gigantism): Rapid growth and unusual height; possibly, blindness.
	Adrenal insufficiency *Inadequate production of steroid hormones by the adrenal gland*	Loss of weight and appetite; fatigue; weakness; darkening of the skin; abdominal pain; diarrhea; indigestion; nausea and vomiting; constipation; lack of sex drive; dizziness when rising from sitting or lying position.
	Amyotrophic lateral sclerosis *Progressive degeneration of nerve cells of the central nervous system*	Progressive loss of strength and coordination in the limbs; muscle twitching and cramps that begin in the hands and spread to the arms, shoulders, and legs; stiff, clumsy gait; swallowing, breathing, or speaking difficulty; weight loss; drooling; involuntary laughing or crying.
	Cirrhosis *Chronic damage to the cells of the liver*	No symptoms in early stages; loss of weight and appetite; nausea; swollen legs, ankles and abdomen; itching; jaundice; black stools; vomiting blood; fatigue; impotence; memory loss; confusion.
	Coronary artery disease *Blockage in the arteries supplying blood to the heart muscle*	Initially, asymptomatic. In later stages, dull chest pain that may spread to the neck or the arms usually exacerbated by physical exertion and alleviated with rest; heart palpitations; shortness of breath.
	Cushing's syndrome	Red, oval-shaped face; humped upper back and obese trunk; acne; purple stretch marks on the abdomen, thighs, and breasts; thin and easily bruised skin; easily fractured bones; depression or euphoria; insomnia; fatigue; muscle weakness; hirsutism (in women).
	Depression	Persistent feelings of sadness, apathy, or hopelessness; diminished interest in activities; loss of or unusual increase in appetite and weight; insomnia or drowsiness; difficulty concentrating; agitation.
	Diabetes mellitus *Insufficiency of or resistance to insulin*	Fatigue; excessive thirst; frequent urination; weight loss despite increased appetite; blurred vision; numbness and tingling of feet and hands; impotence.
	Erectile dysfunction	Inability to achieve or maintain an erection, despite sexual desire.

Erectile dysfunction Impotence *continued*

Associated Symptoms	Possible Diagnosis	Distinguishing Features
	Hemochromatosis *An excess accumulation of iron in the liver, pancreas, heart, testes, skin, and other organs*	A bronze or slate-grey tone to skin that is normally fair; chronic abdominal pain; heart palpitations; joint pain; drowsiness. In men, a decrease in the size of the testes, loss of sexual desire, and impotence.
	Hyperprolactinemia *Overproduction of the hormone prolactin by the pituitary gland*	Symptoms may vary depending on gender; in women: cessation of menstrual periods, decreased menstrual flow, excess facial hair; in men: erectile dysfunction, infertility, decreased libido, enlarged breasts; in men and women: abnormal production of breast milk, headaches, decreased vision.
	Hypopituitarism *Underactivity of the pituitary gland*	Intolerance to cold; chronic headaches; decreased sex drive; fatigue; dizziness; fine wrinkles around the eyes and mouth; dry skin; extreme thirst and excessive urination; loss of appetite; vaginal dryness; absence of milk production in new mothers; in men, reduced muscular strength, shrinking of the testes, and loss of body hair; growth retardation in children and adolescents.
	Hypothyroidism *Underactivity of the thyroid gland*	Unexplained weight gain; fatigue; muscle weakness; cramps; dry skin; hair loss; deepening of the voice; intolerance for cold; constipation; chest pain; insomnia; puffiness around eyes; loss of sex drive; depression; menstrual abnormalities; possible swelling in the neck.
	Multiple sclerosis *Gradual degeneration of the protective sheaths surrounding the nerves within the brain and spinal cord*	Symptoms may appear suddenly and then disappear; persistent symptoms may take years to develop and include numbness or tingling in any part of the body, weakness in the extremities, an unsteady walk, slurred speech, urinary incontinence, fatigue, depression, temporary loss of vision, double or blurred vision, mental confusion, and memory loss.
	Peripheral neuropathies *Degeneration of the nerves that supply the extremities*	Tingling or numbness commonly beginning in the hands and feet and gradually spreading toward the center of the body; sensitive skin; muscle weakness; possibly, pain in the hands and feet; lack of coordination; shooting pains exacerbated by touch or changes in temperature; breathing difficulty; urinary or fecal incontinence.
	Peripheral vascular disease *Narrowing of blood vessels in the legs or arms*	Muscle pain on one or both legs that occurs with exercise and subsides with rest; possible pain in the fingers, arms, buttocks, lower back, or the arch of the foot; impotence. Severe symptoms include: muscle pain at rest that intensifies at night; discolored or blue toes; cold or numb feet; open sores; heightened sensitivity to cold; weak or absent pulse in the affected limb; scaly or hairless skin over the affected area.

Erectile dysfunction Impotence *continued*

Associated Symptoms	Possible Diagnosis	Distinguishing Features
	Prostate cancer	Difficulty urinating; frequent urination with decreased urine output; pain in the pelvic area and lower back; painful ejaculation or bowel movements; impotence.
	Prostatitis *Inflammation of the prostate gland*	Burning during urination; urgent and frequent urination; fever and chills; discharge from the penis; lower abdominal and back pain; blood in the urine.
	Renal failure, chronic *Persistent, mild kidney failure*	Asymptomatic in early stages. Possibly, mental confusion; shortness of breath; abdominal pain; decreased sex drive; fatigue; muscle and bone pain; numbness in the legs and feet; headache; impaired mental acuity; bad breath.
	Spinal cord trauma	Severe pain and swelling in the affected area; loss of sensation, muscle weakness, or paralysis below the site of the injury; urinary or fecal incontinence or retention; impotence; breathing difficulty; shock.
	Spinal tumor	Progressive numbness, tingling, and muscle weakness; fecal or urinary incontinence; persistent back pain.
	Syphilis	Initially, painless, ulcerated, red sore on the genitals, mouth, or rectum; swollen glands in the neck, armpit, or groin; rash with small, red, scaly bumps; fever; headache. If left untreated, damage to heart valves leading to congestive heart failure; mental deterioration; loss of balance; seizures; dementia; personality changes.

Eye discharge

Associated Symptoms	Possible Diagnosis	Distinguishing Features
	Anaphylaxis	Itching and hives; swelling of the eyes, lips, and tongue; weakness or faintness; tightening in the chest or throat; wheezing; shortness of breath; profuse sweating; palpitations; sudden, intense distress; feelings of impending doom; stomach cramps; nausea, vomiting, or diarrhea; bluish tinge (cyanosis) to the skin, lips, and nail beds due to oxygen insufficiency.
	Bell's palsy *Paralysis of muscles on one side of the face*	Drooping muscles and weakness on one side of the face resulting in a distorted smile or an expressionless look; drooping brow, tearing and an inability to close the affected eyelid; drooling; possibly, ear pain on the affected side of the face; possibly, changes in taste perception; increased sensitivity to noise.
	Blepharitis *Inflammation of the eyelids*	Red, irritated, scaly eyelids; burning sensation and feeling of grittiness in the eye. Crusted lids in the morning.
	Carcinoid tumors and carcinoid syndrome	May be asymptomatic; flushing or redness of the face and neck; gas and profuse diarrhea; abdominal cramping; watery, swollen eyes; shortness of breath or wheezing.
	Common cold	Nasal congestion; watery eyes; sneezing; sore throat; cough; muscle aches; mild headache; listlessness; possibly, low-grade fever.
	Conjunctivitis *Pinkeye*	Itching and redness in the affected eye; discharge from the eye, clear or pus-filled; excessive tearing; aversion to bright lights; possibly, swollen eyelids.
	Corneal ulcers and infections	Severe eye pain; blurred vision; increased tear production; aversion to light.
	Headache, cluster	Persistent pain in or around one eye; redness and tearing of one eye; nasal congestion on the same side of the face as the affected eye.
	Measles	Cough; fever; watery nasal discharge; loss of appetite; red, watering eyes; sore throat; body aches; red, slightly itchy rash that gradually spreads all over the body.
	Scleritis and episcleritis *Inflammation of the sclera, the white of the eye*	Dull eye pain; redness in the white of the eye; possibly, blurred vision; aversion to light; excessive tearing.
	Styes	Small, possibly painful, pus-filled abscess on the eyelid; watering of the eye; feeling of something in the eye.

Eye discharge *continued*

Associated Symptoms	Possible Diagnosis	Distinguishing Features
	Uveitis and iritis *Inflammation of the uvea, a group of structures in the eye including the iris*	Moderate to severe eye pain; aversion to light; redness in the eye; excessive tearing; blurred vision; spots in the field of vision.

Eye pain

Associated Symptoms	Possible Diagnosis	Distinguishing Features
with eye discharge or excessive tearing	Blepharitis *Inflammation of the eyelids*	Red, irritated, scaly eyelids; burning sensation and feeling of grittiness in the eye. Crusted lids in the morning.
	Conjunctivitis *Pinkeye*	Itching and redness in the affected eye; discharge from the eye, clear or pus-filled; excessive tearing; aversion to bright lights; possibly, swollen eyelids.
	Corneal ulcers and infections	Severe eye pain; blurred vision; increased tear production; aversion to light.
	Headache, cluster	Persistent pain in or around one eye; redness and tearing of one eye; nasal congestion on the same side of the face as the affected eye.
	Measles	Cough; fever; watery nasal discharge; loss of appetite; red, watering eyes; sore throat; body aches; red, slightly itchy rash that gradually spreads all over the body.
	Scleritis and episcleritis *Inflammation of the sclera, the white of the eye*	Dull eye pain; redness in the white of the eye; possibly, blurred vision; aversion to light; excessive tearing.
	Styes	Small, possibly painful, pus-filled abscess on the eyelid; watering of the eye; feeling of something in the eye.
	Uveitis and iritis *Inflammation of the uvea, a group of structures in the eye including the iris*	Moderate to severe eye pain; aversion to light; redness in the eye; excessive tearing; blurred vision; spots in the field of vision.
without eye discharge or excessive tearing	Chlamydia *Contagious, infectious disease caused by chlamydia, a group of microorganisms*	Usually asymptomatic; possibly, pain or burning during urination, watery discharge from the penis or vagina, swelling of the testicles, breathing difficulty, cough, high fever, inflammation of the inner lining of the eyelids and the membrane covering the whites of the eyes.
	Eye cancers	Often initially asymptomatic. In later stages, gradual blurring and loss of vision, bulging eyes. Possibly, crossed eyes, change in eye color, or a tumor visible through the pupil. Painful red eye.
	Glaucoma	Often initially asymptomatic. In later stages, the symptoms of closed-angle glaucoma include: the appearance of halos and rainbows around lights; dilated pupil in the affected eye; severe headache and eye pain; possibly, nausea and vomiting. Open-angle glaucoma symptoms include: blurred vision and a gradual loss of peripheral vision.

Eye pain *continued*

Associated Symptoms	Possible Diagnosis	Distinguishing Features
without eye discharge or excessive tearing *continued*	Headache, migraine	Throbbing pain in the temple which spreads to the side of the head; nausea; vomiting. Pain may be preceded by blurred or impaired vision with bright spots and zig-zag patterns.
	Hyphema *Blood within the eye*	Visible bleeding within the front portion of the eye in and around the iris; impaired vision.
	Neuralgia *Pain due to nerve damage or irritation*	Symptoms vary depending on the area affected and include: recurring episodes of sharp pain on one side of the lips, gums, cheek, or chin; radiating pain around the eyes; a burning pain along the path of a nerve encircling the torso. Pain may last from a few seconds to several minutes and always affects the same location. Attacks may occur several times a day for weeks with asymptomatic periods of weeks or months in between and may be triggered by touching or blowing on the affected area. Mouth pain may be exacerbated by talking, eating, or swallowing.
	Optic neuritis	Sudden, partial loss of vision, usually in the central portion of the field of vision; blurred vision; pain in affected eye.
	Sinusitis *Inflammation of the mucous membranes lining the sinuses*	Throbbing pain above or below one or both eyes that intensifies when bending the head forward or coughing; nasal congestion; loss of sense of smell; often, pus-like nasal discharge; possible dental pain in the upper jaw; fever.
	Sjögren's syndrome	Dry, itching, burning eyes; sensation of a foreign body under the eyelids; dry mouth; difficulty swallowing; vaginal dryness; dry skin; frequent dental cavities; joint pain; swelling of glands (parotids) in front of the ears; Raynaud's phenomenon.

Eye redness

Associated Symptoms	Possible Diagnosis	Distinguishing Features
	Allergic rhinitis *Hay fever*	Nasal congestion; frequent sneezing; itchy eyes, nose, and throat.
	Anaphylaxis	Itching and hives; swelling of the eyes, lips, and tongue; weakness or faintness; tightening in the chest or throat; wheezing; shortness of breath; profuse sweating; palpitations; sudden, intense distress; feelings of impending doom; stomach cramps; nausea, vomiting, or diarrhea; bluish tinge (cyanosis) to the skin, lips, and nail beds due to oxygen insufficiency.
	Conjunctivitis *Pinkeye*	Itching and redness in the affected eye; discharge from the eye, clear or pus-filled; excessive tearing; aversion to bright lights; possibly, swollen eyelids.
	Corneal ulcers and infections	Severe eye pain; blurred vision; increased tear production; aversion to light.
	Crohn's disease *Inflammation of the lining of the small intestine*	Episodes of abdominal pain or cramps in lower abdomen; nausea; diarrhea; loss of weight and appetite; possibly, fever; rectal bleeding or blood in stools; fatigue; anal fissures; joint pains; inflammation of the eyes.
	Glaucoma	Often initially asymptomatic. In later stages, the symptoms of closed-angle glaucoma include: the appearance of halos and rainbows around lights; dilated pupil in the affected eye; severe headache and eye pain; possibly, nausea and vomiting. Open-angle glaucoma symptoms include: blurred vision and a gradual loss of peripheral vision.
	Headache, cluster	Persistent pain in or around one eye; redness and tearing of one eye; nasal congestion on the same side of the face as the affected eye.
	Hyphema *Blood within the eye*	Visible bleeding within the front portion of the eye in and around the iris; impaired vision.
	Meningitis *Inflammation of the membranes covering the brain and spinal cord*	Severe headache; nausea and vomiting; sensitivity to light; stiffness in the neck; possible red skin rash; fever; mental confusion; drowsiness; loss of consciousness; seizures.
	Sarcoidosis *Accumulation of inflammatory cells in the lymph nodes and other tissues throughout the body*	Often no symptoms. Swollen lymph nodes in the neck or armpits; muscle aches; fever; breathing difficulty; possibly, purple rash on the face; reddish or brownish skin spots on the forearms, face, or legs; numbness; joint pain or stiffness; a painful, red eye; blurred vision; loss of appetite and weight.

Eye redness *continued*

Associated Symptoms	Possible Diagnosis	Distinguishing Features
	Scleritis and episcleritis *Inflammation of the sclera,* *the white of the eye*	Dull eye pain; redness in the white of the eye; possibly, blurred vision; aversion to light; copious tearing.
	Toxic shock syndrome	Lethargy; conjunctivitis; confusion; sudden high fever accompanied by nausea, watery diarrhea, sore throat, and headache. Red rash on the palms and soles of the feet, which, after a week or two, begins to peel.
	Uveitis and iritis *Inflammation of the uvea,* *a group of structures in the* *eye including the iris*	Moderate to severe eye pain; aversion to light; redness in the eye; excessive tearing; blurred vision; spots in the field of vision.
	Whooping cough	Initially, mild cough, sneezing, nasal congestion, and irritated eyes. Within approximately two weeks, cough becomes severe and persistent, and is accompanied by characteristic high-pitched "whooping" sound during inhalation; loss of appetite; listlessness; vomiting or choking spells. Most common among young children.

Eyeballs bulging/protruding

Associated Symptoms	Possible Diagnosis	Distinguishing Features
	Anaphylaxis	Itching and hives; swelling of the eyes, lips, and tongue; weakness or faintness; tightening in the chest or throat; wheezing; shortness of breath; profuse sweating; palpitations; sudden, intense distress; feelings of impending doom; stomach cramps; nausea, vomiting, or diarrhea; bluish tinge (cyanosis) to the skin, lips, and nail beds due to oxygen insufficiency.
	Carcinoid tumors and carcinoid syndrome	May be asymptomatic; flushing or redness of the face and neck; gas and profuse diarrhea; abdominal cramping; watery, swollen eyes; shortness of breath or wheezing.
	Eye cancers	Often initially asymptomatic. In later stages, gradual blurring and loss of vision, bulging eyes. Possibly, crossed eyes, change in eye color, or a tumor visible through the pupil. Painful red eye.
	Hyperthyroidism *Overactivity of the thyroid gland*	Protruding eyes; weight loss despite increased appetite; intolerance to heat; excessive perspiration; nervousness or restlessness; possibly, swelling in the neck (goiter); palpitations; tremor; diarrhea.
	Scleritis and episcleritis *Inflammation of the sclera, the white of the eye*	Dull eye pain; redness in the white of the eye; possibly, blurred vision; aversion to light; excessive tearing.

Eyelid drooping

Associated Symptoms	Possible Diagnosis	Distinguishing Features
	Botulism	Difficulty swallowing and speaking; nausea; vomiting; blurred or double vision.
	Hypothyroidism *Underactivity of the thyroid gland*	Unexplained weight gain; fatigue; muscle weakness; cramps; dry skin; hair loss; deepening of the voice; intolerance for cold; constipation; chest pain; insomnia; puffiness around eyes; loss of sex drive; depression; menstrual abnormalities; possible swelling in the neck.
	Myasthenia gravis *Nerve degeneration causing gradual loss of voluntary muscle control*	Drooping eyelids; double or blurred vision; muscle weakness especially in the face, throat, and neck; chewing and swallowing difficulties; possible breathing difficulty. Slurred, nasal-sounding speech.

Eyes, dry

Associated Symptoms	Possible Diagnosis	Distinguishing Features
	Corneal ulcers and infections	Severe eye pain; blurred vision; increased tear production; aversion to light.
	Rheumatoid arthritis	Fatigue and weakness; joint pain, stiffness, and inflammation, especially in the hands, feet, and arms; joint deformity; dry mouth; dry, painful eyes. Morning stiffness.
	Sjögren's syndrome	Dry, itching, burning eyes; sensation of a foreign body under the eyelids; dry mouth; difficulty swallowing; vaginal dryness; dry skin; frequent dental cavities; joint pain; swelling of glands (parotids) in front of the ears; Raynaud's phenomenon.

Eyes, tearing or watering also see Eye discharge

Associated Symptoms	Possible Diagnosis	Distinguishing Features
	Bell's palsy *Paralysis of muscles on one side of the face*	Drooping muscles and weakness on one side of the face resulting in a distorted smile or an expressionless look; drooping brow, tearing and an inability to close the affected eyelid; drooling; possibly, ear pain on the affected side of the face or changes in taste perception; increased sensitivity to noise.
	Common cold	Nasal congestion; watery eyes; sneezing; sore throat; cough; muscle aches; mild headache; listlessness; possibly, low-grade fever.
	Conjunctivitis *Pinkeye*	Itching and redness in the affected eye; discharge from the eye, clear or pus-filled; excessive tearing; aversion to bright lights; possibly, swollen eyelids.
	Corneal ulcers and infections	Severe eye pain; blurred vision; increased tear production; aversion to light.
	Headache, cluster	Persistent pain in or around one eye; redness and tearing of one eye; nasal congestion on the same side of the face as the affected eye.
	Measles	Cough; fever; watery nasal discharge; loss of appetite; red, watering eyes; sore throat; body aches; red, slightly itchy rash that gradually spreads all over the body.
	Scleritis and episcleritis *Inflammation of the sclera, the white of the eye*	Dull eye pain; redness in the white of the eye; possibly, blurred vision; aversion to light; excessive tearing.
	Uveitis and iritis *Inflammation of the uvea, a group of structures in the eye including the iris*	Moderate to severe eye pain; aversion to light; redness in the eye; excessive tearing; blurred vision; spots in the field of vision.

Facial pain

Associated Symptoms	Possible Diagnosis	Distinguishing Features
	Impacted teeth	Gum pain; unpleasant taste in mouth, especially when biting down; red, swollen gums around the affected tooth; headache or jaw ache; possibly, bad breath.
	Jaw dislocation or fracture	Inability to close the jaw normally; painful, swollen, or numb jaw; misalignment of teeth; speaking difficulty; possible breathing difficulty.
	Multiple sclerosis *Gradual degeneration of the protective sheaths surrounding the nerves within the brain and spinal cord*	Symptoms may appear suddenly and then disappear; persistent symptoms may take years to develop and include numbness or tingling in any part of the body, weakness in the extremities, an unsteady walk, slurred speech, urinary incontinence, fatigue, depression, temporary loss of vision, double or blurred vision, mental confusion, and memory loss.
	Neuralgia *Pain due to nerve damage or irritation*	Symptoms vary depending on the area affected and include: recurring episodes of sharp pain on one side of the lips, gums, cheek, or chin; radiating pain around the eyes; a burning pain along the path of a nerve encircling the torso. Pain may last from a few seconds to several minutes and always affects the same location. Attacks may occur several times a day for weeks with asymptomatic periods of weeks or months in between and may be triggered by touching or blowing on the affected area. Mouth pain may be exacerbated by talking, eating, or swallowing.
	Rosacea *Redness, swelling, and blemishes around the nose, cheeks, and forehead*	Facial flushing; stinging, burning, or feeling of skin pulled tight across face; bumps, blemishes, and swelling of nose and cheeks; severe swelling or enlargement of the nose.
	Sinusitis *Inflammation of the mucous membranes lining the sinuses*	Throbbing pain above or below one or both eyes that intensifies when bending the head forward or coughing; nasal congestion; loss of sense of smell; often, pus-like nasal discharge; possible dental pain in the upper jaw; fever.
	Temporomandibular joint syndrome	Pain in the joints connecting the jaw to the skull; headache; tender jaw muscles; dull facial pain; clicking noise when opening or closing the mouth; pain when yawning and chewing. Jaw may temporarily lock in position.
	Tooth abscess	Persistent tooth pain; pain when biting or chewing; difficulty swallowing; swollen glands in the neck; earache; fever; possibly, foul taste in the mouth or bad breath.

Faintness or fainting

Associated Symptoms	Possible Diagnosis	Distinguishing Features
with shortness of breath	Anaphylaxis	Itching and hives; swelling of the eyes, lips, and tongue; weakness or faintness; tightening in the chest or throat; wheezing; shortness of breath; profuse sweating; palpitations; sudden, intense distress; feelings of impending doom; stomach cramps; nausea, vomiting, or diarrhea; bluish tinge (cyanosis) to the skin, lips, and nail beds due to oxygen insufficiency.
	Anemia, aplastic	Fatigue and weakness; shortness of breath; heart palpitations; pallor; bleeding gums; nosebleeds; tendency to bruise easily; small red dots under the skin (petechiae). Increased susceptibility to infection.
	Anemia, folic acid deficiency	Fatigue and weakness; pallor; shortness of breath, heart palpitations, or noticeably rapid heartbeat on exertion; sore, red, and glazed looking tongue; loss of weight and appetite; nausea and diarrhea; abdominal distention.
	Anemia, hemolytic	Fatigue and weakness; shortness of breath on exertion; pallor; heart palpitations; jaundice and dark urine.
	Anemia, iron deficiency	Fatigue and weakness; pallor; shortness of breath and heart palpitations on exertion; irritability or inability to concentrate; sore tongue or tiny cracks at the corners of the mouth; black, tarry or bloody stools; unusual craving for dirt, paint, or ice.
	Anemia, pernicious	Fatigue; inability to concentrate; sore, red tongue; weakness; dizziness; pallor; shortness of breath on exertion; palpitations; numbness and tingling in extremities; incoordination; headache; loss of weight and appetite; possibly, jaundice.
	Cardiac arrhythmias *Irregularities in the heartbeat*	Frequently, asymptomatic; possibly; heart palpitations; lightheadedness; shortness of breath; sudden weakness; loss of consciousness.
	Cardiomyopathy *Disease of the heart muscle causing a reduction in the force of heart contractions*	Fatigue; chest pain and palpitations; shortness of breath; swelling of the legs; wheezing; cough.
	Chronic obstructive pulmonary disease	Shortness of breath; wheezing; persistent, mucus-producing cough, especially in the morning; possibly, chest pain, swollen legs and ankles.
	Congestive heart failure	Shortness of breath; fatigue; need to sleep on several pillows; weakness; cough; heart palpitations; swelling in the legs, ankles, and abdomen; frequent urination at night; indigestion; nausea and vomiting; loss of appetite.

Faintness or fainting *continued*

Associated Symptoms	Possible Diagnosis	Distinguishing Features
with shortness of breath *continued*	Mitral valve prolapse *A deformity in the heart's mitral valve possibly causing it to leak*	Usually asymptomatic. Possible palpitations, shortness of breath, dizziness, fainting, or fatigue.
	Valvular heart disease	Depends on which heart valve is affected. Often asymptomatic. Possibly, fatigue and weakness; dizziness; chest pain; shortness of breath; heart palpitations; fainting; edema; stroke from embolism to the brain.
without shortness of breath	Adrenal insufficiency *Inadequate production of steroid hormones by the adrenal gland*	Loss of weight and appetite; fatigue; weakness; darkening of the skin; abdominal pain; diarrhea; indigestion; nausea and vomiting; constipation; lack of sex drive; dizziness when rising from sitting or lying position.
	Aortic aneurysm *A sac-like ballooning at a weak spot in the wall of the aorta, the body's primary artery*	Usually asymptomatic; occasionally, severe abdominal and back pain; chest pain; swallowing difficulty; dizziness and fainting; hoarseness; cough.
	Brain hemorrhage	Sudden loss of consciousness; sudden, severe headache; mental confusion; stiff neck; nausea and vomiting; paralysis on one side of the face or body; weakness and dizziness; loss of speech; blurred or double vision; dilated pupils.
	Concussion	Brief loss of consciousness following a blow to the head. Occasionally causes nausea and vomiting.
	Heatstroke	Sudden dizziness; weakness; headache; hot, dry, red skin which later turns grey; high body temperature; muscle cramps; confusion; seizures; loss of consciousness.
	Hemochromatosis *An excess accumulation of iron in the liver, pancreas, heart, testes, skin, and other organs*	A bronze or slate-grey tone to skin that is normally fair; chronic abdominal pain; heart palpitations; joint pain; drowsiness. In men, a decrease in the size of the testes, loss of sexual desire, and impotence.
	Hypoglycemia *Low blood sugar*	Anxiety; hunger; trembling; headache; palpitations; perspiration; confusion; irritability; loss of coordination; possibly, double vision, seizures, or coma.
	Hypothermia *Low body temperature (below 94°)*	Shivering; pallor; puffy face; fatigue and confusion; slow, shallow breathing; muscle stiffness; normally warm areas of the body are cold; loss of consciousness.
	Inguinal hernia *Displaced loop of intestine in the inguinal canal, a tubular passage through the abdominal wall*	A swelling in the groin area that may recede when lying down; pain at the site of the swelling, especially when lifting a heavy object; swelling of the scrotum. Nausea, vomiting, loss of appetite, and abdominal pain if intestine becomes obstructed.

Faintness or fainting *continued*

Associated Symptoms	Possible Diagnosis	Distinguishing Features
without shortness of breath *continued*	Meningitis *Inflammation of the membranes covering the brain and spinal cord*	Severe headache; nausea and vomiting; sensitivity to light; stiffness in the neck; possible red skin rash; fever; mental confusion; drowsiness; loss of consciousness; seizures.
	Seizures	Involuntary twitching or jerking; muscle rigidity; loss of consciousness; confusion; drooling; hallucinations.
	Testicular torsion *Twisting of the spermatic cord*	Severe pain and swelling on one side of the scrotum; skin on the scrotum may appear red or purple; light-headedness or fainting; possibly, abdominal pain, nausea and vomiting.
	Transient ischemic attack *Temporary blockage in an artery supplying the brain*	Weakness or numbness in a limb; slurred speech; short-lived, temporary partial blindness; numbness and tingling; speech difficulties; confusion; dizziness.

Fatigue

Associated Symptoms	Possible Diagnosis	Distinguishing Features
	Acromegaly *Overproduction of growth hormone by the pituitary gland*	In adults (acromegaly): Gradual thickening of the bones of the face, jaw, and the extremities in adults; oily skin; severe headache; excessive hair growth; excessive perspiration; joint pains. In children (in which the disease is called gigantism): Rapid growth and unusual height; possibly, blindness.
	Adrenal insufficiency *Inadequate production of steroid hormones by the adrenal gland*	Loss of weight and appetite; fatigue; weakness; darkening of the skin; abdominal pain; diarrhea; indigestion; nausea and vomiting; constipation; lack of sex drive; dizziness when rising from sitting or lying position.
	Cirrhosis *Chronic damage to the cells of the liver*	No symptoms in early stages; loss of weight and appetite; nausea; swollen legs, ankles and abdomen; itching; jaundice; black stools; vomiting blood; fatigue; impotence; memory loss; confusion.
	Colorectal cancer *A growth of malignant cells in the colon or rectum*	Change in bowel habits; diarrhea; constipation; narrow stools; bloody or dark stools; lower abdominal pain; bloating; cramps; gas; loss of weight and appetite; fatigue and heart palpitations due to anemia.
	Cushing's syndrome	Red, oval-shaped face; humped upper back and obese trunk; acne; purple stretch marks on the abdomen, thighs, and breasts; thin and easily bruised skin; easily fractured bones; depression or euphoria; insomnia; fatigue; muscle weakness; hirsutism (in women).
	Depression	Persistent feelings of sadness, apathy, or hopelessness; diminished interest in activities; loss of or unusual increase in appetite and weight; insomnia or drowsiness; difficulty concentrating; agitation.
	Diabetes mellitus *Insufficiency of or resistance to insulin*	Fatigue; excessive thirst; frequent urination; weight loss despite increased appetite; blurred vision; numbness and tingling of feet and hands; impotence.
	Fibromyalgia	Muscle aches, pains, and stiffness; specific points on the body that feel sore when pressed; fatigue; headaches; feeling unrefreshed upon awakening in the morning.
	Hyperthyroidism *Overactivity of the thyroid gland*	Protruding eyes; weight loss despite increased appetite; intolerance to heat; excessive perspiration; nervousness or restlessness; possibly, swelling in the neck (goiter); palpitations; tremor; diarrhea.

Fatigue *continued*

Associated Symptoms	Possible Diagnosis	Distinguishing Features
	Hypopituitarism *Underactivity of the pituitary gland*	Intolerance to cold; chronic headaches; decreased sex drive; fatigue; dizziness; fine wrinkles around the eyes and mouth; dry skin; extreme thirst and excessive urination; loss of appetite; vaginal dryness; absence of milk production in new mothers; in men, reduced muscular strength, shrinking of the testes, and loss of body hair; growth retardation in children and adolescents.
	Hypothyroidism *Underactivity of the thyroid gland*	Unexplained weight gain; fatigue; muscle weakness; cramps; dry skin; hair loss; deepening of the voice; intolerance for cold; constipation; chest pain; insomnia; puffiness around eyes; loss of sex drive; depression; menstrual abnormalities; possible swelling in the neck.
	Insomnia	Difficulty falling asleep or staying asleep; daytime fatigue; irritability.
	Malabsorption, digestive *A failure of the small intestine to absorb nutrients in the diet*	Diarrhea; weight loss; yellowish, foul-smelling stools; abdominal cramps, gas, and bloating; weakness and lethargy.
	Multiple sclerosis *Gradual degeneration of the protective sheaths surrounding the nerves within the brain and spinal cord*	Symptoms may appear suddenly and then disappear; persistent symptoms may take years to develop and include numbness or tingling in any part of the body, weakness in the extremities, an unsteady walk, slurred speech, urinary incontinence, fatigue, depression, temporary loss of vision, double or blurred vision, mental confusion, and memory loss.
	Pancreatic cancer	Often, no symptoms until far advanced. Upper abdominal pain which spreads to the back; loss of weight and appetite; jaundice; nausea, vomiting, and indigestion; diarrhea; fatigue; depression.
	Renal failure, acute *Severe kidney failure*	Initially, decreased urine output, weight gain and swelling due to edema, loss of appetite, nausea and vomiting, fatigue. If untreated, confusion, seizures, and drowsiness.
	Rheumatoid arthritis	Fatigue and weakness; joint pain, stiffness, and inflammation, especially in the hands, feet, and arms; joint deformity; dry mouth; dry, painful eyes. Morning stiffness.

Fatigue *continued*

Associated Symptoms	Possible Diagnosis	Distinguishing Features
	Scleroderma	Shiny, tight, and hardened skin, especially on the fingers, arms, and face; hands or feet may successively turn blue, white, and red upon exposure to cold (Raynaud's phenomenon); swallowing difficulty; bloating after eating; weight loss; shortness of breath on exertion; high blood pressure; symptoms of renal failure. Possibly, heartburn, muscle aches and weakness, joint pain, fever, or fatigue.
	Sjögren's syndrome	Dry, itching, burning eyes; sensation of a foreign body under the eyelids; dry mouth; difficulty swallowing; vaginal dryness; dry skin; frequent dental cavities; joint pain; swelling of glands (parotids) in front of the ears; Raynaud's phenomenon.
	Sleep apnea *Recurrent episodes of breathing cessation during sleep*	Loud snoring; morning fatigue and headache; sleep disturbances; daytime sleepiness; difficulty concentrating; memory loss. Most common among overweight men.
with breathing difficulty/shortness of breath	Amyloidosis *Accumulation of amyloid, a waxy substance, in tissues and organs*	Symptoms vary greatly depending on the body parts affected and may include fatigue and weakness; weight loss; heart palpitations; shortness of breath; swelling of the legs; difficulty swallowing due to swelling of the tongue; diarrhea; abdominal pain; raised spots on the armpits, groin, face, and neck; numbness or tingling of the hands or feet; dizziness on standing; joint pains.
	Anemia, aplastic	Fatigue and weakness; shortness of breath; heart palpitations; pallor; bleeding gums; nosebleeds; tendency to bruise easily; small red dots under the skin (petechiae). Increased susceptibility to infection.
	Anemia, folic acid deficiency	Fatigue and weakness; pallor; shortness of breath, heart palpitations, or noticeably rapid heartbeat on exertion; sore, red, and glazed looking tongue; loss of weight and appetite; nausea and diarrhea; abdominal distention.
	Anemia, hemolytic	Fatigue and weakness; shortness of breath on exertion; pallor; heart palpitations; jaundice and dark urine.
	Anemia, iron deficiency	Fatigue and weakness; pallor; shortness of breath and heart palpitations on exertion; irritability or inability to concentrate; sore tongue or tiny cracks at the corners of the mouth; black, tarry or bloody stools; unusual craving for dirt, paint, or ice.

Fatigue *continued*

Associated Symptoms	Possible Diagnosis	Distinguishing Features
with breathing difficulty/shortness of breath *continued*	Anemia, pernicious	Fatigue; inability to concentrate; sore, red tongue; weakness; dizziness; pallor; shortness of breath on exertion; palpitations; numbness and tingling in extremities; incoordination; headache; loss of weight and appetite; possibly, jaundice.
	Cardiomyopathy *Disease of the heart muscle causing a reduction in the force of heart contractions*	Fatigue; chest pain and palpitations; shortness of breath; swelling of the legs; wheezing; cough.
	Chronic obstructive pulmonary disease	Shortness of breath; wheezing; persistent, mucus-producing cough, especially in the morning; possibly, chest pain, swollen legs and ankles.
	Congestive heart failure	Shortness of breath; fatigue; need to sleep on several pillows; weakness; cough; heart palpitations; swelling in the legs, ankles, and abdomen; frequent urination at night; indigestion; nausea and vomiting; loss of appetite.
	Hypothermia *Low body temperature (below 94°)*	Shivering; pallor; puffy face; fatigue and confusion; slow, shallow breathing; muscle stiffness; normally warm areas of the body are cold; loss of consciousness.
	Lung cancer	Persistent cough; wheezing; shortness of breath; chest pain; fatigue; weight loss.
	Mitral valve prolapse *A deformity in the heart's mitral valve possibly causing it to leak*	Usually asymptomatic. Possible palpitations, shortness of breath, dizziness, fainting, or fatigue.
	Multiple myeloma *Production of malignant plasma cells in the bone marrow*	Bone pain, especially progressive, constant back pain that intensifies with movement; unexplained bone fractures; fatigue; pallor; shortness of breath; increased bleeding, such as bleeding gums or nosebleeds; easily bruised skin; increased susceptibility to infection; headache; vision disturbances; loss of height.
	Myasthenia gravis *Nerve degeneration causing gradual loss of voluntary muscle control*	Drooping eyelids; double or blurred vision; muscle weakness especially in the face, throat, and neck; chewing and swallowing difficulties; possible breathing difficulty. Slurred, nasal-sounding speech.
	Myelofibrosis *An increase of fibrous scar tissue within the bone marrow*	Weakness and fatigue; abdominal fullness; a tendency to bleed easily; bone pain; pallor; shortness of breath during physical exertion; increased susceptibility to bruising and infections; weight loss.

Fatigue *continued*

Associated Symptoms	Possible Diagnosis	Distinguishing Features
with breathing difficulty/shortness of breath *continued*	Myocarditis *Inflammation of the heart muscle*	Fatigue; shortness of breath; heart palpitations; fever; edema; rarely, continuous pressure or vague pain in the chest.
	Nephrotic syndrome *Damage to the filtering units of the kidneys*	Swelling in the ankles and around the eyes; weight gain, due to fluid retention throughout the body; shortness of breath; passing only small amounts of urine that has an unusually foamy appearance; fatigue; diarrhea; loss of appetite.
	Pericarditis *Inflammation of the membrane surrounding the heart*	Sharp chest pain that may spread to the neck and shoulders; pain may be relieved by sitting up and leaning forward; swollen legs and abdomen; breathing difficulty; chills; fever; fatigue.
	Polycythemia vera *An overproduction of red and white blood cells and platelets*	Headache; ringing in the ears; blurred vision; flushed skin; itching; dizziness; fatigue; night sweats; frequent nose bleeds and bruises.
	Renal failure, chronic *Persistent, mild kidney failure*	Asymptomatic in early stages. Possibly, mental confusion; shortness of breath; abdominal pain; decreased sex drive; fatigue; muscle and bone pain; numbness in the legs and feet; headache; impaired mental acuity; bad breath.
	Sarcoidosis *Accumulation of inflammatory cells in the lymph nodes and other tissues throughout the body*	Often no symptoms. Swollen lymph nodes in the neck or armpits; muscle aches; fever; breathing difficulty; possibly, purple rash on the face; reddish or brownish skin spots on the forearms, face, or legs; numbness; joint pain or stiffness; a painful, red eye; blurred vision; loss of appetite and weight.
	Septic shock *Severe drop in blood pressure due to the presence of microorganisms or their toxins in the bloodstream*	Nausea and vomiting; prostration; diarrhea; sudden high fever; chills; rapid breathing; mental confusion or agitation; decreased urine output; severe fatigue; rapid heartbeat.
	Valvular heart disease	Depends on which heart valve is affected. Often asymptomatic. Possibly, fatigue and weakness; dizziness; chest pain; shortness of breath; heart palpitations; fainting; edema; stroke from embolism to the brain.
with fever	AIDS *Acquired immunodeficiency syndrome*	Recurrent infections affecting the skin and respiratory system; cough; shortness of breath; loss of appetite; weight loss; fatigue; diarrhea; fever; dementia; malignant skin lesions; swollen lymph glands throughout the body; purplish skin nodules; memory loss; confusion; personality changes.

Fatigue *continued*

Associated Symptoms	Possible Diagnosis	Distinguishing Features
with fever *continued*	Chronic fatigue syndrome	Severe fatigue made worse by exercise; recurrent flu-like symptoms; persistent sore throat; low-grade fever; muscle and joint aches; headache; painful, swollen lymph nodes; depression and mental confusion; memory loss; sleep difficulties.
	Crohn's disease *Inflammation of the lining of the small intestine*	Episodes of abdominal pain or cramps in lower abdomen; nausea; diarrhea; loss of weight and appetite; possibly, fever; rectal bleeding or blood in stools; fatigue; anal fissures; joint pains; inflammation of the eyes.
	Encephalitis *Inflammation of the brain*	Initially, headache and fever followed by confusion, hallucinations, and paralysis on one side of the body; memory loss; difficulty with speech and eye movements; drowsiness; possible coma or epileptic seizures; loss of hearing; sensitivity to light; stiff neck.
	Hepatitis, acute viral	Fever; fatigue; loss of appetite; aching muscles and joints; abdominal pain or discomfort; jaundice; dark urine and pale stools.
	Hepatitis, chronic	Fatigue; nausea; vomiting; loss of appetite; jaundice; dark urine; clay-colored stools; depression; pain or discomfort in the upper right abdomen; abdominal swelling; fever; in women, cessation of menstruation, acne, and the appearance of male pattern facial hair.
	Infectious arthritis	Pain, swelling, stiffness, and redness, usually in one joint. Fever. Severity varies from a mild ache to severe, debilitating pain and eventual joint deformity.
	Kidney cancer	Blood in the urine; abdominal and lower back pain; low-grade fever; loss of weight and appetite.
	Kidney infection *Pyelonephritis*	Sudden fever and shaking chills; severe fatigue; burning and frequent urination; cloudy or bloody urine; pain in the abdomen, back, or flanks, sometimes severe; nausea and vomiting.
	Leukemias	Symptoms vary depending on the type of leukemia and may include: loss of appetite and weight; increased bruising and bleeding; bone pain, especially in the legs; abdominal pain and distention; nausea; heart palpitations; severe fatigue; pallor; breathing difficulty; fever; night sweats; headache; enlarged lymph nodes; joint pains (due to gout).

Fatigue *continued*

Associated Symptoms	Possible Diagnosis	Distinguishing Features
with fever *continued*	Liver tumors	Pain or discomfort in the upper right portion of the abdomen; abdominal swelling; loss of weight and appetite; nausea and vomiting; fever; excessive perspiration; jaundice; pallor; severe fatigue.
	Lyme disease	A small red bump, surrounded by a concentric bulls-eye-like red rash with a pale center. Over the following month: fever and chills; extreme fatigue; headaches. Symptoms may progress over several months or years and may include: palpitations; joint or muscle pain; and chronic joint inflammation, especially in the knees.
	Pneumonia	High fever; shortness of breath; cough with sputum; chest pain; fatigue.
	Rheumatoid arthritis, juvenile	Fever; rash; abdominal pain; weight loss; swelling, stiffness, and pain in the affected joints; enlarged lymph glands; fatigue; pallor; red, painful eyes.
	Systemic lupus erythematosus *Inflammation of connective tissues throughout the body*	Red, blotchy, butterfly-shaped rash on the cheeks and bridge of the nose; fatigue; fever; loss of appetite and weight; nausea; joint and abdominal pain; headaches; blurred vision; increased sensitivity to sun exposure; depression; psychosis; mental confusion.
	Tuberculosis	Often, asymptomatic. Possibly, low-grade fever; excessive perspiration; cough producing sputum or blood; weight loss; chronic fatigue; chest pain; shortness of breath; night sweats.

Fever

Associated Symptoms	Possible Diagnosis	Distinguishing Features
with breathing difficulty/shortness of breath	Esophageal rupture *A tear in the esophagus, the passageway from the mouth to the stomach*	Chest pain; rapid, shallow breathing; excessive perspiration; fever.
	Septic shock *Severe drop in blood pressure due to the presence of microorganisms or their toxins in the bloodstream*	Nausea and vomiting; prostration; diarrhea; sudden high fever; chills; rapid breathing; mental confusion or agitation; decreased urine output; severe fatigue; rapid heartbeat.
with cough/breathing difficulty	Bronchitis, acute	Shortness of breath; persistent cough producing yellow or green sputum; possibly, chest pain; wheezing; fever.
	Empyema *Collection of pus in any body cavity, usually between the membranes covering the lungs*	Chest pain exacerbated by deep inhalation; shortness of breath; dry cough; fever and chills; exhaustion; weight loss; night sweats; abdominal pain and jaundice.
	Epiglottitis *Inflammation of the epiglottis, the flap of tissue lying behind the tongue*	Sore throat; sudden fever; breathing difficulty which may become severe within hours of onset; pain or difficulty swallowing; muffled speech; hoarseness; drooling.
	Influenza *Flu*	Chills, muscle aches, and loss of appetite followed by a cough, sore throat, nasal congestion, and fever; possible chest pain.
	Legionnaire's disease	Dry cough progressing to one with blood-streaked sputum; high fever; chills; breathing difficulty; chest pain; headache; muscle aches; diarrhea; nausea; vomiting; mental confusion and disorientation.
	Lung abscess	Cough producing foul-smelling sputum; bad breath; fever; chills; weight loss; possible chest pain.
	Pericarditis *Inflammation of the membrane surrounding the heart*	Sharp chest pain that may spread to the neck and shoulders; pain may be relieved by sitting up and leaning forward; swollen legs and abdomen; breathing difficulty; chills; fever; fatigue.
	Pleurisy *Inflammation of the membranes lining the lungs and chest cavity*	Sudden chest pain worse on inspiration that may also radiate into the shoulder or abdomen; rapid breathing; coughing; sneezing; possibly, fever.
	Pneumonia	High fever; shortness of breath; cough with sputum; chest pain; fatigue.

Fever *continued*

Associated Symptoms	Possible Diagnosis	Distinguishing Features
with cough/breathing difficulty *continued*	Tuberculosis	Often, asymptomatic. Possibly, low-grade fever; excessive perspiration; cough producing sputum or blood; weight loss; chronic fatigue; chest pain; shortness of breath; night sweats.
	Whooping cough	Initially, mild cough, sneezing, nasal congestion, and irritated eyes. Within approximately two weeks, cough becomes severe and persistent, and is accompanied by characteristic high-pitched "whooping" sound during inhalation; loss of appetite; listlessness; vomiting or choking spells. Most common among young children.
with diarrhea	Amebiasis *Parasitic infection*	Usually asymptomatic; possibly, diarrhea; loose stools may contain mucus and blood; abdominal cramps; fatigue; weight loss; gas and flatulence. In severe cases, large amount of bloody stools daily; fever, nausea and vomiting, and abdominal tenderness.
	Crohn's disease *Inflammation of the lining of the small intestine*	Episodes of abdominal pain or cramps in lower abdomen; nausea; diarrhea; loss of weight and appetite; possibly, fever; rectal bleeding or blood in stools; fatigue; anal fissures; joint pains; inflammation of the eyes.
	Dysentery, bacillary	Watery diarrhea that may contain mucus or blood; rectal pain upon defecation; abdominal pain; rapid dehydration and weight loss; nausea and vomiting.
	Megacolon, toxic *Distention of the colon*	Severe constipation; abdominal bloating; loss of weight and appetite; possible diarrhea; in newborns, failure to pass a stool within 48 hours after birth; in children, slow growth from infancy to age five.
with dizziness	Ear infection, middle *Inflammation of the middle ear*	Earache; deafness; ringing in the ear; possibly, a discharge of pus from the ear; fever; dizziness.
	Ear infection, outer	Redness and itching of the ear canal; discharge from the ear; ear pain; possibly, temporary loss of hearing.
with genitourinary symptoms	Bladder cancer	Blood in the urine; painful and frequent urination; pelvic pain; feeling of pressure in the back; persistent fever.
	Epididymitis *Inflammation of the coiled sperm conduit that rests on each testicle*	Severe pain and swelling at the back of a testicle; possibly, redness and swelling of the scrotum; burning on urination.

Fever *continued*

Associated Symptoms	Possible Diagnosis	Distinguishing Features
with genitourinary symptoms *continued*	Kidney infection *Pyelonephritis*	Sudden fever and shaking chills; severe fatigue; burning and frequent urination; cloudy or bloody urine; pain in the abdomen, back, or flanks, sometimes severe; nausea and vomiting.
	Orchitis *Inflammation of a testicle*	Swelling and severe pain in the affected testicle; possible bloody discharge in the semen; pain during intercourse; fever.
	Prostatitis *Inflammation of the prostate gland*	Burning during urination; urgent and frequent urination; fever and chills; discharge from the penis; lower abdominal and back pain; blood in the urine.
	Urethritis *Infection of the urethra, the passageway that drains urine from the bladder*	Frequent and painful urination; blood in the urine; yellow, pus-filled discharge; possible difficulty passing urine; urinary urgency; pain during intercourse; in men, painful ejaculation.
with low-grade fever	Appendicitis, acute	Pain near the navel, spreading to the lower right abdomen; nausea and vomiting; constipation; possibly diarrhea; low-grade fever; loss of appetite.
	Common cold	Nasal congestion; watery eyes; sneezing; sore throat; cough; muscle aches; mild headache; listlessness; possibly, low-grade fever.
	Intestinal obstruction	Abdominal pain and cramps; nausea; vomiting; weakness; gas; bloating; possible diarrhea; progressive constipation culminating in inability to pass stools or gas.
	Pancreatitis *Inflammation of the pancreas*	Sudden, extreme abdominal pain; nausea and vomiting; weakness; fever; clammy skin; abdominal bloating and tenderness.
	Pelvic inflammatory disease	Initially, lower pelvic pain; pain during intercourse; irregular menstrual bleeding; vaginal discharge with abnormal color or odor; low-grade fever; chills; frequent urination; fatigue; loss of appetite; later, severe abdominal pain and high fever.
	Scleroderma	Shiny, tight, and hardened skin, especially on the fingers, arms, and face; hands or feet may successively turn blue, white, and red upon exposure to cold (Raynaud's phenomenon); swallowing difficulty; bloating after eating; weight loss; shortness of breath on exertion; high blood pressure; symptoms of renal failure. Possibly, heartburn, muscle aches and weakness, joint pain, fever, or fatigue.

Fever *continued*

Associated Symptoms	Possible Diagnosis	Distinguishing Features
with low-grade fever *continued*	Sinusitis *Inflammation of the mucous membranes lining the sinuses*	Throbbing pain above or below one or both eyes that intensifies when bending the head forward or coughing; nasal congestion; loss of sense of smell; often, pus-like nasal discharge; possible dental pain in the upper jaw; fever.
	Tetanus	Often, lockjaw; stiffness and, later, muscle spasms in the neck and face; drooling; abdominal and back pain; extreme perspiration; swallowing difficulty; possible convulsions; fever.
with nausea/vomiting	Brain abscess	Headaches; drowsiness; nausea and vomiting; fever; seizures; possible partial paralysis; confusion; speaking difficulty.
	Encephalitis *Inflammation of the brain*	Initially, headache and fever followed by confusion, hallucinations, and paralysis on one side of the body; memory loss; difficulty with speech and eye movements; drowsiness; possible coma or epileptic seizures; loss of hearing; sensitivity to light; stiff neck.
	Food poisoning	Symptoms vary greatly depending on the type and extent of poisoning and may include nausea, vomiting, diarrhea, bloody stools, abdominal pain, and collapse.
	Hepatitis, acute viral	Fever; fatigue; loss of appetite; aching muscles and joints; abdominal pain or discomfort; jaundice; dark urine and pale stools.
	Liver tumors	Pain or discomfort in the upper right portion of the abdomen; abdominal swelling; loss of weight and appetite; nausea and vomiting; fever; excessive perspiration; jaundice; pallor; severe fatigue.
	Meningitis *Inflammation of the membranes covering the brain and spinal cord*	Severe headache; nausea and vomiting; sensitivity to light; stiffness in the neck; possible red skin rash; fever; mental confusion; drowsiness; loss of consciousness; seizures.
	Mesenteric ischemia *A blood clot blocking blood flow to the intestine*	Severe abdominal cramping, usually around the navel, that is exacerbated by eating and alleviated by fasting. Possibly, bloody stools.
	Peritonitis *Inflammation of the abdominal membrane*	Sudden abdominal pain, rigidity, and swelling; chills and fever; weakness; rapid heartbeat; nausea and vomiting; extreme thirst; low urine output.

Fever *continued*

Associated Symptoms	Possible Diagnosis	Distinguishing Features
with nausea/vomiting *continued*	Trichinosis *Parasitic infestation*	Initially, crampy abdominal pain, diarrhea, vomiting, and fever, followed within one to two weeks by swelling around the eyes, muscle aches and tenderness, fever, and weakness. Possibly, coughing up of bloody phlegm; delirium; coma; heart failure symptoms.
with rash/spots	Infectious arthritis	Pain, swelling, stiffness, and redness, usually in one joint. Fever. Severity varies from a mild ache to severe, debilitating pain and eventual joint deformity.
	Lyme disease	A small red bump, surrounded by a concentric bulls-eye-like red rash with a pale center. Over the following month: fever and chills; extreme fatigue; headaches. Symptoms may progress over several months or years and may include: palpitations; joint or muscle pain; and chronic joint inflammation, especially in the knees.
	Measles	Cough; fever; watery nasal discharge; loss of appetite; red, watering eyes; sore throat; body aches; red, slightly itchy rash that gradually spreads all over the body.
	Rheumatic fever	Initially, a sore throat that gets better followed, one to six weeks later, by lethargy and fever. Possibly, swollen joints, rash, abdominal pain, involuntary jerky movements, emotional instability.
	Rocky Mountain spotted fever	Within a week after exposure, high fever, loss of appetite, headache, muscle aches, nausea and vomiting; dry cough; sensitivity to light. Within six days, the appearance of small pink spots on wrists and ankles, eventually spreading over the entire body, where they then grow, darken in color, and bleed.
	Roseola *Infectious disease primarily affecting children*	Abrupt onset of high fever that usually subsides within four to five days, at which time a rash appears on the torso, and spreads to the limbs, neck, and face. Sore throat; swollen lymph nodes in neck.
	Rubella *German Measles*	Rash on the face that spreads to the torso and limbs; enlargement of lymph nodes in neck; usually preceded by headache, fever, and runny nose.
	Toxic shock syndrome	Lethargy; conjunctivitis; confusion; sudden high fever accompanied by nausea, watery diarrhea, sore throat, and headache. Red rash on the palms and soles of the feet, which, after a week or two, begins to peel.

Fever *continued*

Associated Symptoms	Possible Diagnosis	Distinguishing Features
with rash/spots *continued*	Typhoid fever	Headache; fever, loss of appetite; abdominal pain and tenderness; extreme weakness; constipation followed by diarrhea; drowsiness, stupor, or coma; raised, pink skin eruptions on the chest and abdomen; joint aches; sore throat.
without sweating	Heatstroke	Sudden dizziness; weakness; headache; hot, dry, red skin which later turns grey; high body temperature; muscle cramps; confusion; seizures; loss of consciousness.
with swollen lymph nodes/glands	AIDS *Acquired immunodeficiency syndrome*	Recurrent infections affecting the skin and respiratory system; cough; shortness of breath; loss of appetite; weight loss; fatigue; diarrhea; fever; dementia; malignant skin lesions; swollen lymph glands throughout the body; purplish skin nodules; memory loss; confusion; personality changes.
	Chronic fatigue syndrome	Severe fatigue made worse by exercise; recurrent flu-like symptoms; persistent sore throat; low-grade fever; muscle and joint aches; headache; painful, swollen lymph nodes; depression and mental confusion; memory loss; sleep difficulties.
	Leukemias	Symptoms vary depending on the type of leukemia and may include: loss of appetite and weight; increased bruising and bleeding; bone pain, especially in the legs; abdominal pain and distention; nausea; heart palpitations; severe fatigue; pallor; breathing difficulty; fever; night sweats; headache; enlarged lymph nodes; joint pains (due to gout).
	Lymphoma, Hodgkin's *Cancer of the lymph nodes and lymphoid tissue*	Painless swelling of the lymph nodes usually in the neck or armpits; loss of appetite; night sweats.
	Lymphoma, non-Hodgkin's *Cancer of the lymph nodes and lymphoid tissue*	Painless swelling of lymph nodes in the neck or groin; possible abdominal pain, vomiting of blood, headache.
	Mononucleosis, infectious	Headache; high fever; swollen glands in the neck, groin, and armpits; severe sore throat; swallowing difficulty.
	Mumps	Pain in the ear, below the ear, and in the jaw; swollen glands in the neck; headache; pain on swallowing and chewing; sore muscles; joint pain; loss of appetite. Testicular swelling and tenderness in adults.

Fever *continued*

Associated Symptoms	Possible Diagnosis	Distinguishing Features
with swollen lymph nodes/glands *continued*	Peritonsillar abscess *A collection of pus between the tonsils and surrounding tissue due to infection*	Sore throat; severe pain when swallowing; fever; headache; impaired speech; drooling; swollen glands in the neck.
	Pharyngitis *Inflammation of the pharynx, the part of the throat between the mouth and the esophagus*	Sore or red throat; speaking and swallowing difficulties; sensitive, swollen glands in the neck; fever; headache; possible earache.
	Sarcoidosis *Accumulation of inflammatory cells in the lymph nodes and other tissues throughout the body*	Often no symptoms. Swollen lymph nodes in the neck or armpits; muscle aches; fever; breathing difficulty; possibly, purple rash on the face; reddish or brownish skin spots on the forearms, face, or legs; numbness; joint pain or stiffness; a painful, red eye; blurred vision; loss of appetite and weight.
	Thyroiditis, subacute *Inflammation of the thyroid gland*	Pain in the front of the neck and, often, the ear; possibly fever, weight loss, and fatigue; general feeling of being unwell (malaise); discomfort on swallowing.
	Tonsillitis	Sore, inflamed throat; swallowing difficulty; headache; swollen glands in the neck; fever; loss of voice. In children, nausea, vomiting, and abdominal pain.
	Tooth abscess	Persistent tooth pain; pain when biting or chewing; difficulty swallowing; swollen glands in the neck; earache; fever; possibly, foul taste in the mouth or bad breath.
with violent, shaking chills	Malaria	Initially, severe chills and shivering. In later stages, extremely high fever followed by a period of profuse perspiration as fever subsides; headache, sometimes severe; vomiting.

Fingernail abnormalities

Associated Symptoms	Possible Diagnosis	Distinguishing Features
	Chronic obstructive pulmonary disease	Shortness of breath; wheezing; persistent, mucus-producing cough, especially in the morning; possibly, chest pain, swollen legs and ankles.
	Congestive heart failure	Shortness of breath; fatigue; need to sleep on several pillows; weakness; cough; heart palpitations; swelling in the legs, ankles, and abdomen; frequent urination at night; indigestion; nausea and vomiting; loss of appetite.
	Eczema *Inflammation of the skin*	Itching skin; thickened patches of skin; possibly, with oozing and crusting; in infants, rash on the face, inner elbows, or behind the knees that turns scaly and develops small red pimples that leak; swollen legs (stasis dermatitis).
	Lung cancer	Persistent cough; wheezing; shortness of breath; chest pain; fatigue; weight loss.
	Pleurisy and pleural effusion *Inflammation of the membranes lining the lungs and chest cavity*	Sudden chest pain worse on inspiration that may also radiate into the shoulder or abdomen; rapid breathing; coughing; sneezing; possibly, fever.
	Psoriasis	Slightly raised patches of skin with red borders and white-silver scales; joint pain and stiffness; itching; pitted nails.
	Pulmonary edema *An accumulation of fluid in the lungs*	Severe shortness of breath; rapid breathing; pallor; excessive perspiration; bluish nails and lips; cough with frothy sputum; wheezing; anxiety and restlessness.

Flatulence

Associated Symptoms	Possible Diagnosis	Distinguishing Features
	Amebiasis *Parasitic infection*	Usually asymptomatic; possibly, diarrhea; loose stools may contain mucus and blood; abdominal cramps; fatigue; weight loss; gas and flatulence. In severe cases, large amount of bloody stools daily; fever, nausea and vomiting, and abdominal tenderness.
	Carcinoid tumors and carcinoid syndrome	May be asymptomatic; flushing or redness of the face and neck; gas and profuse diarrhea; abdominal cramping; watery, swollen eyes; shortness of breath or wheezing.
	Cirrhosis *Chronic damage to the cells of the liver*	No symptoms in early stages; loss of weight and appetite; nausea; swollen legs, ankles and abdomen; itching; jaundice; black stools; vomiting blood; fatigue; impotence; memory loss; confusion.
	Colorectal cancer *A growth of malignant cells in the colon or rectum*	Change in bowel habits; diarrhea; constipation; narrow stools; bloody or dark stools; lower abdominal pain; bloating; cramps; gas; loss of weight and appetite; fatigue and heart palpitations due to anemia.
	Crohn's disease *Inflammation of the lining of the small intestine*	Episodes of abdominal pain or cramps in lower abdomen; nausea; diarrhea; loss of weight and appetite; possibly, fever; rectal bleeding or blood in stools; fatigue; anal fissures; joint pains; inflammation of the eyes.
	Gallbladder disorders	Moderate to severe pain in the upper right side of the abdomen, chest, upper back, or right shoulder. Pain often follows the ingestion of high-fat foods and is episodic, lasting 20 minutes to several hours. Nausea and vomiting; low-grade fever; belching; heartburn; gas; possibly, jaundice, pale stools, and itchy skin.
	Intestinal obstruction	Abdominal pain and cramps; nausea; vomiting; weakness; gas; bloating; possible diarrhea; progressive constipation culminating in inability to pass stools or gas.
	Irritable bowel syndrome	Cramps in the middle or to one side of the lower abdomen that are usually relieved with bowel movements; nausea; bloating; gas; alternating diarrhea and constipation.
	Lactose intolerance *Difficulty digesting milk and dairy products*	Abdominal cramps; diarrhea; nausea; bloating; flatulence.
	Malabsorption, digestive *A failure of the small intestine to absorb nutrients in the diet*	Diarrhea; weight loss; yellowish, foul-smelling stools; abdominal cramps, gas, and bloating; weakness and lethargy.

Foot pain

Associated Symptoms	Possible Diagnosis	Distinguishing Features
	Ankylosing spondylitis *Inflammation of the joints between the spine and the pelvis*	Initially, pain and stiffness in the lower back and hips that becomes worse after resting; neck or chest pain; possible pain in the hip, knee, and ankle joints; pain in the heel of the foot; eye pain; blurred vision.
	Bunions	Painful, bony lump at the side of the base of the big toe; foot pain and stiffness; redness and swelling at the base of the big toe.
	Bursitis *Inflammation of the bursas, the lubricant-filled sacs in and around the joints*	Pain and swelling around a joint, usually the elbow, knee, or shoulder; painful movement in the affected joint; possibly, fever.
	Corns and calluses	Area of thickened skin on the foot; pain in the affected area.
	Dislocations/subluxations	Deformity of the affected joint; joint pain and tenderness; difficulty moving a joint; swelling and stiffness within 30 minutes after joint injury.
	Gout	Most commonly affects the joints of the big toe. Affected joints are red, swollen, hot, and severely painful. In late stages, joint deformity. Kidney stones.
	Hammer toe and mallet toe	A toe, usually the second digit, next to the big toe, that is clenched into a painful, claw-like position, or a toe with an end joint that curls under itself. A painful corn on top of the bent joint or at the tip of the affected toe.
	Infectious arthritis	Pain, swelling, stiffness, and redness, usually in one joint. Fever. Severity varies from a mild ache to severe, debilitating pain and eventual joint deformity.
	Osteoarthritis *Degeneration of the cartilage that lines the joints*	Pain, swelling, and stiffness in one or more joints; enlargement and distortion of affected joints.
	Osteomalacia and Rickets *Softening and weakening of the bones, usually due to poor calcification*	Bone pain, especially in the neck, legs, hips and ribs. Muscle weakness, numbness, or spasms in the hands, feet, and throat; increased susceptibility to bone fractures.
	Osteomyelitis *Infection of bone and bone marrow*	Fever; severe pain in the affected bone; inflammation and swelling of the skin over the affected area; deformity. In children, arrested growth of the affected bone.

Foot pain *continued*

Associated Symptoms	Possible Diagnosis	Distinguishing Features
	Peripheral neuropathies *Degeneration of the nerves that supply the extremities*	Tingling or numbness commonly beginning in the hands and feet and gradually spreading toward the center of the body; sensitive skin; muscle weakness; possibly, pain in the hands and feet; lack of coordination; shooting pains exacerbated by touch or changes in temperature; breathing difficulty; urinary or fecal incontinence.
	Peripheral vascular disease *Narrowing of blood vessels in the legs or arms*	Muscle pain on one or both legs that occurs with exercise and subsides with rest; possible pain in the fingers, arms, buttocks, lower back, or the arch of the foot; impotence. Severe symptoms include: muscle pain at rest that intensifies at night; discolored or blue toes; cold or numb feet; open sores; heightened sensitivity to cold; weak or absent pulse in the affected limb; scaly or hairless skin over the affected area.
	Plantar fasciitis *Inflammation of the ligament between the front of the heel bone and base of the toes*	Heel pain, especially when running or walking; possibly, tenderness and swelling in the heel.
	Plantar warts *Hard, rough-surfaced growth on the foot occurring singularly or in groups*	Body weight causes wart to grow into skin surface rather than being raised, giving it the appearance of a callous. Pain when putting weight on the foot.
	Rheumatoid arthritis	Fatigue and weakness; joint pain, stiffness, and inflammation, especially in the hands, feet, and arms; joint deformity; dry mouth; dry, painful eyes. Morning stiffness.
	Rheumatoid arthritis, juvenile	Fever; rash; abdominal pain; weight loss; swelling, stiffness, and pain in the affected joints; enlarged lymph glands; fatigue; pallor; red, painful eyes.
	Sprains and strains	Swelling, pain or tenderness in the affected joints; impaired joint function.
	Tendinitis *Inflammation of a tendon*	Pain over a tendon anywhere in the body; if involved tendon is near or part of a joint, restricted movement of the joint.
	Varicose veins	Blue or purplish, knotted veins, usually in the legs; itching or discomfort in the affected area; swollen feet and ankles. Possible scaly skin, muscle cramps, or skin ulcers.

Gait abnormalities

Associated Symptoms	Possible Diagnosis	Distinguishing Features
	Acoustic neuroma *A benign tumor in the cells covering the auditory nerve*	Gradual hearing loss; ringing in the ear; headache; numbness in the face; unsteady walk. In later stages, swallowing and speaking difficulties; possibly, slight paralysis.
	Amyotrophic lateral sclerosis *Progressive degeneration of nerve cells of the central nervous system*	Progressive loss of strength and coordination in the limbs; muscle twitching and cramps that begin in the hands and spread to the arms, shoulders, and legs; stiff, clumsy gait; swallowing, breathing, or speaking difficulty; weight loss; drooling; involuntary laughing or crying.
	Multiple sclerosis *Gradual degeneration of the protective sheaths surrounding the nerves within the brain and spinal cord*	Symptoms may appear suddenly and then disappear; persistent symptoms may take years to develop and include numbness or tingling in any part of the body, weakness in the extremities, an unsteady walk, slurred speech, urinary incontinence, fatigue, depression, temporary loss of vision, double or blurred vision, mental confusion, and memory loss.
	Muscular dystrophy	Symptoms depend on type of muscular dystrophy and may include: Progressive muscle wasting, weakness, and loss of mobility; lack of coordination; muscular and skeletal deformities including curvature of the spine with protruding abdomen; waddling gait; cataracts; frontal baldness; gonadal atrophy.
	Osteoarthritis *Degeneration of the cartilage that lines the joints*	Pain, swelling, and stiffness in one or more joints; enlargement and distortion of affected joints.
	Parkinson's disease *Degeneration of the basal ganglia, a cluster of nerve cells in the brain*	Tremors in the hands; stiffness and weakness; impaired voluntary movement; shuffling gait; stooped posture; unblinking, fixed expression; possibly, slow, hesitant speech; difficulty swallowing; drooling; depression. Tremors occur at rest (not with voluntary movements) and disappear during sleep.
	Poliomyelitis *Polio*	Low fever; sore throat; headache; nausea and vomiting. In severe cases, paralysis without loss of sensation; stiff neck and back; twitching; swallowing and breathing difficulty; drooling.
	Rheumatic fever	Initially, a sore throat that gets better followed, one to six weeks later, by lethargy and fever. Possibly, swollen joints, rash, abdominal pain, involuntary jerky movements, emotional instability.

Gait abnormalities *continued*

Associated Symptoms	Possible Diagnosis	Distinguishing Features
	Rheumatoid arthritis	Fatigue and weakness; joint pain, stiffness, and inflammation, especially in the hands, feet, and arms; joint deformity; dry mouth; dry, painful eyes. Morning stiffness.
	Schizophrenia	Delusions; hallucinations; rambling, nonsensical, or minimal speech; extremely disorganized behavior; inappropriate emotional responses or emotional detachment; lack of willful movement.
	Spinal cord trauma	Severe pain and swelling in the affected area; loss of sensation, muscle weakness, or paralysis below the site of the injury; urinary or fecal incontinence or retention; impotence; breathing difficulty; shock.
	Spinal tumor	Progressive numbness, tingling, and muscle weakness; fecal or urinary incontinence; persistent back pain.
	Spondylosis, cervical *Arthritis of the vertebral disks in the neck*	Neck pain and stiffness that spreads to the shoulders, upper arms, hands, or back of the head; numbness or tingling in the arms, hands, and fingers; weakness in the arms and legs; unsteady gait; possible loss of bladder or bowel control.
	Stroke	Symptoms vary with the location of brain injury. Sudden onset of weakness, paralysis, or loss of sensation, usually on one side of the body; a sudden heaviness in a limb; speech abnormalities; headache; vision disturbances; dizziness; confusion; coma; urinary and fecal incontinence.

Gas

Associated Symptoms	Possible Diagnosis	Distinguishing Features
	Amebiasis *Parasitic infection*	Usually asymptomatic; possibly, diarrhea; loose stools may contain mucus and blood; abdominal cramps; fatigue; weight loss; gas and flatulence. In severe cases, large amount of bloody stools daily; fever, nausea and vomiting, and abdominal tenderness.
	Carcinoid tumors and carcinoid syndrome	May be asymptomatic; flushing or redness of the face and neck; gas and profuse diarrhea; abdominal cramping; watery, swollen eyes; shortness of breath or wheezing.
	Cirrhosis *Chronic damage to the cells of the liver*	No symptoms in early stages; loss of weight and appetite; nausea; swollen legs, ankles and abdomen; itching; jaundice; black stools; vomiting blood; fatigue; impotence; memory loss; confusion.
	Colorectal cancer *A growth of malignant cells in the colon or rectum*	Change in bowel habits; diarrhea; constipation; narrow stools; bloody or dark stools; lower abdominal pain; bloating; cramps; gas; loss of weight and appetite; fatigue and heart palpitations due to anemia.
	Crohn's disease *Inflammation of the lining of the small intestine*	Episodes of abdominal pain or cramps in lower abdomen; nausea; diarrhea; loss of weight and appetite; possibly, fever; rectal bleeding or blood in stools; fatigue; anal fissures; joint pains; inflammation of the eyes.
	Gallbladder disorders	Moderate to severe pain in the upper right side of the abdomen, chest, upper back, or right shoulder. Pain often follows the ingestion of high-fat foods and is episodic, lasting 20 minutes to several hours. Nausea and vomiting; low-grade fever; belching; heartburn; gas; possibly, jaundice, pale stools, and itchy skin.
	Intestinal obstruction	Abdominal pain and cramps; nausea; vomiting; weakness; gas; bloating; possible diarrhea; progressive constipation culminating in inability to pass stools or gas.
	Irritable bowel syndrome	Cramps in the middle or to one side of the lower abdomen that are usually relieved with bowel movements; nausea; bloating; gas; alternating diarrhea and constipation.
	Lactose intolerance *Difficulty digesting milk and dairy products*	Abdominal cramps; diarrhea; nausea; bloating; flatulence.
	Malabsorption, digestive *A failure of the small intestine to absorb nutrients in the diet*	Diarrhea; weight loss; yellowish, foul-smelling stools; abdominal cramps, gas, and bloating; weakness and lethargy.

Genital lesions

Associated Symptoms	Possible Diagnosis	Distinguishing Features
	Candidiasis *Fungal infection of the mouth, genitals, or mucous membranes*	Thick, white discharge from the vagina; itching and irritation in the vaginal area; pain while urinating or during intercourse; in men, inflammation of the head of the penis; possibly, yellow raised patches in the mouth.
	Genital herpes	Approximately one week after infection, itching, burning, soreness, and small blisters in the genital area. Blisters later burst, leaving painful ulcers which heal 10 to 20 days later. Possibly, enlarged, painful lymph nodes in the groin; fever, headache, and cold sores around the mouth. In women, pain during urination.
	Genital warts	Small, red, round or flat, itchy bumps on or around the vagina, anus, penis, or perineum (area between the anus and genitals) developing between eight and 18 months after infection. Several warts may grow together into a cauliflower shape.
	Penile cancer	Sore, ulcer, or wart-like lump on the penis, usually near the head, possibly painful; bleeding or unusual discharge from the penis. Possibly, pain during urination, or enlarged lymph nodes in the groin.
	Ringworm *Fungal skin infection*	A rash with distinct, advancing borders and clear centers; affected areas may have abnormally dark pigmentation; itching; scaly patches of skin; bald patches on scalp; Athlete's foot; red, swollen finger- and toenails.
	Scabies	Tiny, grey, scaly blisters—usually on the wrists, genitals, armpits, or between the fingers—that rupture easily when scratched; severe itching; red lumps or rashes may develop.
	Syphilis	Initially, painless, ulcerated, red sore on the genitals, mouth, or rectum; swollen glands in the neck, armpit, or groin; rash with small, red, scaly bumps; fever; headache. If left untreated, damage to heart valves leading to congestive heart failure; mental deterioration; loss of balance; seizures; dementia; personality changes.
	Vaginal cancer	Vaginal itching; bleeding after intercourse or between menstrual periods; abnormal vaginal discharge; lesions with thick, raised edges; possibly rectal bleeding; discomfort when urinating or defecating; pain during intercourse; urinary frequency and urgency.

Genital pain

Associated Symptoms	Possible Diagnosis	Distinguishing Features
	Candidiasis *Fungal infection of the mouth, genitals, or mucous membranes*	Thick, white discharge from the vagina; itching and irritation in the vaginal area; pain while urinating or during intercourse; in men, inflammation of the head of the penis; possibly, yellow raised patches in the mouth.
	Cervical disorders, non-malignant	Vaginal discharge; vaginal burning and itching; vaginal bleeding after intercourse, between periods, or after bowel movements.
	Endometriosis *The migration of the uterine lining to other reproductive or abdominal organs*	Pain in the lower abdomen, vagina, and lower back beginning just prior to menses and intensifying after blood flow has ceased; heavy bleeding during periods; pain during intercourse; diarrhea; constipation; pain during bowel movements; bleeding from the rectum; bloody urine during menses; nausea and vomiting prior to menses; infertility.
	Epididymitis *Inflammation of the coiled sperm conduit that rests on each testicle*	Severe pain and swelling at the back of a testicle; possibly, redness and swelling of the scrotum; burning on urination.
	Gonorrhea	Burning pain during urination; yellowish, pus-like discharge from the penis or vagina; redness or swelling at the infection site; abnormal vaginal bleeding.
	Orchitis *Inflammation of a testicle*	Swelling and severe pain in the affected testicle; possible bloody discharge in the semen; pain during intercourse; fever.
	Pelvic inflammatory disease	Initially, lower pelvic pain; pain during intercourse; irregular menstrual bleeding; vaginal discharge with abnormal color or odor; low-grade fever; chills; frequent urination; fatigue; loss of appetite; later, severe abdominal pain and high fever.
	Prostatitis *Inflammation of the prostate gland*	Burning during urination; urgent and frequent urination; fever and chills; discharge from the penis; lower abdominal and back pain; blood in the urine.
	Testicular torsion *Twisting of the spermatic cord*	Severe pain and swelling on one side of the scrotum; skin on the scrotum may appear red or purple; lightheadedness or fainting; possibly, abdominal pain, nausea and vomiting.
	Vaginitis *Inflammation of the vagina*	Vaginal irritation, itching, and discharge; painful intercourse and minor postcoital bleeding. In later stages, vaginal pain.

Growth/sore that does not heal

Associated Symptoms	Possible Diagnosis	Distinguishing Features
	Basal cell skin cancer	Small, flat, waxy, or pearly bump, usually on the face, ears, or neck or back; skin blemish that grows steadily over a period of weeks without healing, developing into a shallow ulcer with a moist center and raised edges that doesn't heal.
	Hemophilia	Profuse bleeding from minor injuries and tooth extractions; internal bleeding that may cause blood in the urine; bleeding into joints; symptoms of stroke due to intracerebral bleeding; possibly, extensive bruising.
	Melanoma *Skin cancer*	Change in the appearance of an existing mole including enlargement, bleeding, change in color, development of a black edge. Itching.
	Oral cancers	Sore in the mouth that bleeds and does not heal; lump in the cheek; white or red patch on the gums; swallowing and chewing difficulties; numbness of the tongue; swelling of the jaw.
	Peripheral vascular disease *Narrowing of blood vessels in the legs or arms*	Muscle pain on one or both legs that occurs with exercise and subsides with rest; possible pain in the fingers, arms, buttocks, lower back, or the arch of the foot; impotence. Severe symptoms include: muscle pain at rest that intensifies at night; discolored or blue toes; cold or numb feet; open sores; heightened sensitivity to cold; weak or absent pulse in the affected limb; scaly or hairless skin over the affected area.
	Varicose veins	Blue or purplish, knotted veins, usually in the legs; itching or discomfort in the affected area; swollen feet and ankles. Possible scaly skin, muscle cramps, or skin ulcers.

Gum swelling

Associated Symptoms	Possible Diagnosis	Distinguishing Features
	Gingivitis	Red-purple gums that are swollen, shiny, and bleed easily; bad breath.
	Impacted teeth	Gum pain; unpleasant taste in mouth, especially when biting down; red, swollen gums around the affected tooth; headache or jaw ache; possibly, bad breath.
	Oral cancers	Sore in the mouth that bleeds and does not heal; lump in the cheek; white or red patch on the gums; swallowing and chewing difficulties; numbness of the tongue; swelling of the jaw.
	Periodontitis *Inflammation of the tissues supporting the teeth*	Red, swollen, painful gums that bleed easily; loose teeth; bad breath; possible pus discharge.
	Tongue disorders	Symptoms vary depending on the specific disorder and include: dark or bright red, black, or dark brown tongue; sore, swollen, or smooth tongue; hair-like growths on the tongue; adjacent areas of the mouth may be inflamed; ulcers or raised, white patches on the tongue; excessive salivation; swallowing difficulty; bad breath.
	Tooth abscess	Persistent tooth pain; pain when biting or chewing; difficulty swallowing; swollen glands in the neck; earache; fever; possibly, foul taste in the mouth or bad breath.
	Tooth decay	Tooth pain, especially after eating sweet or sour foods; tooth sensitivity to hot and cold; bad breath; unpleasant taste in the mouth.
	Trench mouth	Grayish film on the gums; red, swollen, painful, bleeding gums; bad breath; bad taste in the mouth; pain on swallowing or speaking; excessive salivation.

Hair growth in women, unusual

Associated Symptoms	Possible Diagnosis	Distinguishing Features
	Hepatitis, chronic	Fatigue; nausea; vomiting; loss of appetite; jaundice; dark urine; clay-colored stools; depression; pain or discomfort in the upper right abdomen; abdominal swelling; fever; in women, cessation of menstruation, acne, and the appearance of male pattern facial hair.
	Hyperprolactinemia *Overproduction of the hormone prolactin by the pituitary gland*	Symptoms may vary depending on gender; in women: cessation of menstrual periods, decreased menstrual flow, excess facial hair; in men: erectile dysfunction, infertility, decreased libido, enlarged breasts; in men and women: abnormal production of breast milk, headaches, decreased vision.
	Ovarian cancer	Often asymptomatic until widespread. Possibly, abdominal swelling or discomfort, nausea, and vomiting. In advanced stages, excessive hair growth, unexplained weight loss, abnormal menstrual bleeding or post-menopausal bleeding; urinary frequency.
	Ovarian cysts	In many cases, no symptoms. Painless swelling in the lower abdomen; possibly, pain during intercourse; brown vaginal discharge; lack of or heavier than usual menstrual periods; vomiting; unusual hair growth on face or body.
	Polycystic ovaries	Absent or unpredictable menstrual periods; infertility; excessive hair growth with a male pattern of distribution; obesity; acne.

Hair loss

Associated Symptoms	Possible Diagnosis	Distinguishing Features
	Alopecia *Hair loss*	Gradual loss of hair from the head or any other hair-bearing area of the body.
	Hypopituitarism *Underactivity of the pituitary gland*	Intolerance to cold; chronic headaches; decreased sex drive; fatigue; dizziness; fine wrinkles around the eyes and mouth; dry skin; extreme thirst and excessive urination; loss of appetite; vaginal dryness; absence of milk production in new mothers; in men, reduced muscular strength, shrinking of the testes, and loss of body hair; growth retardation in children and adolescents.
	Hypothyroidism *Underactivity of the thyroid gland*	Unexplained weight gain; fatigue; muscle weakness; cramps; dry skin; hair loss; deepening of the voice; intolerance for cold; constipation; chest pain; insomnia; puffiness around eyes; loss of sex drive; depression; menstrual abnormalities; possible swelling in the neck.
	Ringworm *Fungal skin infection*	A rash with distinct, advancing borders and clear centers; affected areas may have abnormally dark pigmentation; itching; scaly patches of skin; bald patches on scalp; Athlete's foot; red, swollen finger- and toenails.
	Systemic lupus erythematosus *Inflammation of connective tissues throughout the body*	Red, blotchy, butterfly-shaped rash on the cheeks and bridge of the nose; fatigue; fever; loss of appetite and weight; nausea; joint and abdominal pain; headaches; blurred vision; increased sensitivity to sun exposure; depression; psychosis; mental confusion.

Hallucinations

Associated Symptoms	Possible Diagnosis	Distinguishing Features
	Alzheimer's disease	Symptoms vary greatly in different individuals. Initially, minor forgetfulness gradually developing into severe, short-term memory loss, disorientation, an inability to concentrate, and sudden mood and personality changes. In later stages, severe confusion, possible hallucinations or paranoid delusions, loss of social and sexual inhibitions, impaired judgment, anxiety, depression, agitation and combativeness, wandering and getting lost, inability to write, urinary and fecal incontinence.
	Encephalitis *Inflammation of the brain*	Initially, headache and fever followed by confusion, hallucinations, and paralysis on one side of the body; memory loss; difficulty with speech and eye movements; drowsiness; possible coma or epileptic seizures; loss of hearing; sensitivity to light; stiff neck.
	Heatstroke	Sudden dizziness; weakness; headache; hot, dry, red skin which later turns grey; high body temperature; muscle cramps; confusion; seizures; loss of consciousness.
	Schizophrenia	Delusions; hallucinations; rambling, nonsensical, or minimal speech; extremely disorganized behavior; inappropriate emotional responses or emotional detachment; lack of willful movement.
	Seizures	Involuntary twitching or jerking; muscle rigidity; loss of consciousness; confusion; drooling; hallucinations.

Hand pain

Associated Symptoms	Possible Diagnosis	Distinguishing Features
	Bone cancer	Pain, tenderness, and swelling in the affected bones and joints, often intensifying at night; a noticeable tumor or mass; increased susceptibility to bone fractures.
	Carpal tunnel syndrome	Numbness, tingling, and pain in the hand and wrist, often intensifying at night; weakness of the fingers and hand.
	Dislocations/subluxations	Deformity of the affected joint; joint pain and tenderness; difficulty moving a joint; swelling and stiffness within 30 minutes after joint injury.
	Dupuytren's contracture	Inability to straighten one or more fingers or toes, usually the ring and little fingers; hard nodule on the palm of the hand; puckering of the skin on the hand.
	Ganglion	A round swelling or cyst under the skin, usually on the wrist, which may feel soft and rubbery or hard and solid. Possible pain or tenderness in the lump, especially when the wrist is extended or flexed.
	Osteoarthritis *Degeneration of the cartilage that lines the joints*	Pain, swelling, and stiffness in one or more joints; enlargement and distortion of affected joints.
	Osteomalacia and Rickets *Softening or weakening of the bones, usually due to poor calcification*	Bone pain, especially in the neck, legs, hips and ribs. Muscle weakness, numbness, or spasms in the hands, feet, and throat; increased susceptibility to bone fractures.
	Osteomyelitis *Infection of bone and bone marrow*	Fever; severe pain in the affected bone; inflammation and swelling of the skin over the affected area; deformity. In children, arrested growth of the affected bone.
	Osteoporosis *Loss of bone mass due to calcium depletion*	Backache; easily fractured bones, especially in the wrists, hips, and spine; gradual loss of height; stooped or hunched posture.
	Rheumatoid arthritis	Fatigue; weakness; joint pain, stiffness, and inflammation, especially in the hands, feet, and arms; joint deformity; dry mouth; dry, painful eyes. Morning stiffness.
	Rheumatoid arthritis, juvenile	Fever; rash; abdominal pain; weight loss; swelling, stiffness, and pain in the affected joints; enlarged lymph glands; fatigue; pallor; red, painful eyes.
	Sprains and strains	Swelling, pain or tenderness in the affected joints; impaired joint function.
	Tendinitis *Inflammation of a tendon*	Pain over a tendon anywhere in the body; if involved tendon is near or part of a joint, restricted movement of the joint.

Headache

Associated Symptoms	Possible Diagnosis	Distinguishing Features
	Acoustic neuroma *A benign tumor in the cells covering the auditory nerve*	Gradual hearing loss; ringing in the ear; headache; numbness in the face; unsteady walk. In later stages, swallowing and speaking difficulties; possibly, slight paralysis.
	Acromegaly *Overproduction of growth hormone by the pituitary gland*	In adults (acromegaly): Gradual thickening of the bones of the face, jaw, and the extremities in adults; oily skin; severe headache; excessive hair growth; excessive perspiration; joint pains. In children (in which the disease is called gigantism): Rapid growth and unusual height; possibly, blindness.
	Anemia, aplastic	Fatigue and weakness; shortness of breath; heart palpitations; pallor; bleeding gums; nosebleeds; tendency to bruise easily; small red dots under the skin (petechiae). Increased susceptibility to infection.
	Anemia, folic acid deficiency	Fatigue and weakness; pallor; shortness of breath, heart palpitations, or noticeably rapid heartbeat on exertion; sore, red, and glazed looking tongue; loss of weight and appetite; nausea and diarrhea; abdominal distention.
	Anemia, hemolytic	Fatigue and weakness; shortness of breath on exertion; pallor; heart palpitations; jaundice and dark urine.
	Anemia, iron deficiency	Fatigue and weakness; pallor; shortness of breath and heart palpitations on exertion; irritability or inability to concentrate; sore tongue or tiny cracks at the corners of the mouth; black, tarry or bloody stools; unusual craving for dirt, paint, or ice.
	Anemia, pernicious	Fatigue; inability to concentrate; sore, red tongue; weakness; dizziness; pallor; shortness of breath on exertion; palpitations; numbness and tingling in extremities; incoordination; headache; loss of weight and appetite; possibly, jaundice.
	Brain tumors	Headaches that become more severe when reclining; nausea and vomiting; memory loss; double vision; muscle weakness; numbness, tingling, or partial paralysis; vision loss; speech disturbances; seizures; drowsiness.
	Cholesteatoma *Infected cyst in the eardrum or middle ear*	Hearing loss; discharge of pus from ear; headaches and earaches; weakness of facial muscles; dizziness.
	Fibromyalgia	Muscle aches, pains, and stiffness; specific points on the body that feel sore when pressed; fatigue; headaches; feeling unrefreshed upon awakening in the morning.

Headache *continued*

Associated Symptoms	Possible Diagnosis	Distinguishing Features
	Glaucoma	Often initially asymptomatic. In later stages, the symptoms of closed-angle glaucoma include: the appearance of halos and rainbows around lights; dilated pupil in the affected eye; severe headache and eye pain; possibly, nausea and vomiting. Open-angle glaucoma symptoms include: blurred vision and a gradual loss of peripheral vision.
	Headache, cluster	Persistent pain in or around one eye; redness and tearing of one eye; nasal congestion on the same side of the face as the affected eye.
	Headache, migraine	Throbbing pain in the temple which spreads to the side of the head; nausea; vomiting. Pain may be preceded by blurred or impaired vision with bright spots and zig-zag patterns.
	Headache, tension	Dull, persistent pain in the forehead, temples, or back of the neck. Sensation of constricting band encircling the head.
	Hydrocephalus *Overaccumulation of cerebrospinal fluid, the liquid surrounding the brain*	In infants, an enlarged head, rigidity of the legs, irritability, projectile vomiting, drowsiness, seizures, and lethargy. In older persons, headache, vomiting, loss of coordination, deterioration of mental faculties, speech difficulty, and loss of appetite.
	Hyperprolactinemia *Overproduction of the hormone prolactin by the pituitary gland*	Symptoms may vary depending on gender; in women: cessation of menstrual periods, decreased menstrual flow, excess facial hair; in men: erectile dysfunction, infertility, decreased libido, enlarged breasts; in men and women: abnormal production of breast milk, headaches, decreased vision.
	Hypertension	Usually asymptomatic except in severe cases. Possibly, headache, easy fatigability, palpitations, chest pain, blurred vision, dizziness, nose bleeds, and confusion.
	Hypoglycemia *Low blood sugar*	Anxiety; hunger; trembling; headache; palpitations; perspiration; confusion; irritability; loss of coordination; possibly, double vision, seizures, or coma.
	Hypopituitarism *Underactivity of the pituitary gland*	Intolerance to cold; chronic headaches; decreased sex drive; fatigue; dizziness; fine wrinkles around the eyes and mouth; dry skin; extreme thirst and excessive urination; loss of appetite; vaginal dryness; absence of milk production in new mothers; in men, reduced muscular strength, shrinking of the testes, and loss of body hair; growth retardation in children and adolescents.

Headache *continued*

Associated Symptoms	Possible Diagnosis	Distinguishing Features
	Impacted teeth	Gum pain; unpleasant taste in mouth, especially when biting down; red, swollen gums around the affected tooth; headache or jaw ache; possibly, bad breath.
	Lymphoma, non–Hodgkin's *Cancer of the lymph nodes and lymphoid tissue*	Painless swelling of lymph nodes in the neck or groin; possible abdominal pain, vomiting of blood, headache.
	Multiple myeloma *Production of malignant plasma cells in the bone marrow*	Bone pain, especially progressive, constant back pain that intensifies with movement; unexplained bone fractures; fatigue; pallor; shortness of breath; increased bleeding, such as bleeding gums or nosebleeds; easily bruised skin; increased susceptibility to infection; headache; vision disturbances; loss of height.
	Mumps	Pain in the ear, below the ear, and in the jaw; swollen glands in the neck; headache; pain on swallowing and chewing; sore muscles; joint pain; loss of appetite. Testicular swelling and tenderness in adults.
	Nasal polyps	Impaired sense of smell; a feeling of fullness in the face; possible nasal discharge, facial pain, or headaches.
	Paget's disease *A weakening, thickening, and deformity of the bones*	Often asymptomatic. Possibly, bone pain or deformity, especially bowing of the legs, bent spine, and facial deformity; unexplained bone fractures; joint pain or stiffness; hearing loss; headaches; ringing in ears.
	Pheochromocytoma *Tumor in central part of the adrenal, the glands above the kidneys*	Headaches, sometimes severe; rapid heartbeat or heart palpitations; excessive perspiration; faintness, especially when standing up; chest pain; abdominal pain; constipation; weight loss; nervousness, irritability, or anxiety; mental confusion or psychosis.
	Polycythemia vera *An overproduction of red and white blood cells and platelets*	Headache; ringing in the ears; blurred vision; flushed skin; itching; dizziness; fatigue; night sweats; frequent nose bleeds and bruises.
	Presbyopia *Loss of elasticity of lens of the eye*	Progressive decrease in the ability to focus on objects at close range; eye strain; possibly headache.
	Refractive disorders	Depending on the specific disorder, blurred vision or an inability to clearly see objects that are either near or far.
	Renal failure, acute *Severe kidney failure*	Initially, decreased urine output, weight gain and swelling due to edema, loss of appetite, nausea and vomiting, fatigue. If untreated, confusion, seizures, and drowsiness.

Headache *continued*

Associated Symptoms	Possible Diagnosis	Distinguishing Features
	Sleep apnea *Recurrent episodes of breathing cessation during sleep*	Loud snoring; morning fatigue and headache; sleep disturbances; daytime sleepiness; difficulty concentrating; memory loss. Most common among overweight men.
	Spondylosis, cervical *Arthritis of the vertebral disks in the neck*	Neck pain and stiffness that spreads to the shoulders, upper arms, hands, or back of the head; numbness or tingling in the arms, hands, and fingers; weakness in the arms and legs; unsteady gait; possible loss of bladder or bowel control.
	Stroke	Symptoms vary with the location of brain injury. Sudden onset of weakness, paralysis, or loss of sensation, usually on one side of the body; a sudden heaviness in a limb; speech abnormalities; headache; vision disturbances; dizziness; confusion; coma; urinary and fecal incontinence.
	Temporomandibular joint syndrome	Pain in the joints connecting the jaw to the skull; headache; tender jaw muscles; dull facial pain; clicking noise when opening or closing the mouth; pain when yawning and chewing. Jaw may temporarily lock in position.
with fever	Brain hemorrhage	Sudden loss of consciousness; sudden, severe headache; mental confusion; stiff neck; nausea and vomiting; paralysis on one side of the face or body; weakness and dizziness; loss of speech; blurred or double vision; dilated pupils.
	Chronic fatigue syndrome	Severe fatigue made worse by exercise; recurrent flu-like symptoms; persistent sore throat; low-grade fever; muscle and joint aches; headache; painful, swollen lymph nodes; depression and mental confusion; memory loss; sleep difficulties.
	Common cold	Nasal congestion; watery eyes; sneezing; sore throat; cough; muscle aches; mild headache; listlessness; possibly, low-grade fever.
	Encephalitis *Inflammation of the brain*	Initially, headache and fever followed by confusion, hallucinations, and paralysis on one side of the body; memory loss; difficulty with speech and eye movements; drowsiness; possible coma or epileptic seizures; loss of hearing; sensitivity to light; stiff neck.

Headache *continued*

Associated Symptoms	Possible Diagnosis	Distinguishing Features
with fever *continued*	Genital herpes	Approximately one week after infection, itching, burning, soreness, and small blisters in the genital area. Blisters later burst, leaving painful ulcers which heal 10 to 20 days later. Possibly, enlarged, painful lymph nodes in the groin; fever, headache, and cold sores around the mouth. In women, pain during urination.
	Heatstroke	Sudden dizziness; weakness; headache; hot, dry, red skin which later turns grey; high body temperature; muscle cramps; confusion; seizures; loss of consciousness.
	Influenza *Flu*	Chills, muscle aches, and loss of appetite followed by a cough, sore throat, nasal congestion, and fever; possible chest pain.
	Lyme disease	A small red bump, surrounded by a concentric bulls-eye-like red rash with a pale center. Over the following month: fever and chills; extreme fatigue; headaches. Symptoms may progress over several months or years and may include: palpitations; joint or muscle pain; and chronic joint inflammation, especially in the knees.
	Mononucleosis, infectious	Headache; high fever; swollen glands in the neck, groin, and armpits; severe sore throat; swallowing difficulty.
	Peritonsillar abscess *A collection of pus between the tonsils and surrounding tissue due to infection*	Sore throat; severe pain when swallowing; fever; headache; impaired speech; drooling; swollen glands in the neck.
	Pharyngitis *Inflammation of the pharynx, the part of the throat between the mouth and the esophagus*	Sore or red throat; speaking and swallowing difficulties; sensitive, swollen glands in the neck; fever; headache; possible earache.
	Rabies	Low-grade fever; headache; loss of appetite; difficulty swallowing; tingling at site of animal bite; intense thirst exacerbated by the inability to drink without violent, painful throat spasms; paralysis of facial muscles; drooling. Agitation and violent behavior, confusion, convulsions, coma.
	Rubella *German Measles*	Rash on the face that spreads to the torso and limbs; enlargement of lymph nodes in neck; usually preceded by headache, fever, and runny nose.

Headache *continued*

Associated Symptoms	Possible Diagnosis	Distinguishing Features
with fever *continued*	Sinusitis *Inflammation of the mucous membranes lining the sinuses*	Throbbing pain above or below one or both eyes that intensifies when bending the head forward or coughing; nasal congestion; loss of sense of smell; often, pus-like nasal discharge; possible dental pain in the upper jaw; fever.
	Syphilis	Initially, painless, ulcerated, red sore on the genitals, mouth, or rectum; swollen glands in the neck, armpit, or groin; rash with small, red, scaly bumps; fever; headache. If left untreated, damage to heart valves leading to congestive heart failure; mental deterioration; loss of balance; seizures; dementia; personality changes.
	Tonsillitis	Sore, inflamed throat; swallowing difficulty; headache; swollen glands in the neck; fever; loss of voice. In children, nausea, vomiting, and abdominal pain.
	Typhoid fever	Headache; fever, loss of appetite; abdominal pain and tenderness; extreme weakness; constipation followed by diarrhea; drowsiness, stupor, or coma; raised, pink skin eruptions on the chest and abdomen; joint aches; sore throat.
with fever and nausea	Brain abscess	Headaches; drowsiness; nausea and vomiting; fever; seizures; possible partial paralysis; confusion; speaking difficulty.
	Glomerulonephritis, acute *Sudden or intense inflammation of the glomeruli, tiny structures that filter blood in the kidneys*	Blood in the urine; passing only small amounts of urine; swelling of the ankles or the tissues around the eyes; shortness of breath; possibly, fatigue, nausea and vomiting, loss of appetite, headaches, back pain, fever, impaired vision.
	Glomerulonephritis, chronic *Persistent inflammation of the glomeruli, tiny structures that filter blood in the kidneys*	Blood in the urine; passing only small amounts of urine; swelling of the legs or ankles; shortness of breath; possibly, fatigue, nausea and vomiting, loss of appetite, itching, headaches, impaired vision.
	Legionnaire's disease	Dry cough progressing to one with blood-streaked sputum; high fever; chills; breathing difficulty; chest pain; headache; muscle aches; diarrhea; nausea; vomiting; mental confusion and disorientation.
	Leukemias	Symptoms vary depending on the type of leukemia and may include: loss of appetite and weight; increased bruising and bleeding; bone pain, especially in the legs; abdominal pain and distention; nausea; heart palpitations; severe fatigue; pallor; breathing difficulty; fever; night sweats; headache; enlarged lymph nodes; joint pains (due to gout).

Headache *continued*

Associated Symptoms	Possible Diagnosis	Distinguishing Features
with fever and nausea *continued*	Malaria	Initially, severe chills and shivering. In later stages, extremely high fever followed by a period of profuse perspiration as fever subsides; headache, sometimes severe; vomiting.
	Meningitis *Inflammation of the membranes covering the brain and spinal cord*	Severe headache; nausea and vomiting; sensitivity to light; stiffness in the neck; possible red skin rash; fever; mental confusion; drowsiness; loss of consciousness; seizures.
	Poliomyelitis *Polio*	Low fever; sore throat; headache; nausea and vomiting. In severe cases, paralysis without loss of sensation; stiff neck and back; twitching; swallowing and breathing difficulty; drooling.
	Rocky Mountain spotted fever	Within a week after exposure, high fever, loss of appetite, headache, muscle aches, nausea and vomiting; dry cough; sensitivity to light. Within six days, the appearance of small pink spots on wrists and ankles, eventually spreading over the entire body, where they then grow, darken in color, and bleed.
	Systemic lupus erythematosus *Inflammation of connective tissues throughout the body*	Red, blotchy, butterfly-shaped rash on the cheeks and bridge of the nose; fatigue; fever; loss of appetite and weight; nausea; joint and abdominal pain; headaches; blurred vision; increased sensitivity to sun exposure; depression; psychosis; mental confusion.
	Toxic shock syndrome	Lethargy; conjunctivitis; confusion; sudden high fever accompanied by nausea, watery diarrhea, sore throat, and headache. Red rash on the palms and soles of the feet, which, after a week or two, begins to peel.

Hearing loss

Associated Symptoms	Possible Diagnosis	Distinguishing Features
with ear pain	Cholesteatoma *Infected cyst in the eardrum or middle ear*	Hearing loss; discharge of pus from ear; headaches and earaches; weakness of facial muscles; dizziness.
	Ear drum, perforated	Earache or sudden pain in the ear; partial hearing loss; slight bleeding or discharge from the ear; ringing or buzzing in the affected ear.
	Ear infection, middle *Inflammation of the middle ear*	Earache; deafness; ringing in the ear; possibly, a discharge of pus from the ear; fever; dizziness.
	Ear infection, outer	Redness and itching of the ear canal; discharge from the ear; ear pain; possibly, temporary loss of hearing.
without ear pain	Acoustic neuroma *A benign tumor in the cells covering the auditory nerve*	Gradual hearing loss; ringing in the ear; headache; numbness in the face; unsteady walk. In later stages, swallowing and speaking difficulties; possibly, slight paralysis.
	Labyrinthitis *Inflammation of the semicircular canals of the inner ear*	Severe dizziness, loss of balance, jerky movements of the eyes; nausea and vomiting; ringing in the ears. In later stages, possible hearing loss.
	Ménière's disease *Dysfunction of structures in the inner ear*	Sudden attack of severe vertigo; nausea and vomiting; impaired sense of balance; ringing in the ears; hearing loss in the affected ear. Jerky movements of the eyes.
	Otosclerosis *An overgrowth of bone in the middle ear*	Progressive hearing loss; ringing in the ears; dizziness. Hearing is more distinct when background noise is present.
	Paget's disease *A weakening, thickening, and deformity of the bones*	Often asymptomatic. Possibly, bone pain or deformity, especially bowing of the legs, bent spine, and facial deformity; unexplained bone fractures; joint pain or stiffness; hearing loss; headaches; ringing in ears.
	Presbycusis *Loss of hearing due to age*	Progressive inability to hear well in the presence of background noise; difficulty understanding speech.

Heartburn

Associated Symptoms	Possible Diagnosis	Distinguishing Features
	Cirrhosis *Chronic damage to the cells of the liver*	No symptoms in early stages; loss of weight and appetite; nausea; swollen legs, ankles and abdomen; itching; jaundice; black stools; vomiting blood; fatigue; impotence; memory loss; confusion.
	Esophageal cancer	Swallowing difficulty and pain; weight loss; drooling; possibly, vomiting or coughing up of bloody mucus, regurgitation of food; chest pain; repeated respiratory infections.
	Esophageal stricture *Narrowing of the esophagus, the passageway from the mouth to the stomach*	Sudden or gradual decrease in the ability to swallow solid food or liquids; chest pain after eating; regurgitation of food and liquids; increased salivation; weight loss. Aspiration into lungs can cause cough, wheezing, shortness of breath.
	Gallbladder disorders	Moderate to severe pain in the upper right side of the abdomen, chest, upper back, or right shoulder. Pain often follows the ingestion of high-fat foods and is episodic, lasting 20 minutes to several hours. Nausea and vomiting; low-grade fever; belching; heartburn; gas; possibly, jaundice, pale stools, and itchy skin.
	Gastroesophageal reflux *Heartburn*	Burning sensation in the middle of the chest; pain and difficulty swallowing; slight regurgitation of stomach's contents into the mouth, especially when reclining or bending forward; mild abdominal pain.
	Peptic ulcer	Intermittent, burning or gnawing pain in the upper abdomen or lower chest; indigestion; loss of appetite and weight. Pain may be relieved by eating or antacids. Possible nausea and vomiting. Black, tarry stools, vomiting blood.
	Scleroderma	Shiny, tight, and hardened skin, especially on the fingers, arms, and face; hands or feet may successively turn blue, white, and red upon exposure to cold (Raynaud's phenomenon); swallowing difficulty; bloating after eating; weight loss; shortness of breath on exertion; high blood pressure; symptoms of renal failure. Possibly, heartburn, muscle aches and weakness, joint pain, fever, or fatigue.

Hip pain

Associated Symptoms	Possible Diagnosis	Distinguishing Features
	Bone cancer	Pain, tenderness, and swelling in the affected bones and joints, often intensifying at night; a noticeable tumor or mass; increased susceptibility to bone fractures.
	Bursitis *Inflammation of the bursas, the lubricant-filled sacs in and around the joints*	Pain and swelling around a joint, usually the elbow, knee, or shoulder; painful movement in the affected joint; possibly, fever.
	Dislocations/subluxations	Deformity of the affected joint; joint pain and tenderness; difficulty moving a joint; swelling and stiffness within 30 minutes after joint injury.
	Infectious arthritis	Pain, swelling, stiffness, and redness, usually in one joint. Fever. Severity varies from a mild ache to severe, debilitating pain and eventual joint deformity.
	Obesity	Symptoms such as chest pain or shortness of breath from heart disease, knee or hip pain, or abdominal pain from gallstones all result from the complications of obesity.
	Osteoarthritis *Degeneration of the cartilage that lines the joints*	Pain, swelling, and stiffness in one or more joints; enlargement and distortion of affected joints.
	Osteomalacia and Rickets *Softening and weakening of the bones, usually due to poor calcification*	Bone pain, especially in the neck, legs, hips and ribs. Muscle weakness, numbness, or spasms in the hands, feet, and throat; increased susceptibility to bone fractures.
	Osteomyelitis *Infection of bone and bone marrow*	Fever; severe pain in the affected bone; inflammation and swelling of the skin over the affected area; deformity. In children, arrested growth of the affected bone.
	Osteoporosis *Loss of bone mass due to calcium depletion*	Backache; easily fractured bones, especially in the wrists, hips, and spine; gradual loss of height; stooped or hunched posture.
	Rheumatoid arthritis	Fatigue and weakness; joint pain, stiffness, and inflammation, especially in the hands, feet, and arms; joint deformity; dry mouth; dry, painful eyes. Morning stiffness.
	Rheumatoid arthritis, juvenile	Fever; rash; abdominal pain; weight loss; swelling, stiffness, and pain in the affected joints; enlarged lymph glands; fatigue; pallor; red, painful eyes.
	Sprains and strains	Swelling, pain or tenderness in the affected joints; impaired joint function.

Hip pain *continued*

Associated Symptoms	Possible Diagnosis	Distinguishing Features
	Tendinitis *Inflammation of a tendon*	Pain over a tendon anywhere in the body; if involved tendon is near or part of a joint, restricted movement of the joint.
	Thrombophlebitis *Inflammation associated with a blood clot*	Redness, swelling, pain, and tenderness in the affected area; most often occurs in the leg; swelling of the leg; prominent superficial veins around affected area; possibly, fever.

Hoarseness

Associated Symptoms	Possible Diagnosis	Distinguishing Features
	Hypothyroidism *Underactivity of the thyroid gland*	Unexplained weight gain; fatigue; muscle weakness; cramps; dry skin; hair loss; deepening of the voice; intolerance for cold; constipation; chest pain; insomnia; puffiness around eyes; loss of sex drive; depression; menstrual abnormalities; possible swelling in the neck.
	Laryngeal cancer	Initially, hoarseness, sore throat, and swallowing difficulty; later, pain when swallowing; swelling in the neck.
	Laryngitis	Hoarseness that often progresses to loss of the voice; throat pain; dry cough; possible fever.
	Pharyngitis *Inflammation of the pharynx, the part of the throat between the mouth and the esophagus*	Sore or red throat; speaking and swallowing difficulties; sensitive, swollen glands in the neck; fever; headache; possible earache.
	Rheumatoid arthritis, juvenile	Fever; rash; abdominal pain; weight loss; swelling, stiffness, and pain in the affected joints; enlarged lymph glands; fatigue; pallor; red, painful eyes.
	Sjögren's syndrome	Dry, itching, burning eyes; sensation of a foreign body under the eyelids; dry mouth; difficulty swallowing; vaginal dryness; dry skin; frequent dental cavities; joint pain; swelling of glands (parotids) in front of the ears; Raynaud's phenomenon.
	Tuberculosis	Often, asymptomatic. Possibly, low-grade fever; excessive perspiration; cough producing sputum or blood; weight loss; chronic fatigue; chest pain; shortness of breath; night sweats.

Hunger, unusual Polyphagia

Associated Symptoms	Possible Diagnosis	Distinguishing Features
	Anemia, iron deficiency	Fatigue and weakness; pallor; shortness of breath and heart palpitations on exertion; irritability or inability to concentrate; sore tongue or tiny cracks at the corners of the mouth; black, tarry or bloody stools; unusual craving for dirt, paint, or ice.
	Bipolar disorder *Manic-depressive illness*	Symptoms vary depending on phase of the disorder; mania: inflated self-esteem, elation, euphoria, grandiosity, increased activity, and a decreased need for sleep; depression: persistent feelings of sadness, apathy, or hopelessness; diminished interest in activities; loss of appetite and weight or unusual increase in appetite and weight; insomnia or drowsiness; difficulty concentrating; agitation in older patients.
	Depression	Persistent feelings of sadness, apathy, or hopelessness; diminished interest in activities; loss of or unusual increase in appetite and weight; insomnia or drowsiness; difficulty concentrating; agitation.
	Diabetes mellitus *Insufficiency of or resistance to insulin*	Fatigue; excessive thirst; frequent urination; weight loss despite increased appetite; blurred vision; numbness and tingling of feet and hands; impotence.
	Hyperthyroidism *Overactivity of the thyroid gland*	Protruding eyes; weight loss despite increased appetite; intolerance to heat; excessive perspiration; nervousness or restlessness; possibly, swelling in the neck (goiter); palpitations; tremor; diarrhea.
	Hypoglycemia *Low blood sugar*	Anxiety; hunger; trembling; headache; palpitations; perspiration; confusion; irritability; loss of coordination; possibly, double vision, seizures, or coma.
	Tapeworm infestation	Often asymptomatic. Unexplained weight loss; presence of white eggs or ribbon-like segments of worm in the stool, bedding, or clothing; symptoms of pernicious anemia.

Incontinence, fecal

Associated Symptoms	Possible Diagnosis	Distinguishing Features
	Alzheimer's disease	Symptoms vary greatly in different individuals. Initially, minor forgetfulness gradually developing into severe, short-term memory loss, disorientation, an inability to concentrate, and sudden mood and personality changes. In later stages, severe confusion, possible hallucinations or paranoid delusions, loss of social and sexual inhibitions, impaired judgment, anxiety, depression, agitation and combativeness, wandering and getting lost, inability to write, urinary and fecal incontinence.
	Brain tumors	Headaches that become more severe when reclining; nausea and vomiting; memory loss; double vision; muscle weakness; numbness, tingling, or partial paralysis; vision loss; speech disturbances; seizures; drowsiness.
	Colitis, ulcerative *Inflammation of the lining of the colon*	Pain on the left side of the abdomen that lessens after bowel movements; bloody diarrhea; pain in the rectal area; possibly, fever, rapid heartbeat, nausea and vomiting, loss of appetite, dehydration with severe attacks.
	Multiple sclerosis *Gradual degeneration of the protective sheaths surrounding the nerves within the brain and spinal cord*	Symptoms may appear suddenly and then disappear; persistent symptoms may take years to develop and include numbness or tingling in any part of the body, weakness in the extremities, an unsteady walk, slurred speech, urinary incontinence, fatigue, depression, temporary loss of vision, double or blurred vision, mental confusion, and memory loss.
	Peripheral neuropathies *Degeneration of the nerves that supply the extremities*	Tingling or numbness commonly beginning in the hands and feet and gradually spreading toward the center of the body; sensitive skin; muscle weakness; possibly, pain in the hands and feet; lack of coordination; shooting pains exacerbated by touch or changes in temperature; breathing difficulty; urinary or fecal incontinence.
	Spinal cord trauma	Severe pain and swelling in the affected area; loss of sensation, muscle weakness, or paralysis below the site of the injury; urinary or fecal incontinence or retention; impotence; breathing difficulty; shock.
	Spinal tumor	Progressive numbness, tingling, and muscle weakness; fecal or urinary incontinence; persistent back pain.
	Stroke	Symptoms vary with the location of brain injury. Sudden onset of weakness, paralysis, or loss of sensation, usually on one side of the body; a sudden heaviness in a limb; speech abnormalities; headache; vision disturbances; dizziness; confusion; coma; urinary and fecal incontinence.

Incontinence, urinary

Associated Symptoms	Possible Diagnosis	Distinguishing Features
	Alzheimer's disease	Symptoms vary greatly in different individuals. Initially, minor forgetfulness gradually developing into severe, short-term memory loss, disorientation, an inability to concentrate, and sudden mood and personality changes. In later stages, severe confusion, possible hallucinations or paranoid delusions, loss of social and sexual inhibitions, impaired judgment, anxiety, depression, agitation and combativeness, wandering and getting lost, inability to write, urinary and fecal incontinence.
	Irritable bladder	Sudden, urgent need to urinate; frequent urination.
	Multiple sclerosis *Gradual degeneration of the protective sheaths surrounding the nerves within the brain and spinal cord*	Symptoms may appear suddenly and then disappear; persistent symptoms may take years to develop and include numbness or tingling in any part of the body, weakness in the extremities, an unsteady walk, slurred speech, urinary incontinence, fatigue, depression, temporary loss of vision, double or blurred vision, mental confusion, and memory loss.
	Neurogenic bladder *Inability to control passage of urine due to damage to nerves to the bladder*	Inability to control urine flow which may involuntarily release in large volumes or in a continuous dribbling. Bed-wetting during sleep; feeling the need to urinate though no urine is passed; pain or burning during urination.
	Peripheral neuropathies *Degeneration of the nerves that supply the extremities*	Tingling or numbness commonly beginning in the hands and feet and gradually spreading toward the center of the body; sensitive skin; muscle weakness; possibly, pain in the hands and feet; lack of coordination; shooting pains exacerbated by touch or changes in temperature; breathing difficulty; urinary or fecal incontinence.
	Prostate cancer	Difficulty urinating; frequent urination with decreased urine output; pain in the pelvic area and lower back; painful ejaculation or bowel movements; impotence.
	Seizures	Involuntary twitching or jerking; muscle rigidity; loss of consciousness; confusion; drooling; hallucinations.
	Spinal cord trauma	Severe pain and swelling in the affected area; loss of sensation, muscle weakness, or paralysis below the site of the injury; urinary or fecal incontinence or retention; impotence; breathing difficulty; shock.
	Spinal tumor	Progressive numbness, tingling, and muscle weakness; fecal or urinary incontinence; persistent back pain.

Incontinence, urinary *continued*

Associated Symptoms	Possible Diagnosis	Distinguishing Features
	Stroke	Symptoms vary with the location of brain injury. Sudden onset of weakness, paralysis, or loss of sensation, usually on one side of the body; a sudden heaviness in a limb; speech abnormalities; headache; vision disturbances; dizziness; confusion; coma; urinary and fecal incontinence.
	Urinary incontinence	Uncontrollable, involuntary release of urine, either in large volumes or a continuous dribble. May be increased by coughing, sneezing, laughing, or with any activity involving contraction of the abdominal muscles.
with blood in urine	Bladder infection *Cystitis*	Burning during urination; frequent and urgent urination with only small amounts of urine passed; blood in the urine; lower abdominal pain; low-grade fever; pain during sexual intercourse and, in men, during ejaculation.
	Kidney infection *Pyelonephritis*	Sudden fever and shaking chills; severe fatigue; burning and frequent urination; cloudy or bloody urine; pain in the abdomen, back, or flanks, sometimes severe; nausea and vomiting.

Indigestion

Associated Symptoms	Possible Diagnosis	Distinguishing Features
	Adrenal insufficiency *Inadequate production of steroid hormones by the adrenal gland*	Loss of weight and appetite; fatigue; weakness; darkening of the skin; abdominal pain; diarrhea; indigestion; nausea and vomiting; constipation; lack of sex drive; dizziness when rising from sitting or lying position.
	Carcinoid tumors and carcinoid syndrome	May be asymptomatic; flushing or redness of the face and neck; gas and profuse diarrhea; abdominal cramping; watery, swollen eyes; shortness of breath or wheezing.
	Cirrhosis *Chronic damage to the cells of the liver*	No symptoms in early stages; loss of weight and appetite; nausea; swollen legs, ankles and abdomen; itching; jaundice; black stools; vomiting blood; fatigue; impotence; memory loss; confusion.
	Colitis, ulcerative *Inflammation of the lining of the colon*	Pain on the left side of the abdomen that lessens after bowel movements; bloody diarrhea; pain in the rectal area; possibly, fever, rapid heartbeat, nausea and vomiting, loss of appetite, dehydration with severe attacks.
	Congestive heart failure	Shortness of breath; fatigue; need to sleep on several pillows; weakness; cough; heart palpitations; swelling in the legs, ankles, and abdomen; frequent urination at night; indigestion; nausea and vomiting; loss of appetite.
	Crohn's disease *Inflammation of the lining of the small intestine*	Episodes of abdominal pain or cramps in lower abdomen; nausea; diarrhea; loss of weight and appetite; possibly, fever; rectal bleeding or blood in stools; fatigue; anal fissures; joint pains; inflammation of the eyes.
	Gastroesophageal reflux *Heartburn*	Burning sensation in the middle of the chest; pain and difficulty swallowing; slight regurgitation of stomach's contents into the mouth, especially when reclining or bending forward; mild abdominal pain.
	Hepatitis, acute viral	Fever; fatigue; loss of appetite; aching muscles and joints; abdominal pain or discomfort; jaundice; dark urine and pale stools.
	Hepatitis, chronic	Fatigue; nausea; vomiting; loss of appetite; jaundice; dark urine; clay-colored stools; depression; pain or discomfort in the upper right abdomen; abdominal swelling; fever; in women, cessation of menstruation, acne, and the appearance of male pattern facial hair.
	Hyperparathyroidism *Overactivity of the parathyroid glands*	Increased susceptibility to bone fractures; depression; indigestion; increased thirst and urine output; fatigue, lethargy; somnolence; muscle weakness; nausea and vomiting; loss of appetite; weight loss.

Indigestion *continued*

Associated Symptoms	Possible Diagnosis	Distinguishing Features
	Intestinal obstruction	Abdominal pain and cramps; nausea; vomiting; weakness; gas; bloating; possible diarrhea; progressive constipation culminating in inability to pass stools or gas.
	Lactose intolerance *Difficulty digesting milk and dairy products*	Abdominal cramps; diarrhea; nausea; bloating; flatulence.
	Malabsorption, digestive *A failure of the small intestine to absorb nutrients in the diet*	Diarrhea; weight loss; yellowish, foul-smelling stools; abdominal cramps, gas, and bloating; weakness and lethargy.
	Pancreatic cancer	Often, no symptoms until far advanced. Upper abdominal pain which spreads to the back; loss of weight and appetite; jaundice; nausea, vomiting, and indigestion; diarrhea; fatigue; depression.
	Pancreatitis *Inflammation of the pancreas*	Sudden, extreme abdominal pain; nausea and vomiting; weakness; fever; clammy skin; abdominal bloating and tenderness.
	Peptic ulcer	Intermittent, burning or gnawing pain in the upper abdomen or lower chest; indigestion; loss of appetite and weight. Pain may be relieved by eating or antacids. Possible nausea and vomiting. Black, tarry stools, vomiting blood.

Insomnia

Associated Symptoms	Possible Diagnosis	Distinguishing Features
	Anxiety states	Sudden attacks of unreasonable fear and panic; rapid heartbeat or palpitations; perspiration; dry mouth; irritability; muscle tension; trembling; shortness of breath; restlessness; poor concentration; insomnia; fatigue; weakness.
	Bipolar disorder *Manic-depressive illness*	Symptoms vary depending on phase of the disorder; mania: inflated self-esteem, elation, euphoria, grandiosity, increased activity, and a decreased need for sleep; depression: persistent feelings of sadness, apathy, or hopelessness; diminished interest in activities; loss of appetite and weight or unusual increase in appetite and weight; insomnia or drowsiness; difficulty concentrating; agitation in older patients.
	Chronic fatigue syndrome	Severe fatigue made worse by exercise; recurrent flu-like symptoms; persistent sore throat; low-grade fever; muscle and joint aches; headache; painful, swollen lymph nodes; depression and mental confusion; memory loss; sleep difficulties.
	Cushing's syndrome	Red, oval-shaped face; humped upper back and obese trunk; acne; purple stretch marks on the abdomen, thighs, and breasts; thin and easily bruised skin; easily fractured bones; depression or euphoria; insomnia; fatigue; muscle weakness; hirsutism (in women).
	Depression	Persistent feelings of sadness, apathy, or hopelessness; diminished interest in activities; loss of or unusual increase in appetite and weight; insomnia or drowsiness; difficulty concentrating; agitation.
	Fibromyalgia	Muscle aches, pains, and stiffness; specific points on the body that feel sore when pressed; fatigue; headaches; feeling unrefreshed upon awakening in the morning.
	Hyperthyroidism *Overactivity of the thyroid gland*	Protruding eyes; weight loss despite increased appetite; intolerance to heat; excessive perspiration; nervousness or restlessness; possibly, swelling in the neck (goiter); palpitations; tremor; diarrhea.
	Hypothyroidism *Underactivity of the thyroid gland*	Unexplained weight gain; fatigue; muscle weakness; cramps; dry skin; hair loss; deepening of the voice; intolerance for cold; constipation; chest pain; insomnia; puffiness around eyes; loss of sex drive; depression; menstrual abnormalities; possible swelling in the neck.
	Insomnia	Difficulty falling asleep or staying asleep; daytime fatigue; irritability.

Itching skin/scalp

Associated Symptoms	Possible Diagnosis	Distinguishing Features
with rash/red skin/ marks on skin	Breast cancer	Lump or swelling, usually painless, in the breast or under the armpit; flattening, dimpling, indentation, redness, or scaliness of the breast; itching sensation in the nipple; change in size or symmetry of the breasts; breast pain.
	Chiggers *Parasitic infestation*	Itchy patches of red skin. Itching may persist for weeks.
	Dermatomyositis *Inflammation of the muscles and skin*	Red rash on the neck, upper torso, and upper arms and legs; purple discoloration and swelling of the eyelids; areas of thickened skin; muscle weakness and stiffness, usually in the shoulders and pelvis; cold hands and feet; speaking or swallowing difficulty; weight loss.
	Eczema *Inflammation of the skin*	Itching skin; thickened patches of skin; possibly, with oozing and crusting; in infants, rash on the face, inner elbows, or behind the knees that turns scaly and develops small red pimples that leak; swollen legs (stasis dermatitis).
	Herpes zoster *Shingles*	A sensitive band of skin on one side of the body that becomes severely painful and develops slightly raised red spots that blister, dry and crust over. Pain may persist for months or years after skin has healed.
	Lice	Intense itching, usually on hair-covered areas; visible nits (eggs) on hair shafts; red bite marks; visible lice on clothing.
	Melanoma *Skin cancer*	Change in the appearance of an existing mole including enlargement, bleeding, change in color, development of a black edge. Itching.
	Polycythemia vera *An overproduction of red and white blood cells and platelets*	Headache; ringing in the ears; blurred vision; flushed skin; itching; dizziness; fatigue; night sweats; frequent nose bleeds and bruises.
	Psoriasis	Slightly raised patches of skin with red borders and white-silver scales; joint pain and stiffness; itching; pitted nails.
	Ringworm *Fungal skin infection*	A rash with distinct, advancing borders and clear centers; affected areas may have abnormally dark pigmentation; itching; scaly patches of skin; bald patches on scalp; Athlete's foot; red, swollen finger- and toenails.

Itching skin/scalp *continued*

Associated Symptoms	Possible Diagnosis	Distinguishing Features
with rash/red skin/ marks on skin *continued*	Scabies	Tiny, grey, scaly blisters—usually on the wrists, genitals, armpits, or between the fingers—that rupture easily when scratched; severe itching; red lumps or rashes may develop.
without rash/ red skin/ marks on skin	Anaphylaxis	Itching and hives; swelling of the eyes, lips, and tongue; weakness or faintness; tightening in the chest or throat; wheezing; shortness of breath; profuse sweating; palpitations; sudden, intense distress; feelings of impending doom; stomach cramps; nausea, vomiting, or diarrhea; bluish tinge (cyanosis) to the skin, lips, and nail beds due to oxygen insufficiency.
	Anemia, aplastic	Fatigue and weakness; shortness of breath; heart palpitations; pallor; bleeding gums; nosebleeds; tendency to bruise easily; small red dots under the skin (petechiae). Increased susceptibility to infection.
	Anemia, folic acid deficiency	Fatigue and weakness; pallor; shortness of breath, heart palpitations, or noticeably rapid heartbeat on exertion; sore, red, and glazed looking tongue; loss of weight and appetite; nausea and diarrhea; abdominal distention.
	Anemia, hemolytic	Fatigue and weakness; shortness of breath on exertion; pallor; heart palpitations; jaundice and dark urine.
	Anemia, iron deficiency	Fatigue and weakness; pallor; shortness of breath and heart palpitations on exertion; irritability or inability to concentrate; sore tongue or tiny cracks at the corners of the mouth; black, tarry or bloody stools; unusual craving for dirt, paint, or ice.
	Anemia, pernicious	Fatigue; inability to concentrate; sore, red tongue; weakness; dizziness; pallor; shortness of breath on exertion; palpitations; numbness and tingling in extremities; incoordination; headache; loss of weight and appetite; possibly, jaundice.
	Cirrhosis *Chronic damage to the cells of the liver*	No symptoms in early stages; loss of weight and appetite; nausea; swollen legs, ankles and abdomen; itching; jaundice; black stools; vomiting blood; fatigue; impotence; memory loss; confusion.
	Glomerulonephritis, acute *Sudden or intense inflammation of the glomeruli, tiny structures that filter blood in the kidneys*	Blood in the urine; passing only small amounts of urine; swelling of the ankles or the tissues around the eyes; shortness of breath; possibly, fatigue, nausea, vomiting, loss of appetite, headaches, back pain, fever, impaired vision.

Itching skin/scalp *continued*

Associated Symptoms	Possible Diagnosis	Distinguishing Features
without rash/ red skin/ marks on skin *continued*	Glomerulonephritis, chronic *Persistent inflammation of the glomeruli, tiny structures that filter blood in the kidneys*	Blood in the urine; passing only small amounts of urine; swelling of the legs or ankles; shortness of breath; possibly, fatigue, nausea and vomiting, loss of appetite, itching, headaches, impaired vision.
	Leukemias	Symptoms vary depending on the type of leukemia and may include: loss of appetite and weight; increased bruising and bleeding; bone pain, especially in the legs; abdominal pain and distention; nausea; heart palpitations; severe fatigue; pallor; breathing difficulty; fever; night sweats; headache; enlarged lymph nodes; joint pains (due to gout).
	Lymphoma, Hodgkin's *Cancer of the lymph nodes and lymphoid tissue*	Painless swelling of the lymph nodes usually in the neck or armpits; loss of appetite; night sweats.
	Renal failure, chronic *Persistent, mild kidney failure*	Asymptomatic in early stages. Possibly, mental confusion; shortness of breath; abdominal pain; decreased sex drive; fatigue; muscle and bone pain; numbness in the legs and feet; headache; impaired mental acuity; bad breath.
	Sjögren's syndrome	Dry, itching, burning eyes; sensation of a foreign body under the eyelids; dry mouth; difficulty swallowing; vaginal dryness; dry skin; frequent dental cavities; joint pain; swelling of glands (parotids) in front of the ears; Raynaud's phenomenon.
	Varicose veins	Blue or purplish, knotted veins, usually in the legs; itching or discomfort in the affected area; swollen feet and ankles. Possible scaly skin, muscle cramps, or skin ulcers.

Jaundice, skin/eyes

Associated Symptoms	Possible Diagnosis	Distinguishing Features
	Anemia, pernicious	Fatigue; inability to concentrate; sore, red tongue; weakness; dizziness; pallor; shortness of breath on exertion; palpitations; numbness and tingling in extremities; incoordination; headache; loss of weight and appetite; possibly, jaundice.
	Cirrhosis *Chronic damage to the cells of the liver*	No symptoms in early stages; loss of weight and appetite; nausea; swollen legs, ankles and abdomen; itching; jaundice; black stools; vomiting blood; fatigue; impotence; memory loss; confusion.
	Empyema *Collection of pus in any body cavity, usually between the membranes covering the lungs*	Chest pain exacerbated by deep inhalation; shortness of breath; dry cough; fever and chills; exhaustion; weight loss; night sweats; abdominal pain and jaundice.
	Gallbladder disorders	Moderate to severe pain in the upper right side of the abdomen, chest, upper back, or right shoulder. Pain often follows the ingestion of high-fat foods and is episodic, lasting 20 minutes to several hours. Nausea and vomiting; low-grade fever; belching; heartburn; gas; possibly, jaundice, pale stools, and itchy skin.
	Hepatitis, acute viral	Fever; fatigue; loss of appetite; aching muscles and joints; abdominal pain or discomfort; jaundice; dark urine and pale stools.
	Hepatitis, chronic	Fatigue; nausea; vomiting; loss of appetite; jaundice; dark urine; clay-colored stools; depression; pain or discomfort in the upper right abdomen; abdominal swelling; fever; in women, cessation of menstruation, acne, and the appearance of male pattern facial hair.
	Liver tumors	Pain or discomfort in the upper right portion of the abdomen; abdominal swelling; loss of weight and appetite; nausea and vomiting; fever; excessive perspiration; jaundice; pallor; severe fatigue.
	Pancreatic cancer	Often, no symptoms until far advanced. Upper abdominal pain which spreads to the back; loss of weight and appetite; jaundice; nausea, vomiting, and indigestion; diarrhea; fatigue; depression.
	Pancreatitis *Inflammation of the pancreas*	Sudden, extreme abdominal pain; nausea and vomiting; weakness; fever; clammy skin; abdominal bloating and tenderness.
	Reye's syndrome *Childhood disease marked by brain and liver damage*	Following recovery from an upper respiratory infection, nausea and vomiting; memory loss; confusion or delirium; possible seizures; drowsiness; lethargy.

Jaw pain

Associated Symptoms	Possible Diagnosis	Distinguishing Features
	Impacted teeth	Gum pain; unpleasant taste in mouth, especially when biting down; red, swollen gums around the affected tooth; headache or jaw ache; possibly, bad breath.
	Jaw dislocation or fracture	Inability to close the jaw normally; painful, swollen, or numb jaw; misalignment of teeth; speaking difficulty; possible breathing difficulty.
	Mumps	Pain in the ear, below the ear, and in the jaw; swollen glands in the neck; headache; pain on swallowing and chewing; sore muscles; joint pain; loss of appetite. Testicular swelling and tenderness in adults.
	Myocardial infarction *Heart attack*	Sudden chest pain or pressure that may spread to the arm, shoulder and jaw; excessive perspiration; shortness of breath. Possible nausea and vomiting.
	Neuralgia *Pain due to nerve damage or irritation*	Symptoms vary depending on the area affected and include: recurring episodes of sharp pain on one side of the lips, gums, cheek, or chin; radiating pain around the eyes; a burning pain along the path of a nerve encircling the torso. Pain may last from a few seconds to several minutes and always affects the same location. Attacks may occur several times a day for weeks with asymptomatic periods of weeks or months in between and may be triggered by touching or blowing on the affected area. Mouth pain may be exacerbated by talking, eating, or swallowing.
	Oral cancers	Sore in the mouth that bleeds and does not heal; lump in the cheek; white or red patch on the gums; swallowing and chewing difficulties; numbness of the tongue; swelling of the jaw.
	Osteomyelitis *Infection of bone and bone marrow*	Fever; severe pain in the affected bone; inflammation and swelling of the skin over the affected area; deformity. In children, arrested growth of the affected bone.
	Rheumatoid arthritis	Fatigue and weakness; joint pain, stiffness, and inflammation, especially in the hands, feet, and arms; joint deformity; dry mouth; dry, painful eyes. Morning stiffness.
	Sinusitis *Inflammation of the mucous membranes lining the sinuses*	Throbbing pain above or below one or both eyes that intensifies when bending the head forward or coughing; nasal congestion; loss of sense of smell; often, pus-like nasal discharge; possible dental pain in the upper jaw; fever.

Jaw pain *continued*

Associated Symptoms	Possible Diagnosis	Distinguishing Features
	Temporomandibular joint syndrome	Pain in the joints connecting the jaw to the skull; headache; tender jaw muscles; dull facial pain; clicking noise when opening or closing the mouth; pain when yawning and chewing. Jaw may temporarily lock in position.
	Tetanus	Often, lockjaw; stiffness and, later, muscle spasms in the neck and face; drooling; abdominal and back pain; extreme perspiration; swallowing difficulty; possible convulsions; fever.
	Thyroiditis *Inflammation of the thyroid gland*	Pain in the front of the neck and, often, the ear; possibly fever, weight loss, and fatigue; general feeling of being unwell (malaise); discomfort on swallowing.
	Tooth abscess	Persistent tooth pain; pain when biting or chewing; difficulty swallowing; swollen glands in the neck; earache; fever; possibly, foul taste in the mouth or bad breath.
	Tooth decay	Tooth pain, especially after eating sweet or sour foods; tooth sensitivity to hot and cold; bad breath; unpleasant taste in the mouth.

Joint pain

Associated Symptoms	Possible Diagnosis	Distinguishing Features
with fever	Gout	Most commonly affects the joints of the big toe. Affected joints are red, swollen, hot, and severely painful. In late stages, joint deformity. Kidney stones.
	Hepatitis, acute viral	Fever; fatigue; loss of appetite; aching muscles and joints; abdominal pain or discomfort; jaundice; dark urine and pale stools.
	Infectious arthritis	Pain, swelling, stiffness, and redness, usually in one joint. Fever. Severity varies from a mild ache to severe, debilitating pain and eventual joint deformity.
	Influenza *Flu*	Chills, muscle aches, and loss of appetite followed by a cough, sore throat, nasal congestion, and fever; possible chest pain.
	Lyme disease	A small red bump, surrounded by a concentric bulls-eye-like red rash with a pale center. Over the following month: fever and chills; extreme fatigue; headaches. Symptoms may progress over several months or years and may include: palpitations; joint or muscle pain; and chronic joint inflammation, especially in the knees.
	Mumps	Pain in the ear, below the ear, and in the jaw; swollen glands in the neck; headache; pain on swallowing and chewing; sore muscles; joint pain; loss of appetite. Testicular swelling and tenderness in adults.
	Osteomyelitis *Infection of bone and bone marrow*	Fever; severe pain in the affected bone; inflammation and swelling of the skin over the affected area; deformity. In children, arrested growth of the affected bone.
	Rheumatic fever	Initially, a sore throat that gets better followed, one to six weeks later, by lethargy and fever. Possibly, swollen joints, rash, abdominal pain, involuntary jerky movements, emotional instability.
	Rheumatoid arthritis	Fatigue and weakness; joint pain, stiffness, and inflammation, especially in the hands, feet, and arms; joint deformity; dry mouth; dry, painful eyes. Morning stiffness.
	Rheumatoid arthritis, juvenile	Fever; rash; abdominal pain; weight loss; swelling, stiffness, and pain in the affected joints; enlarged lymph glands; fatigue; pallor; red, painful eyes.

Joint pain *continued*

Associated Symptoms	Possible Diagnosis	Distinguishing Features
with fever *continued*	Sarcoidosis *Accumulation of inflammatory cells in the lymph nodes and other tissues throughout the body*	Often no symptoms. Swollen lymph nodes in the neck or armpits; muscle aches; fever; breathing difficulty; possibly, purple rash on the face; reddish or brownish skin spots on the forearms, face, or legs; numbness; joint pain or stiffness; a painful, red eye; blurred vision; loss of appetite and weight.
	Scleroderma	Shiny, tight, and hardened skin, especially on the fingers, arms, and face; hands or feet may successively turn blue, white, and red upon exposure to cold (Raynaud's phenomenon); swallowing difficulty; bloating after eating; weight loss; shortness of breath on exertion; high blood pressure; symptoms of renal failure. Possibly, heartburn, muscle aches and weakness, joint pain, fever, or fatigue.
	Syphilis	Initially, painless, ulcerated, red sore on the genitals, mouth, or rectum; swollen glands in the neck, armpit, or groin; rash with small, red, scaly bumps; fever; headache. If left untreated, damage to heart valves leading to congestive heart failure; mental deterioration; loss of balance; seizures; dementia; personality changes.
	Systemic lupus erythematosus *Inflammation of connective tissues throughout the body*	Red, blotchy, butterfly-shaped rash on the cheeks and bridge of the nose; fatigue; fever; loss of appetite and weight; nausea; joint and abdominal pain; headaches; blurred vision; increased sensitivity to sun exposure; depression; psychosis; mental confusion.
	Tendinitis *Inflammation of a tendon*	Pain over a tendon anywhere in the body; if involved tendon is near or part of a joint, restricted movement of the joint.
without fever	Acromegaly *Overproduction of growth hormone by the pituitary gland*	In adults (acromegaly): Gradual thickening of the bones of the face, jaw, and the extremities in adults; oily skin; severe headache; excessive hair growth; excessive perspiration; joint pains. In children (in which the disease is called gigantism): Rapid growth and unusual height; possibly, blindness.
	Ankylosing spondylitis *Inflammation of the joints between the spine and the pelvis*	Initially, pain and stiffness in the lower back and hips that becomes worse after resting; neck or chest pain; possible pain in the hip, knee, and ankle joints; pain in the heel of the foot; eye pain; blurred vision.
	Bone cancer	Pain, tenderness, and swelling in the affected bones and joints, often intensifying at night; a noticeable tumor or mass; increased susceptibility to bone fractures.

Joint pain *continued*

Associated Symptoms	Possible Diagnosis	Distinguishing Features
without fever *continued*	Bursitis *Inflammation of the bursas, the lubricant-filled sacs in and around the joints*	Pain and swelling around a joint, usually the elbow, knee, or shoulder; painful movement in the affected joint; possibly, fever.
	Dislocations/subluxations	Deformity of the affected joint; joint pain and tenderness; difficulty moving a joint; swelling and stiffness within 30 minutes after joint injury.
	Hemochromatosis *An excess accumulation of iron in the liver, pancreas, heart, testes, skin, and other organs*	A bronze or slate-grey tone to skin that is normally fair; chronic abdominal pain; heart palpitations; joint pain; drowsiness. In men, a decrease in the size of the testes, loss of sexual desire, and impotence.
	Hemophilia	Profuse bleeding from minor injuries and tooth extractions; internal bleeding that may cause blood in the urine; bleeding into joints; symptoms of stroke due to intracerebral bleeding; possibly, extensive bruising.
	Hyperparathyroidism *Overactivity of the parathyroid glands*	Increased susceptibility to bone fractures; depression; indigestion; increased thirst and urine output; fatigue, lethargy; somnolence; muscle weakness; nausea and vomiting; loss of appetite; weight loss.
	Osteoarthritis *Degeneration of the cartilage that lines the joints*	Pain, swelling, and stiffness in one or more joints; enlargement and distortion of affected joints.
	Paget's disease *A weakening, thickening, and deformity of the bones*	Often asymptomatic. Possibly, bone pain or deformity, especially bowing of the legs, bent spine, and facial deformity; unexplained bone fractures; joint pain or stiffness; hearing loss; headaches; ringing in ears.
	Psoriasis	Slightly raised patches of skin with red borders and white-silver scales; joint pain and stiffness; itching; pitted nails.
	Sjögren's syndrome	Dry, itching, burning eyes; sensation of a foreign body under the eyelids; dry mouth; difficulty swallowing; vaginal dryness; dry skin; frequent dental cavities; joint pain; swelling of glands (parotids) in front of the ears; Raynaud's phenomenon.
	Sprains and strains	Swelling, pain or tenderness in the affected joints; impaired joint function.
	Temporomandibular joint syndrome	Pain in the joints connecting the jaw to the skull; headache; tender jaw muscles; dull facial pain; clicking noise when opening or closing the mouth; pain when yawning and chewing. Jaw may temporarily lock in position.

Knee pain

Associated Symptoms	Possible Diagnosis	Distinguishing Features
	Bone cancer	Pain, tenderness, and swelling in the affected bones and joints, often intensifying at night; a noticeable tumor or mass; increased susceptibility to bone fractures.
	Bursitis *Inflammation of the bursas, the lubricant-filled sacs in and around the joints*	Pain and swelling around a joint, usually the elbow, knee, or shoulder; painful movement in the affected joint; possibly, fever.
	Dislocations/subluxations	Deformity of the affected joint; joint pain and tenderness; difficulty moving a joint; swelling and stiffness within 30 minutes after joint injury.
	Infectious arthritis	Pain, swelling, stiffness, and redness, usually in one joint. Fever. Severity varies from a mild ache to severe, debilitating pain and eventual joint deformity.
	Obesity	Symptoms such as chest pain or shortness of breath from heart disease, knee or hip pain, or abdominal pain from gallstones all result from the complications of obesity.
	Osteoarthritis *Degeneration of the cartilage that lines the joints*	Pain, swelling, and stiffness in one or more joints; enlargement and distortion of affected joints.
	Osteomalacia and Rickets *Softening and weakening of the bones, usually due to poor calcification*	Bone pain, especially in the neck, legs, hips and ribs. Muscle weakness, numbness, or spasms in the hands, feet, and throat; increased susceptibility to bone fractures.
	Osteomyelitis *Infection of bone and bone marrow*	Fever; severe pain in the affected bone; inflammation and swelling of the skin over the affected area; deformity. In children, arrested growth of the affected bone.
	Rheumatoid arthritis	Fatigue and weakness; joint pain, stiffness, and inflammation, especially in the hands, feet, and arms; joint deformity; dry mouth; dry, painful eyes. Morning stiffness.
	Rheumatoid arthritis, juvenile	Fever; rash; abdominal pain; weight loss; swelling, stiffness, and pain in the affected joints; enlarged lymph glands; fatigue; pallor; red, painful eyes.
	Sprains and strains	Swelling, pain or tenderness in the affected joints; impaired joint function.
	Tendinitis *Inflammation of a tendon*	Pain over a tendon anywhere in the body; if involved tendon is near or part of a joint, restricted movement of the joint.

Knee pain *continued*

Associated Symptoms	Possible Diagnosis	Distinguishing Features
	Thrombophlebitis *Inflammation associated with a blood clot*	Redness, swelling, pain, and tenderness in the affected area; most often occurs in the leg; swelling of the leg; prominent superficial veins around affected area; possibly, fever.
	Varicose veins	Blue or purplish, knotted veins, usually in the legs; itching or discomfort in the affected area; swollen feet and ankles. Possible scaly skin, muscle cramps, or skin ulcers.

Leg pain

Associated Symptoms	Possible Diagnosis	Distinguishing Features
	Bone cancer	Pain, tenderness, and swelling in the affected bones and joints, often intensifying at night; a noticeable tumor or mass; increased susceptibility to bone fractures.
	Bursitis *Inflammation of the bursas, the lubricant-filled sacs in and around the joints*	Pain and swelling around a joint, usually the elbow, knee, or shoulder; painful movement in the affected joint; possibly, fever.
	Infectious arthritis	Pain, swelling, stiffness, and redness, usually in one joint. Fever. Severity varies from a mild ache to severe, debilitating pain and eventual joint deformity.
	Lyme disease	A small red bump, surrounded by a concentric bulls-eye-like red rash with a pale center. Over the following month: fever and chills; extreme fatigue; headaches. Symptoms may progress over several months or years and may include: palpitations; joint or muscle pain; and chronic joint inflammation, especially in the knees.
	Osteoarthritis *Degeneration of the cartilage that lines the joints*	Pain, swelling, and stiffness in one or more joints; enlargement and distortion of affected joints.
	Osteomalacia and Rickets *Softening and weakening of the bones, usually due to poor calcification*	Bone pain, especially in the neck, legs, hips and ribs. Muscle weakness, numbness, or spasms in the hands, feet, and throat; increased susceptibility to bone fractures.
	Osteomyelitis *Infection of bone and bone marrow*	Fever; severe pain in the affected bone; inflammation and swelling of the skin over the affected area; deformity. In children, arrested growth of the affected bone.
	Osteoporosis *Loss of bone mass due to calcium depletion*	Backache; easily fractured bones, especially in the wrists, hips, and spine; gradual loss of height; stooped or hunched posture.
	Paget's disease *A weakening, thickening, and deformity of the bones*	Often asymptomatic. Possibly, bone pain or deformity, especially bowing of the legs, bent spine, and facial deformity; unexplained bone fractures; joint pain or stiffness; hearing loss; headaches; ringing in ears.
	Peripheral vascular disease *Narrowing of blood vessels in the legs or arms*	Muscle pain on one or both legs that occurs with exercise and subsides with rest; possible pain in the fingers, arms, buttocks, lower back, or the arch of the foot; impotence. Severe symptoms include: muscle pain at rest that intensifies at night; discolored or blue toes; cold or numb feet; open sores; heightened sensitivity to cold; weak or absent pulse in the affected limb; scaly or hairless skin over the affected area.

Leg pain *continued*

Associated Symptoms	Possible Diagnosis	Distinguishing Features
	Rheumatoid arthritis	Fatigue and weakness; joint pain, stiffness, and inflammation, especially in the hands, feet, and arms; joint deformity; dry mouth; dry, painful eyes. Morning stiffness.
	Rheumatoid arthritis, juvenile	Fever; rash; abdominal pain; weight loss; swelling, stiffness, and pain in the affected joints; enlarged lymph glands; fatigue; pallor; red, painful eyes.
	Shin splints	Pain in the front of the calf that may intensify during walking or running.
	Sprains and strains	Swelling, pain or tenderness in the affected joints; impaired joint function.
	Tendinitis *Inflammation of a tendon*	Pain over a tendon anywhere in the body; if involved tendon is near or part of a joint, restricted movement of the joint.
	Thrombophlebitis *Inflammation associated with a blood clot*	Redness, swelling, pain, and tenderness in the affected area; most often occurs in the leg; swelling of the leg; prominent superficial veins around affected area; possibly, fever.
	Varicose veins	Blue or purplish, knotted veins, usually in the legs; itching or discomfort in the affected area; swollen feet and ankles. Possible scaly skin, muscle cramps, or skin ulcers.

Lethargy

Associated Symptoms	Possible Diagnosis	Distinguishing Features
	Acromegaly *Overproduction of growth hormone by the pituitary gland*	In adults (acromegaly): Gradual thickening of the bones of the face, jaw, and the extremities in adults; oily skin; severe headache; excessive hair growth; excessive perspiration; joint pains. In children (in which the disease is called gigantism): Rapid growth and unusual height; possibly, blindness.
	Adrenal insufficiency *Inadequate production of steroid hormones by the adrenal gland*	Loss of weight and appetite; fatigue; weakness; darkening of the skin; abdominal pain; diarrhea; indigestion; nausea and vomiting; constipation; lack of sex drive; dizziness when rising from sitting or lying position.
	Anemia, aplastic	Fatigue and weakness; shortness of breath; heart palpitations; pallor; bleeding gums; nosebleeds; tendency to bruise easily; small red dots under the skin (petechiae). Increased susceptibility to infection.
	Anemia, folic acid deficiency	Fatigue and weakness; pallor; shortness of breath, heart palpitations, or noticeably rapid heartbeat on exertion; sore, red, and glazed looking tongue; loss of weight and appetite; nausea and diarrhea; abdominal distention.
	Anemia, hemolytic	Fatigue and weakness; shortness of breath on exertion; pallor; heart palpitations; jaundice and dark urine.
	Anemia, iron deficiency	Fatigue and weakness; pallor; shortness of breath and heart palpitations on exertion; irritability or inability to concentrate; sore tongue or tiny cracks at the corners of the mouth; black, tarry or bloody stools; unusual craving for dirt, paint, or ice.
	Anemia, pernicious	Fatigue; inability to concentrate; sore, red tongue; weakness; dizziness; pallor; shortness of breath on exertion; palpitations; numbness and tingling in extremities; incoordination; headache; loss of weight and appetite; possibly, jaundice.
	Anxiety states	Sudden attacks of unreasonable fear and panic; rapid heartbeat or palpitations; perspiration; dry mouth; irritability; muscle tension; trembling; palpitations; shortness of breath; restlessness; poor concentration; insomnia; fatigue; weakness.

Lethargy *continued*

Associated Symptoms	Possible Diagnosis	Distinguishing Features
	Bipolar disorder *Manic-depressive illness*	Symptoms vary depending on phase of the disorder; mania: inflated self-esteem, elation, euphoria, grandiosity, increased activity, and a decreased need for sleep; depression: persistent feelings of sadness, apathy, or hopelessness; diminished interest in activities; loss of appetite and weight or unusual increase in appetite and weight; insomnia or drowsiness; difficulty concentrating; agitation in older patients.
	Congestive heart failure	Shortness of breath; fatigue; need to sleep on several pillows; weakness; cough; heart palpitations; swelling in the legs, ankles, and abdomen; frequent urination at night; indigestion; nausea and vomiting; loss of appetite.
	Depression	Persistent feelings of sadness, apathy, or hopelessness; diminished interest in activities; loss of or unusual increase in appetite and weight; insomnia or drowsiness; difficulty concentrating; agitation.
	Diabetes mellitus *Insufficiency of or resistance to insulin*	Fatigue; excessive thirst; frequent urination; weight loss despite increased appetite; blurred vision; numbness and tingling of feet and hands; impotence.
	Hyperparathyroidism *Overactivity of the parathyroid glands*	Increased susceptibility to bone fractures; depression; indigestion; increased thirst and urine output; fatigue, lethargy; somnolence; muscle weakness; nausea and vomiting; loss of appetite; weight loss.
	Hypothyroidism *Underactivity of the thyroid gland*	Unexplained weight gain; fatigue; muscle weakness; cramps; dry skin; hair loss; deepening of the voice; intolerance for cold; constipation; chest pain; insomnia; puffiness around eyes; loss of sex drive; depression; menstrual abnormalities; possible swelling in the neck.
	Malabsorption, digestive *A failure of the small intestine to absorb nutrients in the diet*	Diarrhea; weight loss; yellowish, foul-smelling stools; abdominal cramps, gas, and bloating; weakness and lethargy.
	Mononucleosis, infectious	Headache; high fever; swollen glands in the neck, groin, and armpits; severe sore throat; swallowing difficulty.
	Reye's syndrome *Childhood disease marked by brain and liver damage*	Following recovery from an upper respiratory infection, nausea and vomiting; memory loss; confusion or delirium; possible seizures; drowsiness; lethargy.
	Rheumatoid arthritis, juvenile	Fever; rash; abdominal pain; weight loss; swelling, stiffness, and pain in the affected joints; enlarged lymph glands; fatigue; pallor; red, painful eyes.

Lethargy *continued*

Associated Symptoms	Possible Diagnosis	Distinguishing Features
	Schizophrenia	Delusions; hallucinations; rambling, nonsensical, or minimal speech; extremely disorganized behavior; inappropriate emotional responses or emotional detachment; lack of willful movement.
	Toxic shock syndrome	Lethargy; conjunctivitis; confusion; sudden high fever accompanied by nausea, watery diarrhea, sore throat, and headache. Red rash on the palms and soles of the feet, which, after a week or two, begins to peel.

Loss of coordination

Associated Symptoms	Possible Diagnosis	Distinguishing Features
	Acoustic neuroma *A benign tumor in the cells covering the auditory nerve*	Gradual hearing loss; ringing in the ear; headache; numbness in the face; unsteady walk. In later stages, swallowing and speaking difficulties; possibly, slight paralysis.
	Amyotrophic lateral sclerosis *Progressive degeneration of nerve cells of the central nervous system*	Progressive loss of strength and coordination in the limbs; muscle twitching and cramps that begin in the hands and spread to the arms, shoulders, and legs; stiff, clumsy gait; swallowing, breathing, or speaking difficulty; weight loss; drooling; involuntary laughing or crying.
	Hydrocephalus *Overaccumulation of cerebrospinal fluid, the liquid surrounding the brain*	In infants, an enlarged head, rigidity of the legs, irritability, projectile vomiting, drowsiness, seizures, and lethargy. In older persons, headache, vomiting, loss of coordination, deterioration of mental faculties, speech difficulty, and loss of appetite.
	Hypoglycemia *Low blood sugar*	Anxiety; hunger; trembling; headache; palpitations; perspiration; confusion; irritability; loss of coordination; possibly, double vision, seizures, or coma.
	Muscular dystrophy	Symptoms depend on type of muscular dystrophy and may include: Progressive muscle wasting, weakness, and loss of mobility; lack of coordination; muscular and skeletal deformities including curvature of the spine with protruding abdomen; waddling gait; cataracts; frontal baldness; gonadal atrophy.
	Myasthenia gravis *Nerve degeneration causing gradual loss of voluntary muscle control*	Drooping eyelids; double or blurred vision; muscle weakness especially in the face, throat, and neck; chewing and swallowing difficulties; possible breathing difficulty. Slurred, nasal-sounding speech.
	Osteoarthritis *Degeneration of the cartilage that lines the joints*	Pain, swelling, and stiffness in one or more joints; enlargement and distortion of affected joints.
	Parkinson's disease *Degeneration of the basal ganglia, a cluster of nerve cells in the brain*	Tremors in the hands; stiffness and weakness; impaired voluntary movement; shuffling gait; stooped posture; unblinking, fixed expression; possibly, slow, hesitant speech; difficulty swallowing; drooling; depression. Tremors occur at rest (not with voluntary movements) and disappear during sleep.

Loss of coordination *continued*

Associated Symptoms	Possible Diagnosis	Distinguishing Features
	Peripheral neuropathies *Degeneration of the nerves* *that supply the extremities*	Tingling or numbness commonly beginning in the hands and feet and gradually spreading toward the center of the body; sensitive skin; muscle weakness; possibly, pain in the hands and feet; lack of coordination; shooting pains exacerbated by touch or changes in temperature; breathing difficulty; urinary or fecal incontinence.
	Poliomyelitis *Polio*	Low fever; sore throat; headache; nausea and vomiting. In severe cases, paralysis without loss of sensation; stiff neck and back; twitching; swallowing and breathing difficulty; drooling.
	Rheumatic fever	Initially, a sore throat that gets better followed, one to six weeks later, by lethargy and fever. Possibly, swollen joints, rash, abdominal pain, involuntary jerky movements, emotional instability.
	Rheumatoid arthritis	Fatigue and weakness; joint pain, stiffness, and inflammation, especially in the hands, feet, and arms; joint deformity; dry mouth; dry, painful eyes. Morning stiffness.
	Schizophrenia	Delusions; hallucinations; rambling, nonsensical, or minimal speech; extremely disorganized behavior; inappropriate emotional responses or emotional detachment; lack of willful movement.
	Seizures	Involuntary twitching or jerking; muscle rigidity; loss of consciousness; confusion; drooling; hallucinations.
	Stroke	Symptoms vary with the location of brain injury. Sudden onset of weakness, paralysis, or loss of sensation, usually on one side of the body; a sudden heaviness in a limb; speech abnormalities; headache; vision disturbances; dizziness; confusion; coma; urinary and fecal incontinence.

Loss of smell

Associated Symptoms	Possible Diagnosis	Distinguishing Features
	Anemia, pernicious	Fatigue; inability to concentrate; sore, red tongue; weakness; dizziness; pallor; shortness of breath on exertion; palpitations; numbness and tingling in extremities; incoordination; headache; loss of weight and appetite; possibly, jaundice.
	Brain tumors	Headaches that become more severe when reclining; nausea and vomiting; memory loss; double vision; muscle weakness; numbness, tingling, or partial paralysis; vision loss; speech disturbances; seizures; drowsiness.
	Diabetes mellitus *Insufficiency of or resistance to insulin*	Fatigue; excessive thirst; frequent urination; weight loss despite increased appetite; blurred vision; numbness and tingling of feet and hands; impotence.
	Nasal polyps	Impaired sense of smell; a feeling of fullness in the face; possible nasal discharge, facial pain, or headaches.

Loss of taste

Associated Symptoms	Possible Diagnosis	Distinguishing Features
	Bell's palsy *Paralysis of muscles on one side of the face*	Drooping muscles and weakness on one side of the face resulting in a distorted smile or an expressionless look; drooping brow, tearing and an inability to close the affected eyelid; drooling; possibly, ear pain on the affected side of the face; possibly, changes in taste perception; increased sensitivity to noise.
	Brain tumors	Headaches that become more severe when reclining; nausea and vomiting; memory loss; double vision; muscle weakness; numbness, tingling, or partial paralysis; vision loss; speech disturbances; seizures; drowsiness.
	Dry mouth	Dry or burning sensation in the mouth; difficulty chewing, swallowing, and speaking; possibly, cracked lips, changes in the tongue's surface, mouth ulcers, changes in taste perception, or tooth decay.
	Headache, migraine	Throbbing pain in the temple which spreads to the side of the head; nausea; vomiting. Pain may be preceded by blurred or impaired vision with bright spots and zig-zag patterns.
	Oral cancers	Sore in the mouth that bleeds and does not heal; lump in the cheek; white or red patch on the gums; swallowing and chewing difficulties; numbness of the tongue; swelling of the jaw.
	Salivary gland disorders	Swollen, painful glands behind the ear or under the tongue; soft, painful, swollen glands in the neck; bitter taste in the mouth; fever; dry mouth; increased number of dental cavities; difficulty swallowing.
	Sjögren's syndrome	Dry, itching, burning eyes; sensation of a foreign body under the eyelids; dry mouth; difficulty swallowing; vaginal dryness; dry skin; frequent dental cavities; joint pain; swelling of glands (parotids) in front of the ears; Raynaud's phenomenon.
	Tongue disorders	Symptoms vary depending on the specific disorder and include: dark or bright red, black, or dark brown tongue; sore, swollen, or smooth tongue; hair-like growths on the tongue; adjacent areas of the mouth may be inflamed; ulcers or raised, white patches on the tongue; excessive salivation; swallowing difficulty; bad breath.

Loss of vision

Associated Symptoms	Possible Diagnosis	Distinguishing Features
	Cataracts	Painless, increasingly blurred vision; appearance of halos around lights; changes in color perception; increased sensitivity to light and glare.
	Eye cancers	Often initially asymptomatic. In later stages, gradual blurring and loss of vision, bulging eyes. Possibly, crossed eyes, change in eye color, or a tumor visible through the pupil. Painful red eye.
	Glaucoma	Often initially asymptomatic. In later stages, the symptoms of closed angle glaucoma include: the appearance of halos and rainbows around lights; dilated pupil in the affected eye; severe headache and eye pain; possibly, nausea and vomiting. Open angle glaucoma symptoms include: blurred vision and a gradual loss of peripheral vision.
	Macular degeneration	Gradual loss of vision in the central portion of the field of vision, interfering with reading or any close work requiring keen near-vision; blurred vision.
	Optic neuritis	Sudden, partial loss of vision, usually in the central portion of the field of vision; blurred vision; pain in affected eye.
	Retinal detachment	Possibly, bright flashes of light in the peripheral vision, blurred vision, shadows or blindness in part of the field of vision.
	Retinal vessel occlusion *Blockage of the retinal arteries and veins*	Sudden blurring or loss of vision in all or a portion of the field of vision in one eye, bleeding in the eye.
	Strabismus *Crossed or misaligned eyes*	Double vision; possible vision loss in one eye associated with loss of depth perception; crossed eyes.
	Uveitis and iritis *Inflammation of the uvea, a group of structures in the eye including the iris*	Moderate to severe eye pain; aversion to light; redness in the eye; excessive tearing; blurred vision; spots in the field of vision.

Loss of voice

Associated Symptoms	Possible Diagnosis	Distinguishing Features
	Amyotrophic lateral sclerosis *Progressive degeneration of nerve cells of the central nervous system*	Progressive loss of strength and coordination in the limbs; muscle twitching and cramps that begin in the hands and spread to the arms, shoulders, and legs; stiff, clumsy gait; swallowing, breathing, or speaking difficulty; weight loss; drooling; involuntary laughing or crying.
	Botulism	Difficulty swallowing and speaking; nausea; vomiting; blurred or double vision.
	Laryngitis	Hoarseness that often progresses to loss of the voice; throat pain; dry cough; possible fever.
	Multiple sclerosis *Gradual degeneration of the protective sheaths surrounding the nerves within the brain and spinal cord*	Symptoms may appear suddenly and then disappear; persistent symptoms may take years to develop and include numbness or tingling in any part of the body, weakness in the extremities, an unsteady walk, slurred speech, urinary incontinence, fatigue, depression, temporary loss of vision, double or blurred vision, mental confusion, and memory loss.
	Myasthenia gravis *Nerve degeneration causing gradual loss of voluntary muscle control*	Drooping eyelids; double or blurred vision; muscle weakness especially in the face, throat, and neck; chewing and swallowing difficulties; possible breathing difficulty. Slurred, nasal-sounding speech.
	Parkinson's disease *Degeneration of the basal ganglia, a cluster of nerve cells in the brain*	Tremors in the hands; stiffness and weakness; impaired voluntary movement; shuffling gait; stooped posture; unblinking, fixed expression; possibly, slow, hesitant speech; difficulty swallowing; drooling; depression. Tremors occur at rest (not with voluntary movements) and disappear during sleep.
	Pharyngitis *Inflammation of the pharynx, the part of the throat between the mouth and the esophagus*	Sore or red throat; speaking and swallowing difficulties; sensitive, swollen glands in the neck; fever; headache; possible earache.
	Stroke	Symptoms vary with the location of brain injury. Sudden onset of weakness, paralysis, or loss of sensation, usually on one side of the body; a sudden heaviness in a limb; speech abnormalities; headache; vision disturbances; dizziness; confusion; coma; urinary and fecal incontinence.

Lump(s) or thickening in the breast

Associated Symptoms	Possible Diagnosis	Distinguishing Features
	Breast cancer	Lump or swelling, usually painless, in the breast or under the armpit; flattening, dimpling, indentation, redness, or scaliness of the breast; itching sensation in the nipple; change in size or symmetry of the breasts; breast pain.
	Fibrocystic breast changes *Benign lumps in the breast*	A lump or swelling, usually painless, anywhere in the breast or underarm, typically located in the upper and outer part of the breast. Pain around the lump, usually more apparent during the week prior to menses. Changes in the size or symmetry of the breasts.

Memory problems

Associated Symptoms	Possible Diagnosis	Distinguishing Features
	AIDS *Acquired immunodeficiency syndrome*	Recurrent infections affecting the skin and respiratory system; cough; shortness of breath; loss of appetite; weight loss; fatigue; diarrhea; fever; dementia; malignant skin lesions; swollen lymph glands throughout the body; purplish skin nodules; memory loss; confusion; personality changes.
	Alzheimer's disease	Symptoms vary greatly in different individuals. Initially, minor forgetfulness gradually developing into severe, short-term memory loss, disorientation, an inability to concentrate, and sudden mood and personality changes. In later stages, severe confusion, possible hallucinations or paranoid delusions, loss of social and sexual inhibitions, impaired judgment, anxiety, depression, agitation and combativeness, wandering and getting lost, inability to write, urinary and fecal incontinence.
	Brain tumors	Headaches that become more severe when reclining; nausea and vomiting; memory loss; double vision; muscle weakness; numbness, tingling, or partial paralysis; vision loss; speech disturbances; seizures; drowsiness.
	Chronic fatigue syndrome	Severe fatigue made worse by exercise; recurrent flu-like symptoms; persistent sore throat; low-grade fever; muscle and joint aches; headache; painful, swollen lymph nodes; depression and mental confusion; memory loss; sleep difficulties.
	Cirrhosis *Chronic damage to the cells of the liver*	No symptoms in early stages; loss of weight and appetite; nausea; swollen legs, ankles and abdomen; itching; jaundice; black stools; vomiting blood; fatigue; impotence; memory loss; confusion.
	Depression	Persistent feelings of sadness, apathy, or hopelessness; diminished interest in activities; loss of or unusual increase in appetite and weight; insomnia or drowsiness; difficulty concentrating; agitation.
	Encephalitis *Inflammation of the brain*	Initially, headache and fever followed by confusion, hallucinations, and paralysis on one side of the body; memory loss; difficulty with speech and eye movements; drowsiness; possible coma or epileptic seizures; loss of hearing; sensitivity to light; stiff neck.
	Hypothermia *Low body temperature (below 94°)*	Shivering; pallor; puffy face; fatigue and confusion; slow, shallow breathing; muscle stiffness; normally warm areas of the body are cold; loss of consciousness.

Memory problems *continued*

Associated Symptoms	Possible Diagnosis	Distinguishing Features
	Multiple sclerosis *Gradual degeneration of the protective sheaths surrounding the nerves within the brain and spinal cord*	Symptoms may appear suddenly and then disappear; persistent symptoms may take years to develop and include numbness or tingling in any part of the body, weakness in the extremities, an unsteady walk, slurred speech, urinary incontinence, fatigue, depression, temporary loss of vision, double or blurred vision, mental confusion, and memory loss.
	Reye's syndrome *Childhood disease marked by brain and liver damage*	Following recovery from an upper respiratory infection, nausea and vomiting; memory loss; confusion or delirium; possible seizures; drowsiness; lethargy.
	Seizures	Involuntary twitching or jerking; muscle rigidity; loss of consciousness; confusion; drooling; hallucinations.
	Stroke	Symptoms vary with the location of brain injury. Sudden onset of weakness, paralysis, or loss of sensation, usually on one side of the body; a sudden heaviness in a limb; speech abnormalities; headache; vision disturbances; dizziness; confusion; coma; urinary and fecal incontinence.
	Systemic lupus erythematosus *Inflammation of connective tissues throughout the body*	Red, blotchy, butterfly-shaped rash on the cheeks and bridge of the nose; fatigue; fever; loss of appetite and weight; nausea; joint and abdominal pain; headaches; blurred vision; increased sensitivity to sun exposure; depression; psychosis; mental confusion.

Menstrual pain

Associated Symptoms	Possible Diagnosis	Distinguishing Features
	Cervical disorders, non-malignant	Vaginal discharge; vaginal burning and itching; vaginal bleeding after intercourse, between periods, or after bowel movements.
	Endometrial polyps *Growths on the lining of the uterus*	Often no symptoms; light bleeding between periods, especially following sexual intercourse; abnormally heavy or prolonged bleeding during menses; pelvic cramps; foul-smelling vaginal discharge.
	Endometriosis *The migration of the uterine lining to other reproductive or abdominal organs*	Pain in the lower abdomen, vagina, and lower back beginning just prior to menses and intensifying after blood flow has ceased; heavy bleeding during periods; pain during intercourse; diarrhea; constipation; pain during bowel movements; bleeding from the rectum; bloody urine during menses; nausea and vomiting prior to menses; infertility.
	Fibroids, uterine *Benign growths of the muscular wall of the uterus*	Heavier or prolonged bleeding during menses; abdominal discomfort; lower back pain; pressure on the bladder and frequent urination; constipation. Possible, sharp, sudden, lower abdominal pain.
	Pelvic inflammatory disease	Initially, lower pelvic pain; pain during intercourse; irregular menstrual bleeding; vaginal discharge with abnormal color or odor; low-grade fever; chills; frequent urination; fatigue; loss of appetite; later, severe abdominal pain and high fever.
	Uterine prolapse	Often asymptomatic. Possibly, difficulty passing urine or stools, pain during intercourse, backache that intensifies when lifting, sensation of heaviness or dragging within the pelvis, painful or heavy menstrual periods, or bleeding between periods. In severe cases, uterus visibly protrudes outside of vagina.

Mouth, dry

Associated Symptoms	Possible Diagnosis	Distinguishing Features
	Anxiety states	Sudden attacks of unreasonable fear and panic; rapid heartbeat or palpitations; perspiration; dry mouth; irritability; muscle tension; trembling; palpitations; shortness of breath; restlessness; poor concentration; insomnia; fatigue; weakness.
	Diarrhea, acute	Loose, watery stools; increased frequency of bowel movements; abdominal cramping and pain. In infants, possibly drowsiness, slack skin, dry, sticky mouth and tongue, or persistent crying.
	Dry mouth	Dry or burning sensation in the mouth; difficulty chewing, swallowing, and speaking; possibly, cracked lips, changes in the tongue's surface, mouth ulcers, changes in taste perception, or tooth decay.
	Rheumatoid arthritis	Fatigue and weakness; joint pain, stiffness, and inflammation, especially in the hands, feet, and arms; joint deformity; dry mouth; dry, painful eyes. Morning stiffness.
	Salivary gland disorders	Swollen, painful glands behind the ear or under the tongue; soft, painful, swollen glands in the neck; bitter taste in the mouth; fever; dry mouth; increased number of dental cavities; difficulty swallowing.
	Sjögren's syndrome	Dry, itching, burning eyes; sensation of a foreign body under the eyelids; dry mouth; difficulty swallowing; vaginal dryness; dry skin; frequent dental cavities; joint pain; swelling of glands (parotids) in front of the ears; Raynaud's phenomenon.

Mouth, sore

Associated Symptoms	Possible Diagnosis	Distinguishing Features
	Anaphylaxis	Itching and hives; swelling of the eyes, lips, and tongue; weakness or faintness; tightening in the chest or throat; wheezing; shortness of breath; profuse sweating; palpitations; sudden, intense distress; feelings of impending doom; stomach cramps; nausea, vomiting, or diarrhea; bluish tinge (cyanosis) to the skin, lips, and nail beds due to oxygen insufficiency.
	Anemia, pernicious	Fatigue; inability to concentrate; sore, red tongue; weakness; dizziness; pallor; shortness of breath on exertion; palpitations; numbness and tingling in extremities; incoordination; headache; loss of weight and appetite; possibly, jaundice.
	Candidiasis *Fungal infection of the mouth, genitals, or mucous membranes*	Thick, white discharge from the vagina; itching and irritation in the vaginal area; pain while urinating or during intercourse; in men, inflammation of the head of the penis; possibly, yellow raised patches in the mouth.
	Canker sores	Small, painful, white or gray, crater-like, red-rimmed ulcers in the gums, tongue, or lips.
	Dry mouth	Dry or burning sensation in the mouth; difficulty chewing, swallowing, and speaking; possibly, cracked lips, changes in the tongue's surface, mouth ulcers, changes in taste perception, or tooth decay.
	Gingivitis	Red-purple gums that are swollen, shiny, and bleed easily; bad breath.
	Impacted teeth	Gum pain; unpleasant taste in mouth, especially when biting down; red, swollen gums around the affected tooth; headache or jaw ache; possibly, bad breath.
	Neuralgia *Pain due to nerve damage or irritation*	Symptoms vary depending on the area affected and include: recurring episodes of sharp pain on one side of the lips, gums, cheek, or chin; radiating pain around the eyes; a burning pain along the path of a nerve encircling the torso. Pain may last from a few seconds to several minutes and always affects the same location. Attacks may occur several times a day for weeks with asymptomatic periods of weeks or months in between and may be triggered by touching or blowing on the affected area. Mouth pain may be exacerbated by talking, eating, or swallowing.
	Oral cancers	Sore in the mouth that bleeds and does not heal; lump in the cheek; white or red patch on the gums; swallowing and chewing difficulties; numbness of the tongue; swelling of the jaw.

Mouth, sore *continued*

Associated Symptoms	Possible Diagnosis	Distinguishing Features
	Oral herpes *Cold sores*	Initially, a tingling sensation or discomfort around the mouth, followed by small, raw, open sores on outside edge of lips; scabbing of sores.
	Salivary gland disorders	Swollen, painful glands behind the ear or under the tongue; soft, painful, swollen glands in the neck; bitter taste in the mouth; fever; dry mouth; increased number of dental cavities; difficulty swallowing.
	Temporomandibular joint syndrome	Pain in the joints connecting the jaw to the skull; headache; tender jaw muscles; dull facial pain; clicking noise when opening or closing the mouth; pain when yawning and chewing. Jaw may temporarily lock in position.
	Tongue disorders	Symptoms vary depending on the specific disorder and include: dark or bright red, black, or dark brown tongue; sore, swollen, or smooth tongue; hair-like growths on the tongue; adjacent areas of the mouth may be inflamed; ulcers or raised, white patches on the tongue; excessive salivation; swallowing difficulty; bad breath.
	Trench mouth	Grayish film on the gums; red, swollen, painful, bleeding gums; bad breath; bad taste in the mouth; pain on swallowing or speaking; excessive salivation.

Movement, slowed

Associated Symptoms	Possible Diagnosis	Distinguishing Features
	Amyotrophic lateral sclerosis *Progressive degeneration of nerve cells of the central nervous system*	Progressive loss of strength and coordination in the limbs; muscle twitching and cramps that begin in the hands and spread to the arms, shoulders, and legs; stiff, clumsy gait; swallowing, breathing, or speaking difficulty; weight loss; drooling; involuntary laughing or crying.
	Botulism	Difficulty swallowing and speaking; nausea; vomiting; blurred or double vision.
	Cardiomyopathy *Disease of the heart muscle causing a reduction in the force of heart contractions*	Fatigue; chest pain and palpitations; shortness of breath; swelling of the legs; wheezing; cough.
	Congestive heart failure	Shortness of breath; fatigue; need to sleep on several pillows; weakness; cough; heart palpitations; swelling in the legs, ankles, and abdomen; frequent urination at night; indigestion; nausea and vomiting; loss of appetite.
	Dermatomyositis *Inflammation of the muscles and skin*	Red rash on the neck, upper torso, and upper arms and legs; purple discoloration and swelling of the eyelids; areas of thickened skin; muscle weakness and stiffness, usually in the shoulders and pelvis; cold hands and feet; speaking or swallowing difficulty; weight loss.
	Dislocations/subluxations	Deformity of the affected joint; joint pain and tenderness; difficulty moving a joint; swelling and stiffness within 30 minutes after joint injury.
	Hypothyroidism *Underactivity of the thyroid gland*	Unexplained weight gain; fatigue; muscle weakness; cramps; dry skin; hair loss; deepening of the voice; intolerance for cold; constipation; chest pain; insomnia; puffiness around eyes; loss of sex drive; depression; menstrual abnormalities; possible swelling in the neck.
	Multiple sclerosis *Gradual degeneration of the protective sheaths surrounding the nerves within the brain and spinal cord*	Symptoms may appear suddenly and then disappear; persistent symptoms may take years to develop and include numbness or tingling in any part of the body, weakness in the extremities, an unsteady walk, slurred speech, urinary incontinence, fatigue, depression, temporary loss of vision, double or blurred vision, mental confusion, and memory loss.
	Muscular dystrophy	Symptoms depend on type of muscular dystrophy and may include: Progressive muscle wasting, weakness, and loss of mobility; lack of coordination; muscular and skeletal deformities including curvature of the spine with protruding abdomen; waddling gait; cataracts; frontal baldness; gonadal atrophy.

Movement, slowed *continued*

Associated Symptoms	Possible Diagnosis	Distinguishing Features
	Myasthenia gravis *Nerve degeneration causing gradual loss of voluntary muscle control*	Drooping eyelids; double or blurred vision; muscle weakness especially in the face, throat, and neck; chewing and swallowing difficulties; possible breathing difficulty. Slurred, nasal-sounding speech.
	Osteoarthritis *Degeneration of the cartilage that lines the joints*	Pain, swelling, and stiffness in one or more joints; enlargement and distortion of affected joints.
	Parkinson's disease *Degeneration of the basal ganglia, a cluster of nerve cells in the brain*	Tremors in the hands; stiffness and weakness; impaired voluntary movement; shuffling gait; stooped posture; unblinking, fixed expression; possibly, slow, hesitant speech; difficulty swallowing; drooling; depression. Tremors occur at rest (not with voluntary movements) and disappear during sleep.
	Rheumatoid arthritis	Fatigue and weakness; joint pain, stiffness, and inflammation, especially in the hands, feet, and arms; joint deformity; dry mouth; dry, painful eyes. Morning stiffness.
	Schizophrenia	Delusions; hallucinations; rambling, nonsensical, or minimal speech; extremely disorganized behavior; inappropriate emotional responses or emotional detachment; lack of willful movement.
	Valvular heart disease	Depends on which heart valve is affected. Often asymptomatic. Possibly, fatigue and weakness; dizziness; chest pain; shortness of breath; heart palpitations; fainting; edema; stroke from embolism to the brain.

Mucus production, excessive

Associated Symptoms	Possible Diagnosis	Distinguishing Features
	Anaphylaxis	Itching and hives; swelling of the eyes, lips, and tongue; weakness or faintness; tightening in the chest or throat; wheezing; shortness of breath; profuse sweating; palpitations; sudden, intense distress; feelings of impending doom; stomach cramps; nausea, vomiting, or diarrhea; bluish tinge (cyanosis) to the skin, lips, and nail beds due to oxygen insufficiency.
	Asthma	Shortness of breath; wheezing; cough; tightness in the chest; possibly, excessive perspiration, rapid heartbeat.
	Bronchiectasis *Lung condition that stretches and distorts the walls of the bronchial tubes*	Cough that produces dark green sputum; bad breath; possibly, shortness of breath; loss of appetite and weight; clubbed fingers.
	Bronchitis, acute	Shortness of breath; persistent cough producing yellow or green sputum; possibly, chest pain; wheezing; fever.
	Chronic obstructive pulmonary disease	Shortness of breath; wheezing; persistent, mucus-producing cough, especially in the morning; possibly, chest pain, swollen legs and ankles.
	Esophageal cancer	Swallowing difficulty and pain; weight loss; drooling; possibly, vomiting or coughing up of bloody mucus, regurgitation of food; chest pain; repeated respiratory infections.
	Influenza *Flu*	Chills, muscle aches, and loss of appetite followed by a cough, sore throat, nasal congestion, and fever; possible chest pain.
	Nasal polyps	Impaired sense of smell; a feeling of fullness in the face; possible nasal discharge, facial pain, or headaches.
	Sinusitis *Inflammation of the mucous membranes lining the sinuses*	Throbbing pain above or below one or both eyes that intensifies when bending the head forward or coughing; nasal congestion; loss of sense of smell; often, pus-like nasal discharge; possible dental pain in the upper jaw; fever.
	Strep infection	Symptoms depend on the location and nature of the specific infection, but may include fever, headaches, swollen lymph glands, fatigue, loss of appetite, nasal discharge, red skin rash.
	Tuberculosis	Often, asymptomatic. Possibly, low-grade fever; excessive perspiration; cough producing sputum or blood; weight loss; chronic fatigue; chest pain; shortness of breath; night sweats.

Muscle aches/pains

Associated Symptoms	Possible Diagnosis	Distinguishing Features
	Carpal tunnel syndrome	Numbness, tingling, and pain in the hand and wrist, often intensifying at night; weakness of the fingers and hand.
	Fibromyalgia	Muscle aches, pains, and stiffness; specific points on the body that feel sore when pressed; fatigue; headaches; feeling unrefreshed upon awakening in the morning.
	Heatstroke	Sudden dizziness; weakness; headache; hot, dry, red skin which later turns grey; high body temperature; muscle cramps; confusion; seizures; loss of consciousness.
	Hyperparathyroidism *Overactivity of the parathyroid glands*	Increased susceptibility to bone fractures; depression; indigestion; increased thirst and urine output; fatigue, lethargy; somnolence; muscle weakness; nausea and vomiting; loss of appetite; weight loss.
	Hypoparathyroidism *Underactivity of the parathyroid glands*	Numbness and tingling and painful, cramp-like spasms of the face, hands, arms, and feet; cataracts; possible seizures.
	Hypothermia *Low body temperature (below 94°)*	Shivering; pallor; puffy face; fatigue and confusion; slow, shallow breathing; muscle stiffness; normally warm areas of the body are cold; loss of consciousness.
	Multiple myeloma *Production of malignant plasma cells in the bone marrow*	Bone pain, especially progressive, constant back pain that intensifies with movement; unexplained bone fractures; fatigue; pallor; shortness of breath; increased bleeding, such as bleeding gums or nosebleeds; easily bruised skin; increased susceptibility to infection; headache; vision disturbances; loss of height.
	Peripheral neuropathies *Degeneration of the nerves that supply the extremities*	Tingling or numbness commonly beginning in the hands and feet and gradually spreading toward the center of the body; sensitive skin; muscle weakness; possibly, pain in the hands and feet; lack of coordination; shooting pains exacerbated by touch or changes in temperature; breathing difficulty; urinary or fecal incontinence.
	Peripheral vascular disease *Narrowing of blood vessels in the legs or arms*	Muscle pain on one or both legs that occurs with exercise and subsides with rest; possible pain in the fingers, arms, buttocks, lower back, or the arch of the foot; impotence. Severe symptoms include: muscle pain at rest that intensifies at night; discolored or blue toes; cold or numb feet; open sores; heightened sensitivity to cold; weak or absent pulse in the affected limb; scaly or hairless skin over the affected area.

Muscle aches/pains *continued*

Associated Symptoms	Possible Diagnosis	Distinguishing Features
	Renal failure, chronic *Persistent, mild kidney failure*	Asymptomatic in early stages. Possibly, mental confusion; shortness of breath; abdominal pain; decreased sex drive; fatigue; muscle and bone pain; numbness in the legs and feet; headache; impaired mental acuity; bad breath.
	Rotator cuff injury	Pain in the shoulder; difficulty raising and lowering the arm; recurring dull ache in the shoulder; pain after sleeping on the shoulder; shoulder weakness.
	Shin splints	Pain in the front of the calf that may intensify during walking or running.
	Sprains and strains	Swelling, pain or tenderness in the affected joints; impaired joint function.
	Tetanus	Often, lockjaw; stiffness and, later, muscle spasms in the neck and face; drooling; abdominal and back pain; extreme perspiration; swallowing difficulty; possible convulsions; fever.
with fever	Chronic fatigue syndrome	Severe fatigue made worse by exercise; recurrent flu-like symptoms; persistent sore throat; low-grade fever; muscle and joint aches; headache; painful, swollen lymph nodes; depression and mental confusion; memory loss; sleep difficulties.
	Common cold	Nasal congestion; watery eyes; sneezing; sore throat; cough; muscle aches; mild headache; listlessness; possibly, low-grade fever.
	Dermatomyositis *Inflammation of the muscles and skin*	Red rash on the neck, upper torso, and upper arms and legs; purple discoloration and swelling of the eyelids; areas of thickened skin; muscle weakness and stiffness, usually in the shoulders and pelvis; cold hands and feet; speaking or swallowing difficulty; weight loss.
	Encephalitis *Inflammation of the brain*	Initially, headache and fever followed by confusion, hallucinations, and paralysis on one side of the body; memory loss; difficulty with speech and eye movements; drowsiness; possible coma or epileptic seizures; loss of hearing; sensitivity to light; stiff neck.
	Hepatitis, acute viral	Fever; fatigue; loss of appetite; aching muscles and joints; abdominal pain or discomfort; jaundice; dark urine and pale stools.
	Influenza *Flu*	Chills, muscle aches, and loss of appetite followed by a cough, sore throat, nasal congestion, and fever; possible chest pain.

Muscle aches/pains *continued*

Associated Symptoms	Possible Diagnosis	Distinguishing Features
with fever *continued*	Legionnaire's disease	Dry cough progressing to one with blood-streaked sputum; high fever; chills; breathing difficulty; chest pain; headache; muscle aches; diarrhea; nausea; vomiting; mental confusion and disorientation.
	Lyme disease	A small red bump, surrounded by a concentric bulls-eye-like red rash with a pale center. Over the following month: fever and chills; extreme fatigue; headaches. Symptoms may progress over several months or years and may include: palpitations; joint or muscle pain; and chronic joint inflammation, especially in the knees.
	Malaria	Initially, severe chills and shivering. In later stages, extremely high fever followed by a period of profuse perspiration as fever subsides; headache, sometimes severe; vomiting.
	Measles	Cough; fever; watery nasal discharge; loss of appetite; red, watering eyes; sore throat; body aches; red, slightly itchy rash that gradually spreads all over the body.
	Mumps	Pain in the ear, below the ear, and in the jaw; swollen glands in the neck; headache; pain on swallowing and chewing; sore muscles; joint pain; loss of appetite. Testicular swelling and tenderness in adults.
	Pancreatitis *Inflammation of the pancreas*	Sudden, extreme abdominal pain; nausea and vomiting; weakness; fever; clammy skin; abdominal bloating and tenderness.
	Pneumonia	High fever; shortness of breath; cough with sputum; chest pain; fatigue.
	Poliomyelitis *Polio*	Low fever; sore throat; headache; nausea and vomiting. In severe cases, paralysis without loss of sensation; stiff neck and back; twitching; swallowing and breathing difficulty; drooling.
	Prostatitis *Inflammation of the prostate gland*	Burning during urination; urgent and frequent urination; fever and chills; discharge from the penis; lower abdominal and back pain; blood in the urine.
	Rocky Mountain spotted fever	Within a week after exposure, high fever, loss of appetite, headache, muscle aches, nausea and vomiting; dry cough; sensitivity to light. Within six days, the appearance of small pink spots on wrists and ankles, eventually spreading over the entire body, where they then grow, darken in color, and bleed.

Muscle aches/pains *continued*

Associated Symptoms	Possible Diagnosis	Distinguishing Features
with fever *continued*	Sarcoidosis *Accumulation of inflammatory cells in the lymph nodes and other tissues throughout the body*	Often no symptoms. Swollen lymph nodes in the neck or armpits; muscle aches; fever; breathing difficulty; possibly, purple rash on the face; reddish or brownish skin spots on the forearms, face, or legs; numbness; joint pain or stiffness; a painful, red eye; blurred vision; loss of appetite and weight.
	Scleroderma	Shiny, tight, and hardened skin, especially on the fingers, arms, and face; hands or feet may successively turn blue, white, and red upon exposure to cold (Raynaud's phenomenon); swallowing difficulty; bloating after eating; weight loss; shortness of breath on exertion; high blood pressure; symptoms of renal failure. Possibly, heartburn, muscle aches and weakness, joint pain, fever, or fatigue.
	Toxic shock syndrome	Lethargy; conjunctivitis; confusion; sudden high fever accompanied by nausea, watery diarrhea, sore throat, and headache. Red rash on the palms and soles of the feet, which, after a week or two, begins to peel.
	Trichinosis *Parasitic infestation*	Initially, crampy abdominal pain, diarrhea, vomiting, and fever, followed within one to two weeks by swelling around the eyes, muscle aches and tenderness, fever, and weakness. Possibly, coughing up of bloody phlegm; delirium; coma; heart failure symptoms.

Muscle cramps

Associated Symptoms	Possible Diagnosis	Distinguishing Features
	Amyotrophic lateral sclerosis *Progressive degeneration of nerve cells of the central nervous system*	Progressive loss of strength and coordination in the limbs; muscle twitching and cramps that begin in the hands and spread to the arms, shoulders, and legs; stiff, clumsy gait; swallowing, breathing, or speaking difficulty; weight loss; drooling; involuntary laughing or crying.
	Dermatomyositis *Inflammation of the muscles and skin*	Red rash on the neck, upper torso, and upper arms and legs; purple discoloration and swelling of the eyelids; areas of thickened skin; muscle weakness and stiffness, usually in the shoulders and pelvis; cold hands and feet; speaking or swallowing difficulty; weight loss.
	Fibromyalgia	Muscle aches, pains, and stiffness; specific points on the body that feel sore when pressed; fatigue; headaches; feeling unrefreshed upon awakening in the morning.
	Heatstroke	Sudden dizziness; weakness; headache; hot, dry, red skin which later turns grey; high body temperature; muscle cramps; confusion; seizures; loss of consciousness.
	Hypothyroidism *Underactivity of the thyroid gland*	Unexplained weight gain; fatigue; muscle weakness; cramps; dry skin; hair loss; deepening of the voice; intolerance for cold; constipation; chest pain; insomnia; puffiness around eyes; loss of sex drive; depression; menstrual abnormalities; possible swelling in the neck.
	Tetanus	Often, lockjaw; stiffness and, later, muscle spasms in the neck and face; drooling; abdominal and back pain; extreme perspiration; swallowing difficulty; possible convulsions; fever.
	Varicose veins	Blue or purplish, knotted veins, usually in the legs; itching or discomfort in the affected area; swollen feet and ankles. Possible scaly skin, muscle cramps, or skin ulcers.

Muscle spasms

Associated Symptoms	Possible Diagnosis	Distinguishing Features
	Amyotrophic lateral sclerosis *Progressive degeneration of nerve cells of the central nervous system*	Progressive loss of strength and coordination in the limbs; muscle twitching and cramps that begin in the hands and spread to the arms, shoulders, and legs; stiff, clumsy gait; swallowing, breathing, or speaking difficulty; weight loss; drooling; involuntary laughing or crying.
	Hypothyroidism *Underactivity of the thyroid gland*	Unexplained weight gain; fatigue; muscle weakness; cramps; dry skin; hair loss; deepening of the voice; intolerance for cold; constipation; chest pain; insomnia; puffiness around eyes; loss of sex drive; depression; menstrual abnormalities; possible swelling in the neck.
	Osteomalacia and Rickets *Softening and weakening of the bones, usually due to poor calcification*	Bone pain, especially in the neck, legs, hips and ribs. Muscle weakness, numbness, or spasms in the hands, feet, and throat; increased susceptibility to bone fractures.
	Parkinson's disease *Degeneration of the basal ganglia, a cluster of nerve cells in the brain*	Tremors in the hands; stiffness and weakness; impaired voluntary movement; shuffling gait; stooped posture; unblinking, fixed expression; possibly, slow, hesitant speech; difficulty swallowing; drooling; depression. Tremors occur at rest (not with voluntary movements) and disappear during sleep.
	Poliomyelitis *Polio*	Low fever; sore throat; headache; nausea and vomiting. In severe cases, paralysis without loss of sensation; stiff neck and back; twitching; swallowing and breathing difficulty; drooling.
	Rabies	Low-grade fever; headache; loss of appetite; difficulty swallowing; tingling at site of animal bite; intense thirst exacerbated by the inability to drink without violent, painful throat spasms; paralysis of facial muscles; drooling. Agitation and violent behavior, confusion, convulsions, coma.
	Seizures	Involuntary twitching or jerking; muscle rigidity; loss of consciousness; confusion; drooling; hallucinations.
	Spinal cord trauma	Severe pain and swelling in the affected area; loss of sensation, muscle weakness, or paralysis below the site of the injury; urinary or fecal incontinence or retention; impotence; breathing difficulty; shock.
	Tetanus	Often, lockjaw; stiffness and, later, muscle spasms in the neck and face; drooling; abdominal and back pain; extreme perspiration; swallowing difficulty; possible convulsions; fever.

Muscle spasticity

Associated Symptoms	Possible Diagnosis	Distinguishing Features
	Amyotrophic lateral sclerosis *Progressive degeneration of nerve cells of the central nervous system*	Progressive loss of strength and coordination in the limbs; muscle twitching and cramps that begin in the hands and spread to the arms, shoulders, and legs; stiff, clumsy gait; swallowing, breathing, or speaking difficulty; weight loss; drooling; involuntary laughing or crying.
	Hypoparathyroidism *Underactivity of the parathyroid glands*	Numbness and tingling and painful, cramp-like spasms of the face, hands, arms, and feet; cataracts; possible seizures.
	Parkinson's disease *Degeneration of the basal ganglia, a cluster of nerve cells in the brain*	Tremors in the hands; stiffness and weakness; impaired voluntary movement; shuffling gait; stooped posture; unblinking, fixed expression; possibly, slow, hesitant speech; difficulty swallowing; drooling; depression. Tremors occur at rest (not with voluntary movements) and disappear during sleep.
	Rabies	Low-grade fever; headache; loss of appetite; difficulty swallowing; tingling at site of animal bite; intense thirst exacerbated by the inability to drink without violent, painful throat spasms; paralysis of facial muscles; drooling. Agitation and violent behavior, confusion, convulsions, coma.
	Seizures	Involuntary twitching or jerking; muscle rigidity; loss of consciousness; confusion; drooling; hallucinations.
	Spinal cord trauma	Severe pain and swelling in the affected area; loss of sensation, muscle weakness, or paralysis below the site of the injury; urinary or fecal incontinence or retention; impotence; breathing difficulty; shock.
	Tetanus	Often, lockjaw; stiffness and, later, muscle spasms in the neck and face; drooling; abdominal and back pain; extreme perspiration; swallowing difficulty; possible convulsions; fever.
	Tics	Recurring, involuntary twitch, usually in the face, shoulders, or arms.

Muscle wasting

Associated Symptoms	Possible Diagnosis	Distinguishing Features
	AIDS *Acquired immunodeficiency syndrome*	Recurrent infections affecting the skin and respiratory system; cough; shortness of breath; loss of appetite; weight loss; fatigue; diarrhea; fever; dementia; malignant skin lesions; swollen lymph glands throughout the body; purplish skin nodules; memory loss; confusion; personality changes.
	Amyotrophic lateral sclerosis *Progressive degeneration of nerve cells of the central nervous system*	Progressive loss of strength and coordination in the limbs; muscle twitching and cramps that begin in the hands and spread to the arms, shoulders, and legs; stiff, clumsy gait; swallowing, breathing, or speaking difficulty; weight loss; drooling; involuntary laughing or crying.
	Hypothyroidism *Underactivity of the thyroid gland*	Unexplained weight gain; fatigue; muscle weakness; cramps; dry skin; hair loss; deepening of the voice; intolerance for cold; constipation; chest pain; insomnia; puffiness around eyes; loss of sex drive; depression; menstrual abnormalities; possible swelling in the neck.
	Multiple sclerosis *Gradual degeneration of the protective sheaths surrounding the nerves within the brain and spinal cord*	Symptoms may appear suddenly and then disappear; persistent symptoms may take years to develop and include numbness or tingling in any part of the body, weakness in the extremities, an unsteady walk, slurred speech, urinary incontinence, fatigue, depression, temporary loss of vision, double or blurred vision, mental confusion, and memory loss.
	Muscular dystrophy	Symptoms depend on type of muscular dystrophy and may include: Progressive muscle wasting, weakness, and loss of mobility; lack of coordination; muscular and skeletal deformities including curvature of the spine with protruding abdomen; waddling gait; cataracts; frontal baldness; gonadal atrophy.
	Osteoarthritis *Degeneration of the cartilage that lines the joints*	Pain, swelling, and stiffness in one or more joints; enlargement and distortion of affected joints.
	Parkinson's disease *Degeneration of the basal ganglia, a cluster of nerve cells in the brain*	Tremors in the hands; stiffness and weakness; impaired voluntary movement; shuffling gait; stooped posture; unblinking, fixed expression; possibly, slow, hesitant speech; difficulty swallowing; drooling; depression. Tremors occur at rest (not with voluntary movements) and disappear during sleep.

Muscle wasting *continued*

Associated Symptoms	Possible Diagnosis	Distinguishing Features
	Peripheral neuropathies *Degeneration of the nerves that supply the extremities*	Tingling or numbness commonly beginning in the hands and feet and gradually spreading toward the center of the body; sensitive skin; muscle weakness; possibly, pain in the hands and feet; lack of coordination; shooting pains exacerbated by touch or changes in temperature; breathing difficulty; urinary or fecal incontinence.
	Poliomyelitis *Polio*	Low fever; sore throat; headache; nausea and vomiting. In severe cases, paralysis without loss of sensation; stiff neck and back; twitching; swallowing and breathing difficulty; drooling.
	Rheumatoid arthritis	Fatigue and weakness; joint pain, stiffness, and inflammation, especially in the hands, feet, and arms; joint deformity; dry mouth; dry, painful eyes. Morning stiffness.
	Spinal cord trauma	Severe pain and swelling in the affected area; loss of sensation, muscle weakness, or paralysis below the site of the injury; urinary or fecal incontinence or retention; impotence; breathing difficulty; shock.
	Spinal tumor	Progressive numbness, tingling, and muscle weakness; fecal or urinary incontinence; persistent back pain.

Muscle weakness

Associated Symptoms	Possible Diagnosis	Distinguishing Features
	Cushing's syndrome	Red, oval-shaped face; humped upper back and obese trunk; acne; purple stretch marks on the abdomen, thighs, and breasts; thin and easily bruised skin; easily fractured bones; depression or euphoria; insomnia; fatigue; muscle weakness; hirsutism (in women).
	Dermatomyositis *Inflammation of the muscles and skin*	Red rash on the neck, upper torso, and upper arms and legs; purple discoloration and swelling of the eyelids; areas of thickened skin; muscle weakness and stiffness, usually in the shoulders and pelvis; cold hands and feet; speaking or swallowing difficulty; weight loss.
	Hyperparathyroidism *Overactivity of the parathyroid glands*	Increased susceptibility to bone fractures; depression; indigestion; increased thirst and urine output; fatigue, lethargy; somnolence; muscle weakness; nausea and vomiting; loss of appetite; weight loss.
	Muscular dystrophy	Symptoms depend on type of muscular dystrophy and may include: Progressive muscle wasting, weakness, and loss of mobility; lack of coordination; muscular and skeletal deformities including curvature of the spine with protruding abdomen; waddling gait; cataracts; frontal baldness; gonadal atrophy.
	Myasthenia gravis *Nerve degeneration causing gradual loss of voluntary muscle control*	Drooping eyelids; double or blurred vision; muscle weakness especially in the face, throat, and neck; chewing and swallowing difficulties; possible breathing difficulty. Slurred, nasal-sounding speech.
	Trichinosis *Parasitic infestation*	Initially, crampy abdominal pain, diarrhea, vomiting, and fever, followed within one to two weeks by swelling around the eyes, muscle aches and tenderness, fever, and weakness. Possibly, coughing up of bloody phlegm; delirium; coma; heart failure symptoms.
with tingling or loss of sensation	Brain tumors	Headaches that become more severe when reclining; nausea and vomiting; memory loss; double vision; muscle weakness; numbness, tingling, or partial paralysis; vision loss; speech disturbances; seizures; drowsiness.
	Multiple sclerosis *Gradual degeneration of the protective sheaths surrounding the nerves within the brain and spinal cord*	Symptoms may appear suddenly and then disappear; persistent symptoms may take years to develop and include numbness or tingling in any part of the body, weakness in the extremities, an unsteady walk, slurred speech, urinary incontinence, fatigue, depression, temporary loss of vision, double or blurred vision, mental confusion, and memory loss.

Muscle weakness *continued*

Associated Symptoms	Possible Diagnosis	Distinguishing Features
with tingling or loss of sensation *continued*	Peripheral neuropathies *Degeneration of the nerves that supply the extremities*	Tingling or numbness commonly beginning in the hands and feet and gradually spreading toward the center of the body; sensitive skin; muscle weakness; possibly, pain in the hands and feet; lack of coordination; shooting pains exacerbated by touch or changes in temperature; breathing difficulty; urinary or fecal incontinence.
	Spinal cord trauma	Severe pain and swelling in the affected area; loss of sensation, muscle weakness, or paralysis below the site of the injury; urinary or fecal incontinence or retention; impotence; breathing difficulty; shock.
	Spinal tumor	Progressive numbness, tingling, and muscle weakness; fecal or urinary incontinence; persistent back pain.
	Spondylosis, cervical *Arthritis of the vertebral disks in the neck*	Neck pain and stiffness that spreads to the shoulders, upper arms, hands, or back of the head; numbness or tingling in the arms, hands, and fingers; weakness in the arms and legs; unsteady gait; possible loss of bladder or bowel control.
with twitching or muscle spasms	Amyotrophic lateral sclerosis *Progressive degeneration of nerve cells of the central nervous system*	Progressive loss of strength and coordination in the limbs; muscle twitching and cramps that begin in the hands and spread to the arms, shoulders, and legs; stiff, clumsy gait; swallowing, breathing, or speaking difficulty; weight loss; drooling; involuntary laughing or crying.
	Hypothyroidism *Underactivity of the thyroid gland*	Unexplained weight gain; fatigue; muscle weakness; cramps; dry skin; hair loss; deepening of the voice; intolerance for cold; constipation; chest pain; insomnia; puffiness around eyes; loss of sex drive; depression; menstrual abnormalities; possible swelling in the neck.
	Parkinson's disease *Degeneration of the basal ganglia, a cluster of nerve cells in the brain*	Tremors in the hands; stiffness and weakness; impaired voluntary movement; shuffling gait; stooped posture; unblinking, fixed expression; possibly, slow, hesitant speech; difficulty swallowing; drooling; depression. Tremors occur at rest (not with voluntary movements) and disappear during sleep.
	Poliomyelitis *Polio*	Low fever; sore throat; headache; nausea and vomiting. In severe cases, paralysis without loss of sensation; stiff neck and back; twitching; swallowing and breathing difficulty; drooling.

Nasal congestion

Associated Symptoms	Possible Diagnosis	Distinguishing Features
	Allergic rhinitis *Hay fever*	Nasal congestion; frequent sneezing; itchy eyes, nose, and throat.
	Common cold	Nasal congestion; watery eyes; sneezing; sore throat; cough; muscle aches; mild headache; listlessness; possibly, low-grade fever.
	Headache, cluster	Persistent pain in or around one eye; redness and tearing of one eye; nasal congestion on the same side of the face as the affected eye.
	Influenza *Flu*	Chills, muscle aches, and loss of appetite followed by a cough, sore throat, nasal congestion, and fever; possible chest pain.
	Pneumonia	High fever; shortness of breath; cough with sputum; chest pain; fatigue.
	Sinusitis *Inflammation of the mucous membranes lining the sinuses*	Throbbing pain above or below one or both eyes that intensifies when bending the head forward or coughing; nasal congestion; loss of sense of smell; often, pus-like nasal discharge; possible dental pain in the upper jaw; fever.
	Whooping cough	Initially, mild cough, sneezing, nasal congestion, and irritated eyes. Within approximately two weeks, cough becomes severe and persistent, and is accompanied by characteristic high-pitched "whooping" sound during inhalation; loss of appetite; listlessness; vomiting or choking spells. Most common among young children.

Nasal discharge, excessive

Associated Symptoms	Possible Diagnosis	Distinguishing Features
	Allergic rhinitis *Hay fever*	Nasal congestion; frequent sneezing; itchy eyes, nose, and throat.
	Common cold	Nasal congestion; watery eyes; sneezing; sore throat; cough; muscle aches; mild headache; listlessness; possibly, low-grade fever.
	Influenza *Flu*	Chills, muscle aches, and loss of appetite followed by a cough, sore throat, nasal congestion, and fever; possible chest pain.
	Measles	Cough; fever; watery nasal discharge; loss of appetite; red, watering eyes; sore throat; body aches; red, slightly itchy rash that gradually spreads all over the body.
	Nasal polyps	Impaired sense of smell; a feeling of fullness in the face; possible nasal discharge, facial pain, or headaches.
	Pneumonia	High fever; shortness of breath; cough with sputum; chest pain; fatigue.
	Rubella *German Measles*	Rash on the face that spreads to the torso and limbs; enlargement of lymph nodes in neck; usually preceded by headache, fever, and runny nose.
	Sinusitis *Inflammation of the mucous membranes lining the sinuses*	Throbbing pain above or below one or both eyes that intensifies when bending the head forward or coughing; nasal congestion; loss of sense of smell; often, pus-like nasal discharge; possible dental pain in the upper jaw; fever.
	Strep infection	Symptoms depend on the location and nature of the specific infection, but may include fever, headaches, swollen lymph glands, fatigue, loss of appetite, nasal discharge, red skin rash.

Nausea and/or vomiting

Associated Symptoms	Possible Diagnosis	Distinguishing Features
	Adrenal insufficiency *Inadequate production of steroid hormones by the adrenal gland*	Loss of weight and appetite; fatigue; weakness; darkening of the skin; abdominal pain; diarrhea; indigestion; nausea and vomiting; constipation; lack of sex drive; dizziness when rising from sitting or lying position.
	Anaphylaxis	Itching and hives; swelling of the eyes, lips, and tongue; weakness or faintness; tightening in the chest or throat; wheezing; shortness of breath; profuse sweating; palpitations; sudden, intense distress; feelings of impending doom; stomach cramps; nausea, vomiting, or diarrhea; bluish tinge (cyanosis) to the skin, lips, and nail beds due to oxygen insufficiency.
	Anemia, folic acid deficiency	Fatigue and weakness; pallor; shortness of breath, heart palpitations, or noticeably rapid heartbeat on exertion; sore, red, and glazed looking tongue; loss of weight and appetite; nausea and diarrhea; abdominal distention.
	Anemia, pernicious	Fatigue; inability to concentrate; sore, red tongue; weakness; dizziness; pallor; shortness of breath on exertion; palpitations; numbness and tingling in extremities; incoordination; headache; loss of weight and appetite; possibly, jaundice.
	Benign paroxysmal positional vertigo	Sudden sensation of spinning that occurs after changing the position of the head; loss of balance; nausea and vomiting.
	Botulism	Difficulty swallowing and speaking; nausea; vomiting; blurred or double vision.
	Cirrhosis *Chronic damage to the cells of the liver*	No symptoms in early stages; loss of weight and appetite; nausea; swollen legs, ankles and abdomen; itching; jaundice; black stools; vomiting blood; fatigue; impotence; memory loss; confusion.
	Congestive heart failure	Shortness of breath; fatigue; need to sleep on several pillows; weakness; cough; heart palpitations; swelling in the legs, ankles, and abdomen; frequent urination at night; indigestion; nausea and vomiting; loss of appetite.
	Coronary artery disease *Blockage in the arteries supplying blood to the heart muscle*	Initially, asymptomatic. In later stages, dull chest pain that may spread to the neck or the arms usually exacerbated by physical exertion and alleviated with rest; heart palpitations; shortness of breath.
	Esophageal cancer	Swallowing difficulty and pain; weight loss; drooling; possibly, vomiting or coughing up of bloody mucus, regurgitation of food; chest pain; repeated respiratory infections.

Nausea and/or vomiting *continued*

Associated Symptoms	Possible Diagnosis	Distinguishing Features
	Hyperparathyroidism *Overactivity of the parathyroid glands*	Increased susceptibility to bone fractures; depression; indigestion; increased thirst and urine output; fatigue, lethargy; somnolence; muscle weakness; nausea and vomiting; loss of appetite; weight loss.
	Kidney infection *Pyelonephritis*	Sudden fever and shaking chills; severe fatigue; burning and frequent urination; cloudy or bloody urine; pain in the abdomen, back, or flanks, sometimes severe; nausea and vomiting.
	Labyrinthitis *Inflammation of the semicircular canals of the inner ear*	Severe dizziness, loss of balance, jerky movements of the eyes; nausea and vomiting; ringing in the ears. In later stages, possible hearing loss.
	Ménière's disease *Dysfunction of structures in the inner ear*	Sudden attack of severe vertigo; nausea and vomiting; impaired sense of balance; ringing in the ears; hearing loss in the affected ear. Jerky movements of the eyes.
	Myocardial infarction *Heart attack*	Sudden chest pain or pressure that may spread to the arm, shoulder and jaw; excessive perspiration; shortness of breath. Possible nausea and vomiting.
	Ovarian cysts	In many cases, no symptoms. Painless swelling in the lower abdomen; possibly, pain during intercourse; brown vaginal discharge; lack of or heavier than usual menstrual periods; vomiting; unusual hair growth on face or body.
	Poliomyelitis *Polio*	Low fever; sore throat; headache; nausea and vomiting. In severe cases, paralysis without loss of sensation; stiff neck and back; twitching; swallowing and breathing difficulty; drooling.
	Renal calculi *Kidney stones*	Intermittent spasms of pain in the back and flanks, radiating through the lower abdomen towards the groin; nausea and vomiting; blood in the urine; urge to urinate but only small amounts of urine are passed.
	Renal failure, acute *Severe kidney failure*	Initially, decreased urine output, weight gain and swelling due to edema, loss of appetite, nausea and vomiting, fatigue. If untreated, confusion, seizures, and drowsiness.
	Reye's syndrome *Childhood disease marked by brain and liver damage*	Following recovery from an upper respiratory infection, nausea and vomiting; memory loss; confusion or delirium; possible seizures; drowsiness; lethargy.

Nausea and/or vomiting *continued*

Associated Symptoms	Possible Diagnosis	Distinguishing Features
	Trichinosis *Parasitic infestation*	Initially, crampy abdominal pain, diarrhea, vomiting, and fever, followed within one to two weeks by swelling around the eyes, muscle aches and tenderness, fever, and weakness. Possibly, coughing up of bloody phlegm; delirium; coma; heart failure symptoms.
with abdominal pain	Adrenal insufficiency *Inadequate production of steroid hormones by the adrenal gland*	Loss of weight and appetite; fatigue; weakness; darkening of the skin; abdominal pain; diarrhea; indigestion; nausea and vomiting; constipation; lack of sex drive; dizziness when rising from sitting or lying position.
	Amebiasis *Parasitic infection*	Usually asymptomatic; possibly, diarrhea; loose stools may contain mucus and blood; abdominal cramps; fatigue; weight loss; gas and flatulence. In severe cases, large amount of bloody stools daily; fever, nausea and vomiting, and abdominal tenderness.
	Disseminated intravascular coagulation *Bleeding disorder marked by excessive and inappropriate blood coagulation*	Abnormal bleeding possibly at several sites at once; vomiting blood; bloody or black stools; abnormal vaginal bleeding; blood in the urine; severe abdominal or back pain; possibly, convulsions, or coma.
	Diverticular disorders *Swellings in the wall of the colon*	Usually no symptoms unless diverticulae become inflamed. Tenderness or pain in the lower left abdomen relieved by passing stools or gas; constipation or diarrhea; blood in the stool; severe, spasmodic abdominal pain that becomes constant; possibly, fever and nausea.
	Dysentery, bacillary	Watery diarrhea that may contain mucus or blood; rectal pain upon defecation; abdominal pain; rapid dehydration and weight loss; nausea and vomiting.
	Endometriosis *The migration of the uterine lining to other reproductive or abdominal organs*	Pain in the lower abdomen, vagina, and lower back beginning just prior to menses and intensifying after blood flow has ceased; heavy bleeding during periods; pain during intercourse; diarrhea; constipation; pain during bowel movements; bleeding from the rectum; bloody urine during menses; nausea and vomiting prior to menses; infertility.
	Gallbladder disorders	Moderate to severe pain in the upper right side of the abdomen, chest, upper back, or right shoulder. Pain often follows the ingestion of high-fat foods and is episodic, lasting 20 minutes to several hours. Nausea and vomiting; low-grade fever; belching; heartburn; gas; possibly, jaundice, pale stools, and itchy skin.

Nausea and/or vomiting *continued*

Associated Symptoms	Possible Diagnosis	Distinguishing Features
with abdominal pain *continued*	Hepatitis, chronic	Fatigue; nausea; vomiting; loss of appetite; jaundice; dark urine; clay-colored stools; depression; pain or discomfort in the upper right abdomen; abdominal swelling; fever; in women, cessation of menstruation, acne, and the appearance of male pattern facial hair.
	Inguinal hernia *Displaced loop of intestine in the inguinal canal, a tubular passage through the abdominal wall*	A swelling in the groin area that may recede when lying down; pain at the site of the swelling, especially when lifting a heavy object; swelling of the scrotum. Nausea, vomiting, loss of appetite, and abdominal pain if intestine becomes obstructed.
	Intestinal obstruction	Abdominal pain and cramps; nausea; vomiting; weakness; gas; bloating; possible diarrhea; progressive constipation culminating in inability to pass stools or gas.
	Irritable bowel syndrome	Cramps in the middle or to one side of the lower abdomen that are usually relieved with bowel movements; nausea; bloating; gas; alternating diarrhea and constipation.
	Kidney cancer	Blood in the urine; abdominal and lower back pain; low-grade fever; loss of weight and appetite.
	Lactose intolerance *Difficulty digesting milk and dairy products*	Abdominal cramps; diarrhea; nausea; bloating; flatulence.
	Liver tumors	Pain or discomfort in the upper right portion of the abdomen; abdominal swelling; loss of weight and appetite; nausea and vomiting; fever; excessive perspiration; jaundice; pallor; severe fatigue.
	Mesenteric ischemia *A blood clot blocking blood flow to the intestine*	Severe abdominal cramping, usually around the navel, that is exacerbated by eating and alleviated by fasting. Possibly, bloody stools.
	Ovarian cancer	Often asymptomatic until widespread. Possibly, abdominal swelling or discomfort, nausea, and vomiting. In advanced stages, excessive hair growth, unexplained weight loss, abnormal menstrual bleeding or post-menopausal bleeding; urinary frequency.
	Pancreatic cancer	Often, no symptoms until far advanced. Upper abdominal pain which spreads to the back; loss of weight and appetite; jaundice; nausea, vomiting, and indigestion; diarrhea; fatigue; depression.

Nausea and/or vomiting *continued*

Associated Symptoms	Possible Diagnosis	Distinguishing Features
with abdominal pain *continued*	Pancreatitis *Inflammation of the pancreas*	Sudden, extreme abdominal pain; nausea and vomiting; weakness; fever; clammy skin; abdominal bloating and tenderness.
	Peptic ulcer	Intermittent, burning or gnawing pain in the upper abdomen or lower chest; indigestion; loss of appetite and weight. Pain may be relieved by eating or antacids. Possible nausea and vomiting. Black, tarry stools, vomiting blood.
	Peritonitis *Inflammation of the abdominal membrane*	Sudden abdominal pain, rigidity, and swelling; chills and fever; weakness; rapid heartbeat; nausea and vomiting; extreme thirst; low urine output.
	Stomach cancer	Discomfort in the upper abdomen; black, tarry stools; vomiting of blood; loss of appetite and weight; vomiting after meals.
	Testicular torsion *Twisting of the spermatic cord*	Severe pain and swelling on one side of the scrotum; skin on the scrotum may appear red or purple; light-headedness or fainting; possibly, abdominal pain, nausea and vomiting.
with abdominal pain and headache	Food poisoning	Symptoms vary greatly depending on the type and extent of poisoning and may include nausea, vomiting, diarrhea, bloody stools, abdominal pain, and collapse.
	Leukemias	Symptoms vary depending on the type of leukemia and may include: loss of appetite and weight; increased bruising and bleeding; bone pain, especially in the legs; abdominal pain and distention; nausea; heart palpitations; severe fatigue; pallor; breathing difficulty; fever; night sweats; headache; enlarged lymph nodes; joint pains (due to gout).
	Systemic lupus erythematosus *Inflammation of connective tissues throughout the body*	Red, blotchy, butterfly-shaped rash on the cheeks and bridge of the nose; fatigue; fever; loss of appetite and weight; nausea; joint and abdominal pain; headaches; blurred vision; increased sensitivity to sun exposure; depression; psychosis; mental confusion.
with headache	Brain abscess	Headaches; drowsiness; nausea and vomiting; fever; seizures; possible partial paralysis; confusion; speaking difficulty.
	Brain tumors	Headaches that become more severe when reclining; nausea and vomiting; memory loss; double vision; muscle weakness; numbness, tingling, or partial paralysis; vision loss; speech disturbances; seizures; drowsiness.

Nausea and/or vomiting *continued*

Associated Symptoms	Possible Diagnosis	Distinguishing Features
with headache *continued*	Concussion	Brief loss of consciousness following a blow to the head. Occasionally causes nausea and vomiting.
	Glaucoma	Often initially asymptomatic. In later stages, the symptoms of closed-angle glaucoma include: the appearance of halos and rainbows around lights; dilated pupil in the affected eye; severe headache and eye pain; possibly, nausea and vomiting. Open-angle glaucoma symptoms include: blurred vision and a gradual loss of peripheral vision.
	Glomerulonephritis, acute *Sudden or intense inflammation of the glomeruli, tiny structures that filter blood in the kidneys*	Blood in the urine; passing only small amounts of urine; swelling of the ankles or the tissues around the eyes; shortness of breath; possibly, fatigue, nausea and vomiting, loss of appetite, headaches, back pain, fever, impaired vision.
	Glomerulonephritis, chronic *Persistent inflammation of the glomeruli, tiny structures that filter blood in the kidneys*	Blood in the urine; passing only small amounts of urine; swelling of the legs or ankles; shortness of breath; possibly, fatigue, nausea and vomiting, loss of appetite, itching, headaches, impaired vision.
	Headache, migraine	Throbbing pain in the temple which spreads to the side of the head; nausea; vomiting. Pain may be preceded by blurred or impaired vision with bright spots and zig-zag patterns.
	Hydrocephalus *Overaccumulation of cerebrospinal fluid, the liquid surrounding the brain*	In infants, an enlarged head, rigidity of the legs, irritability, projectile vomiting, drowsiness, seizures, and lethargy. In older persons, headache, vomiting, loss of coordination, deterioration of mental faculties, speech difficulty, and loss of appetite.
	Legionnaire's disease	Dry cough progressing to one with blood-streaked sputum; high fever; chills; breathing difficulty; chest pain; headache; muscle aches; diarrhea; nausea; vomiting; mental confusion and disorientation.
	Malaria	Initially, severe chills and shivering. In later stages, extremely high fever followed by a period of profuse perspiration as fever subsides; headache, sometimes severe; vomiting.
	Meningitis *Inflammation of the membranes covering the brain and spinal cord*	Severe headache; nausea and vomiting; sensitivity to light; stiffness in the neck; possible red skin rash; fever; mental confusion; drowsiness; loss of consciousness; seizures.

Nausea and/or vomiting *continued*

Associated Symptoms	Possible Diagnosis	Distinguishing Features
with headache *continued*	Rocky Mountain spotted fever	Within a week after exposure, high fever, loss of appetite, headache, muscle aches, nausea and vomiting; dry cough; sensitivity to light. Within six days, the appearance of small pink spots on wrists and ankles, eventually spreading over the entire body, where they then grow, darken in color, and bleed.
	Toxic shock syndrome	Lethargy; conjunctivitis; confusion; sudden high fever accompanied by nausea, watery diarrhea, sore throat, and headache. Red rash on the palms and soles of the feet, which, after a week or two, begins to peel.

Neck pain

Associated Symptoms	Possible Diagnosis	Distinguishing Features
	Ankylosing spondylitis *Inflammation of the joints between the spine and the pelvis*	Initially, pain and stiffness in the lower back and hips that becomes worse after resting; neck or chest pain; possible pain in the hip, knee, and ankle joints; pain in the heel of the foot; eye pain; blurred vision.
	Cervical acceleration/ deceleration injuries *Whiplash*	Pain and stiffness in the neck that usually intensifies 24 hours after a head injury or neck sprain.
	Intervertebral disk, herniated	Severe lower back or neck pain that is exacerbated by movement or lifting heavy objects, sneezing, coughing, straining at stool. Pain, tingling, or numbness in a leg or an arm, usually on one side.
	Meningitis *Inflammation of the membranes covering the brain and spinal cord*	Severe headache; nausea and vomiting; sensitivity to light; stiffness in the neck; possible red skin rash; fever; mental confusion; drowsiness; loss of consciousness; seizures.
	Osteoarthritis *Degeneration of the cartilage that lines the joints*	Pain, swelling, and stiffness in one or more joints; enlargement and distortion of affected joints.
	Osteomalacia and Rickets *Softening and weakening of the bones, usually due to poor calcification*	Bone pain, especially in the neck, legs, hips and ribs. Muscle weakness, numbness, or spasms in the hands, feet, and throat; increased susceptibility to bone fractures.
	Osteomyelitis *Infection of bone and bone marrow*	Fever; severe pain in the affected bone; inflammation and swelling of the skin over the affected area; deformity. In children, arrested growth of the affected bone.
	Osteoporosis *Loss of bone mass due to calcium depletion*	Backache; easily fractured bones, especially in the wrists, hips, and spine; gradual loss of height; stooped or hunched posture.
	Paget's disease *A weakening, thickening, and deformity of the bones*	Often asymptomatic. Possibly, bone pain or deformity, especially bowing of the legs, bent spine, and facial deformity; unexplained bone fractures; joint pain or stiffness; hearing loss; headaches; ringing in ears.
	Rheumatoid arthritis	Fatigue and weakness; joint pain, stiffness, and inflammation, especially in the hands, feet, and arms; joint deformity; dry mouth; dry, painful eyes. Morning stiffness.
	Rheumatoid arthritis, juvenile	Fever; rash; abdominal pain; weight loss; swelling, stiffness, and pain in the affected joints; enlarged lymph glands; fatigue; pallor; red, painful eyes.

Neck pain *continued*

Associated Symptoms	Possible Diagnosis	Distinguishing Features
	Spinal cord trauma	Severe pain and swelling in the affected area; loss of sensation, muscle weakness, or paralysis below the site of the injury; urinary or fecal incontinence or retention; impotence; breathing difficulty; shock.
	Spinal stenosis *Narrowing of the spinal canal due to bony overgrowth*	Numbness, pain, and weakness in the legs and back that is exacerbated by walking and alleviated by sitting.
	Spinal tumor	Progressive numbness, tingling, and muscle weakness; fecal or urinary incontinence; persistent back pain.
	Spondylosis, cervical *Arthritis of the vertebral disks in the neck*	Neck pain and stiffness that spreads to the shoulders, upper arms, hands, or back of the head; numbness or tingling in the arms, hands, and fingers; weakness in the arms and legs; unsteady gait; possible loss of bladder or bowel control.
	Sprains and strains	Swelling, pain or tenderness in the affected joints; impaired joint function.

Night blindness

Associated Symptoms	Possible Diagnosis	Distinguishing Features
	Cataracts	Painless, increasingly blurred vision; appearance of halos around lights; changes in color perception; increased sensitivity to light and glare.
	Glaucoma	Often initially asymptomatic. In later stages, the symptoms of closed angle glaucoma include: the appearance of halos and rainbows around lights; dilated pupil in the affected eye; severe headache and eye pain; possibly, nausea and vomiting. Open angle glaucoma symptoms include: blurred vision and a gradual loss of peripheral vision.
	Malabsorption, digestive *A failure of the small intestine to absorb nutrients in the diet*	Diarrhea; weight loss; yellowish, foul-smelling stools; abdominal cramps, gas, and bloating; weakness and lethargy.

Night sweats

Associated Symptoms	Possible Diagnosis	Distinguishing Features
	AIDS *Acquired immunodeficiency syndrome*	Recurrent infections affecting the skin and respiratory system; cough; shortness of breath; loss of appetite; weight loss; fatigue; diarrhea; fever; dementia; malignant skin lesions; swollen lymph glands throughout the body; purplish skin nodules; memory loss; confusion; personality changes.
	Empyema *Collection of pus in any body cavity, usually between the membranes covering the lungs*	Chest pain exacerbated by deep inhalation; shortness of breath; dry cough; fever and chills; exhaustion; weight loss; night sweats; abdominal pain and jaundice.
	Leukemias	Symptoms vary depending on the type of leukemia and may include: loss of appetite and weight; increased bruising and bleeding; bone pain, especially in the legs; abdominal pain and distention; nausea; heart palpitations; severe fatigue; pallor; breathing difficulty; fever; night sweats; headache; enlarged lymph nodes; joint pains (due to gout).
	Lymphoma, Hodgkin's *Cancer of the lymph nodes and lymphoid tissue*	Painless swelling of the lymph nodes usually in the neck or armpits; loss of appetite; night sweats.
	Lymphoma, non-Hodgkin's *Cancer of the lymph nodes and lymphoid tissue*	Painless swelling of lymph nodes in the neck or groin; possible abdominal pain, vomiting of blood, headache.
	Polycythemia vera *An overproduction of red and white blood cells and platelets*	Headache; ringing in the ears; blurred vision; flushed skin; itching; dizziness; fatigue; night sweats; frequent nose bleeds and bruises.
	Tuberculosis	Often, asymptomatic. Possibly, low-grade fever; excessive perspiration; cough producing sputum or blood; weight loss; chronic fatigue; chest pain; shortness of breath; night sweats.

Nipple discharge

Associated Symptoms	Possible Diagnosis	Distinguishing Features
	Breast cancer	Lump or swelling, usually painless, in the breast or under the armpit; flattening, dimpling, indentation, redness, or scaliness of the breast; itching sensation in the nipple; change in size or symmetry of the breasts; breast pain.
	Fibrocystic breast changes *Benign lumps in the breast*	A lump or swelling, usually painless, anywhere in the breast or underarm, typically located in the upper and outer part of the breast. Pain around the lump, usually more apparent during the week prior to menses. Changes in the size or symmetry of the breasts.
	Hyperprolactinemia *Overproduction of the hormone prolactin by the pituitary gland*	Symptoms may vary depending on gender; in women: cessation of menstrual periods, decreased menstrual flow, excess facial hair; in men: erectile dysfunction, infertility, decreased libido, enlarged breasts; in men and women: abnormal production of breast milk, headaches, decreased vision.
	Hypothyroidism *Underactivity of the thyroid gland*	Unexplained weight gain; fatigue; muscle weakness; cramps; dry skin; hair loss; deepening of the voice; intolerance for cold; constipation; chest pain; insomnia; puffiness around eyes; loss of sex drive; depression; menstrual abnormalities; possible swelling in the neck.

Nosebleeds

Associated Symptoms	Possible Diagnosis	Distinguishing Features
	Anemia, aplastic	Fatigue and weakness; shortness of breath; heart palpitations; pallor; bleeding gums; nosebleeds; tendency to bruise easily; small red dots under the skin (petechiae). Increased susceptibility to infection.
	Cirrhosis *Chronic damage to the cells of the liver*	No symptoms in early stages; loss of weight and appetite; nausea; swollen legs, ankles and abdomen; itching; jaundice; black stools; vomiting blood; fatigue; impotence; memory loss; confusion.
	Hemophilia	Profuse bleeding from minor injuries and tooth extractions; internal bleeding that may cause blood in the urine; bleeding into joints; symptoms of stroke due to intracerebral bleeding; possibly, extensive bruising.
	Hypertension	Usually asymptomatic except in severe cases. Possibly, headache, easy fatigability, palpitations, chest pain, blurred vision, dizziness, nose bleeds, and confusion.
	Leukemias	Symptoms vary depending on the type of leukemia and may include: loss of appetite and weight; increased bruising and bleeding; bone pain, especially in the legs; abdominal pain and distention; nausea; heart palpitations; severe fatigue; pallor; breathing difficulty; fever; night sweats; headache; enlarged lymph nodes; joint pains (due to gout).
	Platelet function disorders	Minor bleeding in the mouth or just beneath the surface of the skin, often appearing as clusters of small, pinpoint-sized red specks; frequent nosebleeds; easy bruising; prolonged menstrual periods; fatigue; pallor; dark-colored stools.
	Polycythemia vera *An overproduction of red and white blood cells and platelets*	Headache; ringing in the ears; blurred vision; flushed skin; itching; dizziness; fatigue; night sweats; frequent nose bleeds and bruises.
	Sinusitis *Inflammation of the mucous membranes lining the sinuses*	Throbbing pain above or below one or both eyes that intensifies when bending the head forward or coughing; nasal congestion; loss of sense of smell; often, pus-like nasal discharge; possible dental pain in the upper jaw; fever.
	Von Willebrand's disease *Chronic bleeding disorder*	Frequent nosebleeds; excessive bleeding from cuts; bleeding gums; easy bruising; abnormal or excessive menstrual bleeding; blood in the stool.

Numbness or tingling sensation Paresthesia

Associated Symptoms	Possible Diagnosis	Distinguishing Features
	Anemia, pernicious	Fatigue; inability to concentrate; sore, red tongue; weakness; dizziness; pallor; shortness of breath on exertion; palpitations; numbness and tingling in extremities; incoordination; headache; loss of weight and appetite; possibly, jaundice.
	Brain tumors	Headaches that become more severe when reclining; nausea and vomiting; memory loss; double vision; muscle weakness; numbness, tingling, or partial paralysis; vision loss; speech disturbances; seizures; drowsiness.
	Carpal tunnel syndrome	Numbness, tingling, and pain in the hand and wrist, often intensifying at night; weakness of the fingers and hand.
	Cervical acceleration/ deceleration injuries *Whiplash*	Pain and stiffness in the neck that usually intensifies 24 hours after a head injury or neck sprain.
	Diabetes mellitus *Insufficiency of or resistance to insulin*	Fatigue; excessive thirst; frequent urination; weight loss despite increased appetite; blurred vision; numbness and tingling of feet and hands; impotence.
	Herpes zoster *Shingles*	A sensitive band of skin on one side of the body that becomes severely painful and develops slightly raised red spots that blister, dry and crust over. Pain may persist for months or years after skin has healed.
	Intervertebral disk, herniated	Severe lower back or neck pain that is exacerbated by movement or lifting heavy objects, sneezing, coughing, straining at stool. Pain, tingling, or numbness in a leg or an arm, usually on one side.
	Multiple sclerosis *Gradual degeneration of the protective sheaths surrounding the nerves within the brain and spinal cord*	Symptoms may appear suddenly and then disappear; persistent symptoms may take years to develop and include numbness or tingling in any part of the body, weakness in the extremities, an unsteady walk, slurred speech, urinary incontinence, fatigue, depression, temporary loss of vision, double or blurred vision, mental confusion, and memory loss.
	Peripheral neuropathies *Degeneration of the nerves that supply the extremities*	Tingling or numbness commonly beginning in the hands and feet and gradually spreading toward the center of the body; sensitive skin; muscle weakness; possibly, pain in the hands and feet; lack of coordination; shooting pains exacerbated by touch or changes in temperature; breathing difficulty; urinary or fecal incontinence.

Numbness or tingling sensation Paresthesia *continued*

Associated Symptoms	Possible Diagnosis	Distinguishing Features
	Rabies	Low-grade fever; headache; loss of appetite; difficulty swallowing; tingling at site of animal bite; intense thirst exacerbated by the inability to drink without violent, painful throat spasms; paralysis of facial muscles; drooling. Agitation and violent behavior, confusion, convulsions, coma.
	Renal failure, chronic *Persistent, mild kidney failure*	Asymptomatic in early stages. Possibly, mental confusion; shortness of breath; abdominal pain; decreased sex drive; fatigue; muscle and bone pain; numbness in the legs and feet; headache; impaired mental acuity; bad breath.
	Sarcoidosis *Accumulation of inflammatory cells in the lymph nodes and other tissues throughout the body*	Often no symptoms. Swollen lymph nodes in the neck or armpits; muscle aches; fever; breathing difficulty; possibly, purple rash on the face; reddish or brownish skin spots on the forearms, face, or legs; numbness; joint pain or stiffness; a painful, red eye; blurred vision; loss of appetite and weight.
	Spinal cord trauma	Severe pain and swelling in the affected area; loss of sensation, muscle weakness, or paralysis below the site of the injury; urinary or fecal incontinence or retention; impotence; breathing difficulty; shock.
	Spinal stenosis *Narrowing of the spinal canal due to bony overgrowth*	Numbness, pain, and weakness in the legs and back that is exacerbated by walking and alleviated by sitting.
	Spinal tumor	Progressive numbness, tingling, and muscle weakness; fecal or urinary incontinence; persistent back pain.
	Spondylosis, cervical *Arthritis of the vertebral disks in the neck*	Neck pain and stiffness that spreads to the shoulders, upper arms, hands, or back of the head; numbness or tingling in the arms, hands, and fingers; weakness in the arms and legs; unsteady gait; possible loss of bladder or bowel control.
	Systemic lupus erythematosus *Inflammation of connective tissues throughout the body*	Red, blotchy, butterfly-shaped rash on the cheeks and bridge of the nose; fatigue; fever; loss of appetite and weight; nausea; joint and abdominal pain; headaches; blurred vision; increased sensitivity to sun exposure; depression; psychosis; mental confusion.
	Transient ischemic attack *Temporary blockage in an artery supplying the brain*	Weakness or numbness in a limb; slurred speech; short-lived, temporary partial blindness; numbness and tingling; speech difficulties; confusion; dizziness.

Painful urination

Associated Symptoms	Possible Diagnosis	Distinguishing Features
	Bladder cancer	Blood in the urine; painful and frequent urination; pelvic pain; feeling of pressure in the back; persistent fever.
	Bladder infection *Cystitis*	Burning during urination; frequent and urgent urination with only small amounts of urine passed; blood in the urine; lower abdominal pain; low-grade fever; pain during sexual intercourse and, in men, during ejaculation.
	Bladder stones	Interruption of urine stream; inability to urinate except in certain positions; frequent and urgent urination with only small amounts of urine passed; blood in the urine; pain in the genitals, lower back, or abdomen; low-grade fever.
	Candidiasis *Fungal infection of the mouth, genitals, or mucous membranes*	Thick, white discharge from the vagina; itching and irritation in the vaginal area; pain while urinating or during intercourse; in men, inflammation of the head of the penis; possibly, yellow raised patches in the mouth.
	Epididymitis *Inflammation of the coiled sperm conduit that rests on each testicle*	Severe pain and swelling at the back of a testicle; possibly, redness and swelling of the scrotum; burning on urination.
	Genital herpes	Approximately one week after infection, itching, burning, soreness, and small blisters in the genital area. Blisters later burst, leaving painful ulcers which heal 10 to 20 days later. Possibly, enlarged, painful lymph nodes in the groin; fever, headache, and cold sores around the mouth. In women, pain during urination.
	Gonorrhea	Burning pain during urination; yellowish, pus-like discharge from the penis or vagina; redness or swelling at the infection site; abnormal vaginal bleeding.
	Kidney cysts	Pain or tenderness in the lower back or abdomen; blood in the urine. In infants, symmetrical, protruding masses visible in the flanks.
	Kidney infection *Pyelonephritis*	Sudden fever and shaking chills; severe fatigue; burning and frequent urination; cloudy or bloody urine; pain in the abdomen, back, or flanks, sometimes severe; nausea and vomiting.
	Pelvic inflammatory disease	Initially, lower pelvic pain; pain during intercourse; irregular menstrual bleeding; vaginal discharge with abnormal color or odor; low-grade fever; chills; frequent urination; fatigue; loss of appetite; later, severe abdominal pain and high fever.

Painful urination *continued*

Associated Symptoms	Possible Diagnosis	Distinguishing Features
	Prostate cancer	Difficulty urinating; frequent urination with decreased urine output; pain in the pelvic area and lower back; painful ejaculation or bowel movements; impotence.
	Prostatic hyperplasia, benign *Prostate enlargement*	Slow or delayed urination; dribbling urine; the need to urinate several times during the night; possibly, pain during urination; blood in the urine.
	Prostatitis *Inflammation of the prostate gland*	Burning during urination; urgent and frequent urination; fever and chills; discharge from the penis; lower abdominal and back pain; blood in the urine.
	Renal calculi *Kidney stones*	Intermittent spasms of pain in the back and flanks, radiating through the lower abdomen towards the groin; nausea and vomiting; blood in the urine; urge to urinate but only small amounts of urine are passed.
	Urethritis *Infection of the urethra,* *the passageway that drains* *urine from the bladder*	Frequent and painful urination; blood in the urine; yellow, pus-filled discharge; possible difficulty passing urine; urinary urgency; pain during intercourse; in men, painful ejaculation.
	Vaginitis *Inflammation of the vagina*	Vaginal irritation, itching, and discharge; painful intercourse and minor postcoital bleeding. In later stages, vaginal pain.

Pallor Paleness

Associated Symptoms	Possible Diagnosis	Distinguishing Features
	Anemia, aplastic	Fatigue and weakness; shortness of breath; heart palpitations; pallor; bleeding gums; nosebleeds; tendency to bruise easily; small red dots under the skin (petechiae). Increased susceptibility to infection.
	Anemia, folic acid deficiency	Fatigue and weakness; pallor; shortness of breath, heart palpitations, or noticeably rapid heartbeat on exertion; sore, red, and glazed looking tongue; loss of weight and appetite; nausea and diarrhea; abdominal distention.
	Anemia, hemolytic	Fatigue and weakness; shortness of breath on exertion; pallor; heart palpitations; jaundice and dark urine.
	Anemia, iron deficiency	Fatigue and weakness; pallor; shortness of breath and heart palpitations on exertion; irritability or inability to concentrate; sore tongue or tiny cracks at the corners of the mouth; black, tarry or bloody stools; unusual craving for dirt, paint, or ice.
	Anemia, pernicious	Fatigue; inability to concentrate; sore, red tongue; weakness; dizziness; pallor; shortness of breath on exertion; palpitations; numbness and tingling in extremities; incoordination; headache; loss of weight and appetite; possibly, jaundice.
	Hypothermia *Low body temperature (below 94°)*	Shivering; pallor; puffy face; fatigue and confusion; slow, shallow breathing; muscle stiffness; normally warm areas of the body are cold; loss of consciousness.
	Leukemias	Symptoms vary depending on the type of leukemia and may include: loss of appetite and weight; increased bruising and bleeding; bone pain, especially in the legs; abdominal pain and distention; nausea; heart palpitations; severe fatigue; pallor; breathing difficulty; fever; night sweats; headache; enlarged lymph nodes; joint pains (due to gout).
	Liver tumors	Pain or discomfort in the upper right portion of the abdomen; abdominal swelling; loss of weight and appetite; nausea and vomiting; fever; excessive perspiration; jaundice; pallor; severe fatigue.
	Malabsorption, digestive *A failure of the small intestine to absorb nutrients in the diet*	Diarrhea; weight loss; yellowish, foul-smelling stools; abdominal cramps, gas, and bloating; weakness and lethargy.

Pallor Paleness *continued*

Associated Symptoms	Possible Diagnosis	Distinguishing Features
	Multiple myeloma *Production of malignant plasma cells in the bone marrow*	Bone pain, especially progressive, constant back pain that intensifies with movement; unexplained bone fractures; fatigue; pallor; shortness of breath; increased bleeding, such as bleeding gums or nosebleeds; easily bruised skin; increased susceptibility to infection; headache; vision disturbances; loss of height.
	Myelofibrosis *An increase of fibrous scar tissue within the bone marrow*	Weakness and fatigue; abdominal fullness; a tendency to bleed easily; bone pain; pallor; shortness of breath during physical exertion; increased susceptibility to bruising and infections; weight loss.
	Platelet function disorders	Minor bleeding in the mouth or just beneath the surface of the skin, often appearing as clusters of small, pinpoint-sized red specks; frequent nosebleeds; easy bruising; prolonged menstrual periods; fatigue; pallor; dark-colored stools.
	Pulmonary edema *An accumulation of fluid in the lungs*	Severe shortness of breath; rapid breathing; pallor; excessive perspiration; bluish nails and lips; cough with frothy sputum; wheezing; anxiety and restlessness.
	Rheumatoid arthritis, juvenile	Fever; rash; abdominal pain; weight loss; swelling, stiffness, and pain in the affected joints; enlarged lymph glands; fatigue; pallor; red, painful eyes.

Palpitations

Associated Symptoms	Possible Diagnosis	Distinguishing Features
with shortness of breath	Amyloidosis *Accumulation of amyloid, a waxy substance, in tissues and organs*	Symptoms vary greatly depending on the body parts affected and may include fatigue and weakness; weight loss; heart palpitations; shortness of breath; swelling of the legs; difficulty swallowing due to swelling of the tongue; diarrhea; abdominal pain; raised spots on the armpits, groin, face, and neck; numbness or tingling of the hands or feet; dizziness on standing; joint pains.
	Anemia, aplastic	Fatigue and weakness; shortness of breath; heart palpitations; pallor; bleeding gums; nosebleeds; tendency to bruise easily; small red dots under the skin (petechiae). Increased susceptibility to infection.
	Anemia, folic acid deficiency	Fatigue and weakness; pallor; shortness of breath, heart palpitations, or noticeably rapid heartbeat on exertion; sore, red, and glazed looking tongue; loss of weight and appetite; nausea and diarrhea; abdominal distention.
	Anemia, hemolytic	Fatigue and weakness; shortness of breath on exertion; pallor; heart palpitations; jaundice and dark urine.
	Anemia, iron deficiency	Fatigue and weakness; pallor; shortness of breath and heart palpitations on exertion; irritability or inability to concentrate; sore tongue or tiny cracks at the corners of the mouth; black, tarry or bloody stools; unusual craving for dirt, paint, or ice.
	Anemia, pernicious	Fatigue; inability to concentrate; sore, red tongue; weakness; dizziness; pallor; shortness of breath on exertion; palpitations; numbness and tingling in extremities; incoordination; headache; loss of weight and appetite; possibly, jaundice.
	Anxiety states	Sudden attacks of unreasonable fear and panic; rapid heartbeat or palpitations; perspiration; dry mouth; irritability; muscle tension; trembling; palpitations; shortness of breath; restlessness; poor concentration; insomnia; fatigue; weakness.
	Cardiac arrhythmias *Irregularities in the heartbeat*	Frequently, asymptomatic; possibly; heart palpitations; light-headedness; shortness of breath; sudden weakness; loss of consciousness.
	Cardiomyopathy *Disease of the heart muscle causing a reduction in the force of heart contractions*	Fatigue; chest pain and palpitations; shortness of breath; swelling of the legs; wheezing; cough.

Palpitations *continued*

Associated Symptoms	Possible Diagnosis	Distinguishing Features
with shortness of breath *continued*	Congestive heart failure	Shortness of breath; fatigue; need to sleep on several pillows; weakness; cough; heart palpitations; swelling in the legs, ankles, and abdomen; frequent urination at night; indigestion; nausea and vomiting; loss of appetite.
	Leukemias	Symptoms vary depending on the type of leukemia and may include: loss of appetite and weight; increased bruising and bleeding; bone pain, especially in the legs; abdominal pain and distention; nausea; heart palpitations; severe fatigue; pallor; breathing difficulty; fever; night sweats; headache; enlarged lymph nodes; joint pains (due to gout).
	Mitral valve prolapse *A deformity in the heart's mitral valve possibly causing it to leak*	Usually asymptomatic. Possible palpitations, shortness of breath, dizziness, fainting, or fatigue.
	Myocarditis *Inflammation of the heart muscle*	Fatigue; shortness of breath; heart palpitations; fever; edema; rarely, continuous pressure or vague pain in the chest.
	Valvular heart disease	Depends on which heart valve is affected. Often asymptomatic. Possibly, fatigue and weakness; dizziness; chest pain; shortness of breath; heart palpitations; fainting; edema; stroke from embolism to the brain.
without shortness of breath	Colorectal cancer *A growth of malignant cells in the colon or rectum*	Change in bowel habits; diarrhea; constipation; narrow stools; bloody or dark stools; lower abdominal pain; bloating; cramps; gas; loss of weight and appetite; fatigue and heart palpitations due to anemia.
	Hemochromatosis *An excess accumulation of iron in the liver, pancreas, heart, testes, skin, and other organs*	A bronze or slate-grey tone to skin that is normally fair; chronic abdominal pain; heart palpitations; joint pain; drowsiness. In men, a decrease in the size of the testes, loss of sexual desire, and impotence.
	Hypertension	Usually asymptomatic except in severe cases. Possibly, headache, easy fatigability, palpitations, chest pain, blurred vision, dizziness, nose bleeds, and confusion.
	Hyperthyroidism *Overactivity of the thyroid gland*	Protruding eyes; weight loss despite increased appetite; intolerance to heat; excessive perspiration; nervousness or restlessness; possibly, swelling in the neck (goiter); palpitations; tremor; diarrhea.
	Hypoglycemia *Low blood sugar*	Anxiety; hunger; trembling; headache; palpitations; perspiration; confusion; irritability; loss of coordination; possibly, double vision, seizures, or coma.

Palpitations *continued*

Associated Symptoms	Possible Diagnosis	Distinguishing Features
without shortness of breath *continued*	Lyme disease	A small red bump, surrounded by a concentric bulls-eye-like red rash with a pale center. Over the following month: fever and chills; extreme fatigue; headaches. Symptoms may progress over several months or years and may include: palpitations; joint or muscle pain; and chronic joint inflammation, especially in the knees.
	Pheochromocytoma *Tumor in central part of the adrenal, the glands above the kidneys*	Headaches, sometimes severe; rapid heartbeat or heart palpitations; excessive perspiration; faintness, especially when standing up; chest pain; abdominal pain; constipation; weight loss; nervousness, irritability, or anxiety; mental confusion or psychosis.

Paralysis

Associated Symptoms	Possible Diagnosis	Distinguishing Features
with headache	Brain abscess	Headaches; drowsiness; nausea and vomiting; fever; seizures; possible partial paralysis; confusion; speaking difficulty.
	Brain hemorrhage	Sudden loss of consciousness; sudden, severe headache; mental confusion; stiff neck; nausea and vomiting; paralysis on one side of the face or body; weakness and dizziness; loss of speech; blurred or double vision; dilated pupils.
	Brain tumors	Headaches that become more severe when reclining; nausea and vomiting; memory loss; double vision; muscle weakness; numbness, tingling, or partial paralysis; vision loss; speech disturbances; seizures; drowsiness.
	Encephalitis *Inflammation of the brain*	Initially, headache and fever followed by confusion, hallucinations, and paralysis on one side of the body; memory loss; difficulty with speech and eye movements; drowsiness; possible coma or epileptic seizures; loss of hearing; sensitivity to light; stiff neck.
	Multiple sclerosis *Gradual degeneration of the protective sheaths surrounding the nerves within the brain and spinal cord*	Symptoms may appear suddenly and then disappear; persistent symptoms may take years to develop and include numbness or tingling in any part of the body, weakness in the extremities, an unsteady walk, slurred speech, urinary incontinence, fatigue, depression, temporary loss of vision, double or blurred vision, mental confusion, and memory loss.
	Poliomyelitis *Polio*	Low fever; sore throat; headache; nausea and vomiting. In severe cases, paralysis without loss of sensation; stiff neck and back; twitching; swallowing and breathing difficulty; drooling.
	Rabies	Low-grade fever; headache; loss of appetite; difficulty swallowing; tingling at site of animal bite; intense thirst exacerbated by the inability to drink without violent, painful throat spasms; paralysis of facial muscles; drooling. Agitation and violent behavior, confusion, convulsions, coma.
	Stroke	Symptoms vary with the location of brain injury. Sudden onset of weakness, paralysis, or loss of sensation, usually on one side of the body; a sudden heaviness in a limb; speech abnormalities; headache; vision disturbances; dizziness; confusion; coma; urinary and fecal incontinence.

Paralysis *continued*

Associated Symptoms	Possible Diagnosis	Distinguishing Features
with headache *continued*	Transient ischemic attack *Temporary blockage in an artery supplying the brain*	Weakness or numbness in a limb; slurred speech; short-lived, temporary partial blindness; numbness and tingling; speech difficulties; confusion; dizziness.
without headache	Amyotrophic lateral sclerosis *Progressive degeneration of nerve cells of the central nervous system*	Progressive loss of strength and coordination in the limbs; muscle twitching and cramps that begin in the hands and spread to the arms, shoulders, and legs; stiff, clumsy gait; swallowing, breathing, or speaking difficulty; weight loss; drooling; involuntary laughing or crying.
	Bell's palsy *Paralysis of muscles on one side of the face*	Drooping muscles and weakness on one side of the face resulting in a distorted smile or an expressionless look; drooping brow, tearing and an inability to close the affected eyelid; drooling; possibly, ear pain on the affected side of the face; possibly, changes in taste perception; increased sensitivity to noise.
	Botulism	Difficulty swallowing and speaking; nausea; vomiting; blurred or double vision.
	Myasthenia gravis *Nerve degeneration causing gradual loss of voluntary muscle control*	Drooping eyelids; double or blurred vision; muscle weakness especially in the face, throat, and neck; chewing and swallowing difficulties; possible breathing difficulty. Slurred, nasal-sounding speech.
	Parkinson's disease *Degeneration of the basal ganglia, a cluster of nerve cells in the brain*	Tremors in the hands; stiffness and weakness; impaired voluntary movement; shuffling gait; stooped posture; unblinking, fixed expression; possibly, slow, hesitant speech; difficulty swallowing; drooling; depression. Tremors occur at rest (not with voluntary movements) and disappear during sleep.
	Peripheral neuropathies *Degeneration of the nerves that supply the extremities*	Tingling or numbness commonly beginning in the hands and feet and gradually spreading toward the center of the body; sensitive skin; muscle weakness; possibly, pain in the hands and feet; lack of coordination; shooting pains exacerbated by touch or changes in temperature; breathing difficulty; urinary or fecal incontinence.
	Seizures	Involuntary twitching or jerking; muscle rigidity; loss of consciousness; confusion; drooling; hallucinations.
	Spinal cord trauma	Severe pain and swelling in the affected area; loss of sensation, muscle weakness, or paralysis below the site of the injury; urinary or fecal incontinence or retention; impotence; breathing difficulty; shock.

Paralysis *continued*

Associated Symptoms	Possible Diagnosis	Distinguishing Features
without headache *continued*	Spinal tumor	Progressive numbness, tingling, and muscle weakness; fecal or urinary incontinence; persistent back pain.
	Syphilis	Initially, painless, ulcerated, red sore on the genitals, mouth, or rectum; swollen glands in the neck, armpit, or groin; rash with small, red, scaly bumps; fever; headache. If left untreated, damage to heart valves leading to congestive heart failure; mental deterioration; loss of balance; seizures; dementia; personality changes.

Postnasal drip

Associated Symptoms	Possible Diagnosis	Distinguishing Features
	Allergic rhinitis *Hay fever*	Nasal congestion; frequent sneezing; itchy eyes, nose, and throat.
	Common cold	Nasal congestion; watery eyes; sneezing; sore throat; cough; muscle aches; mild headache; listlessness; possibly, low-grade fever.
	Sinusitis *Inflammation of the mucous membranes lining the sinuses*	Throbbing pain above or below one or both eyes that intensifies when bending the head forward or coughing; nasal congestion; loss of sense of smell; often, pus-like nasal discharge; possible dental pain in the upper jaw; fever.
	Strep infection	Symptoms depend on the location and nature of the specific infection, but may include fever, headaches, swollen lymph glands, fatigue, loss of appetite, nasal discharge, red skin rash.

Posture or height changes

Associated Symptoms	Possible Diagnosis	Distinguishing Features
	Acromegaly *Overproduction of growth hormone by the pituitary gland*	In adults (acromegaly): Gradual thickening of the bones of the face, jaw, and the extremities in adults; oily skin; severe headache; excessive hair growth; excessive perspiration; joint pains. In children (in which the disease is called gigantism): Rapid growth and unusual height; possibly, blindness.
	Amyotrophic lateral sclerosis *Progressive degeneration of nerve cells of the central nervous system*	Progressive loss of strength and coordination in the limbs; muscle twitching and cramps that begin in the hands and spread to the arms, shoulders, and legs; stiff, clumsy gait; swallowing, breathing, or speaking difficulty; weight loss; drooling; involuntary laughing or crying.
	Ankylosing spondylitis *Inflammation of the joints between the spine and the pelvis*	Initially, pain and stiffness in the lower back and hips that becomes worse after resting; neck or chest pain; possible pain in the hip, knee, and ankle joints; pain in the heel of the foot; eye pain; blurred vision.
	Bone cancer	Pain, tenderness, and swelling in the affected bones and joints, often intensifying at night; a noticeable tumor or mass; increased susceptibility to bone fractures.
	Bursitis *Inflammation of the bursas, the lubricant-filled sacs in and around the joints*	Pain and swelling around a joint, usually the elbow, knee, or shoulder; painful movement in the affected joint; possibly, fever.
	Multiple myeloma *Production of malignant plasma cells in the bone marrow*	Bone pain, especially progressive, constant back pain that intensifies with movement; unexplained bone fractures; fatigue; pallor; shortness of breath; increased bleeding, such as bleeding gums or nosebleeds; easily bruised skin; increased susceptibility to infection; headache; vision disturbances; loss of height.
	Muscular dystrophy	Symptoms depend on type of muscular dystrophy and may include: Progressive muscle wasting, weakness, and loss of mobility; lack of coordination; muscular and skeletal deformities including curvature of the spine with protruding abdomen; waddling gait; cataracts; frontal baldness; gonadal atrophy.
	Osteoporosis *Loss of bone mass due to calcium depletion*	Backache; easily fractured bones, especially in the wrists, hips, and spine; gradual loss of height; stooped or hunched posture.
	Scoliosis	Gradual bending of the spine to one side or into an S-shape; shoulders and hips may appear uneven; noticeable hump of the upper back; noticeable flatness of the lower back with loss of normal curve.

Pupils, constricted

Associated Symptoms	Possible Diagnosis	Distinguishing Features
	Corneal ulcers and infections	Severe eye pain; blurred vision; increased tear production; aversion to light.
	Headache, cluster	Persistent pain in or around one eye; redness and tearing of one eye; nasal congestion on the same side of the face as the affected eye.
	Uveitis and iritis *Inflammation of the uvea, a group of structures in the eye including the iris*	Moderate to severe eye pain; aversion to light; redness in the eye; excessive tearing; blurred vision; spots in the field of vision.

Pupils, dilated

Associated Symptoms	Possible Diagnosis	Distinguishing Features
	Anxiety states	Sudden attacks of unreasonable fear and panic; rapid heartbeat or palpitations; perspiration; dry mouth; irritability; muscle tension; trembling; palpitations; shortness of breath; restlessness; poor concentration; insomnia; fatigue; weakness.
	Botulism	Difficulty swallowing and speaking; nausea; vomiting; blurred or double vision.
	Glaucoma	Often initially asymptomatic. In later stages, the symptoms of closed-angle glaucoma include: the appearance of halos and rainbows around lights; dilated pupil in the affected eye; severe headache and eye pain; possibly, nausea and vomiting. Open-angle glaucoma symptoms include: blurred vision and a gradual loss of peripheral vision.
	Heatstroke	Sudden dizziness; weakness; headache; hot, dry, red skin which later turns grey; high body temperature; muscle cramps; confusion; seizures; loss of consciousness.

Rash

Associated Symptoms	Possible Diagnosis	Distinguishing Features
	Anaphylaxis	Itching and hives; swelling of the eyes, lips, and tongue; weakness or faintness; tightening in the chest or throat; wheezing; shortness of breath; profuse sweating; palpitations; sudden, intense distress; feelings of impending doom; stomach cramps; nausea, vomiting, or diarrhea; bluish tinge (cyanosis) to the skin, lips, and nail beds due to oxygen insufficiency.
	Eczema *Inflammation of the skin*	Itching skin; thickened patches of skin; possibly, with oozing and crusting; in infants, rash on the face, inner elbows, or behind the knees that turns scaly and develops small red pimples that leak; swollen legs (stasis dermatitis).
	Psoriasis	Slightly raised patches of skin with red borders and white-silver scales; joint pain and stiffness; itching; pitted nails.
	Ringworm *Fungal skin infection*	A rash with distinct, advancing borders and clear centers; affected areas may have abnormally dark pigmentation; itching; scaly patches of skin; bald patches on scalp; Athlete's foot; red, swollen finger- and toenails.
	Rosacea *Redness, swelling, and blemishes around the nose, cheeks, and forehead*	Facial flushing; stinging, burning, or feeling of skin pulled tight across face; bumps, blemishes, and swelling of nose and cheeks; severe swelling or enlargement of the nose.
	Scabies	Tiny, grey, scaly blisters—usually on the wrists, genitals, armpits, or between the fingers—that rupture easily when scratched; severe itching; red lumps or rashes may develop.
with fever	Dermatomyositis *Inflammation of the muscles and skin*	Red rash on the neck, upper torso, and upper arms and legs; purple discoloration and swelling of the eyelids; areas of thickened skin; muscle weakness and stiffness, usually in the shoulders and pelvis; cold hands and feet; speaking or swallowing difficulty; weight loss.
	Herpes zoster *Shingles*	A sensitive band of skin on one side of the body that becomes severely painful and develops slightly raised red spots that blister, dry and crust over. Pain may persist for months or years after skin has healed.
	Lyme disease	A small red bump, surrounded by a concentric bulls-eye-like red rash with a pale center. Over the following month: fever and chills; extreme fatigue; headaches. Symptoms may progress over several months or years and may include: palpitations; joint or muscle pain; and chronic joint inflammation, especially in the knees.

Rash *continued*

Associated Symptoms	Possible Diagnosis	Distinguishing Features
with fever *continued*	Measles	Cough; fever; watery nasal discharge; loss of appetite; red, watering eyes; sore throat; body aches; red, slightly itchy rash that gradually spreads all over the body.
	Meningitis *Inflammation of the membranes covering the brain and spinal cord*	Severe headache; nausea and vomiting; sensitivity to light; stiffness in the neck; possible red skin rash; fever; mental confusion; drowsiness; loss of consciousness; seizures.
	Rheumatic fever	Initially, a sore throat that gets better followed, one to six weeks later, by lethargy and fever. Possibly, swollen joints, rash, abdominal pain, involuntary jerky movements, emotional instability.
	Rheumatoid arthritis, juvenile	Fever; rash; abdominal pain; weight loss; swelling, stiffness, and pain in the affected joints; enlarged lymph glands; fatigue; pallor; red, painful eyes.
	Rocky Mountain spotted fever	Within a week after exposure, high fever, loss of appetite, headache, muscle aches, nausea and vomiting; dry cough; sensitivity to light. Within six days, the appearance of small pink spots on wrists and ankles, eventually spreading over the entire body, where they then grow, darken in color, and bleed.
	Roseola *Infectious disease primarily affecting children*	Abrupt onset of high fever that usually subsides within four to five days, at which time a rash appears on the torso, and spreads to the limbs, neck, and face. Sore throat; swollen lymph nodes in neck.
	Rubella *German Measles*	Rash on the face that spreads to the torso and limbs; enlargement of lymph nodes in neck; usually preceded by headache, fever, and runny nose.
	Sarcoidosis *Accumulation of inflammatory cells in the lymph nodes and other tissues throughout the body*	Often no symptoms. Swollen lymph nodes in the neck or armpits; muscle aches; fever; breathing difficulty; possibly, purple rash on the face; reddish or brownish skin spots on the forearms, face, or legs; numbness; joint pain or stiffness; a painful, red eye; blurred vision; loss of appetite and weight.
	Syphilis	Initially, painless, ulcerated, red sore on the genitals, mouth, or rectum; swollen glands in the neck, armpit, or groin; rash with small, red, scaly bumps; fever; headache. If left untreated, damage to heart valves leading to congestive heart failure; mental deterioration; loss of balance; seizures; dementia; personality changes.

Rash *continued*

Associated Symptoms	Possible Diagnosis	Distinguishing Features
with fever *continued*	Systemic lupus erythematosus *Inflammation of connective tissues throughout the body*	Red, blotchy, butterfly-shaped rash on the cheeks and bridge of the nose; fatigue; fever; loss of appetite and weight; nausea; joint and abdominal pain; headaches; blurred vision; increased sensitivity to sun exposure; depression; psychosis; mental confusion.
	Toxic shock syndrome	Lethargy; conjunctivitis; confusion; sudden high fever accompanied by nausea, watery diarrhea, sore throat, and headache. Red rash on the palms and soles of the feet, which, after a week or two, begins to peel.
	Typhoid fever	Headache; fever, loss of appetite; abdominal pain and tenderness; extreme weakness; constipation followed by diarrhea; drowsiness, stupor, or coma; raised, pink skin eruptions on the chest and abdomen; joint aches; sore throat.

Rectal bleeding

Associated Symptoms	Possible Diagnosis	Distinguishing Features
	Amebiasis *Parasitic infection*	Usually asymptomatic; possibly, diarrhea; loose stools may contain mucus and blood; abdominal cramps; fatigue; weight loss; gas and flatulence. In severe cases, large amount of bloody stools daily; fever, nausea and vomiting, and abdominal tenderness.
	Amyloidosis *Accumulation of amyloid, a waxy substance, in tissues and organs*	Symptoms vary greatly depending on the body parts affected and may include fatigue and weakness; weight loss; heart palpitations; shortness of breath; swelling of the legs; difficulty swallowing due to swelling of the tongue; diarrhea; abdominal pain; raised spots on the armpits, groin, face, and neck; numbness or tingling of the hands or feet; dizziness on standing; joint pains.
	Anal fissures	Rectal pain or burning during and immediately after bowel movements; blood in the stool or on toilet paper; rectal itching.
	Colitis, ulcerative *Inflammation of the lining of the colon*	Pain on the left side of the abdomen that lessens after bowel movements; bloody diarrhea; pain in the rectal area; possibly, fever, rapid heartbeat, nausea and vomiting, loss of appetite, dehydration with severe attacks.
	Colon Polyps	Rectal bleeding; blood in the stool; abdominal pain; change in bowel habits.
	Colorectal cancer *A growth of malignant cells in the colon or rectum*	Change in bowel habits; diarrhea; constipation; narrow stools; bloody or dark stools; lower abdominal pain; bloating; cramps; gas; loss of weight and appetite; fatigue and heart palpitations due to anemia.
	Crohn's disease *Inflammation of the lining of the small intestine*	Episodes of abdominal pain or cramps in lower abdomen; nausea; diarrhea; loss of weight and appetite; possibly, fever; rectal bleeding or blood in stools; fatigue; anal fissures; joint pains; inflammation of the eyes.
	Diverticular disorders *Swellings in the wall of the colon*	Usually no symptoms unless diverticulae become inflamed. Tenderness or pain in the lower left abdomen relieved by passing stools or gas; constipation or diarrhea; blood in the stool; severe, spasmodic abdominal pain that becomes constant; possibly, fever and nausea.
	Dysentery, bacillary	Watery diarrhea that may contain mucus or blood; rectal pain upon defecation; abdominal pain; rapid dehydration and weight loss; nausea and vomiting.
	Food poisoning	Symptoms vary greatly depending on the type and extent of poisoning and may include nausea, vomiting, diarrhea, bloody stools, abdominal pain, and collapse.

Rectal bleeding *continued*

Associated Symptoms	Possible Diagnosis	Distinguishing Features
	Hemophilia	Profuse bleeding from minor injuries and tooth extractions; internal bleeding that may cause blood in the urine; bleeding into joints; symptoms of stroke due to intracerebral bleeding; possibly, extensive bruising.
	Hemorrhoids	Pain during defecation; anal itching; mucus discharge from the anus. Bright, red blood on toilet paper, stool, or in toilet bowl after a bowel movement.
	Mesenteric ischemia *A blood clot blocking blood flow to the intestine*	Severe abdominal cramping, usually around the navel, that is exacerbated by eating and alleviated by fasting. Possibly, bloody stools.
	Proctitis *Inflammation of the rectum*	Soreness in the rectal area; mucus discharge from the anus; constipation; painful bowel movements; possibly, rectal bleeding.
	Vaginal cancer	Vaginal itching; bleeding after intercourse or between menstrual periods; abnormal vaginal discharge; lesions with thick, raised edges; possibly rectal bleeding; discomfort when urinating or defecating; pain during intercourse; urinary frequency and urgency.
	Von Willebrand's disease *Chronic bleeding disorder*	Frequent nosebleeds; excessive bleeding from cuts; bleeding gums; easy bruising; abnormal or excessive menstrual bleeding; blood in the stool.

Rectal itching

Associated Symptoms	Possible Diagnosis	Distinguishing Features
	Anal fissures	Rectal pain or burning during and immediately after bowel movements; blood in the stool or on toilet paper; rectal itching.
	Candidiasis *Fungal infection of the mouth, genitals, or mucous membranes*	Thick, white discharge from the vagina; itching and irritation in the vaginal area; pain while urinating or during intercourse; in men, inflammation of the head of the penis; possibly, yellow raised patches in the mouth.
	Hemorrhoids	Pain during defecation; anal itching; mucus discharge from the anus. Bright, red blood on toilet paper, stool, or in toilet bowl after a bowel movement.
	Pinworms	Anal itching, often at night; irritability; fidgetiness; restless sleep.
	Proctitis *Inflammation of the rectum*	Soreness in the rectal area; mucus discharge from the anus; constipation; painful bowel movements; possibly, rectal bleeding.

Rectal pain

Associated Symptoms	Possible Diagnosis	Distinguishing Features
	Anal fissures	Rectal pain or burning during and immediately after bowel movements; blood in the stool or on toilet paper; rectal itching.
	Colitis, ulcerative *Inflammation of the lining of the colon*	Pain on the left side of the abdomen that lessens after bowel movements; bloody diarrhea; pain in the rectal area; possibly, fever, rapid heartbeat, nausea and vomiting, loss of appetite, dehydration with severe attacks.
	Constipation, chronic	Infrequent and possibly painful bowel movements; straining during bowel movements; hard, dry stool; abdominal swelling; continued sensation of fullness after evacuating bowels.
	Crohn's disease *Inflammation of the lining of the small intestine*	Episodes of abdominal pain or cramps in lower abdomen; nausea; diarrhea; loss of weight and appetite; possibly, fever; rectal bleeding or blood in stools; fatigue; anal fissures; joint pains; inflammation of the eyes.
	Dysentery, bacillary	Watery diarrhea that may contain mucus or blood; rectal pain upon defecation; abdominal pain; rapid dehydration and weight loss; nausea and vomiting.
	Hemorrhoids	Pain during defecation; anal itching; mucus discharge from the anus. Bright, red blood on toilet paper, stool, or in toilet bowl after a bowel movement.
	Proctitis *Inflammation of the rectum*	Soreness in the rectal area; mucus discharge from the anus; constipation; painful bowel movements; possibly, rectal bleeding.
	Prostate cancer	Difficulty urinating; frequent urination with decreased urine output; pain in the pelvic area and lower back; painful ejaculation or bowel movements; impotence.
	Prostatitis *Inflammation of the prostate gland*	Burning during urination; urgent and frequent urination; fever and chills; discharge from the penis; lower abdominal and back pain; blood in the urine.

Seizures

Associated Symptoms	Possible Diagnosis	Distinguishing Features
	Brain abscess	Headaches; drowsiness; nausea and vomiting; fever; seizures; possible partial paralysis; confusion; speaking difficulty.
	Brain tumors	Headaches that become more severe when reclining; nausea and vomiting; memory loss; double vision; muscle weakness; numbness, tingling, or partial paralysis; vision loss; speech disturbances; seizures; drowsiness.
	Diabetes mellitus *Insufficiency of or resistance to insulin*	Fatigue; excessive thirst; frequent urination; weight loss despite increased appetite; blurred vision; numbness and tingling of feet and hands; impotence.
	Disseminated intravascular coagulation *Bleeding disorder marked by excessive and inappropriate blood coagulation*	Abnormal bleeding possibly at several sites at once; vomiting blood; bloody or black stools; abnormal vaginal bleeding; blood in the urine; severe abdominal or back pain; possibly, convulsions, or coma.
	Encephalitis *Inflammation of the brain*	Initially, headache and fever followed by confusion, hallucinations, and paralysis on one side of the body; memory loss; difficulty with speech and eye movements; drowsiness; possible coma or epileptic seizures; loss of hearing; sensitivity to light; stiff neck.
	Heatstroke	Sudden dizziness; weakness; headache; hot, dry, red skin which later turns grey; high body temperature; muscle cramps; confusion; seizures; loss of consciousness.
	Hydrocephalus *Overaccumulation of cerebrospinal fluid, the liquid surrounding the brain*	In infants, an enlarged head, rigidity of the legs, irritability, projectile vomiting, drowsiness, seizures, and lethargy. In older persons, headache, vomiting, loss of coordination, deterioration of mental faculties, speech difficulty, and loss of appetite.
	Hypoglycemia *Low blood sugar*	Anxiety; hunger; trembling; headache; palpitations; perspiration; confusion; irritability; loss of coordination; possibly, double vision, seizures, or coma.
	Hypoparathyroidism *Underactivity of the parathyroid glands*	Numbness and tingling and painful, cramp-like spasms of the face, hands, arms, and feet; cataracts; possible seizures.
	Leukemias	Symptoms vary depending on the type of leukemia and may include: loss of appetite and weight; increased bruising and bleeding; bone pain, especially in the legs; abdominal pain and distention; nausea; heart palpitations; severe fatigue; pallor; breathing difficulty; fever; night sweats; headache; enlarged lymph nodes; joint pains (due to gout).

Seizures *continued*

Associated Symptoms	Possible Diagnosis	Distinguishing Features
	Meningitis *Inflammation of the membranes covering the brain and spinal cord*	Severe headache; nausea and vomiting; sensitivity to light; stiffness in the neck; possible red skin rash; fever; mental confusion; drowsiness; loss of consciousness; seizures.
	Multiple sclerosis *Gradual degeneration of the protective sheaths surrounding the nerves within the brain and spinal cord*	Symptoms may appear suddenly and then disappear; persistent symptoms may take years to develop and include numbness or tingling in any part of the body, weakness in the extremities, an unsteady walk, slurred speech, urinary incontinence, fatigue, depression, temporary loss of vision, double or blurred vision, mental confusion, and memory loss.
	Renal failure, acute *Severe kidney failure*	Initially, decreased urine output, weight gain and swelling due to edema, loss of appetite, nausea and vomiting, fatigue. If untreated, confusion, seizures, and drowsiness.
	Renal failure, chronic *Persistent, mild kidney failure*	Asymptomatic in early stages. Possibly, mental confusion; shortness of breath; abdominal pain; decreased sex drive; fatigue; muscle and bone pain; numbness in the legs and feet; headache; impaired mental acuity; bad breath.
	Reye's syndrome *Childhood disease marked by brain and liver damage*	Following recovery from an upper respiratory infection, nausea and vomiting; memory loss; confusion or delirium; possible seizures; drowsiness; lethargy.
	Sarcoidosis *Accumulation of inflammatory cells in the lymph nodes and other tissues throughout the body*	Often no symptoms. Swollen lymph nodes in the neck or armpits; muscle aches; fever; breathing difficulty; possibly, purple rash on the face; reddish or brownish skin spots on the forearms, face, or legs; numbness; joint pain or stiffness; a painful, red eye; blurred vision; loss of appetite and weight.
	Seizures	Involuntary twitching or jerking; muscle rigidity; loss of consciousness; confusion; drooling; hallucinations.
	Tetanus	Often, lockjaw; stiffness and, later, muscle spasms in the neck and face; drooling; abdominal and back pain; extreme perspiration; swallowing difficulty; possible convulsions; fever.

Sensitivity to light, increased

Associated Symptoms	Possible Diagnosis	Distinguishing Features
	Cataracts	Painless, increasingly blurred vision; appearance of halos around lights; changes in color perception; increased sensitivity to light and glare.
	Conjunctivitis *Pinkeye*	Itching and redness in the affected eye; discharge from the eye, clear or pus-filled; excessive tearing; aversion to bright lights; possibly, swollen eyelids.
	Corneal ulcers and infections	Severe eye pain; blurred vision; increased tear production; aversion to light.
	Headache, migraine	Throbbing pain in the temple which spreads to the side of the head; nausea; vomiting. Pain may be preceded by blurred or impaired vision with bright spots and zig-zag patterns.
	Meningitis *Inflammation of the membranes covering the brain and spinal cord*	Severe headache; nausea and vomiting; sensitivity to light; stiffness in the neck; possible red skin rash; fever; mental confusion; drowsiness; loss of consciousness; seizures.
	Scleritis and episcleritis *Inflammation of the sclera, the white of the eye*	Dull eye pain; redness in the white of the eye; possibly, blurred vision; aversion to light; copious tearing.
	Uveitis and iritis *Inflammation of the uvea, a group of structures in the eye including the iris*	Moderate to severe eye pain; aversion to light; redness in the eye; excessive tearing; blurred vision; spots in the field of vision.

Sexual intercourse, painful Dyspareunia

Associated Symptoms	Possible Diagnosis	Distinguishing Features
	Bladder infection *Cystitis*	Burning during urination; frequent and urgent urination with only small amounts of urine passed; blood in the urine; lower abdominal pain; low-grade fever; pain during sexual intercourse and, in men, during ejaculation.
	Candidiasis *Fungal infection of the mouth, genitals, or mucous membranes*	Thick, white discharge from the vagina; itching and irritation in the vaginal area; pain while urinating or during intercourse; in men, inflammation of the head of the penis; possibly, yellow raised patches in the mouth.
	Dyspareunia *Pain during sexual intercourse*	Pain occurs primarily during sexual activity. May include any type of discomfort from a burning sensation in the genitals to lower back pain.
	Endometriosis *The migration of the uterine lining to other reproductive or abdominal organs*	Pain in the lower abdomen, vagina, and lower back beginning just prior to menses and intensifying after blood flow has ceased; heavy bleeding during periods; pain during intercourse; diarrhea; constipation; pain during bowel movements; bleeding from the rectum; bloody urine during menses; nausea and vomiting prior to menses; infertility.
	Epididymitis *Inflammation of the coiled sperm conduit that rests on each testicle*	Severe pain and swelling at the back of a testicle; possibly, redness and swelling of the scrotum; burning on urination.
	Genital herpes	Approximately one week after infection, itching, burning, soreness, and small blisters in the genital area. Blisters later burst, leaving painful ulcers which heal 10 to 20 days later. Possibly, enlarged, painful lymph nodes in the groin; fever, headache, and cold sores around the mouth. In women, pain during urination.
	Gonorrhea	Burning pain during urination; yellowish, pus-like discharge from the penis or vagina; redness or swelling at the infection site; abnormal vaginal bleeding.
	Orchitis *Inflammation of a testicle*	Swelling and severe pain in the affected testicle; possible bloody discharge in the semen; pain during intercourse; fever.
	Ovarian cysts	In many cases, no symptoms. Painless swelling in the lower abdomen; possibly, pain during intercourse; brown vaginal discharge; lack of or heavier than usual menstrual periods; vomiting; unusual hair growth on face or body.

Sexual intercourse, painful Dyspareunia *continued*

Associated Symptoms	Possible Diagnosis	Distinguishing Features
	Pelvic inflammatory disease	Initially, lower pelvic pain; pain during intercourse; irregular menstrual bleeding; vaginal discharge with abnormal color or odor; low-grade fever; chills; frequent urination; fatigue; loss of appetite; later, severe abdominal pain and high fever.
	Penile cancer	Sore, ulcer, or wart-like lump on the penis, usually near the head, possibly painful; bleeding or unusual discharge from the penis. Possibly, pain during urination, or enlarged lymph nodes in the groin.
	Prostatitis *Inflammation of the prostate gland*	Burning during urination; urgent and frequent urination; fever and chills; discharge from the penis; lower abdominal and back pain; blood in the urine.
	Urethritis *Infection of the urethra, the passageway that drains urine from the bladder*	Frequent and painful urination; blood in the urine; yellow, pus-filled discharge; possible difficulty passing urine; urinary urgency; pain during intercourse; in men, painful ejaculation.
	Uterine prolapse	Often asymptomatic. Possibly, difficulty passing urine or stools, pain during intercourse, backache that intensifies when lifting, sensation of heaviness or dragging within the pelvis, painful or heavy menstrual periods, or bleeding between periods. In severe cases, uterus visibly protrudes outside of vagina.
	Vaginitis *Inflammation of the vagina*	Vaginal irritation, itching, and discharge; painful intercourse and minor postcoital bleeding. In later stages, vaginal pain.

Shakiness

Associated Symptoms	Possible Diagnosis	Distinguishing Features
	Brain tumors	Headaches that become more severe when reclining; nausea and vomiting; memory loss; double vision; muscle weakness; numbness, tingling, or partial paralysis; vision loss; speech disturbances; seizures; drowsiness.
	Essential tremor	Involuntary rhythmic shaking of the hands and arms and, less frequently, the head, tongue, larynx, eyelids, or other parts of the body. Tremors intensify during emotional stress and voluntary movements, and cease during periods of rest or sleep. Shaky handwriting; quavering voice.
	Hyperthyroidism *Overactivity of the thyroid gland*	Protruding eyes; weight loss despite increased appetite; intolerance to heat; excessive perspiration; nervousness or restlessness; possibly, swelling in the neck (goiter); palpitations; tremor; diarrhea.
	Hypoglycemia *Low blood sugar*	Anxiety; hunger; trembling; headache; palpitations; perspiration; confusion; irritability; loss of coordination; possibly, double vision, seizures, or coma.
	Parkinson's disease *Degeneration of the basal ganglia, a cluster of nerve cells in the brain*	Tremors in the hands; stiffness and weakness; impaired voluntary movement; shuffling gait; stooped posture; unblinking, fixed expression; possibly, slow, hesitant speech; difficulty swallowing; drooling; depression. Tremors occur at rest (not with voluntary movements) and disappear during sleep.

Shoulder pain

Associated Symptoms	Possible Diagnosis	Distinguishing Features
	Bone cancer	Pain, tenderness, and swelling in the affected bones and joints, often intensifying at night; a noticeable tumor or mass; increased susceptibility to bone fractures.
	Bursitis *Inflammation of the bursas, the lubricant-filled sacs in and around the joints*	Pain and swelling around a joint, usually the elbow, knee, or shoulder; painful movement in the affected joint; possibly, fever.
	Dislocations/subluxations	Deformity of the affected joint; joint pain and tenderness; difficulty moving a joint; swelling and stiffness within 30 minutes after joint injury.
	Infectious arthritis	Pain, swelling, stiffness, and redness, usually in one joint. Fever. Severity varies from a mild ache to severe, debilitating pain and eventual joint deformity.
	Myocardial infarction *Heart attack*	Sudden chest pain or pressure that may spread to the arm, shoulder and jaw; excessive perspiration; shortness of breath. Possible nausea and vomiting.
	Osteoarthritis *Degeneration of the cartilage that lines the joints*	Pain, swelling, and stiffness in one or more joints; enlargement and distortion of affected joints.
	Osteomyelitis *Infection of bone and bone marrow*	Fever; severe pain in the affected bone; inflammation and swelling of the skin over the affected area; deformity. In children, arrested growth of the affected bone.
	Pneumothorax *Accumulation of air between the two membranes lining the lungs and the chest cavity*	Chest pain that may radiate into the abdomen or shoulder; shortness of breath; dry cough.
	Rheumatoid arthritis	Fatigue and weakness; joint pain, stiffness, and inflammation, especially in the hands, feet, and arms; joint deformity; dry mouth; dry, painful eyes. Morning stiffness.
	Rheumatoid arthritis, juvenile	Fever; rash; abdominal pain; weight loss; swelling, stiffness, and pain in the affected joints; enlarged lymph glands; fatigue; pallor; red, painful eyes.
	Rotator cuff injury	Pain in the shoulder; difficulty raising and lowering the arm; recurring dull ache in the shoulder; pain after sleeping on the shoulder; shoulder weakness.

Shoulder pain *continued*

Associated Symptoms	Possible Diagnosis	Distinguishing Features
	Spondylosis, cervical *Arthritis of the vertebral disks in the neck*	Neck pain and stiffness that spreads to the shoulders, upper arms, hands, or back of the head; numbness or tingling in the arms, hands, and fingers; weakness in the arms and legs; unsteady gait; possible loss of bladder or bowel control.
	Tendinitis *Inflammation of a tendon*	Pain over a tendon anywhere in the body; if involved tendon is near or part of a joint, restricted movement of the joint.

Skin, clammy

Associated Symptoms	Possible Diagnosis	Distinguishing Features
	Anxiety states	Sudden attacks of unreasonable fear and panic; rapid heartbeat or palpitations; perspiration; dry mouth; irritability; muscle tension; trembling; palpitations; shortness of breath; restlessness; poor concentration; insomnia; fatigue; weakness.
	Hypoglycemia *Low blood sugar*	Anxiety; hunger; trembling; headache; palpitations; perspiration; confusion; irritability; loss of coordination; possibly, double vision, seizures, or coma.
	Peripheral vascular disease *Narrowing of blood vessels in the legs or arms*	Muscle pain on one or both legs that occurs with exercise and subsides with rest; possible pain in the fingers, arms, buttocks, lower back, or the arch of the foot; impotence. Severe symptoms include: muscle pain at rest that intensifies at night; discolored or blue toes; cold or numb feet; open sores; heightened sensitivity to cold; weak or absent pulse in the affected limb; scaly or hairless skin over the affected area.

Skin, dry

Associated Symptoms	Possible Diagnosis	Distinguishing Features
	Eczema *Inflammation of the skin*	Itching skin; thickened patches of skin; possibly, with oozing and crusting; in infants, rash on the face, inner elbows, or behind the knees that turns scaly and develops small red pimples that leak; swollen legs (stasis dermatitis).
	Heatstroke	Sudden dizziness; weakness; headache; hot, dry, red skin which later turns grey; high body temperature; muscle cramps; confusion; seizures; loss of consciousness.
	Hypopituitarism *Underactivity of the pituitary gland*	Intolerance to cold; chronic headaches; decreased sex drive; fatigue; dizziness; fine wrinkles around the eyes and mouth; dry skin; extreme thirst and excessive urination; loss of appetite; vaginal dryness; absence of milk production in new mothers; in men, reduced muscular strength, shrinking of the testes, and loss of body hair; growth retardation in children and adolescents.
	Hypothyroidism *Underactivity of the thyroid gland*	Unexplained weight gain; fatigue; muscle weakness; cramps; dry skin; hair loss; deepening of the voice; intolerance for cold; constipation; chest pain; insomnia; puffiness around eyes; loss of sex drive; depression; menstrual abnormalities; possible swelling in the neck.
	Psoriasis	Slightly raised patches of skin with red borders and white-silver scales; joint pain and stiffness; itching; pitted nails.
	Scleroderma	Shiny, tight, and hardened skin, especially on the fingers, arms, and face; hands or feet may successively turn blue, white, and red upon exposure to cold (Raynaud's phenomenon); swallowing difficulty; bloating after eating; weight loss; shortness of breath on exertion; high blood pressure; symptoms of renal failure. Possibly, heartburn, muscle aches and weakness, joint pain, fever, or fatigue.
	Sjögren's syndrome	Dry, itching, burning eyes; sensation of a foreign body under the eyelids; dry mouth; difficulty swallowing; vaginal dryness; dry skin; frequent dental cavities; joint pain; swelling of glands (parotids) in front of the ears; Raynaud's phenomenon.

Skin, mottled

Associated Symptoms	Possible Diagnosis	Distinguishing Features
	Melanoma *Skin cancer*	Change in the appearance of an existing mole including enlargement, bleeding, change in color, development of a black edge. Itching.
	Peripheral vascular disease *Narrowing of blood vessels in the legs or arms*	Muscle pain on one or both legs that occurs with exercise and subsides with rest; possible pain in the fingers, arms, buttocks, lower back, or the arch of the foot; impotence. Severe symptoms include: muscle pain at rest that intensifies at night; discolored or blue toes; cold or numb feet; open sores; heightened sensitivity to cold; weak or absent pulse in the affected limb; scaly or hairless skin over the affected area.
	Polycythemia vera *An overproduction of red and white blood cells and platelets*	Headache; ringing in the ears; blurred vision; flushed skin; itching; dizziness; fatigue; night sweats; frequent nose bleeds and bruises.
	Rheumatoid arthritis	Fatigue and weakness; joint pain, stiffness, and inflammation, especially in the hands, feet, and arms; joint deformity; dry mouth; dry, painful eyes. Morning stiffness.
	Rheumatoid arthritis, juvenile	Fever; rash; abdominal pain; weight loss; swelling, stiffness, and pain in the affected joints; enlarged lymph glands; fatigue; pallor; red, painful eyes.
	Systemic lupus erythematosus *Inflammation of connective tissues throughout the body*	Red, blotchy, butterfly-shaped rash on the cheeks and bridge of the nose; fatigue; fever; loss of appetite and weight; nausea; joint and abdominal pain; headaches; blurred vision; increased sensitivity to sun exposure; depression; psychosis; mental confusion.
	Vitiligo *Loss of skin pigmentation*	White or abnormally pale patches of skin, usually on the face, hands, armpits, and groin.

Skin, red

Associated Symptoms	Possible Diagnosis	Distinguishing Features
	Anaphylaxis	Itching and hives; swelling of the eyes, lips, and tongue; weakness or faintness; tightening in the chest or throat; wheezing; shortness of breath; profuse sweating; palpitations; sudden, intense distress; feelings of impending doom; stomach cramps; nausea, vomiting, or diarrhea; bluish tinge (cyanosis) to the skin, lips, and nail beds due to oxygen insufficiency.
	Candidiasis *Fungal infection of the mouth, genitals, or mucous membranes*	Thick, white discharge from the vagina; itching and irritation in the vaginal area; pain while urinating or during intercourse; in men, inflammation of the head of the penis; possibly, yellow raised patches in the mouth.
	Carcinoid tumors and carcinoid syndrome	May be asymptomatic; flushing or redness of the face and neck; gas and profuse diarrhea; abdominal cramping; watery, swollen eyes; shortness of breath or wheezing.
	Cirrhosis *Chronic damage to the cells of the liver*	No symptoms in early stages; loss of weight and appetite; nausea; swollen legs, ankles and abdomen; itching; jaundice; black stools; vomiting blood; fatigue; impotence; memory loss; confusion.
	Dermatomyositis *Inflammation of the muscles and skin*	Red rash on the neck, upper torso, and upper arms and legs; purple discoloration and swelling of the eyelids; areas of thickened skin; muscle weakness and stiffness, usually in the shoulders and pelvis; cold hands and feet; speaking or swallowing difficulty; weight loss.
	Frostbite	Initially, prickling sensation or numbness in affected area. White or bluish-gray skin that is hard and numb. Thawed skin becomes red, swollen, painful, and blistered. In severe cases, shivering; slurred speech; memory loss.
	Heatstroke	Sudden dizziness; weakness; headache; hot, dry, red skin which later turns grey; high body temperature; muscle cramps; confusion; seizures; loss of consciousness.
	Psoriasis	Slightly raised patches of skin with red borders and white-silver scales; joint pain and stiffness; itching; pitted nails.
	Rheumatoid arthritis	Fatigue and weakness; joint pain, stiffness, and inflammation, especially in the hands, feet, and arms; joint deformity; dry mouth; dry, painful eyes. Morning stiffness.

Skin, red *continued*

Associated Symptoms	Possible Diagnosis	Distinguishing Features
	Ringworm *Fungal skin infection*	A rash with distinct, advancing borders and clear centers; affected areas may have abnormally dark pigmentation; itching; scaly patches of skin; bald patches on scalp; Athlete's foot; red, swollen finger- and toenails.
	Rosacea *Redness, swelling, and blemishes around the nose, cheeks, and forehead*	Facial flushing; stinging, burning, or feeling of skin pulled tight across face; bumps, blemishes, and swelling of nose and cheeks; severe swelling or enlargement of the nose.
	Roseola *Infectious disease primarily affecting children*	Abrupt onset of high fever that usually subsides within four to five days, at which time a rash appears on the torso, and spreads to the limbs, neck, and face. Sore throat; swollen lymph nodes in neck.
	Rubella *German Measles*	Rash on the face that spreads to the torso and limbs; enlargement of lymph nodes in neck; usually preceded by headache, fever, and runny nose.
Systemic lupus erythematosus *Inflammation of connective tissues throughout the body*		Red, blotchy, butterfly-shaped rash on the cheeks and bridge of the nose; fatigue; fever; loss of appetite and weight; nausea; joint and abdominal pain; headaches; blurred vision; increased sensitivity to sun exposure; depression; psychosis; mental confusion.
Toxic shock syndrome		Lethargy; conjunctivitis; confusion; sudden high fever accompanied by nausea, watery diarrhea, sore throat, and headache. Red rash on the palms and soles of the feet, which, after a week or two, begins to peel.

Skin, scaly

Associated Symptoms	Possible Diagnosis	Distinguishing Features
	Eczema *Inflammation of the skin*	Itching skin; thickened patches of skin; possibly, with oozing and crusting; in infants, rash on the face, inner elbows, or behind the knees that turns scaly and develops small red pimples that leak; swollen legs (stasis dermatitis).
	Lymphoma, non–Hodgkin's *Cancer of the lymph nodes and lymphoid tissue*	Painless swelling of lymph nodes in the neck or groin; possible abdominal pain, vomiting of blood, headache.
	Peripheral vascular disease *Narrowing of blood vessels in the legs or arms*	Muscle pain on one or both legs that occurs with exercise and subsides with rest; possible pain in the fingers, arms, buttocks, lower back, or the arch of the foot; impotence. Severe symptoms include: muscle pain at rest that intensifies at night; discolored or blue toes; cold or numb feet; open sores; heightened sensitivity to cold; weak or absent pulse in the affected limb; scaly or hairless skin over the affected area.
	Psoriasis	Slightly raised patches of skin with red borders and white-silver scales; joint pain and stiffness; itching; pitted nails.
	Ringworm *Fungal skin infection*	A rash with distinct, advancing borders and clear centers; affected areas may have abnormally dark pigmentation; itching; scaly patches of skin; bald patches on scalp; Athlete's foot; red, swollen finger- and toenails.
	Scabies	Tiny, grey, scaly blisters—usually on the wrists, genitals, armpits, or between the fingers—that rupture easily when scratched; severe itching; red lumps or rashes may develop.
	Sjögren's syndrome	Dry, itching, burning eyes; sensation of a foreign body under the eyelids; dry mouth; difficulty swallowing; vaginal dryness; dry skin; frequent dental cavities; joint pain; swelling of glands (parotids) in front of the ears; Raynaud's phenomenon.
	Systemic lupus erythematosus *Inflammation of connective tissues throughout the body*	Red, blotchy, butterfly-shaped rash on the cheeks and bridge of the nose; fatigue; fever; loss of appetite and weight; nausea; joint and abdominal pain; headaches; blurred vision; increased sensitivity to sun exposure; depression; psychosis; mental confusion.
	Varicose veins	Blue or purplish, knotted veins, usually in the legs; itching or discomfort in the affected area; swollen feet and ankles. Possible scaly skin, muscle cramps, or skin ulcers.

Sneezing

Associated Symptoms	Possible Diagnosis	Distinguishing Features
	Allergic rhinitis *Hay fever*	Nasal congestion; frequent sneezing; itchy eyes, nose, and throat.
	Anaphylaxis	Itching and hives; swelling of the eyes, lips, and tongue; weakness or faintness; tightening in the chest or throat; wheezing; shortness of breath; profuse sweating; palpitations; sudden, intense distress; feelings of impending doom; stomach cramps; nausea, vomiting, or diarrhea; bluish tinge (cyanosis) to the skin, lips, and nail beds due to oxygen insufficiency.
	Common cold	Nasal congestion; watery eyes; sneezing; sore throat; cough; muscle aches; mild headache; listlessness; possibly, low-grade fever.
	Pleurisy and Pleural effusion *Inflammation of the membranes lining the lungs and chest cavity*	Sudden chest pain worse on inspiration that may also radiate into the shoulder or abdomen; rapid breathing; coughing; sneezing; possibly, fever.
	Whooping cough	Initially, mild cough, sneezing, nasal congestion, and irritated eyes. Within approximately two weeks, cough becomes severe and persistent, and is accompanied by characteristic high-pitched "whooping" sound during inhalation; loss of appetite; listlessness; vomiting or choking spells. Most common among young children.

Snoring, heavy

Associated Symptoms	Possible Diagnosis	Distinguishing Features
	Common cold	Nasal congestion; watery eyes; sneezing; sore throat; cough; muscle aches; mild headache; listlessness; possibly, low-grade fever.
	Obesity	Symptoms such as chest pain or shortness of breath from heart disease, knee or hip pain, or abdominal pain from gallstones all result from the complications of obesity.
	Sinusitis *Inflammation of the mucous membranes lining the sinuses*	Throbbing pain above or below one or both eyes that intensifies when bending the head forward or coughing; nasal congestion; loss of sense of smell; often, pus-like nasal discharge; possible dental pain in the upper jaw; fever.
	Sleep apnea *Recurrent episodes of breathing cessation during sleep*	Loud snoring; morning fatigue and headache; sleep disturbances; daytime sleepiness; difficulty concentrating; memory loss. Most common among overweight men.

Sore throat

Associated Symptoms	Possible Diagnosis	Distinguishing Features
with cough	Chronic fatigue syndrome	Severe fatigue made worse by exercise; recurrent flu-like symptoms; persistent sore throat; low-grade fever; muscle and joint aches; headache; painful, swollen lymph nodes; depression and mental confusion; memory loss; sleep difficulties.
	Common cold	Nasal congestion; watery eyes; sneezing; sore throat; cough; muscle aches; mild headache; listlessness; possibly, low-grade fever.
	Influenza *Flu*	Chills, muscle aches, and loss of appetite followed by a cough, sore throat, nasal congestion, and fever; possible chest pain.
	Laryngeal cancer	Initially, hoarseness, sore throat, and swallowing difficulty; later, pain when swallowing; swelling in the neck.
	Laryngitis	Hoarseness that often progresses to loss of the voice; throat pain; dry cough; possible fever.
	Measles	Cough; fever; watery nasal discharge; loss of appetite; red, watering eyes; sore throat; body aches; red, slightly itchy rash that gradually spreads all over the body.
without cough	Epiglottitis *Inflammation of the epiglottis, the flap of tissue lying behind the tongue*	Sore throat; sudden fever; breathing difficulty which may become severe within hours of onset; pain or difficulty swallowing; muffled speech; hoarseness; drooling.
	Gingivitis	Red-purple gums that are swollen, shiny, and bleed easily; bad breath.
	Mononucleosis, infectious	Headache; high fever; swollen glands in the neck, groin, and armpits; severe sore throat; swallowing difficulty.
	Peritonsillar abscess *A collection of pus between the tonsils and surrounding tissue due to infection*	Sore throat; severe pain when swallowing; fever; headache; impaired speech; drooling; swollen glands in the neck.
	Pharyngitis *Inflammation of the pharynx, the part of the throat between the mouth and the esophagus*	Sore or red throat; speaking and swallowing difficulties; sensitive, swollen glands in the neck; fever; headache; possible earache.
	Poliomyelitis *Polio*	Low fever; sore throat; headache; nausea and vomiting. In severe cases, paralysis without loss of sensation; stiff neck and back; twitching; swallowing and breathing difficulty; drooling.

Sore throat *continued*

Associated Symptoms	Possible Diagnosis	Distinguishing Features
without cough *continued*	Roseola *Infectious disease primarily affecting children*	Abrupt onset of high fever that usually subsides within four to five days, at which time a rash appears on the torso, and spreads to the limbs, neck, and face. Sore throat; swollen lymph nodes in neck.
	Sinusitis *Inflammation of the mucous membranes lining the sinuses*	Throbbing pain above or below one or both eyes that intensifies when bending the head forward or coughing; nasal congestion; loss of sense of smell; often, pus-like nasal discharge; possible dental pain in the upper jaw; fever.
	Strep infection	Symptoms depend on the location and nature of the specific infection, but may include fever, headaches, swollen lymph glands, fatigue, loss of appetite, nasal discharge, red skin rash.
	Tonsillitis	Sore, inflamed throat; swallowing difficulty; headache; swollen glands in the neck; fever; loss of voice. In children, nausea, vomiting, and abdominal pain.

Sore tongue

Associated Symptoms	Possible Diagnosis	Distinguishing Features
	Anemia, folic acid deficiency	Fatigue and weakness; pallor; shortness of breath, heart palpitations, or noticeably rapid heartbeat on exertion; sore, red, and glazed looking tongue; loss of weight and appetite; nausea and diarrhea; abdominal distention.
	Anemia, iron deficiency	Fatigue and weakness; pallor; shortness of breath and heart palpitations on exertion; irritability or inability to concentrate; sore tongue or tiny cracks at the corners of the mouth; black, tarry or bloody stools; unusual craving for dirt, paint, or ice.
	Anemia, pernicious	Fatigue; inability to concentrate; sore, red tongue; weakness; dizziness; pallor; shortness of breath on exertion; palpitations; numbness and tingling in extremities; incoordination; headache; loss of weight and appetite; possibly, jaundice.
	Canker sores	Small, painful, white or gray, crater-like, red-rimmed ulcers in the gums, tongue, or lips.
	Dry mouth	Dry or burning sensation in the mouth; difficulty chewing, swallowing, and speaking; possibly, cracked lips, changes in the tongue's surface, mouth ulcers, changes in taste perception, or tooth decay.
	Salivary gland disorders	Swollen, painful glands behind the ear or under the tongue; soft, painful, swollen glands in the neck; bitter taste in the mouth; fever; dry mouth; increased number of dental cavities; difficulty swallowing.
	Tongue disorders	Symptoms vary depending on the specific disorder and include: dark or bright red, black, or dark brown tongue; sore, swollen, or smooth tongue; hair-like growths on the tongue; adjacent areas of the mouth may be inflamed; ulcers or raised, white patches on the tongue; excessive salivation; swallowing difficulty; bad breath.

Speaking difficulty

Associated Symptoms	Possible Diagnosis	Distinguishing Features
with numbness/ paralysis	Amyotrophic lateral sclerosis *Progressive degeneration of nerve cells of the central nervous system*	Progressive loss of strength and coordination in the limbs; muscle twitching and cramps that begin in the hands and spread to the arms, shoulders, and legs; stiff, clumsy gait; swallowing, breathing, or speaking difficulty; weight loss; drooling; involuntary laughing or crying.
	Brain abscess	Headaches; drowsiness; nausea; vomiting; fever; seizures; possible partial paralysis; confusion; speaking difficulty.
	Brain hemorrhage	Sudden loss of consciousness; sudden, severe headache; mental confusion; stiff neck; nausea and vomiting; paralysis on one side of the face or body; weakness and dizziness; loss of speech; blurred or double vision; dilated pupils.
	Brain tumors	Headaches that become more severe when reclining; nausea and vomiting; memory loss; double vision; muscle weakness; numbness, tingling, or partial paralysis; vision loss; speech disturbances; seizures; drowsiness.
	Encephalitis *Inflammation of the brain*	Initially, headache and fever followed by confusion, hallucinations, and paralysis on one side of the body; memory loss; difficulty with speech and eye movements; drowsiness; possible coma or epileptic seizures; loss of hearing; sensitivity to light; stiff neck.
	Hypothermia *Low body temperature (below 94°)*	Shivering; pallor; puffy face; fatigue and confusion; slow, shallow breathing; muscle stiffness; normally warm areas of the body are cold; loss of consciousness.
	Multiple sclerosis *Gradual degeneration of the protective sheaths surrounding the nerves within the brain and spinal cord*	Symptoms may appear suddenly and then disappear; persistent symptoms may take years to develop and include numbness or tingling in any part of the body, weakness in the extremities, an unsteady walk, slurred speech, urinary incontinence, fatigue, depression, temporary loss of vision, double or blurred vision, mental confusion, and memory loss.
	Stroke	Symptoms vary with the location of brain injury. Sudden onset of weakness, paralysis, or loss of sensation, usually on one side of the body; a sudden heaviness in a limb; speech abnormalities; headache; vision disturbances; dizziness; confusion; coma; urinary and fecal incontinence.
	Transient ischemic attack *Temporary blockage in an artery supplying the brain*	Weakness or numbness in a limb; slurred speech; short-lived, temporary partial blindness; numbness and tingling; speech difficulties; confusion; dizziness.

Speaking difficulty *continued*

Associated Symptoms	Possible Diagnosis	Distinguishing Features
without numbness/ paralysis	Botulism	Difficulty swallowing and speaking; nausea; vomiting; blurred or double vision.
	Concussion	Brief loss of consciousness following a blow to the head. Occasionally causes nausea and vomiting.
	Dermatomyositis *Inflammation of the muscles and skin*	Red rash on the neck, upper torso, and upper arms and legs; purple discoloration and swelling of the eyelids; areas of thickened skin; muscle weakness and stiffness, usually in the shoulders and pelvis; cold hands and feet; speaking or swallowing difficulty; weight loss.
	Dry mouth	Dry or burning sensation in the mouth; difficulty chewing, swallowing, and speaking; possibly, cracked lips, changes in the tongue's surface, mouth ulcers, changes in taste perception, or tooth decay.
	Epiglottitis *Inflammation of the epiglottis, the flap of tissue lying behind the tongue*	Sore throat; sudden fever; breathing difficulty which may become severe within hours of onset; pain or difficulty swallowing; muffled speech; hoarseness; drooling.
	Hydrocephalus *Overaccumulation of cerebrospinal fluid, the liquid surrounding the brain*	In infants, an enlarged head, rigidity of the legs, irritability, projectile vomiting, drowsiness, seizures, and lethargy. In older persons, headache, vomiting, loss of coordination, deterioration of mental faculties, speech difficulty, and loss of appetite.
	Jaw dislocation or fracture	Inability to close the jaw normally; painful, swollen, or numb jaw; misalignment of teeth; speaking difficulty; possible breathing difficulty.
	Myasthenia gravis *Nerve degeneration causing gradual loss of voluntary muscle control*	Drooping eyelids; double or blurred vision; muscle weakness especially in the face, throat, and neck; chewing and swallowing difficulties; possible breathing difficulty. Slurred, nasal-sounding speech.
	Parkinson's disease *Degeneration of the basal ganglia, a cluster of nerve cells in the brain*	Tremors in the hands; stiffness and weakness; impaired voluntary movement; shuffling gait; stooped posture; unblinking, fixed expression; possibly, slow, hesitant speech; difficulty swallowing; drooling; depression. Tremors occur at rest (not with voluntary movements) and disappear during sleep.
	Peritonsillar abscess *A collection of pus between the tonsils and surrounding tissue due to infection*	Sore throat; severe pain when swallowing; fever; headache; impaired speech; drooling; swollen glands in the neck.

Speaking difficulty *continued*

Associated Symptoms	Possible Diagnosis	Distinguishing Features
without numbness/ paralysis *continued*	Schizophrenia	Delusions; hallucinations; rambling, nonsensical, or minimal speech; extremely disorganized behavior; inappropriate emotional responses or emotional detachment; lack of willful movement.
	Tongue disorders	Symptoms vary depending on the specific disorder and include: dark or bright red, black, or dark brown tongue; sore, swollen, or smooth tongue; hair-like growths on the tongue; adjacent areas of the mouth may be inflamed; ulcers or raised, white patches on the tongue; excessive salivation; swallowing difficulty; bad breath.

Stool, abnormal appearance

Associated Symptoms	Possible Diagnosis	Distinguishing Features
	Amebiasis *Parasitic infection*	Usually asymptomatic; possibly, diarrhea; loose stools may contain mucus and blood; abdominal cramps; fatigue; weight loss; gas and flatulence. In severe cases, large amount of bloody stools daily; fever, nausea and vomiting, and abdominal tenderness.
	Anemia, iron deficiency	Fatigue and weakness; pallor; shortness of breath and heart palpitations on exertion; irritability or inability to concentrate; sore tongue or tiny cracks at the corners of the mouth; black, tarry or bloody stools; unusual craving for dirt, paint, or ice.
	Cirrhosis *Chronic damage to the cells of the liver*	No symptoms in early stages; loss of weight and appetite; nausea; swollen legs, ankles and abdomen; itching; jaundice; black stools; vomiting blood; fatigue; impotence; memory loss; confusion.
	Colorectal cancer *A growth of malignant cells in the colon or rectum*	Change in bowel habits; diarrhea; constipation; narrow stools; bloody or dark stools; lower abdominal pain; bloating; cramps; gas; loss of weight and appetite; fatigue and heart palpitations due to anemia.
	Constipation, chronic	Infrequent and possibly painful bowel movements; straining during bowel movements; hard, dry stool; abdominal swelling; continued sensation of fullness after evacuating bowels.
	Diarrhea, acute	Loose, watery stools; increased frequency of bowel movements; abdominal cramping and pain. In infants, possibly drowsiness, slack skin, dry, sticky mouth and tongue, or persistent crying.
	Disseminated intravascular coagulation *Bleeding disorder marked by excessive and inappropriate blood coagulation*	Abnormal bleeding possibly at several sites at once; vomiting blood; bloody or black stools; abnormal vaginal bleeding; blood in the urine; severe abdominal or back pain; possibly, convulsions, or coma.
	Gallbladder disorders	Moderate to severe pain in the upper right side of the abdomen, chest, upper back, or right shoulder. Pain often follows the ingestion of high-fat foods and is episodic, lasting 20 minutes to several hours. Nausea and vomiting; low-grade fever; belching; heartburn; gas; possibly, jaundice, pale stools, and itchy skin.
	Hepatitis, acute viral	Fever; fatigue; loss of appetite; aching muscles and joints; abdominal pain or discomfort; jaundice; dark urine and pale stools.

Stool, abnormal appearance *continued*

Associated Symptoms	Possible Diagnosis	Distinguishing Features
	Hepatitis, chronic	Fatigue; nausea; vomiting; loss of appetite; jaundice; dark urine; clay-colored stools; depression; pain or discomfort in the upper right abdomen; abdominal swelling; fever; in women, cessation of menstruation, acne, and the appearance of male pattern facial hair.
	Malabsorption, digestive *A failure of the small intestine* *to absorb nutrients in the diet*	Diarrhea; weight loss; yellowish, foul-smelling stools; abdominal cramps, gas, and bloating; weakness and lethargy.
	Peptic ulcer	Intermittent, burning or gnawing pain in the upper abdomen or lower chest; indigestion; loss of appetite and weight. Pain may be relieved by eating or antacids. Possible nausea and vomiting. Black, tarry stools, vomiting blood.
	Platelet function disorders	Minor bleeding in the mouth or just beneath the surface of the skin, often appearing as clusters of small, pinpoint-sized red specks; frequent nosebleeds; easy bruising; prolonged menstrual periods; fatigue; pallor; dark-colored stools.
	Stomach cancer	Discomfort in the upper abdomen; black, tarry stools; vomiting of blood; loss of appetite and weight; vomiting after meals.
	Tapeworm infestation	Often asymptomatic. Unexplained weight loss; presence of white eggs or ribbon-like segments of worm in the stool, bedding, or clothing; symptoms of pernicious anemia.

Swallowing difficulty

Associated Symptoms	Possible Diagnosis	Distinguishing Features
	Amyloidosis *Accumulation of amyloid, a waxy substance, in tissues and organs*	Symptoms vary greatly depending on the body parts affected and may include fatigue and weakness; weight loss; heart palpitations; shortness of breath; swelling of the legs; difficulty swallowing due to swelling of the tongue; diarrhea; abdominal pain; raised spots on the armpits, groin, face, and neck; numbness or tingling of the hands or feet; dizziness on standing; joint pains.
	Aortic aneurysm *A sac-like ballooning at a weak spot in the wall of the aorta, the body's primary artery*	Usually asymptomatic; occasionally, severe abdominal and back pain; chest pain; swallowing difficulty; dizziness and fainting; hoarseness; cough.
	Botulism	Difficulty swallowing and speaking; nausea; vomiting; blurred or double vision.
	Dermatomyositis *Inflammation of the muscles and skin*	Red rash on the neck, upper torso, and upper arms and legs; purple discoloration and swelling of the eyelids; areas of thickened skin; muscle weakness and stiffness, usually in the shoulders and pelvis; cold hands and feet; speaking or swallowing difficulty; weight loss.
	Dry mouth	Dry or burning sensation in the mouth; difficulty chewing, swallowing, and speaking; possibly, cracked lips, changes in the tongue's surface, mouth ulcers, changes in taste perception, or tooth decay.
	Epiglottitis *Inflammation of the epiglottis, the flap of tissue lying behind the tongue*	Sore throat; sudden fever; breathing difficulty which may become severe within hours of onset; pain or difficulty swallowing; muffled speech; hoarseness; drooling.
	Esophageal cancer	Swallowing difficulty and pain; weight loss; drooling; possibly, vomiting or coughing up of bloody mucus, regurgitation of food; chest pain; repeated respiratory infections.
	Gastroesophageal reflux *Heartburn*	Burning sensation in the middle of the chest; pain and difficulty swallowing; slight regurgitation of stomach's contents into the mouth, especially when reclining or bending forward; mild abdominal pain.
	Goiter *A swelling of the thyroid gland*	A swelling in the neck that can vary from a small lump to a huge growth. Possible breathing or swallowing difficulties. Can be associated with symptoms of hyper- or hypothyroidism.
	Laryngeal cancer	Initially, hoarseness, sore throat, and swallowing difficulty; later, pain when swallowing; swelling in the neck.

Swallowing difficulty *continued*

Associated Symptoms	Possible Diagnosis	Distinguishing Features
	Laryngitis	Hoarseness that often progresses to loss of the voice; throat pain; dry cough; possible fever.
	Neuralgia *Pain due to nerve damage or irritation*	Symptoms vary depending on the area affected and include: recurring episodes of sharp pain on one side of the lips, gums, cheek, or chin; radiating pain around the eyes; a burning pain along the path of a nerve encircling the torso. Pain may last from a few seconds to several minutes and always affects the same location. Attacks may occur several times a day for weeks with asymptomatic periods of weeks or months in between and may be triggered by touching or blowing on the affected area. Mouth pain may be exacerbated by talking, eating, or swallowing.
	Oral cancers	Sore in the mouth that bleeds and does not heal; lump in the cheek; white or red patch on the gums; swallowing and chewing difficulties; numbness of the tongue; swelling of the jaw.
	Parkinson's disease *Degeneration of the basal ganglia, a cluster of nerve cells in the brain*	Tremors in the hands; stiffness and weakness; impaired voluntary movement; shuffling gait; stooped posture; unblinking, fixed expression; possibly, slow, hesitant speech; difficulty swallowing; drooling; depression. Tremors occur at rest (not with voluntary movements) and disappear during sleep.
	Sjögren's syndrome	Dry, itching, burning eyes; sensation of a foreign body under the eyelids; dry mouth; difficulty swallowing; vaginal dryness; dry skin; frequent dental cavities; joint pain; swelling of glands (parotids) in front of the ears; Raynaud's phenomenon.
	Stomach cancer	Discomfort in the upper abdomen; black, tarry stools; vomiting of blood; loss of appetite and weight; vomiting after meals.
	Tetanus	Often, lockjaw; stiffness and, later, muscle spasms in the neck and face; drooling; abdominal and back pain; extreme perspiration; swallowing difficulty; possible convulsions; fever.
	Thyroid cancer	Painless lump in the front of the neck; possibly, swallowing or breathing difficulty; hoarseness or loss of voice; enlarged lymph nodes in the neck.
	Thyroid nodules	Usually painless lump in the front of the neck; possibly, breathing or swallowing difficulty.

Swallowing difficulty *continued*

Associated Symptoms	Possible Diagnosis	Distinguishing Features
	Thyroiditis *Inflammation of the thyroid gland*	Pain in the front of the neck and, often, the ear; possibly fever, weight loss, and fatigue; general feeling of being unwell (malaise); discomfort on swallowing.
	Tongue disorders	Symptoms vary depending on the specific disorder and include: dark or bright red, black, or dark brown tongue; sore, swollen, or smooth tongue; hair-like growths on the tongue; adjacent areas of the mouth may be inflamed; ulcers or raised, white patches on the tongue; excessive salivation; swallowing difficulty; bad breath.
	Tooth abscess	Persistent tooth pain; pain when biting or chewing; difficulty swallowing; swollen glands in the neck; earache; fever; possibly, foul taste in the mouth or bad breath.
	Wilson's disease *An accumulation of copper in the liver, brain, and other tissues*	Anemia; fluid accumulation in the abdomen; vomiting blood; progressive intellectual impairment; tremor; weakness; walking difficulty; rigidity of limbs; personality changes; speech difficulties; dementia.
with headache	Mononucleosis, infectious	Headache; high fever; swollen glands in the neck, groin, and armpits; severe sore throat; swallowing difficulty.
	Mumps	Pain in the ear, below the ear, and in the jaw; swollen glands in the neck; headache; pain on swallowing and chewing; sore muscles; joint pain; loss of appetite. Testicular swelling and tenderness in adults.
	Peritonsillar abscess *A collection of pus between the tonsils and surrounding tissue due to infection*	Sore throat; severe pain when swallowing; fever; headache; impaired speech; drooling; swollen glands in the neck.
	Pharyngitis *Inflammation of the pharynx, the part of the throat between the mouth and the esophagus*	Sore or red throat; speaking and swallowing difficulties; sensitive, swollen glands in the neck; fever; headache; possible earache.
	Poliomyelitis *Polio*	Low fever; sore throat; headache; nausea and vomiting. In severe cases, paralysis without loss of sensation; stiff neck and back; twitching; swallowing and breathing difficulty; drooling.
	Rabies	Low-grade fever; headache; loss of appetite; difficulty swallowing; tingling at site of animal bite; intense thirst exacerbated by the inability to drink without violent, painful throat spasms; paralysis of facial muscles; drooling. Agitation and violent behavior, confusion, convulsions, coma.

Swallowing difficulty *continued*

Associated Symptoms	Possible Diagnosis	Distinguishing Features
with headache *continued*	Strep infection	Symptoms depend on the location and nature of the specific infection, but may include fever, headaches, swollen lymph glands, fatigue, loss of appetite, nasal discharge, red skin rash.
	Tonsillitis	Sore, inflamed throat; swallowing difficulty; headache; swollen glands in the neck; fever; loss of voice. In children, nausea, vomiting, and abdominal pain.
with shortness of breath	Amyotrophic lateral sclerosis *Progressive degeneration of nerve cells of the central nervous system*	Progressive loss of strength and coordination in the limbs; muscle twitching and cramps that begin in the hands and spread to the arms, shoulders, and legs; stiff, clumsy gait; swallowing, breathing, or speaking difficulty; weight loss; drooling; involuntary laughing or crying.
	Anaphylaxis	Itching and hives; swelling of the eyes, lips, and tongue; weakness or faintness; tightening in the chest or throat; wheezing; shortness of breath; profuse sweating; palpitations; sudden, intense distress; feelings of impending doom; stomach cramps; nausea, vomiting, or diarrhea; bluish tinge (cyanosis) to the skin, lips, and nail beds due to oxygen insufficiency.
	Esophageal stricture *Narrowing of the esophagus, the passageway from the mouth to the stomach*	Sudden or gradual decrease in the ability to swallow solid food or liquids; chest pain after eating; regurgitation of food and liquids; increased salivation; weight loss. Aspiration into lungs can cause cough, wheezing, shortness of breath.
	Myasthenia gravis *Nerve degeneration causing gradual loss of voluntary muscle control*	Drooping eyelids; double or blurred vision; muscle weakness especially in the face, throat, and neck; chewing and swallowing difficulties; possible breathing difficulty. Slurred, nasal-sounding speech.
	Scleroderma	Shiny, tight, and hardened skin, especially on the fingers, arms, and face; hands or feet may successively turn blue, white, and red upon exposure to cold (Raynaud's phenomenon); swallowing difficulty; bloating after eating; weight loss; shortness of breath on exertion; high blood pressure; symptoms of renal failure. Possibly, heartburn, muscle aches and weakness, joint pain, fever, or fatigue.

Sweating, profuse

Associated Symptoms	Possible Diagnosis	Distinguishing Features
with shortness of breath *continued*	Anxiety states	Sudden attacks of unreasonable fear and panic; rapid heartbeat or palpitations; perspiration; dry mouth; irritability; muscle tension; trembling; palpitations; shortness of breath; restlessness; poor concentration; insomnia; fatigue; weakness.
	Congestive heart failure	Shortness of breath; fatigue; need to sleep on several pillows; weakness; cough; heart palpitations; swelling in the legs, ankles, and abdomen; frequent urination at night; indigestion; nausea and vomiting; loss of appetite.
	Empyema *Collection of pus in any body cavity, usually between the membranes covering the lungs*	Chest pain exacerbated by deep inhalation; shortness of breath; dry cough; fever and chills; exhaustion; weight loss; night sweats; abdominal pain and jaundice.
	Lung abscess	Cough producing foul-smelling sputum; bad breath; fever; chills; weight loss; possible chest pain.
	Myocardial infarction *Heart attack*	Sudden chest pain or pressure that may spread to the arm, shoulder and jaw; excessive perspiration; shortness of breath. Possible nausea and vomiting.
	Pneumonia	High fever; shortness of breath; cough with sputum; chest pain; fatigue.
without shortness of breath	Acromegaly *Overproduction of growth hormone by the pituitary gland*	In adults (acromegaly): Gradual thickening of the bones of the face, jaw, and the extremities in adults; oily skin; severe headache; excessive hair growth; excessive perspiration; joint pains. In children (in which the disease is called gigantism): Rapid growth and unusual height; possibly, blindness.
	AIDS *Acquired immunodeficiency syndrome*	Recurrent infections affecting the skin and respiratory system; cough; shortness of breath; loss of appetite; weight loss; fatigue; diarrhea; fever; dementia; malignant skin lesions; swollen lymph glands throughout the body; purplish skin nodules; memory loss; confusion; personality changes.
	Hyperthyroidism *Overactivity of the thyroid gland*	Protruding eyes; weight loss despite increased appetite; intolerance to heat; excessive perspiration; nervousness or restlessness; possibly, swelling in the neck (goiter); palpitations; tremor; diarrhea.
	Hypoglycemia *Low blood sugar*	Anxiety; hunger; trembling; headache; palpitations; perspiration; confusion; irritability; loss of coordination; possibly, double vision, seizures, or coma.

Sweating, profuse *continued*

Associated Symptoms	Possible Diagnosis	Distinguishing Features
without shortness of breath *continued*	Malaria	Initially, severe chills and shivering. In later stages, extremely high fever followed by a period of profuse perspiration as fever subsides; headache, sometimes severe; vomiting.
	Ménière's disease *Dysfunction of structures in the inner ear*	Sudden attack of severe vertigo; nausea and vomiting; impaired sense of balance; ringing in the ears; hearing loss in the affected ear. Jerky movements of the eyes.
	Pheochromocytoma *Tumor in central part of the adrenal, the glands above the kidneys*	Headaches, sometimes severe; rapid heartbeat or heart palpitations; excessive perspiration; faintness, especially when standing up; chest pain; abdominal pain; constipation; weight loss; nervousness, irritability, or anxiety; mental confusion or psychosis.
	Renal vein thrombosis *Blood clot in the vein leaving the kidney*	Severe lower back and flank pain, swelling of legs and face from edema.
	Tetanus	Often, lockjaw; stiffness and, later, muscle spasms in the neck and face; drooling; abdominal and back pain; extreme perspiration; swallowing difficulty; possible convulsions; fever.
	Tuberculosis	Often, asymptomatic. Possibly, low-grade fever; excessive perspiration; cough producing sputum or blood; weight loss; chronic fatigue; chest pain; shortness of breath; night sweats.

Swelling, face and neck

Associated Symptoms	Possible Diagnosis	Distinguishing Features
	Acromegaly *Overproduction of growth hormone by the pituitary gland*	In adults (acromegaly): Gradual thickening of the bones of the face, jaw, and the extremities in adults; oily skin; severe headache; excessive hair growth; excessive perspiration; joint pains. In children (in which the disease is called gigantism): Rapid growth and unusual height; possibly, blindness.
	Anaphylaxis	Itching and hives; swelling of the eyes, lips, and tongue; weakness or faintness; tightening in the chest or throat; wheezing; shortness of breath; profuse sweating; palpitations; sudden, intense distress; feelings of impending doom; stomach cramps; nausea, vomiting, or diarrhea; bluish tinge (cyanosis) to the skin, lips, and nail beds due to oxygen insufficiency.
	Cushing's syndrome	Red, oval-shaped face; humped upper back and obese trunk; acne; purple stretch marks on the abdomen, thighs, and breasts; thin and easily bruised skin; easily fractured bones; depression or euphoria; insomnia; fatigue; muscle weakness; hirsutism (in women).
	Glomerulonephritis, acute *Sudden or intense inflammation of the glomeruli, tiny structures that filter blood in the kidneys*	Blood in the urine; passing only small amounts of urine; swelling of the ankles or the tissues around the eyes; shortness of breath; possibly, fatigue, nausea and vomiting, loss of appetite, headaches, back pain, fever, impaired vision.
	Glomerulonephritis, chronic *Persistent inflammation of the glomeruli, tiny structures that filter blood in the kidneys*	Blood in the urine; passing only small amounts of urine; swelling of the legs or ankles; shortness of breath; possibly, fatigue, nausea and vomiting, loss of appetite, itching, headaches, impaired vision.
	Goiter *A swelling of the thyroid gland*	A swelling in the neck that can vary from a small lump to a huge growth. Possible breathing or swallowing difficulties. Can be associated with symptoms of hyper- or hypothyroidism.
	Hyperthyroidism *Overactivity of the thyroid gland*	Protruding eyes; weight loss despite increased appetite; intolerance to heat; excessive perspiration; nervousness or restlessness; possibly, swelling in the neck (goiter); palpitations; tremor; diarrhea.
	Hypothermia *Low body temperature (below 94°)*	Shivering; pallor; puffy face; fatigue and confusion; slow, shallow breathing; muscle stiffness; normally warm areas of the body are cold; loss of consciousness.

Swelling, face and neck *continued*

Associated Symptoms	Possible Diagnosis	Distinguishing Features
	Hypothyroidism *Underactivity of the thyroid gland*	Unexplained weight gain; fatigue; muscle weakness; cramps; dry skin; hair loss; deepening of the voice; intolerance for cold; constipation; chest pain; insomnia; puffiness around eyes; loss of sex drive; depression; menstrual abnormalities; possible swelling in the neck.
	Laryngeal cancer	Initially, hoarseness, sore throat, and swallowing difficulty; later, pain when swallowing; swelling in the neck.
	Mumps	Pain in the ear, below the ear, and in the jaw; swollen glands in the neck; headache; pain on swallowing and chewing; sore muscles; joint pain; loss of appetite. Testicular swelling and tenderness in adults.
	Nephrotic syndrome *Damage to the filtering units of the kidneys*	Swelling in the ankles and around the eyes; weight gain, due to fluid retention throughout the body; shortness of breath; passing only small amounts of urine that has an unusually foamy appearance; fatigue; diarrhea; loss of appetite.
	Renal vein thrombosis *Blood clot in the vein leaving the kidney*	Severe lower back and flank pain, swelling of legs and face from edema.
	Thyroid cancer	Painless lump in the front of the neck; possibly, swallowing or breathing difficulty; hoarseness or loss of voice; enlarged lymph nodes in the neck.
	Thyroid nodules	Usually painless lump in the front of the neck; possibly, breathing or swallowing difficulty.
	Trichinosis *Parasitic infestation*	Initially, crampy abdominal pain, diarrhea, vomiting, and fever, followed within one to two weeks by swelling around the eyes, muscle aches and tenderness, fever, and weakness. Possibly, coughing up of bloody phlegm; delirium; coma; heart failure symptoms.

Swelling, legs/ankles/feet

Associated Symptoms	Possible Diagnosis	Distinguishing Features
	Cirrhosis *Chronic damage to the cells of the liver*	No symptoms in early stages; loss of weight and appetite; nausea; swollen legs, ankles and abdomen; itching; jaundice; black stools; vomiting blood; fatigue; impotence; memory loss; confusion.
	Eczema *Inflammation of the skin*	Itching skin; thickened patches of skin; possibly, with oozing and crusting; in infants, rash on the face, inner elbows, or behind the knees that turns scaly and develops small red pimples that leak; swollen legs (stasis dermatitis).
	Gout	Most commonly affects the joints of the big toe. Affected joints are red, swollen, hot, and severely painful. In late stages, joint deformity. Kidney stones.
	Renal failure, acute *Severe kidney failure*	Initially, decreased urine output, weight gain and swelling due to edema, loss of appetite, nausea, vomiting, fatigue. If untreated, confusion, seizures, and drowsiness.
	Renal failure, chronic *Persistent, mild kidney failure*	Asymptomatic in early stages. Possibly, mental confusion; shortness of breath; abdominal pain; decreased sex drive; fatigue; muscle and bone pain; numbness in the legs and feet; headache; impaired mental acuity; bad breath.
	Sprains and strains	Swelling, pain or tenderness in the affected joints; impaired joint function.
	Varicose veins	Blue or purplish, knotted veins, usually in the legs; itching or discomfort in the affected area; swollen feet and ankles. Possible scaly skin, muscle cramps, or skin ulcers.
with breathing difficulty/shortness of breath	Amyloidosis *Accumulation of amyloid, a waxy substance, in tissues and organs*	Symptoms vary greatly depending on the body parts affected and may include fatigue and weakness; weight loss; heart palpitations; shortness of breath; swelling of the legs; difficulty swallowing due to swelling of the tongue; diarrhea; abdominal pain; raised spots on the armpits, groin, face, and neck; numbness or tingling of the hands or feet; dizziness on standing; joint pains.
	Cardiomyopathy *Disease of the heart muscle causing a reduction in the force of heart contractions*	Fatigue; chest pain and palpitations; shortness of breath; swelling of the legs; wheezing; cough.
	Chronic obstructive pulmonary disease	Shortness of breath; wheezing; persistent, mucus-producing cough, especially in the morning; possibly, chest pain, swollen legs and ankles.

Swelling, legs/ankles/feet *continued*

Associated Symptoms	Possible Diagnosis	Distinguishing Features
with breathing difficulty/shortness of breath *continued*	Congestive heart failure	Shortness of breath; fatigue; need to sleep on several pillows; weakness; cough; heart palpitations; swelling in the legs, ankles, and abdomen; frequent urination at night; indigestion; nausea and vomiting; loss of appetite.
	Glomerulonephritis, acute *Sudden or intense inflammation of the glomeruli, tiny structures that filter blood in the kidneys*	Blood in the urine; passing only small amounts of urine; swelling of the ankles or the tissues around the eyes; shortness of breath; possibly, fatigue, nausea and vomiting, loss of appetite, headaches, back pain, fever, impaired vision.
	Glomerulonephritis, chronic *Persistent inflammation of the glomeruli, tiny structures that filter blood in the kidneys*	Blood in the urine; passing only small amounts of urine; swelling of the legs or ankles; shortness of breath; possibly, fatigue, nausea and vomiting, loss of appetite, itching, headaches, impaired vision.
	Kidney cysts	Pain or tenderness in the lower back or abdomen; blood in the urine. In infants, symmetrical, protruding masses visible in the flanks.
	Nephrotic syndrome *Damage to the filtering units of the kidneys*	Swelling in the ankles and around the eyes; weight gain, due to fluid retention throughout the body; shortness of breath; passing only small amounts of urine that has an unusually foamy appearance; fatigue; diarrhea; loss of appetite.
	Pericarditis *Inflammation of the membrane surrounding the heart*	Sharp chest pain that may spread to the neck and shoulders; pain may be relieved by sitting up and leaning forward; swollen legs and abdomen; breathing difficulty; chills; fever; fatigue.
	Systemic lupus erythematosus *Inflammation of connective tissues throughout the body*	Red, blotchy, butterfly-shaped rash on the cheeks and bridge of the nose; fatigue; fever; loss of appetite and weight; nausea; joint and abdominal pain; headaches; blurred vision; increased sensitivity to sun exposure; depression; psychosis; mental confusion.
	Valvular heart disease	Depends on which heart valve is affected. Often asymptomatic. Possibly, fatigue and weakness; dizziness; chest pain; shortness of breath; heart palpitations; fainting; edema; stroke from embolism to the brain.

Swollen glands

Associated Symptoms	Possible Diagnosis	Distinguishing Features
	AIDS *Acquired immunodeficiency syndrome*	Recurrent infections affecting the skin and respiratory system; cough; shortness of breath; loss of appetite; weight loss; fatigue; diarrhea; fever; dementia; malignant skin lesions; swollen lymph glands throughout the body; purplish skin nodules; memory loss; confusion; personality changes.
	Canker sores	Small, painful, white or gray, crater-like, red-rimmed ulcers in the gums, tongue, or lips.
	Chronic fatigue syndrome	Severe fatigue made worse by exercise; recurrent flu-like symptoms; persistent sore throat; low-grade fever; muscle and joint aches; headache; painful, swollen lymph nodes; depression and mental confusion; memory loss; sleep difficulties.
	Leukemias	Symptoms vary depending on the type of leukemia and may include: loss of appetite and weight; increased bruising and bleeding; bone pain, especially in the legs; abdominal pain and distention; nausea; heart palpitations; severe fatigue; pallor; breathing difficulty; fever; night sweats; headache; enlarged lymph nodes; joint pains (due to gout).
	Lymphoma, Hodgkin's *Cancer of the lymph nodes and lymphoid tissue*	Painless swelling of the lymph nodes usually in the neck or armpits; loss of appetite; night sweats.
	Lymphoma, non-Hodgkin's *Cancer of the lymph nodes and lymphoid tissue*	Painless swelling of lymph nodes in the neck or groin; possible abdominal pain, vomiting of blood, headache.
	Mononucleosis, infectious	Headache; high fever; swollen glands in the neck, groin, and armpits; severe sore throat; swallowing difficulty.
	Mumps	Pain in the ear, below the ear, and in the jaw; swollen glands in the neck; headache; pain on swallowing and chewing; sore muscles; joint pain; loss of appetite. Testicular swelling and tenderness in adults.
	Peritonsillar abscess *A collection of pus between the tonsils and surrounding tissue due to infection*	Sore throat; severe pain when swallowing; fever; headache; impaired speech; drooling; swollen glands in the neck.
	Pharyngitis *Inflammation of the pharynx, the part of the throat between the mouth and the esophagus*	Sore or red throat; speaking and swallowing difficulties; sensitive, swollen glands in the neck; fever; headache; possible earache.

Swollen glands *continued*

Associated Symptoms	Possible Diagnosis	Distinguishing Features
	Rheumatoid arthritis, juvenile	Fever; rash; abdominal pain; weight loss; swelling, stiffness, and pain in the affected joints; enlarged lymph glands; fatigue; pallor; red, painful eyes.
	Rubella *German Measles*	Rash on the face that spreads to the torso and limbs; enlargement of lymph nodes in neck; usually preceded by headache, fever, and runny nose.
	Salivary gland disorders	Swollen, painful glands behind the ear or under the tongue; soft, painful, swollen glands in the neck; bitter taste in the mouth; fever; dry mouth; increased number of dental cavities; difficulty swallowing.
	Strep infection	Symptoms depend on the location and nature of the specific infection, but may include fever, headaches, swollen lymph glands, fatigue, loss of appetite, nasal discharge, red skin rash.
	Syphilis	Initially, painless, ulcerated, red sore on the genitals, mouth, or rectum; swollen glands in the neck, armpit, or groin; rash with small, red, scaly bumps; fever; headache. If left untreated, damage to heart valves leading to congestive heart failure; mental deterioration; loss of balance; seizures; dementia; personality changes.
	Tonsillitis	Sore, inflamed throat; swallowing difficulty; headache; swollen glands in the neck; fever; loss of voice. In children, nausea, vomiting, and abdominal pain.
	Tooth abscess	Persistent tooth pain; pain when biting or chewing; difficulty swallowing; swollen glands in the neck; earache; fever; possibly, foul taste in the mouth or bad breath.

Testicles, painful or swollen

Associated Symptoms	Possible Diagnosis	Distinguishing Features
	Epididymitis *Inflammation of the coiled sperm conduit that rests on each testicle*	Severe pain and swelling at the back of a testicle; possibly, redness and swelling of the scrotum; burning on urination.
	Mumps	Pain in the ear, below the ear, and in the jaw; swollen glands in the neck; headache; pain on swallowing and chewing; sore muscles; joint pain; loss of appetite. Testicular swelling and tenderness in adults.
	Orchitis *Inflammation of a testicle*	Swelling and severe pain in the affected testicle; possible bloody discharge in the semen; pain during intercourse; fever.
	Renal calculi *Kidney stones*	Intermittent spasms of pain in the back and flanks, radiating through the lower abdomen towards the groin; nausea and vomiting; blood in the urine; urge to urinate but only small amounts of urine are passed.
	Testicular cancer	Firm, usually painless mass, usually in one testicle. In later stages, a dull ache in the groin or lower abdomen may occur. Possibly, male breast development. In advanced cases, swollen lymph glands; abdominal or back pain; weight loss; breathing difficulty.
	Testicular torsion *Twisting of the spermatic cord*	Severe pain and swelling on one side of the scrotum; skin on the scrotum may appear red or purple; light-headedness or fainting; possibly, abdominal pain, nausea and vomiting.
	Varicocele *Varicose veins in the scrotum*	Visibly enlarged, twisted veins in the scrotum; swelling around the testicles, usually on the left side, that may subside when reclining; sensation of heaviness or dragging in the groin; possibly, scrotal pain or discomfort.

Thirst, excessive

Associated Symptoms	Possible Diagnosis	Distinguishing Features
	Diabetes insipidus *Insufficient amounts of antidiuretic hormone, leading to excessive urination and possible dehydration*	Extreme thirst; copious urination. When fluid intake is insufficient, confusion, stupor and coma.
	Diabetes mellitus *Insufficiency of or resistance to insulin*	Fatigue; excessive thirst; frequent urination; weight loss despite increased appetite; blurred vision; numbness and tingling of feet and hands; impotence.
	Hypopituitarism *Underactivity of the pituitary gland*	Intolerance to cold; chronic headaches; decreased sex drive; fatigue; dizziness; fine wrinkles around the eyes and mouth; dry skin; extreme thirst and excessive urination; loss of appetite; vaginal dryness; absence of milk production in new mothers; in men, reduced muscular strength, shrinking of the testes, and loss of body hair; growth retardation in children and adolescents.
	Peritonitis *Inflammation of the abdominal membrane*	Sudden abdominal pain, rigidity, and swelling; chills and fever; weakness; rapid heartbeat; nausea and vomiting; extreme thirst; low urine output.
	Rabies	Low-grade fever; headache; loss of appetite; difficulty swallowing; tingling at site of animal bite; intense thirst exacerbated by the inability to drink without violent, painful throat spasms; paralysis of facial muscles; drooling. Agitation and violent behavior, confusion, convulsions, coma.

Toothache

Associated Symptoms	Possible Diagnosis	Distinguishing Features
	Gingivitis	Red-purple gums that are swollen, shiny, and bleed easily; bad breath.
	Impacted teeth	Gum pain; unpleasant taste in mouth, especially when biting down; red, swollen gums around the affected tooth; headache or jaw ache; possibly, bad breath.
	Neuralgia *Pain due to nerve damage or irritation*	Symptoms vary depending on the area affected and include: recurring episodes of sharp pain on one side of the lips, gums, cheek, or chin; radiating pain around the eyes; a burning pain along the path of a nerve encircling the torso. Pain may last from a few seconds to several minutes and always affects the same location. Attacks may occur several times a day for weeks with asymptomatic periods of weeks or months in between and may be triggered by touching or blowing on the affected area. Mouth pain may be exacerbated by talking, eating, or swallowing.
	Salivary gland disorders	Swollen, painful glands behind the ear or under the tongue; soft, painful, swollen glands in the neck; bitter taste in the mouth; fever; dry mouth; increased number of dental cavities; difficulty swallowing.
	Sinusitis *Inflammation of the mucous membranes lining the sinuses*	Throbbing pain above or below one or both eyes that intensifies when bending the head forward or coughing; nasal congestion; loss of sense of smell; often, pus-like nasal discharge; possible dental pain in the upper jaw; fever.
	Sjögren's syndrome	Dry, itching, burning eyes; sensation of a foreign body under the eyelids; dry mouth; difficulty swallowing; vaginal dryness; dry skin; frequent dental cavities; joint pain; swelling of glands (parotids) in front of the ears; Raynaud's phenomenon.
	Tooth abscess	Persistent tooth pain; pain when biting or chewing; difficulty swallowing; swollen glands in the neck; earache; fever; possibly, foul taste in the mouth or bad breath.
	Tooth decay	Tooth pain, especially after eating sweet or sour foods; tooth sensitivity to hot and cold; bad breath; unpleasant taste in the mouth.

Tremors

Associated Symptoms	Possible Diagnosis	Distinguishing Features
	Anxiety states	Sudden attacks of unreasonable fear and panic; rapid heartbeat or palpitations; perspiration; dry mouth; irritability; muscle tension; trembling; palpitations; shortness of breath; restlessness; poor concentration; insomnia; fatigue; weakness.
	Essential tremor	Involuntary rhythmic shaking of the hands and arms and, less frequently, the head, tongue, larynx, eyelids, or other parts of the body. Tremors intensify during emotional stress and voluntary movements, and cease during periods of rest or sleep. Shaky handwriting; quavering voice.
	Hyperthyroidism *Overactivity of the thyroid gland*	Protruding eyes; weight loss despite increased appetite; intolerance to heat; excessive perspiration; nervousness or restlessness; possibly, swelling in the neck (goiter); palpitations; tremor; diarrhea.
	Multiple sclerosis *Gradual degeneration of the protective sheaths surrounding the nerves within the brain and spinal cord*	Symptoms may appear suddenly and then disappear; persistent symptoms may take years to develop and include numbness or tingling in any part of the body, weakness in the extremities, an unsteady walk, slurred speech, urinary incontinence, fatigue, depression, temporary loss of vision, double or blurred vision, mental confusion, and memory loss.
	Parkinson's disease *Degeneration of the basal ganglia, a cluster of nerve cells in the brain*	Tremors in the hands; stiffness and weakness; impaired voluntary movement; shuffling gait; stooped posture; unblinking, fixed expression; possibly, slow, hesitant speech; difficulty swallowing; drooling; depression. Tremors occur at rest (not with voluntary movements) and disappear during sleep.

Twitching/tics

Associated Symptoms	Possible Diagnosis	Distinguishing Features
with confusion/ memory loss	Brain abscess	Headaches; drowsiness; nausea and vomiting; fever; seizures; possible partial paralysis; confusion; speaking difficulty.
	Brain tumors	Headaches that become more severe when reclining; nausea and vomiting; memory loss; double vision; muscle weakness; numbness, tingling, or partial paralysis; vision loss; speech disturbances; seizures; drowsiness.
	Encephalitis *Inflammation of the brain*	Initially, headache and fever followed by confusion, hallucinations, and paralysis on one side of the body; memory loss; difficulty with speech and eye movements; drowsiness; possible coma or epileptic seizures; loss of hearing; sensitivity to light; stiff neck.
	Hydrocephalus *Overaccumulation of cerebrospinal fluid, the liquid surrounding the brain*	In infants, an enlarged head, rigidity of the legs, irritability, projectile vomiting, drowsiness, seizures, and lethargy. In older persons, headache, vomiting, loss of coordination, deterioration of mental faculties, speech difficulty, and loss of appetite.
	Renal failure, acute *Severe kidney failure*	Initially, decreased urine output, weight gain and swelling due to edema, loss of appetite, nausea and vomiting, fatigue. If untreated, confusion, seizures, and drowsiness.
	Reye's syndrome *Childhood disease marked by brain and liver damage*	Following recovery from an upper respiratory infection, nausea and vomiting; memory loss; confusion or delirium; possible seizures; drowsiness; lethargy.
	Seizures	Involuntary twitching or jerking; muscle rigidity; loss of consciousness; confusion; drooling; hallucinations.
without confusion/ memory loss	Amyotrophic lateral sclerosis *Progressive degeneration of nerve cells of the central nervous system*	Progressive loss of strength and coordination in the limbs; muscle twitching and cramps that begin in the hands and spread to the arms, shoulders, and legs; stiff, clumsy gait; swallowing, breathing, or speaking difficulty; weight loss; drooling; involuntary laughing or crying.
	Hypoparathyroidism *Underactivity of the parathyroid glands*	Numbness and tingling and painful, cramp-like spasms of the face, hands, arms, and feet; cataracts; possible seizures.
	Hypothyroidism *Underactivity of the thyroid gland*	Unexplained weight gain; fatigue; muscle weakness; cramps; dry skin; hair loss; deepening of the voice; intolerance for cold; constipation; chest pain; insomnia; puffiness around eyes; loss of sex drive; depression; menstrual abnormalities; possible swelling in the neck.

Twitching/tics *continued*

Associated Symptoms	Possible Diagnosis	Distinguishing Features
without confusion/ memory loss *continued*	Leukemias	Symptoms vary depending on the type of leukemia and may include: loss of appetite and weight; increased bruising and bleeding; bone pain, especially in the legs; abdominal pain and distention; nausea; heart palpitations; severe fatigue; pallor; breathing difficulty; fever; night sweats; headache; enlarged lymph nodes; joint pains (due to gout).
	Neuralgia *Pain due to nerve damage or irritation*	Symptoms vary depending on the area affected and include: recurring episodes of sharp pain on one side of the lips, gums, cheek, or chin; radiating pain around the eyes; a burning pain along the path of a nerve encircling the torso. Pain may last from a few seconds to several minutes and always affects the same location. Attacks may occur several times a day for weeks with asymptomatic periods of weeks or months in between and may be triggered by touching or blowing on the affected area. Mouth pain may be exacerbated by talking, eating, or swallowing.
	Parkinson's disease *Degeneration of the basal ganglia, a cluster of nerve cells in the brain*	Tremors in the hands; stiffness and weakness; impaired voluntary movement; shuffling gait; stooped posture; unblinking, fixed expression; possibly, slow, hesitant speech; difficulty swallowing; drooling; depression. Tremors occur at rest (not with voluntary movements) and disappear during sleep.
	Poliomyelitis *Polio*	Low fever; sore throat; headache; nausea and vomiting. In severe cases, paralysis without loss of sensation; stiff neck and back; twitching; swallowing and breathing difficulty; drooling.
	Rheumatic fever	Initially, a sore throat that gets better followed, one to six weeks later, by lethargy and fever. Possibly, swollen joints, rash, abdominal pain, involuntary jerky movements, emotional instability.
	Schizophrenia	Delusions; hallucinations; rambling, nonsensical, or minimal speech; extremely disorganized behavior; inappropriate emotional responses or emotional detachment; lack of willful movement.
	Tetanus	Often, lockjaw; stiffness and, later, muscle spasms in the neck and face; drooling; abdominal and back pain; extreme perspiration; swallowing difficulty; possible convulsions; fever.
	Tics	Recurring, involuntary twitch, usually in the face, shoulders, or arms.

Urinary frequency

Associated Symptoms	Possible Diagnosis	Distinguishing Features
	Bladder cancer	Blood in the urine; painful and frequent urination; pelvic pain; feeling of pressure in the back; persistent fever.
	Bladder infection *Cystitis*	Burning during urination; frequent and urgent urination with only small amounts of urine passed; blood in the urine; lower abdominal pain; low-grade fever; pain during sexual intercourse and, in men, during ejaculation.
	Congestive heart failure	Shortness of breath; fatigue; need to sleep on several pillows; weakness; cough; heart palpitations; swelling in the legs, ankles, and abdomen; frequent urination at night; indigestion; nausea and vomiting; loss of appetite.
	Diabetes insipidus *Insufficient amounts of antidiuretic hormone, leading to excessive urination and possible dehydration*	Extreme thirst; copious urination. When fluid intake is insufficient, confusion, stupor and coma.
	Diabetes mellitus *Insufficiency of or resistance to insulin*	Fatigue; excessive thirst; frequent urination; weight loss despite increased appetite; blurred vision; numbness and tingling of feet and hands; impotence.
	Fibroids, uterine *Benign growths of the muscular wall of the uterus*	Heavier or prolonged bleeding during menses; abdominal discomfort; lower back pain; pressure on the bladder and frequent urination; constipation. Possible, sharp, sudden, lower abdominal pain.
	Hypopituitarism *Underactivity of the pituitary gland*	Intolerance to cold; chronic headaches; decreased sex drive; fatigue; dizziness; fine wrinkles around the eyes and mouth; dry skin; extreme thirst and excessive urination; loss of appetite; vaginal dryness; absence of milk production in new mothers; in men, reduced muscular strength, shrinking of the testes, and loss of body hair; growth retardation in children and adolescents.
	Irritable bladder	Sudden, urgent need to urinate; frequent urination.
	Kidney infection *Pyelonephritis*	Sudden fever and shaking chills; severe fatigue; burning and frequent urination; cloudy or bloody urine; pain in the abdomen, back, or flanks, sometimes severe; nausea and vomiting.
	Neurogenic bladder *Inability to control passage of urine due to damage to nerves to the bladder*	Inability to control urine flow which may involuntarily release in large volumes or in a continuous dribbling. Bed-wetting during sleep; feeling the need to urinate though no urine is passed; pain or burning during urination.

Urinary frequency *continued*

Associated Symptoms	Possible Diagnosis	Distinguishing Features
	Pelvic inflammatory disease	Initially, lower pelvic pain; pain during intercourse; irregular menstrual bleeding; vaginal discharge with abnormal color or odor; low-grade fever; chills; frequent urination; fatigue; loss of appetite; later, severe abdominal pain and high fever.
	Prostate cancer	Difficulty urinating; frequent urination with decreased urine output; pain in the pelvic area and lower back; painful ejaculation or bowel movements; impotence.
	Prostatic hyperplasia, benign *Prostate enlargement*	Slow or delayed urination; dribbling urine; the need to urinate several times during the night; possibly, pain during urination; blood in the urine.
	Prostatitis *Inflammation of the prostate gland*	Burning during urination; urgent and frequent urination; fever and chills; discharge from the penis; lower abdominal and back pain; blood in the urine.
	Urethritis *Infection of the urethra, the passageway that drains urine from the bladder*	Frequent and painful urination; blood in the urine; yellow, pus-filled discharge; possible difficulty passing urine; urinary urgency; pain during intercourse; in men, painful ejaculation.
	Uterine prolapse	Often asymptomatic. Possibly, difficulty passing urine or stools, pain during intercourse, backache that intensifies when lifting, sensation of heaviness or dragging within the pelvis, painful or heavy menstrual periods, or bleeding between periods. In severe cases, uterus visibly protrudes outside of vagina.

Urinary pain

Associated Symptoms	Possible Diagnosis	Distinguishing Features
	Bladder cancer	Blood in the urine; painful and frequent urination; pelvic pain; feeling of pressure in the back; persistent fever.
	Bladder infection *Cystitis*	Burning during urination; frequent and urgent urination with only small amounts of urine passed; blood in the urine; lower abdominal pain; low-grade fever; pain during sexual intercourse and, in men, during ejaculation.
	Candidiasis *Fungal infection of the mouth, genitals, or mucous membranes*	Thick, white discharge from the vagina; itching and irritation in the vaginal area; pain while urinating or during intercourse; in men, inflammation of the head of the penis; possibly, yellow raised patches in the mouth.
	Chlamydia *Contagious, infectious disease caused by chlamydia, a group of microorganisms*	Usually asymptomatic; possibly, pain or burning during urination, watery discharge from the penis or vagina, swelling of the testicles, breathing difficulty, cough, high fever, inflammation of the inner lining of the eyelids and the membrane covering the whites of the eyes.
	Epididymitis *Inflammation of the coiled sperm conduit that rests on each testicle*	Severe pain and swelling at the back of a testicle; possibly, redness and swelling of the scrotum; burning on urination.
	Genital herpes	Approximately one week after infection, itching, burning, soreness, and small blisters in the genital area. Blisters later burst, leaving painful ulcers which heal 10 to 20 days later. Possibly, enlarged, painful lymph nodes in the groin; fever, headache, and cold sores around the mouth. In women, pain during urination.
	Gonorrhea	Burning pain during urination; yellowish, pus-like discharge from the penis or vagina; redness or swelling at the infection site; abnormal vaginal bleeding.
	Kidney infection *Pyelonephritis*	Sudden fever and shaking chills; severe fatigue; burning and frequent urination; cloudy or bloody urine; pain in the abdomen, back, or flanks, sometimes severe; nausea and vomiting.
	Neurogenic bladder *Inability to control passage of urine due to damage to nerves to the bladder*	Inability to control urine flow which may involuntarily release in large volumes or in a continuous dribbling. Bed-wetting during sleep; feeling the need to urinate though no urine is passed; pain or burning during urination.
	Penile cancer	Sore, ulcer, or wart-like lump on the penis, usually near the head, possibly painful; bleeding or unusual discharge from the penis. Possibly, pain during urination, or enlarged lymph nodes in the groin.

Urinary pain *continued*

Associated Symptoms	Possible Diagnosis	Distinguishing Features
	Prostatic hyperplasia, benign *Prostate enlargement*	Slow or delayed urination; dribbling urine; the need to urinate several times during the night; possibly, pain during urination; blood in the urine.
	Prostatitis *Inflammation of the prostate gland*	Burning during urination; urgent and frequent urination; fever and chills; discharge from the penis; lower abdominal and back pain; blood in the urine.
	Urethritis *Infection of the urethra,* *the passageway that drains* *urine from the bladder*	Frequent and painful urination; blood in the urine; yellow, pus-filled discharge; possible difficulty passing urine; urinary urgency; pain during intercourse; in men, painful ejaculation.
	Vaginal cancer	Vaginal itching; bleeding after intercourse or between menstrual periods; abnormal vaginal discharge; lesions with thick, raised edges; possibly rectal bleeding; discomfort when urinating or defecating; pain during intercourse; urinary frequency and urgency.
	Vaginitis *Inflammation of the vagina*	Vaginal irritation, itching, and discharge; painful intercourse and minor postcoital bleeding. In later stages, vaginal pain.

Urinary urgency

Associated Symptoms	Possible Diagnosis	Distinguishing Features
	Bladder cancer	Blood in the urine; painful and frequent urination; pelvic pain; feeling of pressure in the back; persistent fever.
	Bladder infection *Cystitis*	Burning during urination; frequent and urgent urination with only small amounts of urine passed; blood in the urine; lower abdominal pain; low-grade fever; pain during sexual intercourse and, in men, during ejaculation.
	Bladder stones	Interruption of urine stream; inability to urinate except in certain positions; frequent and urgent urination with only small amounts of urine passed; blood in the urine; pain in the genitals, lower back, or abdomen; low-grade fever.
	Fibroids, uterine *Benign growths of the muscular wall of the uterus*	Heavier or prolonged bleeding during menses; abdominal discomfort; lower back pain; pressure on the bladder and frequent urination; constipation. Possible, sharp, sudden, lower abdominal pain.
	Irritable bladder	Sudden, urgent need to urinate; frequent urination.
	Kidney infection *Pyelonephritis*	Sudden fever and shaking chills; severe fatigue; burning and frequent urination; cloudy or bloody urine; pain in the abdomen, back, or flanks, sometimes severe; nausea and vomiting.
	Neurogenic bladder *Inability to control passage of urine due to damage to nerves to the bladder*	Inability to control urine flow which may involuntarily release in large volumes or in a continuous dribbling. Bed-wetting during sleep; feeling the need to urinate though no urine is passed; pain or burning during urination.
	Pelvic inflammatory disease	Initially, lower pelvic pain; pain during intercourse; irregular menstrual bleeding; vaginal discharge with abnormal color or odor; low-grade fever; chills; frequent urination; fatigue; loss of appetite; later, severe abdominal pain and high fever.
	Prostate cancer	Difficulty urinating; frequent urination with decreased urine output; pain in the pelvic area and lower back; painful ejaculation or bowel movements; impotence.
	Prostatitis *Inflammation of the prostate gland*	Burning during urination; urgent and frequent urination; fever and chills; discharge from the penis; lower abdominal and back pain; blood in the urine.
	Urethritis *Infection of the urethra, the passageway that drains urine from the bladder*	Frequent and painful urination; blood in the urine; yellow, pus-filled discharge; possible difficulty passing urine; urinary urgency; pain during intercourse; in men, painful ejaculation.

Urine, abnormal appearance or smell

Associated Symptoms	Possible Diagnosis	Distinguishing Features
with pain during urination	Bladder cancer	Blood in the urine; painful and frequent urination; pelvic pain; feeling of pressure in the back; persistent fever.
	Bladder infection *Cystitis*	Burning during urination; frequent and urgent urination with only small amounts of urine passed; blood in the urine; lower abdominal pain; low-grade fever; pain during sexual intercourse and, in men, during ejaculation.
	Bladder stones	Interruption of urine stream; inability to urinate except in certain positions; frequent and urgent urination with only small amounts of urine passed; blood in the urine; pain in the genitals, lower back, or abdomen; low-grade fever.
	Kidney infection *Pyelonephritis*	Sudden fever and shaking chills; severe fatigue; burning and frequent urination; cloudy or bloody urine; pain in the abdomen, back, or flanks, sometimes severe; nausea and vomiting.
	Prostate cancer	Difficulty urinating; frequent urination with decreased urine output; pain in the pelvic area and lower back; painful ejaculation or bowel movements; impotence.
	Renal calculi *Kidney stones*	Intermittent spasms of pain in the back and flanks, radiating through the lower abdomen towards the groin; nausea and vomiting; blood in the urine; urge to urinate but only small amounts of urine are passed.
	Urethritis *Infection of the urethra, the passageway that drains urine from the bladder*	Frequent and painful urination; blood in the urine; yellow, pus-filled discharge; possible difficulty passing urine; urinary urgency; pain during intercourse; in men, painful ejaculation.
	Vaginitis *Inflammation of the vagina*	Vaginal irritation, itching, and discharge; painful intercourse and minor postcoital bleeding. In later stages, vaginal pain.
without pain during urination	Anemia, hemolytic	Fatigue and weakness; shortness of breath on exertion; pallor; heart palpitations; jaundice and dark urine.
	Appendicitis, acute	Pain near the navel, spreading to the lower right abdomen; nausea and vomiting; constipation; possibly diarrhea; low-grade fever; loss of appetite.
	Cirrhosis *Chronic damage to the cells of the liver*	No symptoms in early stages; loss of weight and appetite; nausea; swollen legs, ankles and abdomen; itching; jaundice; black stools; vomiting blood; fatigue; impotence; memory loss; confusion.

Urine, abnormal appearance or smell *continued*

Associated Symptoms	Possible Diagnosis	Distinguishing Features
without pain during urination *continued*	Glomerulonephritis, acute *Sudden or intense inflammation of the glomeruli, tiny structures that filter blood in the kidneys*	Blood in the urine; passing only small amounts of urine; swelling of the ankles or the tissues around the eyes; shortness of breath; possibly, fatigue, nausea and vomiting, loss of appetite, headaches, back pain, fever, impaired vision.
	Glomerulonephritis, chronic *Persistent inflammation of the glomeruli, tiny structures that filter blood in the kidneys*	Blood in the urine; passing only small amounts of urine; swelling of the legs or ankles; shortness of breath; possibly, fatigue, nausea and vomiting, loss of appetite, itching, headaches, impaired vision.
	Hepatitis, acute viral	Fever; fatigue; loss of appetite; aching muscles and joints; abdominal pain or discomfort; jaundice; dark urine and pale stools.
	Kidney cancer	Blood in the urine; abdominal and lower back pain; low-grade fever; loss of weight and appetite.
	Nephrotic syndrome *Damage to the filtering units of the kidneys*	Swelling in the ankles and around the eyes; weight gain, due to fluid retention throughout the body; shortness of breath; passing only small amounts of urine that has an unusually foamy appearance; fatigue; diarrhea; loss of appetite.
	Pancreatic cancer	Often, no symptoms until far advanced. Upper abdominal pain which spreads to the back; loss of weight and appetite; jaundice; nausea, vomiting, and indigestion; diarrhea; fatigue; depression.
	Systemic lupus erythematosus *Inflammation of connective tissues throughout the body*	Red, blotchy, butterfly-shaped rash on the cheeks and bridge of the nose; fatigue; fever; loss of appetite and weight; nausea; joint and abdominal pain; headaches; blurred vision; increased sensitivity to sun exposure; depression; psychosis; mental confusion.

Vaginal bleeding, abnormal

Associated Symptoms	Possible Diagnosis	Distinguishing Features
	Acromegaly *Overproduction of growth hormone by the pituitary gland*	In adults (acromegaly): Gradual thickening of the bones of the face, jaw, and the extremities in adults; oily skin; severe headache; excessive hair growth; excessive perspiration; joint pains. In children (in which the disease is called gigantism): Rapid growth and unusual height; possibly, blindness.
	Cushing's syndrome	Red, oval-shaped face; humped upper back and obese trunk; acne; purple stretch marks on the abdomen, thighs, and breasts; thin and easily bruised skin; easily fractured bones; depression or euphoria; insomnia; fatigue; muscle weakness; hirsutism (in women).
	Hyperprolactinemia *Overproduction of the hormone prolactin by the pituitary gland*	Symptoms may vary depending on gender; in women: cessation of menstrual periods, decreased menstrual flow, excess facial hair; in men: erectile dysfunction, infertility, decreased libido, enlarged breasts; in men and women: abnormal production of breast milk, headaches, decreased vision.
	Hyperthyroidism *Overactivity of the thyroid gland*	Protruding eyes; weight loss despite increased appetite; intolerance to heat; excessive perspiration; nervousness or restlessness; possibly, swelling in the neck (goiter); palpitations; tremor; diarrhea.
	Hypopituitarism *Underactivity of the pituitary gland*	Intolerance to cold; chronic headaches; decreased sex drive; fatigue; dizziness; fine wrinkles around the eyes and mouth; dry skin; extreme thirst and excessive urination; loss of appetite; vaginal dryness; absence of milk production in new mothers; in men, reduced muscular strength, shrinking of the testes, and loss of body hair; growth retardation in children and adolescents.
	Hypothyroidism *Underactivity of the thyroid gland*	Unexplained weight gain; fatigue; muscle weakness; cramps; dry skin; hair loss; deepening of the voice; intolerance for cold; constipation; chest pain; insomnia; puffiness around eyes; loss of sex drive; depression; menstrual abnormalities; possible swelling in the neck.
	Ovarian cancer	Often asymptomatic until widespread. Possibly, abdominal swelling or discomfort, nausea, and vomiting. In advanced stages, excessive hair growth, unexplained weight loss, abnormal menstrual bleeding or postmenopausal bleeding; urinary frequency.
	Ovarian cysts	In many cases, no symptoms. Painless swelling in the lower abdomen; possibly, pain during intercourse; brown vaginal discharge; lack of or heavier than usual menstrual periods; vomiting; unusual hair growth on face or body.

Vaginal bleeding, abnormal *continued*

Associated Symptoms	Possible Diagnosis	Distinguishing Features
	Platelet function disorders	Minor bleeding in the mouth or just beneath the surface of the skin, often appearing as clusters of small, pinpoint-sized red specks; frequent nosebleeds; easy bruising; prolonged menstrual periods; fatigue; pallor; dark-colored stools.
	Polycystic ovaries	Absent or unpredictable menstrual periods; infertility; excessive hair growth with a male pattern of distribution; obesity; acne.
	Vaginal cancer	Vaginal itching; bleeding after intercourse or between menstrual periods; abnormal vaginal discharge; lesions with thick, raised edges; possibly rectal bleeding; discomfort when urinating or defecating; pain during intercourse; urinary frequency and urgency.
	Von Willebrand's disease *Chronic bleeding disorder*	Frequent nosebleeds; excessive bleeding from cuts; bleeding gums; easy bruising; abnormal or excessive menstrual bleeding; blood in the stool.
with abdominal, back, or vaginal pain	Cervical cancer	Initially, asymptomatic. In later stages, unexpected vaginal bleeding or discharge between periods, after intercourse, or after menopause. If untreated, pelvic pain.
	Cervical disorders, non-malignant	Vaginal discharge; vaginal burning and itching; vaginal bleeding after intercourse, between periods, or after bowel movements.
	Disseminated intravascular coagulation *Bleeding disorder marked by excessive and inappropriate blood coagulation*	Abnormal bleeding possibly at several sites at once; vomiting blood; bloody or black stools; abnormal vaginal bleeding; blood in the urine; severe abdominal or back pain; possibly, convulsions, or coma.
	Endometrial hyperplasia *Thickening of the uterine lining due to an overgrowth of cells*	Vaginal bleeding between menstrual periods; heavy or prolonged bleeding during menses; postmenstrual bleeding.
	Endometrial polyps *Growths on the lining of the uterus*	Often no symptoms; light bleeding between periods, especially following sexual intercourse; abnormally heavy or prolonged bleeding during menses; pelvic cramps; foul-smelling vaginal discharge.
	Endometriosis *The migration of the uterine lining to other reproductive or abdominal organs*	Pain in the lower abdomen, vagina, and lower back beginning just prior to menses and intensifying after blood flow has ceased; heavy bleeding during periods; pain during intercourse; diarrhea; constipation; pain during bowel movements; bleeding from the rectum; bloody urine during menses; nausea and vomiting prior to menses; infertility.

Vaginal bleeding, abnormal *continued*

Associated Symptoms	Possible Diagnosis	Distinguishing Features
with abdominal, back, or vaginal pain *continued*	Fibroids, uterine *Benign growths of the muscular wall of the uterus*	Heavier or prolonged bleeding during menses; abdominal discomfort; lower back pain; pressure on the bladder and frequent urination; constipation. Possible, sharp, sudden, lower abdominal pain.
	Gonorrhea	Burning pain during urination; yellowish, pus-like discharge from the penis or vagina; redness or swelling at the infection site; abnormal vaginal bleeding.
	Hepatitis, chronic	Fatigue; nausea; vomiting; loss of appetite; jaundice; dark urine; clay-colored stools; depression; pain or discomfort in the upper right abdomen; abdominal swelling; fever; in women, cessation of menstruation, acne, and the appearance of male pattern facial hair.
	Pelvic inflammatory disease	Initially, lower pelvic pain; pain during intercourse; irregular menstrual bleeding; vaginal discharge with abnormal color or odor; low-grade fever; chills; frequent urination; fatigue; loss of appetite; later, severe abdominal pain and high fever.
	Uterine cancer	Heavy bleeding during menses; bleeding between menses or after intercourse; postmenopausal bleeding; abnormal vaginal discharge usually watery and blood-streaked; weight loss.
	Uterine prolapse	Often asymptomatic. Possibly, difficulty passing urine or stools, pain during intercourse, backache that intensifies when lifting, sensation of heaviness or dragging within the pelvis, painful or heavy menstrual periods, or bleeding between periods. In severe cases, uterus visibly protrudes outside of vagina.
	Vaginitis *Inflammation of the vagina*	Vaginal irritation, itching, and discharge; painful intercourse and minor postcoital bleeding. In later stages, vaginal pain.

Vaginal discharge, abnormal

Associated Symptoms	Possible Diagnosis	Distinguishing Features
	Candidiasis *Fungal infection of the mouth, genitals, or mucous membranes*	Thick, white discharge from the vagina; itching and irritation in the vaginal area; pain while urinating or during intercourse; in men, inflammation of the head of the penis; possibly, yellow raised patches in the mouth.
	Cervical cancer	Initially, asymptomatic. In later stages, unexpected vaginal bleeding or discharge between periods, after intercourse, or after menopause. If untreated, pelvic pain.
	Cervical disorders, non-malignant	Vaginal discharge; vaginal burning and itching; vaginal bleeding after intercourse, between periods, or after bowel movements.
	Chlamydia *Contagious, infectious disease caused by chlamydia, a group of microorganisms*	Usually asymptomatic; possibly, pain or burning during urination, watery discharge from the penis or vagina, swelling of the testicles, breathing difficulty, cough, high fever, inflammation of the inner lining of the eyelids and the membrane covering the whites of the eyes.
	Endometrial polyps *Growths on the lining of the uterus*	Often no symptoms; light bleeding between periods, especially following sexual intercourse; abnormally heavy or prolonged bleeding during menses; pelvic cramps; foul-smelling vaginal discharge.
	Gonorrhea	Burning pain during urination; yellowish, pus-like discharge from the penis or vagina; redness or swelling at the infection site; abnormal vaginal bleeding.
	Ovarian cysts	In many cases, no symptoms. Painless swelling in the lower abdomen; possibly, pain during intercourse; brown vaginal discharge; lack of or heavier than usual menstrual periods; vomiting; unusual hair growth on face or body.
	Pelvic inflammatory disease	Initially, lower pelvic pain; pain during intercourse; irregular menstrual bleeding; vaginal discharge with abnormal color or odor; low-grade fever; chills; frequent urination; fatigue; loss of appetite; later, severe abdominal pain and high fever.
	Urethritis *Infection of the urethra, the passageway that drains urine from the bladder*	Frequent and painful urination; blood in the urine; yellow, pus-filled discharge; possible difficulty passing urine; urinary urgency; pain during intercourse; in men, painful ejaculation.
	Uterine cancer	Heavy bleeding during menses; bleeding between menses or after intercourse; postmenopausal bleeding; abnormal vaginal discharge usually watery and blood-streaked; weight loss.

Vaginal discharge, abnormal *continued*

Associated Symptoms	Possible Diagnosis	Distinguishing Features
	Vaginal cancer	Vaginal itching; bleeding after intercourse or between menstrual periods; abnormal vaginal discharge; lesions with thick, raised edges; possibly rectal bleeding; discomfort when urinating or defecating; pain during intercourse; urinary frequency and urgency.
	Vaginitis *Inflammation of the vagina*	Vaginal irritation, itching, and discharge; painful intercourse and minor postcoital bleeding. In later stages, vaginal pain.

Vaginal itching

Associated Symptoms	Possible Diagnosis	Distinguishing Features
	Candidiasis *Fungal infection of the mouth, genitals, or mucous membranes*	Thick, white discharge from the vagina; itching and irritation in the vaginal area; pain while urinating or during intercourse; in men, inflammation of the head of the penis; possibly, yellow raised patches in the mouth.
	Genital herpes	Approximately one week after infection, itching, burning, soreness, and small blisters in the genital area. Blisters later burst, leaving painful ulcers which heal 10 to 20 days later. Possibly, enlarged, painful lymph nodes in the groin; fever, headache, and cold sores around the mouth. In women, pain during urination.
	Gonorrhea	Burning pain during urination; yellowish, pus-like discharge from the penis or vagina; redness or swelling at the infection site; abnormal vaginal bleeding.
	Lice	Intense itching, usually on hair-covered areas; visible nits (eggs) on hair shafts; red bite marks; visible lice on clothing.
	Pinworms	Anal itching, often at night; irritability; fidgetiness; restless sleep.
	Vaginal cancer	Vaginal itching; bleeding after intercourse or between menstrual periods; abnormal vaginal discharge; lesions with thick, raised edges; possibly rectal bleeding; discomfort when urinating or defecating; pain during intercourse; urinary frequency and urgency.
	Vaginitis *Inflammation of the vagina*	Vaginal irritation, itching, and discharge; painful intercourse and minor postcoital bleeding. In later stages, vaginal pain.

Visual floaters

Associated Symptoms	Possible Diagnosis	Distinguishing Features
	Refractive disorders	Depending on the specific disorder, blurred vision or an inability to clearly see objects that are either near or far.
	Retinal detachment	Possibly, bright flashes of light in the peripheral vision, blurred vision, shadows or blindness in part of the field of vision.
	Uveitis and iritis *Inflammation of the uvea, a group of structures in the eye including the iris*	Moderate to severe eye pain; aversion to light; redness in the eye; excessive tearing; blurred vision; spots in the field of vision.

Weight gain, unintentional

Associated Symptoms	Possible Diagnosis	Distinguishing Features
	Acromegaly *Overproduction of growth hormone by the pituitary gland*	In adults (acromegaly): Gradual thickening of the bones of the face, jaw, and the extremities in adults; oily skin; severe headache; excessive hair growth; excessive perspiration; joint pains. In children (in which the disease is called gigantism): Rapid growth and unusual height; possibly, blindness.
	Bipolar disorder *Manic-depressive illness*	Symptoms vary depending on phase of the disorder; mania: inflated self-esteem, elation, euphoria, grandiosity, increased activity, and a decreased need for sleep; depression: persistent feelings of sadness, apathy, or hopelessness; diminished interest in activities; loss of appetite and weight or unusual increase in appetite and weight; insomnia or drowsiness; difficulty concentrating; agitation in older patients.
	Congestive heart failure	Shortness of breath; fatigue; need to sleep on several pillows; weakness; cough; heart palpitations; swelling in the legs, ankles, and abdomen; frequent urination at night; indigestion; nausea and vomiting; loss of appetite.
	Depression	Persistent feelings of sadness, apathy, or hopelessness; diminished interest in activities; loss of or unusual increase in appetite and weight; insomnia or drowsiness; difficulty concentrating; agitation.
	Hypothyroidism *Underactivity of the thyroid gland*	Unexplained weight gain; fatigue; muscle weakness; cramps; dry skin; hair loss; deepening of the voice; intolerance for cold; constipation; chest pain; insomnia; puffiness around eyes; loss of sex drive; depression; menstrual abnormalities; possible swelling in the neck.
	Nephrotic syndrome *Damage to the filtering units of the kidneys*	Swelling in the ankles and around the eyes; weight gain, due to fluid retention throughout the body; shortness of breath; passing only small amounts of urine that has an unusually foamy appearance; fatigue; diarrhea; loss of appetite.
	Obesity	Symptoms such as chest pain or shortness of breath from heart disease, knee or hip pain, or abdominal pain from gallstones all result from the complications of obesity.
	Renal failure, acute *Severe kidney failure*	Initially, decreased urine output, weight gain and swelling due to edema, loss of appetite, nausea and vomiting, fatigue. If untreated, confusion, seizures, and drowsiness.

Weight loss, unintentional

Associated Symptoms	Possible Diagnosis	Distinguishing Features
	AIDS *Acquired immunodeficiency syndrome*	Recurrent infections affecting the skin and respiratory system; cough; shortness of breath; loss of appetite; weight loss; fatigue; diarrhea; fever; dementia; malignant skin lesions; swollen lymph glands throughout the body; purplish skin nodules; memory loss; confusion; personality changes.
	Amyloidosis *Accumulation of amyloid, a waxy substance, in tissues and organs*	Symptoms vary greatly depending on the body parts affected and may include fatigue and weakness; weight loss; heart palpitations; shortness of breath; swelling of the legs; difficulty swallowing due to swelling of the tongue; diarrhea; abdominal pain; raised spots on the armpits, groin, face, and neck; numbness or tingling of the hands or feet; dizziness on standing; joint pains.
	Amyotrophic lateral sclerosis *Progressive degeneration of nerve cells of the central nervous system*	Progressive loss of strength and coordination in the limbs; muscle twitching and cramps that begin in the hands and spread to the arms, shoulders, and legs; stiff, clumsy gait; swallowing, breathing, or speaking difficulty; weight loss; drooling; involuntary laughing or crying.
	Anemia, folic acid deficiency	Fatigue and weakness; pallor; shortness of breath, heart palpitations, or noticeably rapid heartbeat on exertion; sore, red, and glazed looking tongue; loss of weight and appetite; nausea and diarrhea; abdominal distention.
	Anemia, pernicious	Fatigue; inability to concentrate; sore, red tongue; weakness; dizziness; pallor; shortness of breath on exertion; palpitations; numbness and tingling in extremities; incoordination; headache; loss of weight and appetite; possibly, jaundice.
	Bipolar disorder *Manic-depressive illness*	Symptoms vary depending on phase of the disorder; mania: inflated self-esteem, elation, euphoria, grandiosity, increased activity, and a decreased need for sleep; depression: persistent feelings of sadness, apathy, or hopelessness; diminished interest in activities; loss of appetite and weight or unusual increase in appetite and weight; insomnia or drowsiness; difficulty concentrating; agitation in older patients.
	Cirrhosis *Chronic damage to the cells of the liver*	No symptoms in early stages; loss of weight and appetite; nausea; swollen legs, ankles and abdomen; itching; jaundice; black stools; vomiting blood; fatigue; impotence; memory loss; confusion.

Weight loss, unintentional *continued*

Associated Symptoms	Possible Diagnosis	Distinguishing Features
	Depression	Persistent feelings of sadness, apathy, or hopelessness; diminished interest in activities; loss of or unusual increase in appetite and weight; insomnia or drowsiness; difficulty concentrating; agitation.
	Dermatomyositis *Inflammation of the muscles and skin*	Red rash on the neck, upper torso, and upper arms and legs; purple discoloration and swelling of the eyelids; areas of thickened skin; muscle weakness and stiffness, usually in the shoulders and pelvis; cold hands and feet; speaking or swallowing difficulty; weight loss.
	Diabetes mellitus *Insufficiency of or resistance to insulin*	Fatigue; excessive thirst; frequent urination; weight loss despite increased appetite; blurred vision; numbness and tingling of feet and hands; impotence.
	Esophageal cancer	Swallowing difficulty and pain; weight loss; drooling; possibly, vomiting or coughing up of bloody mucus, regurgitation of food; chest pain; repeated respiratory infections.
	Hyperparathyroidism *Overactivity of the parathyroid glands*	Increased susceptibility to bone fractures; depression; indigestion; increased thirst and urine output; fatigue, lethargy; somnolence; muscle weakness; nausea and vomiting; loss of appetite; weight loss.
	Hyperthyroidism *Overactivity of the thyroid gland*	Protruding eyes; weight loss despite increased appetite; intolerance to heat; excessive perspiration; nervousness or restlessness; possibly, swelling in the neck (goiter); palpitations; tremor; diarrhea.
	Hypothyroidism *Underactivity of the thyroid gland*	Unexplained weight gain; fatigue; muscle weakness; cramps; dry skin; hair loss; deepening of the voice; intolerance for cold; constipation; chest pain; insomnia; puffiness around eyes; loss of sex drive; depression; menstrual abnormalities; possible swelling in the neck.
	Lung abscess	Cough producing foul-smelling sputum; bad breath; fever; chills; weight loss; possible chest pain.
	Lung cancer	Persistent cough; wheezing; shortness of breath; chest pain; fatigue; weight loss.
	Lymphoma, Hodgkin's *Cancer of the lymph nodes and lymphoid tissue*	Painless swelling of the lymph nodes usually in the neck or armpits; loss of appetite; night sweats.
	Lymphoma, non-Hodgkin's *Cancer of the lymph nodes and lymphoid tissue*	Painless swelling of lymph nodes in the neck or groin; possible abdominal pain, vomiting of blood, headache.

Weight loss, unintentional *continued*

Associated Symptoms	Possible Diagnosis	Distinguishing Features
	Ovarian cancer	Often asymptomatic until widespread. Possibly, abdominal swelling or discomfort, nausea, and vomiting. In advanced stages, excessive hair growth, unexplained weight loss, abnormal menstrual bleeding or post-menopausal bleeding; urinary frequency.
	Peripheral neuropathies *Degeneration of the nerves that supply the extremities*	Tingling or numbness commonly beginning in the hands and feet and gradually spreading toward the center of the body; sensitive skin; muscle weakness; possibly, pain in the hands and feet; lack of coordination; shooting pains exacerbated by touch or changes in temperature; breathing difficulty; urinary or fecal incontinence.
	Rheumatoid arthritis, juvenile	Fever; rash; abdominal pain; weight loss; swelling, stiffness, and pain in the affected joints; enlarged lymph glands; fatigue; pallor; red, painful eyes.
	Sarcoidosis *Accumulation of inflammatory cells in the lymph nodes and other tissues throughout the body*	Often no symptoms. Swollen lymph nodes in the neck or armpits; muscle aches; fever; breathing difficulty; possibly, purple rash on the face; reddish or brownish skin spots on the forearms, face, or legs; numbness; joint pain or stiffness; a painful, red eye; blurred vision; loss of appetite and weight.
	Scleroderma	Shiny, tight, and hardened skin, especially on the fingers, arms, and face; hands or feet may successively turn blue, white, and red upon exposure to cold (Raynaud's phenomenon); swallowing difficulty; bloating after eating; weight loss; shortness of breath on exertion; high blood pressure; symptoms of renal failure. Possibly, heartburn, muscle aches and weakness, joint pain, fever, or fatigue.
	Systemic lupus erythematosus *Inflammation of connective tissues throughout the body*	Red, blotchy, butterfly-shaped rash on the cheeks and bridge of the nose; fatigue; fever; loss of appetite and weight; nausea; joint and abdominal pain; headaches; blurred vision; increased sensitivity to sun exposure; depression; psychosis; mental confusion.
	Thyroiditis *Inflammation of the thyroid gland*	Pain in the front of the neck and, often, the ear; possibly fever, weight loss, and fatigue; general feeling of being unwell (malaise); discomfort on swallowing.
	Tuberculosis	Often, asymptomatic. Possibly, low-grade fever; excessive perspiration; cough producing sputum or blood; weight loss; chronic fatigue; chest pain; shortness of breath; night sweats.

Weight loss, unintentional *continued*

Associated Symptoms	Possible Diagnosis	Distinguishing Features
with abdominal pain	Adrenal insufficiency *Inadequate production of steroid hormones by the adrenal gland*	Loss of weight and appetite; fatigue; weakness; darkening of the skin; abdominal pain; diarrhea; indigestion; nausea and vomiting; constipation; lack of sex drive; dizziness when rising from sitting or lying position.
	Amebiasis *Parasitic infection*	Usually asymptomatic; possibly, diarrhea; loose stools may contain mucus and blood; abdominal cramps; fatigue; weight loss; gas and flatulence. In severe cases, large amount of bloody stools daily; fever, nausea and vomiting, and abdominal tenderness.
	Colitis, ulcerative *Inflammation of the lining of the colon*	Pain on the left side of the abdomen that lessens after bowel movements; bloody diarrhea; pain in the rectal area; possibly, fever, rapid heartbeat, nausea and vomiting, loss of appetite, dehydration with severe attacks.
	Colorectal cancer *A growth of malignant cells in the colon or rectum*	Change in bowel habits; diarrhea; constipation; narrow stools; bloody or dark stools; lower abdominal pain; bloating; cramps; gas; loss of weight and appetite; fatigue and heart palpitations due to anemia.
	Crohn's disease *Inflammation of the lining of the small intestine*	Episodes of abdominal pain or cramps in lower abdomen; nausea; diarrhea; loss of weight and appetite; possibly, fever; rectal bleeding or blood in stools; fatigue; anal fissures; joint pains; inflammation of the eyes.
	Dysentery, bacillary	Watery diarrhea that may contain mucus or blood; rectal pain upon defecation; abdominal pain; rapid dehydration and weight loss; nausea and vomiting.
	Empyema *Collection of pus in any body cavity, usually between the membranes covering the lungs*	Chest pain exacerbated by deep inhalation; shortness of breath; dry cough; fever and chills; exhaustion; weight loss; night sweats; abdominal pain and jaundice.
	Kidney cancer	Blood in the urine; abdominal and lower back pain; low-grade fever; loss of weight and appetite.
	Leukemias	Symptoms vary depending on the type of leukemia and may include: loss of appetite and weight; increased bruising and bleeding; bone pain, especially in the legs; abdominal pain and distention; nausea; heart palpitations; severe fatigue; pallor; breathing difficulty; fever; night sweats; headache; enlarged lymph nodes; joint pains (due to gout).

Weight loss, unintentional *continued*

Associated Symptoms	Possible Diagnosis	Distinguishing Features
with abdominal pain *continued*	Liver tumors	Pain or discomfort in the upper right portion of the abdomen; abdominal swelling; loss of weight and appetite; nausea and vomiting; fever; excessive perspiration; jaundice; pallor; severe fatigue.
	Malabsorption, digestive *A failure of the small intestine to absorb nutrients in the diet*	Diarrhea; weight loss; yellowish, foul-smelling stools; abdominal cramps, gas, and bloating; weakness and lethargy.
	Pancreatic cancer	Often, no symptoms until far advanced. Upper abdominal pain which spreads to the back; loss of weight and appetite; jaundice; nausea, vomiting, and indigestion; diarrhea; fatigue; depression.
	Pancreatitis *Inflammation of the pancreas*	Sudden, extreme abdominal pain; nausea and vomiting; weakness; fever; clammy skin; abdominal bloating and tenderness.
	Peptic ulcer	Intermittent, burning or gnawing pain in the upper abdomen or lower chest; indigestion; loss of appetite and weight. Pain may be relieved by eating or antacids. Possible nausea and vomiting. Black, tarry stools, vomiting blood.
	Pheochromocytoma *Tumor in central part of the adrenal, the glands above the kidneys*	Headaches, sometimes severe; rapid heartbeat or heart palpitations; excessive perspiration; faintness, especially when standing up; chest pain; abdominal pain; constipation; weight loss; nervousness, irritability, or anxiety; mental confusion or psychosis.
	Stomach cancer	Discomfort in the upper abdomen; black, tarry stools; vomiting of blood; loss of appetite and weight; vomiting after meals.
	Tapeworm infestation	Often asymptomatic. Unexplained weight loss; presence of white eggs or ribbon-like segments of worm in the stool, bedding, or clothing; symptoms of pernicious anemia.
	Trichinosis *Parasitic infestation*	Initially, crampy abdominal pain, diarrhea, vomiting, and fever, followed within one to two weeks by swelling around the eyes, muscle aches and tenderness, fever, and weakness. Possibly, coughing up of bloody phlegm; delirium; coma; heart failure symptoms.
	Uterine cancer	Heavy bleeding during menses; bleeding between menses or after intercourse; postmenopausal bleeding; abnormal vaginal discharge usually watery and blood-streaked; weight loss.

Wheezing

Associated Symptoms	Possible Diagnosis	Distinguishing Features
	Allergic rhinitis *Hay fever*	Nasal congestion; frequent sneezing; itchy eyes, nose, and throat.
	Anaphylaxis	Itching and hives; swelling of the eyes, lips, and tongue; weakness or faintness; tightening in the chest or throat; wheezing; shortness of breath; profuse sweating; palpitations; sudden, intense distress; feelings of impending doom; stomach cramps; nausea, vomiting, or diarrhea; bluish tinge (cyanosis) to the skin, lips, and nail beds due to oxygen insufficiency.
	Asthma	Shortness of breath; wheezing; dry cough; tightness in the chest; possibly, excessive perspiration or rapid heartbeat.
	Bronchiectasis *Lung condition that stretches and distorts the walls of the bronchial tubes*	Cough that produces dark green sputum; bad breath; possibly, shortness of breath; loss of appetite and weight; clubbed fingers.
	Bronchitis, acute	Shortness of breath; persistent cough producing yellow or green sputum; possibly, chest pain; wheezing; fever.
	Carcinoid tumors and carcinoid syndrome	May be asymptomatic; flushing or redness of the face and neck; gas and profuse diarrhea; abdominal cramping; watery, swollen eyes; shortness of breath or wheezing.
	Cardiomyopathy *Disease of the heart muscle causing a reduction in the force of heart contractions*	Fatigue; chest pain and palpitations; shortness of breath; swelling of the legs; wheezing; cough.
	Chronic obstructive pulmonary disease	Shortness of breath; wheezing; persistent, mucus-producing cough, especially in the morning; possibly, chest pain, swollen legs and ankles.
	Congestive heart failure	Shortness of breath; fatigue; need to sleep on several pillows; weakness; cough; heart palpitations; swelling in the legs, ankles, and abdomen; frequent urination at night; indigestion; nausea and vomiting; loss of appetite.
	Croup *Inflammation of the air passages in children*	Barking cough; hoarseness; wheezing; possibly, breathing difficulty; chest discomfort.

Wheezing *continued*

Associated Symptoms	Possible Diagnosis	Distinguishing Features
	Esophageal stricture *Narrowing of the esophagus, the passageway from the mouth to the stomach*	Sudden or gradual decrease in the ability to swallow solid food or liquids; chest pain after eating; regurgitation of food and liquids; increased salivation; weight loss. Aspiration into lungs can cause cough, wheezing, shortness of breath.
	Gastroesophageal reflux *Heartburn*	Burning sensation in the middle of the chest; pain and difficulty swallowing; slight regurgitation of stomach's contents into the mouth, especially when reclining or bending forward; mild abdominal pain.
	Lung cancer	Persistent cough; wheezing; shortness of breath; chest pain; fatigue; weight loss.
	Pneumonia	High fever; shortness of breath; cough with sputum; chest pain; fatigue.
	Pulmonary edema *An accumulation of fluid in the lungs*	Severe shortness of breath; rapid breathing; pallor; excessive perspiration; bluish nails and lips; cough with frothy sputum; wheezing; anxiety and restlessness.
	Pulmonary embolism *A blood clot traveling from legs or heart that lodges in an artery supplying the lungs*	Sudden shortness of breath and severe breathing difficulty; chest pain worse on inspiration; rapid heartbeat; cough, possibly with bloody sputum; wheezing; excessive perspiration.

DISORDERS

In this section, you will find an entry for each of the disorders listed in the "Possible Diagnosis" column of the Symptoms charts in the first half of the book. Each entry offers a brief definition of the disorder, a discussion of its causes and risk factors, a comprehensive list of the symptoms commonly associated with the disorder, prevention tips, diagnostic tests required, how the disorder should be remedied, and when to consult your doctor.

THE EDITORS

Acne

WHAT IS IT?

Acne is characterized by minor, though occasionally severe, skin eruptions due to inflammation around the sebaceous glands. Most prominent on the face, upper chest, and back, the sebaceous glands secrete sebum, a thick, oily substance that lubricates the skin. The male hormones called androgens can trigger overactivity of the sebaceous glands. Acne develops when sebum flow is blocked by skin cells, dried sebum, or bacteria. A complete blockage produces a light-colored bump (whitehead); an incomplete blockage leads to a dark-colored spot (blackhead). Bacteria normally found on the surface of the skin may then infect the whitehead or blackhead, produce pus, and cause an eruption (pimple). In severe cases, which are known as cystic acne, painful purple lumps develop.

Except in cases that cause widespread skin pustules, cysts, or scarring, acne is generally harmless and responsive to treatment. It is most common during adolescence and can cause considerable psychological distress. Eruptions tend to wane by one's 20s, but they may persist. In women, acne may first appear in the 20s or 30s. Unexplained outbreaks of acne in older adults may be a sign of a more serious underlying problem.

WHAT CAUSES IT?

• Hormonal changes (especially excessive androgen secretion) resulting in increased sebum production.
• Hereditary factors.
• Certain drugs or compounds, including oral contraceptives, corticosteroids, or other hormones, as well as barbiturates, iodides, bromides, vitamin B_{12}, antiseizure drugs, and lithium.
• Grease, tar, heavy oils, cosmetics, tight clothing, or anything else that can physically block the pores.
• In adults, underlying medical conditions, including ovary or adrenal gland dysfunction, such as polycystic ovary disease and Cushing's syndrome.
• Other factors including climate changes, stress, and exposure to dioxin.

PREVENTION

• There is no evidence that dietary modifications (such as avoiding chocolate or greasy foods) will reduce the incidence of acne in those so predisposed, although good hygiene may reduce severity.
• Picking or squeezing acne lesions may increase the danger of infection and scarring.

DIAGNOSIS

• Diagnosis can be made upon visual inspection.

HOW TO TREAT IT

• Regular washing of the face with unscented soap to remove excessive oil is recommended. However, overwashing can irritate skin, making acne worse.
• Topical solutions that dry the skin and promote peeling may help eliminate acne over time. Over-the-counter preparations may contain benzoyl peroxide (a potent antibacterial agent), sulfur, or resorcinol.
• In more severe cases, topical or oral antibiotics like tetracycline and erythromycin may be prescribed.
• A synthetic form of vitamin A (tretinoin) can be administered topically to treat blackheads and whiteheads, or given orally for cystic acne. (Oral forms of tretinoin may cause birth defects, and so should not be taken by pregnant women).
• In extreme cases chemical peeling, surgical drainage, or removal of cysts may be warranted.
• Scars can be treated with standard or laser surgery or a resurfacing procedure called dermabrasion.

WHEN TO CALL A DOCTOR

• Consult a doctor or dermatologist to discuss optimal ways to treat acne. 🔺

SYMPTOMS

• Pimples or skin eruptions (blackheads and whiteheads) usually on the face, but also found on the neck, shoulders, back, chest, buttocks, and rarely, upper arms and thighs.
• Clusters of red, inflamed pustules and cysts in more severe cases (cystic acne).
• Thick, firm lumps below the surface of the skin (sebaceous cysts).
• Pockmarks and scarring from chronic acne.

Acoustic Neuroma

WHAT IS IT?

Acoustic neuromas are benign (noncancerous) tumors arising from abnormal growth in the cells of the protective sheath (myelin) that surrounds the eighth cranial nerve (or auditory nerve). These tumors tend to grow very slowly, eventually leading to partial or total hearing loss in the affected ear. If left untreated, the tumor may continue to expand and press on several other cranial nerves, causing dizziness and loss of balance, facial pain (see Neuralgia for more information), or double vision. In some cases an acoustic neuroma grows large enough to involve the brain stem, leading to loss of muscle coordination (cerebellar ataxia) on the affected side of the body. However, most patients seek treatment before such complications occur. Prognosis depends on the size of the tumor but is generally quite favorable. While acoustic neuroma is the most common tumor of cranial nerves and represents about 5 percent of primary brain tumors, it is still a rather uncommon disorder. Incidence is highest among those between the ages of 30 and 50.

WHAT CAUSES IT?

• The cause of acoustic neuromas is unknown, although some studies link the problem to a genetic lack of certain proteins that normally prevent tumor growth in the tissue surrounding nerve fibers.
• A small fraction of cases occur in association with a hereditary disorder called neurofibromatosis, characterized by widespread abnormalities in the nervous system, skin, and bones. Neurofibromatosis can be associated with acoustic neuromas that affect both auditory nerves. (In almost all other cases, neuromas develop only in one auditory nerve.)

PREVENTION

• There is no known way to prevent the development of acoustic neuromas.

DIAGNOSIS

• Patient history and a hearing test (audiogram) may be strongly suggestive of the diagnosis. Evaluation by an otolaryngologist (an ear, nose, and throat specialist) is essential for any signs of hearing loss.
• CT (computed tomography) scans or MRI (magnetic resonance imaging) can confirm the presence of even very small acoustic neuromas.

HOW TO TREAT IT

• The only effective cure for acoustic neuromas is surgical removal of the tumor. Current microsurgery techniques performed by surgeons experienced in using them often yield favorable results, making it possible to preserve hearing for many patients (especially those who had good hearing preoperatively). Occasionally, however, some degree of permanent hearing loss in the affected ear is inevitable, and sometimes the surgery itself can result in weakness in the facial muscles, numbness, or other neurological symptoms owing to unavoidable damage to surrounding nerves.
• Radiation treatment may be an option to surgery for some patients. Though not a cure, the treatment slows tumor growth in the majority of cases.

WHEN TO CALL A DOCTOR

• Consult a doctor regarding any signs of hearing loss. You will most likely be referred to an audiologist or an otolaryngologist for testing and examination. ▲

SYMPTOMS

• Partial or complete hearing loss in one ear (or rarely, in both ears). An inability to hear in one ear when using the telephone is often the first sign.
• Persistent ringing or buzzing in the affected ear (tinnitus).
• Ear pain (in some cases).
• Symptoms that may appear if a tumor affects other nerves or the cerebellum: dizziness and vertigo; facial pain; double vision; loss of muscle coordination on the affected side of the body.

Acromegaly

WHAT IS IT?

One form of hyperpituitarism (overproduction of hormones by the pituitary)—marked by an overproduction of growth hormone by the pituitary gland—is a rare, chronic disorder known as acromegaly in adults and gigantism in children. The pituitary, a peanut-size organ located at the base of the brain, is the most important gland in the body's endocrine, or hormonal, system. It produces a number of essential hormones; one of these, human growth hormone (HGH or somatotropin), is responsible for regulating growth during childhood. Normally, as people reach adulthood, less HGH is produced. Overproduction of HGH in children results in exaggerated height. (The most dramatic case of gigantism on record is a child who grew to a height of nearly nine feet.) When onset of the disorder occurs during adulthood (acromegaly), bones can no longer increase in length but progressively thicken instead. This results in gradual enlargement of the hands, feet, jaw, forehead, nose, and ears and produces the coarse facial features characteristic of the disorder. The internal organs also become abnormally enlarged. Thus, acromegaly often reduces life expectancy and, if left untreated, may lead to blindness, arthritis, infertility, diabetes, high blood pressure, heart valve failure, and coronary artery disease.

WHAT CAUSES IT?

• A benign pituitary tumor (adenoma) is the most common cause of HGH overproduction.
• Rarely, a tumor in the hypothalamus (the region of the brain directly behind the pituitary gland) or elsewhere may overstimulate production of HGH.

PREVENTION

• There is no way to prevent acromegaly.

DIAGNOSIS

• Patient history and physical examination, including visual-field tests.
• Blood tests revealing elevated levels of HGH that are not fully reduced by administration of glucose.
• Measurement of elevated levels of somatomedin-C (IGF-1) in the blood.
• CT (computed tomography) scans and MRI (magnetic resonance imaging) to detect a pituitary tumor.
• X-rays to detect increased bone mass.

HOW TO TREAT IT

• Surgical removal of the underlying tumor is the treatment of choice. It is not uncommon for HGH levels to return to normal within hours of surgery and for soft tissue (but not bony tissue) enlargement to subside rapidly.
• Medications after surgery such as octreotide and sometimes bromocriptine may be prescribed to decrease tumor size and regulate HGH secretion.
• Radiation, alone or following surgery, may be performed to shrink the tumor (or prevent its recurrence).
• In some cases, lifetime hormone replacement therapy with thyroid or adrenal-steroid hormones may be necessary if surgery or radiation damages the remaining pituitary gland.

WHEN TO CALL A DOCTOR

• See a doctor if you or your child develop symptoms of acromegaly or gigantism. 🔺

SYMPTOMS

• In adults: enlarged hands, feet, forehead, and jaw bones; broadened head and neck; coarsened facial features; widely spaced teeth; impotence in men; cessation of menstrual periods (amenorrhea) and excess facial hair (hirsutism) in women.
• In children: excessive height due to abrupt, accelerated growth (not to be confused with normal adolescent growth spurts).
• In both children and adults: fatigue and muscle weakness; profuse sweating; weight gain; oily skin; sinus congestion; increased tongue size; hollow-sounding voice; oversleeping; joint pain; tingling sensations in the hands; sudden mood changes.
• Headaches and impaired vision may occur as tumor growth exerts pressure within the skull.

Adrenal Insufficiency

WHAT IS IT?

Adrenal insufficiency is a relatively rare disorder caused either by destruction of tissue in the portion of the adrenal glands known as the cortex, which normally secretes the corticosteroid hormones (Addison's disease), or by atrophy of the adrenal cortex resulting from a loss of stimulation from the pituitary gland (secondary adrenal failure). Addison's disease produces symptoms only after some 90 percent of the adrenal cortices have been destroyed. Insufficiency of corticosteroids can lead to a number of health problems, including an inability to recover from even a minor infection. Complications such as protracted weakness, shock, or death may result. Adrenal insufficiency may occur at any age and affects both sexes equally. Once invariably fatal, the disorder is now highly treatable since the advent of corticosteroid replacement therapy in the 1950s; thus, a patient's outlook is quite favorable. Steps must be taken, however, to avert adrenal crisis—a sudden, life-threatening steroid deficiency usually brought on by infection, injury, or stress—which requires immediate emergency treatment.

WHAT CAUSES IT?

• Addison's disease results from the destruction of the adrenal cortices. In most cases, no underlying cause

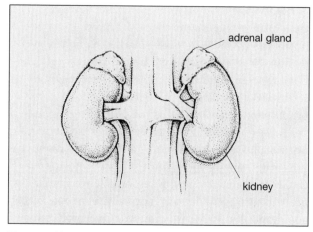

The powerful and crucial corticosteroid hormones are produced in the cortex of the adrenal glands, located atop each kidney.

can be pinpointed, although it often appears to involve an autoimmune disorder (an attack upon healthy tissue by the body's defenses against disease).
• A family history of autoimmune disorders, such as hypothyroidism, is associated with a higher risk of Addison's disease.
• Anticoagulant therapy with medications such as warfarin or heparin can occasionally result in adrenal hemorrhage, leading to destruction of adrenal tissue.
• In a few cases Addison's disease may occur as a complication of certain infections, such as tuberculosis, histoplasmosis, or cytomegalovirus (in AIDS patients).
• Adrenal tissue may be destroyed by metastatic cancer or other disorders (see Amyloidosis and Sarcoidosis for more information).
• Secondary adrenal insufficiency most often results from a pituitary tumor that destroys a part of the pituitary gland or from surgical removal of the pituitary.
• Long-term treatment with steroid hormones leads to atrophy of the adrenal cortex; recovery of adrenal function may take many months after steroid treatment is stopped.

PREVENTION

• There is no way to prevent Addison's disease.

DIAGNOSIS

• Patient history and physical evaluation.
• Blood and urine tests are taken to measure hormone levels.

SYMPTOMS

• Progressive fatigue and weakness.
• Nausea and vomiting.
• Decreased appetite and weight loss.
• Increased pigmentation of skin and mucous membranes (dark freckles, uneven patches of darkened skin, or unusually persistent tanning following sun exposure). This does not occur with secondary adrenal insufficiency.
• Abdominal pain.
• Diarrhea or constipation.
• Dizziness, especially when rising from a lying or sitting position.
• Personality changes, such as increased irritability or restlessness.
• Enhanced senses of smell, taste, or hearing.

Adrenal Insufficiency   *continued*

HOW TO TREAT IT

• Lifelong hormone replacement is the key to treatment. Corticosteroids such as cortisol, prednisone, and dexamethasone are prescribed. Because the drugs promote increased secretion of stomach acid, doses should be taken with meals, milk, or antacids.

• A mineralocorticoid such as fludrocortisone is often needed to help control salt and mineral balance and thus prevent dehydration and hypotension (unusually low blood pressure) in those with Addison's disease.

• The dose of corticosteroids must be increased during stressful times, such as infections, gastrointestinal illness, dental extractions, or surgery.

• Patients should wear or carry medical alert identification with them at all times.

• Adrenal crisis requires emergency medical treatment, which includes intravenous fluid and hydrocortisone infusions.

WHEN TO CALL A DOCTOR

• See a doctor for any persistent unexplained weakness, weight loss, or stomach upset.

• **EMERGENCY** If you have been diagnosed with Addison's disease and experience symptoms of severe lethargy, nausea, vomiting, dizziness, or dehydration, get immediate medical assistance. These may be indications of adrenal crisis.

AIDS Acquired Immunodeficiency Syndrome

WHAT IS IT?

AIDS is the deadly final phase of infection with the human immunodeficiency virus (HIV). The virus, which is carried in blood, semen, and other body fluids, invades and destroys a specific type of white blood cell—the T4 lymphocyte—a chief component of the body's immune system. The virus is spread primarily through sexual contact (mostly heterosexual), needle sharing among drug users, and from an infected woman to her infant.

After initial infection, the virus multiplies over a period of several weeks, sometimes producing fever, fatigue, sore throat, skin rash, and other symptoms resembling a common virus like mononucleosis. Such symptoms tend to last only one or two weeks. The patient may then exhibit no symptoms for five to 10 years or more, although the virus is multiplying constantly and the patient remains infectious. As increasing numbers of T4 lymphocytes are destroyed by the virus, symptoms such as swollen glands, fever, night sweats, diarrhea, and weight loss may appear.

AIDS develops when the immune system becomes severely damaged (a T4 count less than 200 per microliter) and/or when opportunistic infections—normally kept at bay by healthy immune defenses—or unusual types of cancer (such as

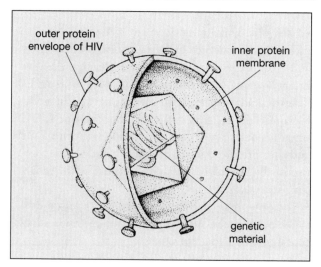

outer protein envelope of HIV

inner protein membrane

genetic material

The outer envelope of the human immunodeficiency virus binds readily with protein receptors on the surface of the immune system's T cells. In this way, the virus's genetic material may enter the T cell and integrate with its genetic material, forever altering the infected cell's genetic code. From this point on, the host cell's protein synthesizing mechanism serves to produce new copies of the virus.

Kaposi's sarcoma or lymphoma) appear. Without treatment, survival after an opportunistic disease is short. Although not a cure, highly potent new drugs to treat HIV have dramatically reduced the rate of death from AIDS. Still, AIDS is a worldwide epidemic, with more than 30 million people infected.

WHAT CAUSES IT?

• AIDS is caused by the human immunodeficiency virus (HIV), which is carried in the body fluids (blood, semen, female genital secretions, saliva, and breast milk) of infected patients. The virus progressively destroys the body's immune defenses, rendering the patient vulnerable to a multitude of potentially deadly secondary infections and cancers.

• HIV is transmitted by exchange of body fluids during sexual contact with an infected partner and by exposure to contaminated blood or blood products, as occurs among intravenous drug users who share needles or hemophiliacs who've received multiple transfusions (improved testing of blood has recently eliminated HIV risk during a transfusion). An infected woman can pass the virus to her infant around the time of delivery or through breast milk. HIV is, however, a very fragile virus and does not

---

SYMPTOMS

• Swollen lymph nodes.
• Persistent fatigue and general feeling of poor health.
• Recurring or prolonged fevers, chills, or night sweats.
• Increased susceptibility to yeast infections (candidiasis), cold sores, fungal infections in the mouth (thrush), and other infections.
• Loss of appetite and unintentional weight loss.
• Cough and breathing problems.
• Changes in bowel habits, such as frequent diarrhea or constipation.
• Outbreaks of skin rashes or discolorations, especially purplish lesions (Kaposi's sarcoma).
• Memory loss, confusion, and personality changes.

AIDS Acquired Immunodeficiency Syndrome *continued*

survive long outside of the body. It is impossible to contract the virus by casual contact such as hugging, dry kissing, or drinking from the same glass as an infected person.

PREVENTION

• HIV infection is preventable by practicing safe sex behaviors, including using condoms (especially those treated with nonoxynol-9 spermicide), and by limiting one's number of sexual partners over a lifetime (short of complete abstinence, an exclusive, mutually monogamous relationship is safest).
• Do not use intravenous drugs; if you do, do not share needles.
• Avoid contact with the blood of others.
• Pregnant women with HIV should take medication to help prevent passing the virus to their child.

DIAGNOSIS

• Patient history and physical examination.
• Blood tests. Presence of antibodies against HIV usually confirms the diagnosis. Measurement of the T4 count indicates the extent of immune system impairment; measurement of viral levels in the blood indicates the risk of disease progression.
• A diagnosis of AIDS is made when one or more opportunistic infections or cancers occur in someone with HIV, or when the T4 count falls below 200 per microliter.

HOW TO TREAT IT

• Although HIV cannot be eradicated, combinations of anti-HIV drugs (protease inhibitors, nucleosides,

and non-nucleosides) stop the virus from replicating and allow the immune system to function more normally.
• Drug treatment should begin when immune function is being compromised and/or viral blood levels are high. Early treatment can prevent damage to the immune system for years. Even patients with late-stage AIDS can experience marked improvement in immune function, accompanied by reduced rates of illness.
• Antibiotics may be prescribed to prevent specific infections from developing.
• Pregnant women should be treated with combination drug therapy, which reduces the spread of HIV to the infant by 70 to 80 percent.
• Vaccines and antibiotics are available to prevent pneumococcal pneumonia and *Pneumocystis carinii* pneumonia, two potentially life-threatening diseases that frequently affect people with AIDS. Other preventive treatments may be employed in certain circumstances.
• Receiving a diagnosis of HIV infection is often emotionally devastating. Psychological counseling, support groups, and outreach from friends and family are invaluable.

WHEN TO CALL A DOCTOR

• Call a doctor if you experience any of the symptoms of HIV or AIDS.
• Be tested if you have any reason to suspect that you have been infected with HIV.
• All pregnant women should consider having an HIV test.

Allergic Rhinitis

WHAT IS IT?

Allergic rhinitis and related nasal or upper respiratory conditions involve inflammation of the mucous membranes in the nasal passages, caused by a hypersensitive response of the immune system to an airborne allergen or irritant. Sneezing, eye irritation, and runny nose are the characteristic symptoms, which may occur seasonally or persist throughout the year. The specific allergens that trigger rhinitis vary from person to person and may include pollen, mold, animal dander, or dust. Symptoms usually first appear between ages 10 and 20, and tend to diminish later in life. Allergic rhinitis is exceedingly common (as many as 25 percent of young adults are afflicted with it) but it is highly treatable.

WHAT CAUSES IT?

• Airborne pollen from various seasonal plants, including grasses, flowers, trees, and ragweed. (Such allergies are commonly referred to as hay fever, although hay is not the cause and fever is not a symptom.)
• Mold spores.
• Animal dander (small scales of dead skin or dried saliva, shed from the hair of certain mammals).
• Household dust, which may contain house dust mites, animal dander, or cockroaches.
• Hereditary factors affecting immune sensitivity.
• Overuse of decongestant sprays.
• A hypersensitivity to medications, including aspirin and other nonsteroidal anti–inflammatory drugs.
• Hormonal disturbances that may occur with pregnancy, oral contraceptive use, or hypothyroidism.

SYMPTOMS

• Frequent sneezing.
• Profuse nasal discharge (usually clear and watery).
• Nasal congestion and itching.
• Red, watering, itching eyes.
• Puffiness and dark circles around the eyes.
• Possible cough or wheezing.
• Impaired sense of taste or smell.
• Itching in the back of the throat.

PREVENTION

• When seasonal allergies flare up, try to stay inside a climate-controlled environment as much as possible, or travel to pollen-free areas. Consider relocating to such areas if symptoms are sufficiently severe.
• If necessary, avoid or isolate furred animals.
• To eliminate dust mites commonly found in bedding, use machine-washable polyester pillows, seal your mattress in a zippered cover, and launder bed linens frequently. Use air filters in bedrooms.

DIAGNOSIS

• Patient history and physical examination.
• Skin tests. The skin is scratched or pricked with a number of needles, each containing a small amount of an allergen; a specific allergen is implicated if the area becomes red or itchy, or a raised welt appears.
• Analysis of nasal secretions.
• Blood tests to reveal a heightened antibody count, indicating an allergic response.

HOW TO TREAT IT

• Antihistamines are the first line of treatment for allergic rhinitis. Many nonprescription varieties are available, although they may cause drowsiness or drying of the mucous membranes. New nonsedating antihistamines are available by prescription—including fexofenadine (Allegra), astemizole (Hismanal), loratadine (Claritin), and cetirizine (Zyrtec).
• Short-term use of decongestants may be beneficial. (Combinations of antihistamines and decongestants are also available.)
• Special eyedrops may be prescribed when eye symptoms persist despite other treatment.
• Inhaled or oral corticosteroids may be prescribed to reduce extreme inflammatory symptoms.
• When all else fails, an allergist may gradually administer increasing amounts of the offending allergen (immunotherapy or allergy shots), which may eventually help desensitize the patient to the allergen.

WHEN TO CALL A DOCTOR

• Call a doctor if allergic rhinitis interferes with normal activities or if over-the-counter antihistamines cause excessive drowsiness (your doctor can prescribe a nonsedating antihistamine).

Alopecia Hair Loss

WHAT IS IT?

Alopecia refers to hair loss of any sort—be it normal male-pattern baldness (MPB) that commonly occurs as men age, or abnormal hair loss associated with certain diseases, hormonal disturbances, or treatments such as chemotherapy. There are two general types of alopecia: scarring and nonscarring. In scarring alopecia, the hair follicles that support the hair shaft are destroyed by an underlying condition, so that hair loss is irreversible. In nonscarring alopecia (which includes MPB and a patchy baldness called alopecia areata), the follicles are preserved, so that regrowth of lost hair remains a possibility. Alopecia has many causes, some of which affect both sexes. Consult a doctor whenever hair loss occurs unexpectedly, in case the cause is pathological in nature.

WHAT CAUSES IT?

• An inherited change that normally occurs with age (MPB); in women, may develop temporarily following pregnancy or after stopping oral contraceptives.
• An autoimmune response (alopecia areata).
• Bacterial or fungal infections (when severe, may cause scarring and permanent hair loss).
• Lupus or scleroderma (scarring alopecia).
• Chemotherapy drugs (diffuse hair loss with temporary complete baldness).
• Other drugs including anticoagulant, anticonvulsant, antidepressant, antihypertensive, antiparkinson, and antithyroid agents (increased rate of hair shedding).

SYMPTOMS

• Male pattern baldness: hairline recession at the temples and thinning hair over the vertex; progressive merging of these areas.
• Female pattern baldness: thinning of hair on top of head with a widened partline; frontal hair margins almost always preserved.
• Alopecia areata (a common type of autoimmune hair loss usually first appearing in children or young adults): coin-size areas of temporary, often recurring, hair loss on the head or elsewhere; rarely, total scalp hair or body hair loss.

• Malnutrition (especially inadequate protein intake), digestive malabsorption, anorexia nervosa, rapid weight loss, or chronic illness.
• Rare congenital and developmental defects.
• Chemical and physical agents, such as acids, bleach, burns, freezing, or radiation (including x-rays and radiotherapy for cancer).
• Poisoning with toxic levels of arsenic, bismuth, boric acid, and vitamin A.

PREVENTION

• Hair shaft breakage may be prevented by not over-processing hair with coloring agents or procedures such as permanent waving or straightening.

DIAGNOSIS

• Alopecia can usually be diagnosed by examination of the characteristic patterns of hair loss.
• More extensive medical tests are warranted when a pathological condition (such as an internal disorder or primary scalp disease) is thought to cause hair loss.

HOW TO TREAT IT

• Any underlying medical condition causing alopecia needs to be diagnosed and treated.
• Treatment for MPB is not necessary, although a number of methods can restore cosmetic appearance.
• The topical medication minoxidil (now available in an extra-strength formulation) often slows the loss of hair and may lead to regrowth of some hair.
• Men may benefit from the prescription oral drug finasteride, which causes some hair growth in most users. (Because finasteride may cause birth defects, it is not prescribed for women).
• Hair gels, permanent waves, wigs, hair weaves, hair transplants, or surgery to reposition existing portions of the scalp are other methods to consider.

WHEN TO CALL A DOCTOR

• Although it is normal to shed 50 to 100 hairs a day, consult your doctor or dermatologist if you notice persistent excess shedding, which may be a symptom of an underlying medical disorder.
• See your doctor if a scalp infection is suspected. Infection can lead to permanent hair loss. 🔺

Alzheimer's Disease

WHAT IS IT?

Alzheimer's disease results from the gradual degeneration of crucial nerve cells (neurons) in the parts of the brain that process cognitive information. Symptoms usually appear very slowly, get progressively worse, and are irreversible. Minor forgetfulness becomes more pronounced; speech deteriorates; and the ability to do everyday things, such as dressing, bathing, and eating, is increasingly difficult. In the final stages, severe mental impairment leads to complete dependence upon caregivers. On average, patients die within 10 years of onset, often from complications such as malnutrition or pneumonia. Alzheimer's disease affects about 6 percent of people over the age of 65, more than 10 percent of those between 75 and 85, and by some estimates, upward of 25 percent of those over 85.

WHAT CAUSES IT?

• Good evidence indicates that a genetic component predisposes some individuals to Alzheimer's disease, but the true cause or causes are unknown. The mechanism of the disease is nonetheless distinctive and is characterized by the death of neurons in certain areas of the cerebral cortex of the brain. This process leads to atrophy in the brain regions where integration of new information and retrieval of memory take place.

• In people with Down syndrome, Alzheimer's disease occurs at an early age.

PREVENTION

• There is no way to prevent Alzheimer's disease.

DIAGNOSIS

• No tests are available to specifically identify Alzheimer's disease; diagnosis is based on patient history (including input from family members) and clinical examination, including a test of mental status. The primary criterion is gradual loss of memory and other cognitive functions. Other disorders that can cause dementia must be ruled out; this may be facilitated by imaging of the brain and various laboratory tests, including:

• MRI (magnetic resonance imaging) or CT (computed tomography) scans of the brain to rule out cancer, subdural hematoma (a collection of blood), adult hydrocephalus (an accumulation of spinal fluid), or multiple small strokes due to vascular disease.

• Blood tests to rule out vitamin deficiencies, endocrine disorders (such as hypothyroidism), syphilis, HIV, and heavy-metal poisoning.

HOW TO TREAT IT

• Donepezil (Aricept) and tacrine (Cognex), inhibitors of the enzyme acetylcholinesterase, provide modest improvement in symptoms of some patients with mild to moderate Alzheimer's disease. Side effects include nausea and loss of appetite.

SYMPTOMS

• Increasing forgetfulness and short-term memory loss.
• Difficulty making decisions.
• Impaired judgment; new difficulty making mathematical calculations or handling money.
• Decreased knowledge of current events.
• Anxiety, withdrawal, and depression as awareness of deficits becomes frightening and embarrassing.
• Language difficulties, including rambling speech, frequent inability to name familiar objects, long pauses to find the right word, and repetition of the same words, phrases, or questions.
• Loss of ability to communicate verbally or to write and understand written language.
• Delusions, hallucinations, paranoia, or irrational accusations.
• Agitation and combativeness.
• Unusual quiet and social withdrawal.
• Wandering or getting lost in familiar places.
• Urinary and fecal incontinence.
• Inappropriate social behavior; indifference to others.
• Failure to recognize friends and family.
• Inability to dress, eat, bathe, or use a bathroom without assistance.
• Walking difficulty or multiple falls.

Alzheimer's Disease   *continued*

• Insomnia, depression, aggression, and other psychological manifestations may be treated with various medications.

• Much of the responsibility to care for a patient with Alzheimer's falls into the hands of the primary caregiver. Supportive counseling, day care, visiting nurses, and eventual inpatient nursing facilities may help to ease the caregiver's burden. Contact your local chapter of the Alzheimer's Association for further information.

WHEN TO CALL A DOCTOR

• Occasional forgetfulness, such as misplacing the car keys, is normal and rarely anything to worry about. However, consult a doctor if you or a family member begins to show increasing signs of memory lapses; becomes lost in a familiar place; loses the ability to do everyday activities; or undergoes a change in personality.

Amebiasis

WHAT IS IT?

Amebiasis is an infection with the parasite *Entamoeba histolytica*. It initially involves the intestine following the consumption of contaminated food or water. Most often, the infected host experiences no symptoms and the infection clears within eight to 12 months. While dwelling in the intestine of the host, the amoeba multiplies, living off of bacteria, food residues, blood cells, and other tissue. Some of these parasites form hard, acid-resistant shells or cysts around themselves. When excreted, these cysts can survive for lengthy periods and are not easily destroyed by hostile environments or water purification systems. If water or food is contaminated with cysts (common in countries where human waste is used as fertilizer), infection may spread. Rare in the United States, amebiasis infects as many as half the inhabitants of some underdeveloped countries.

Serious complications include the formation of a liver abscess that can then rupture into the abdominal cavity (see Peritonitis), the pleural membranes covering the lungs (see Empyema), or the tissues surrounding the heart (see Pericarditis). In rare cases, infection may spread via the bloodstream to the lungs or brain. Amebiasis usually responds quickly and completely to therapy. Relapse and fatality are unlikely with proper treatment, though in developing countries reinfection is common.

WHAT CAUSES IT?

• Infection occurs from ingestion of the fecally excreted, acid-resistant, cystic form of the amoeba. Transmission commonly results from fecal contamination of water or food, which is most prevalent in regions with poor sanitary conditions. Another mode of transmission is oral sex preceded by anal sex.

SYMPTOMS
• Diarrhea, possibly containing blood or mucus.
• Severe abdominal cramping and tenderness.
• Excessive gas.
• Loss of weight.
• High fever.
• Nausea and vomiting (with liver abscess).

• At highest risk for severe illness from amebiasis are those who are malnourished; under two years of age; receiving corticosteroid therapy; pregnant; or who have compromised immune systems.

PREVENTION

• When visiting underdeveloped countries, drink only boiled or purified water (chlorine is ineffective against amoebic cysts; water treated with iodine or globaline tablets is safe, however). In addition, do not eat uncooked vegetables (especially leafy greens, which are often fertilized with human waste) or fruit that is already sliced or peeled. Immunization is not available.

DIAGNOSIS

• Patient history and physical examination are needed.
• Confirmation of the diagnosis requires identification of *E. histolytica* in stool or tissue samples.
• Blood tests may be done to look for antibodies to the parasite.
• An abdominal ultrasound scan may be performed to check for liver abscess.
• Sigmoidoscopy (use of a lighted rectal scope) and a barium enema (use of barium to create a clear image of the intestine on x-ray) may be done to rule out other disorders of the colon that can mimic or occur in conjunction with amebiasis. Tissue biopsies from sigmoidoscopy are sometimes needed to confirm the presence of the amoeba.

HOW TO TREAT IT

• Replacement of fluids, electrolytes (mineral salts), and blood may be needed.
• Several drugs (including diloxanide furoate, tinidazole, iodoquinol, and metronidazole) are used to eliminate the amoeba. Metronidazole is most often used to treat symptomatic disease; iodoquinol helps eradicate cysts in patients with no symptoms.
• A liver abscess may be treated with needle aspiration (removal of pus with a syringe) or may require surgical drainage.

WHEN TO CALL A DOCTOR
• Call a doctor for persistent or recurrent diarrhea.

Amyloidosis

WHAT IS IT?

Amyloidosis is a rare disorder resulting from the buildup of a waxy substance in various organs. The substance (amyloid) is comprised of certain types of protein that, when present in excess amounts in the bloodstream, may seep out into the tissues and solidify. The most common sites for amyloid deposition are the kidneys, heart, skin, gastrointestinal tract, and nervous system. Interference with function of the involved organs, symptoms, and prognosis depend upon the location and the amount of accumulated amyloid protein. In most cases, however, outlook is poor. Kidney failure, congestive heart failure, cardiac arrhythmias, and gastrointestinal bleeding are the major life-threatening complications of amyloidosis.

WHAT CAUSES IT?

• In most cases, amyloidosis is caused by an abnormal protein (beta-amyloid), which is similar to the antibodies normally found in the blood; this condition is known as primary amyloidosis.

• Secondary amyloidosis, which is much more rare, may occur as a complication of certain long-standing inflammatory or infectious diseases, including rheumatoid arthritis and tuberculosis. Again, the culprit is an abnormal protein in the blood that is deposited in the tissues.

• Some forms of amyloidosis, affecting primarily the nerves, are inherited.

• Long-term hemodialysis therapy may lead to amyloidosis.

• Alzheimer's disease is thought to be related to a certain form of amyloidosis.

• Amyloidosis of the heart may develop as a result of old age.

PREVENTION

• There are no known ways to prevent most forms of amyloidosis.

• Effective treatment of infections such as tuberculosis can prevent chronic inflammation that causes secondary amyloidosis.

DIAGNOSIS

• Patient history and physical examination are needed.

• Protein levels in the blood and urine are measured.

• Needle biopsy (removal of a tissue sample for microscopic examination) of abdominal fat is usually performed. Sometimes it is necessary to biopsy the kidney, rectum, or other parts of the body.

HOW TO TREAT IT

• For primary amyloidosis, chemotherapeutic drugs are often given.

• The underlying disorder is treated in secondary amyloidosis.

• Medications may be given to treat the organs affected by amyloidosis.

• Dialysis or kidney transplant may be needed for patients with renal failure.

WHEN TO CALL A DOCTOR

• Amyloidosis can manifest itself in a myriad of ways. See a doctor if you develop unexplained weight loss, severe fatigue, or other symptoms of amyloidosis. ◢

SYMPTOMS

• Weight loss and fatigue are the most common symptoms.

• If the heart is affected: congestive heart failure with excessive accumulation of fluid in the tissues (edema); breathing difficulty; fatigue; heart rhythm disturbances with palpitations.

• If the kidneys are affected: symptoms of kidney failure (see Renal Failure, Chronic).

• If the skin is affected: slightly raised, waxy nodules clustered in the armpits, groin, face, neck, or ears; purple discoloration of the skin.

• Swelling of the tongue often occurs and may interfere with swallowing.

• If the gastrointestinal tract is affected: diarrhea; abdominal pain; blood in stool.

• If the nervous system is affected: dizziness upon standing; numbness or tingling in the hands or feet; inability to sweat; hoarseness.

• If the joints are affected: arthritic pain; morning stiffness.

Amyotrophic Lateral Sclerosis Lou Gehrig's Disease

WHAT IS IT?

Amyotrophic lateral sclerosis (ALS), also known as Lou Gehrig's disease, is a slowly progressive degeneration of the nerve cells of the spinal cord and lower brain stem, resulting in gradual loss of voluntary muscle control. (Sensory nerves and mental function are unaffected.) The disease is eventually fatal as muscles governing breathing, swallowing, and other crucial body functions are affected. Patients live an average of three to five years after the onset of symptoms; most die from respiratory insufficiency or from lung infections that tend to occur when breathing is impaired for long periods of time. ALS generally strikes between the ages of 50 and 70, and affects men slightly more often than women.

WHAT CAUSES IT?

• The cause of ALS is unknown; however, about 5 to 10 percent of cases appear to be inherited.
• Current theories suggest that the neurotransmitter glutamate (which is involved in the sending of nerve signals), free-radicals (unstable oxygen molecules that can damage cells), and the mineral calcium may all play roles in the death of motor nerve cells.

DIAGNOSIS

• No specific tests confirm the diagnosis; patient history and physical examination are needed. Diagnosis is based on clinical manifestations of the disease.
• Special neurological tests such as electromyography (EMG) or magnetic resonance imaging (MRI) may be performed to rule out other possible causes of symptoms.

PREVENTION

• There is no known way to prevent ALS.

HOW TO TREAT IT

• Although there is no cure, several drug treatments are either available or under study. Riluzole is the only Food and Drug Administration-approved drug for ALS; it has a modest effect in prolonging survival. Treatments that show promise include the anticonvulsant drug gabapentin, insulin-like growth factor I (Myotrophin), and certain antioxidants.
• Mechanical devices such as dressing aids and special utensils for eating are available to facilitate various everyday tasks.
• A cane or walker may be helpful for patients with gait impairment.
• Patients should carefully consider the option of using a mechanical respirator in the event that they become unable to breathe unassisted. Artificial ventilation can help some patients survive for years; however, many patients choose not to be kept alive in a state of total paralysis, unable to communicate except with eye movements. It is important to discuss this issue with doctors and family early on, so that decisions about emergency resuscitation may be made in the event of a respiratory crisis.
• Emotional support is crucial. Beyond the help that friends and family provide, a qualified counselor or psychotherapist can be a valuable asset. For assistance, contact the ALS Association or the Muscular Dystrophy Association.

WHEN TO CALL A DOCTOR

• See your doctor at the earliest signs of unexplained muscle weakness or difficulty controlling movement, particularly if speaking, breathing, or swallowing seems to be affected. ▲

SYMPTOMS

• Slow but relentlessly progressive muscle weakness and wasting (atrophy) in the limbs, torso, breathing muscles, throat, and tongue. Weakness usually begins in the limbs.
• Muscle twitching, cramps, stiffness, and easy fatigability.
• Slowed, progressively unintelligible speech.
• Difficulty breathing and swallowing; choking.
• Weight loss, due to both atrophy and swallowing difficulty.
• Involuntary bursts of laughter or crying.
• Changes in gait; eventually, inability to walk.

Anal Fissures

WHAT IS IT?

An anal fissure is a shallow ulceration or tear in the tissue along the anal canal. During bowel movements, irritation of the fissure can trigger a spasm in the anal sphincter, the muscle that surrounds the opening of the anus. Such spasms are often quite painful and may be accompanied by bleeding. This condition is more common among women.

WHAT CAUSES IT?

• Anal fissures are typically caused when large, hard stools tear the lining of the anal canal as they pass.

• Fissures may also occur as a secondary complication to anal surgery, proctitis (inflammation of the rectum), or other disorders.

• The risk of anal fissures increases with constipation, multiple pregnancies, and repeated use of enema nozzles. Also, older people may be more likely to develop anal fissures, owing to age-related changes in the skin as well as increased frequency of constipation. Obesity may lead to increased sweating, which may be an aggravating factor.

PREVENTION

• Eat a high-fiber diet that includes lots of fresh fruits and legumes and whole-grain products.

• Maintain good hygiene in the anal area. Use talcum powder or corn starch to keep the area dry during hot weather.

• Drink plenty of liquids (at least eight glasses of water a day) to soften the stool and help prevent constipation.

• Don't strain during bowel movements.

• Avoid constipating foods and ask your doctor whether any drugs you take may be the cause of constipation.

DIAGNOSIS

• Patient history and physical examination are needed.

• Examination with an anoscope or sigmoidoscope are required to detect the fissure and to rule out other causes of rectal bleeding.

HOW TO TREAT IT

• Most anal fissures heal naturally within a few days (although spasms of the sphincter may aggravate the condition and delay healing).

• A warm sitz bath after a difficult bowel movement may ease painful spasms of the anal sphincter. Apply a nonprescription topical cream, such as zinc oxide or a hemorrhoidal preparation, after the bath.

• Stool softeners may be advised; check with your doctor.

• Nitroglycerin ointment (0.2%) may be prescribed to relieve spasms and promote healing.

• Persistent or recurrent anal fissures may require surgical removal of the fissure or anal dilatation to relieve spasms and relax the anus. Although postoperative healing is usually rapid and complete, fissures may recur.

WHEN TO CALL A DOCTOR

• If symptoms of an anal fissure persist, contact your doctor.

• Blood in the stool can be a warning sign of a more serious condition and should be evaluated by your doctor.

SYMPTOMS

• Sharp or burning rectal pain during and immediately after bowel movements, especially when the stool is hard or bulky.

• Bright red blood in stool or bloody streaks on toilet paper or underwear.

• Rectal itching.

Anaphylaxis

WHAT IS IT?

Anaphylaxis is a severe, life-threatening allergic reaction that affects organ systems throughout the body. It occurs when the immune system becomes sensitized to an allergen (be it a food, drug, insect venom, or anything that elicits an allergic response) and then, upon exposure to the allergen, overreacts, releasing cascades of histamine and other substances that can cause contraction of the intestinal smooth muscles, skin reactions, constriction of the airways, and a precipitous drop in blood pressure that may lead to shock. Immediate medical attention is essential; severe cases may prove fatal even with treatment.

WHAT CAUSES IT?

• An insect sting.
• Ingestion of a food or food additive. Peanuts are the most common cause of food-induced anaphylaxis.
• Injection of a drug, vaccine, or a chemical used in a diagnostic procedure. Penicillin is the most common cause of drug-induced anaphylaxis. Some oral drugs can also trigger the reaction.
• Rarely, symptoms occur without apparent exposure to a known cause.

PREVENTION

• Avoid allergens that have caused an adverse reaction in the past.
• People who have previously had a severe allergic reaction should wear a Medic-Alert bracelet and get a prescription for epinephrine (adrenaline), which halts the allergic reaction and should be carried at all times. An easy-to-use form is the Epi-pen, a spring-loaded device that automatically injects a dose of epinephrine when pressed against the skin (usually the leg). The drug does not substitute for necessary medical treatment but does buy valuable time until help can be found.

DIAGNOSIS

• Diagnosis is indicated by sudden onset of characteristic symptoms, particularly when they appear following exposure to a suspected allergen. Since anaphylaxis is an emergency, immediate treatment supersedes the need for further confirmatory procedures. Tests for the specific allergen may be done after the patient has stabilized.

HOW TO TREAT IT

• Immediate medical treatment is necessary. An injection of the adrenal hormone epinephrine (adrenaline) is necessary to counteract the effect of histamine throughout the body. Doses may need to be repeated every 10 to 20 minutes until the reaction ceases.
• Inhalation of beta-sympathomimetic agents are used to halt asthmatic symptoms.
• If life-threatening breathing obstruction has occurred due to swelling of the larynx, a tube may be placed through the mouth or nose to aid in breathing; in very serious cases a tracheostomy (insertion of a breathing tube through a surgical opening in the throat) may be needed.
• Intravenous fluids containing blood pressure-raising agents are administered if shock occurs.
• Antihistamines (such as diphenhydramine) or corticosteroids (such as prednisone) may be used after the initial crisis has passed to prevent return of symptoms.

WHEN TO CALL A DOCTOR

• **EMERGENCY** An anaphylactic reaction requires immediate medical attention. Call an ambulance or get to an emergency room right away. ⚠

SYMPTOMS

• Itching and hives.
• Swelling of the eyes, lips, and tongue.
• Weakness or faintness.
• Tightening in the chest or throat; wheezing; shortness of breath.
• Profuse sweating.
• Palpitations.
• Sudden, intense distress; feelings of impending doom.
• Stomach cramps, nausea and vomiting, or diarrhea.
• Bluish tinge (cyanosis) to the skin, lips, and nail beds due to oxygen insufficiency.

Anemia, Aplastic

WHAT IS IT?

Aplastic anemia occurs when the bone marrow fails to produce an adequate supply of red blood cells, white blood cells, and platelets. The onset is usually gradual but may be sudden (acute). Low levels of red cells result in weakness, fatigue, pallor, and shortness of breath. Lack of white cells leaves the patient vulnerable to serious infection, while an inadequate number of platelets increases the risk of bleeding. For these reasons, aplastic anemia is potentially life-threatening. In fact, left untreated, severe aplastic anemia is fatal within a year for more than 80 percent of patients. Chances for recovery are best when the disorder is caused by an anticancer drug or a reaction to a medication. Even then, recovery may take six to eight months. This relatively rare disorder is more common among men.

WHAT CAUSES IT?

- In half of all cases, no cause is established.
- Most other cases are due to external causes, including toxic agents (benzene, some solvents, industrial chemicals), certain drugs (such as immunosuppressive and anticancer drugs), and radiation exposure.
- Certain diseases, such as hepatitis or a tumor of the thymus gland, may cause aplastic anemia. Acute leukemia may initially resemble aplastic anemia.
- Risk is increased among those with a family history of a rare disorder called Fanconi's anemia.

PREVENTION

- There is no known way to prevent aplastic anemia, except by avoiding exposure to toxic chemicals, radiation, and drugs known to cause the disorder, such as the antibiotic chloramphenicol or the nonsteroidal anti-inflammatory phenylbutazone.

DIAGNOSIS

- Blood counts indicating a reduction in red cells, white cells, and platelets suggest the presence of aplastic anemia.
- A bone marrow biopsy is necessary to verify the presence of aplastic anemia and its severity.

HOW TO TREAT IT

- For cases of mild to moderate severity, no treatment may be necessary.
- The patient should eliminate exposure to any identifiable potential cause of aplastic anemia. If a medication is the suspected cause, a safer substitute should be used.
- Medications such as antithymocyte globulin, cyclosporine, and cyclophosphamide are available; these are successful in over 50 percent of patients with aplastic anemia of unknown origin.
- Antibiotics are typically given (often intravenously) when fever occurs to ward off infection.
- A bone marrow transplant is the treatment of choice for people under age 55 with severe aplastic anemia, provided a compatible donor can be found. (A twin or other sibling is usually the best choice.)
- For severe cases, a doctor may order periodic transfusions of whole blood or specific blood cells until the bone marrow begins to function properly again. However, transfusions, particularly from family donors, should be avoided, if possible, if bone marrow transplantation is being considered as an option.
- Because of the risk of serious bleeding, the patient should avoid handling sharp instruments, such as razors or knives. To this end, using items such as electric shavers and soft toothbrushes is advised. Aspirin, aspirin-containing products, and alcohol should also be avoided.
- Medicated mouthwash or diluted hydrogen peroxide is often used to ward off mouth infections.

WHEN TO CALL A DOCTOR

- The symptoms of aplastic anemia warrant a doctor's prompt attention. ▲

SYMPTOMS

- Increased susceptibility to infection.
- Ulcers in the mouth, throat, and rectum.
- Unusual bruising or bleeding (including spontaneous unexplained bleeding from the nose, mouth, gums, rectum, or vagina).
- Small red dots (petechiae) under the skin, indicating bleeding; paleness (pallor).
- Weakness, fatigue, and breathlessness.

Anemia, Folic Acid Deficiency

WHAT IS IT?
Folic acid is an essential vitamin for the production of red blood cells. As such, a deficiency in this vitamin can cause anemia. A reduced number of red cells deprives body tissues of an adequate supply of oxygen, resulting in the classic symptoms of anemia (see below). The disorder is particularly common among infants, adolescents during a growth spurt, pregnant or lactating women, the elderly, smokers, alcoholics, and those on fad diets or who suffer from intestinal disorders. It is often accompanied by iron deficiency anemia.

WHAT CAUSES IT?
• Folic acid deficiency is due to either insufficient dietary intake of folic acid or, rarely, an inability of the intestine to absorb folic acid properly.
• Alcoholism interferes with the body's ability to absorb and use folic acid; many alcoholics also have poor diets lacking in folic acid.
• Intestinal disorders such as tropical sprue, celiac disease, inflammatory bowel disease, or bowel resection may impede folic acid absorption.
• The body does not store large amounts of folic acid, and at certain times in the life cycle (such as childhood, pregnancy, and when breastfeeding) the body's demands for it outweigh dietary intake.
• Certain medications (such as anticonvulsants, antibiotics, oral contraceptives, and anticancer drugs) can lead to folic acid deficiency.
• Risk of folic acid deficiency increases in association with certain skin diseases, including psoriasis and exfoliative dermatitis.

SYMPTOMS
• Severe fatigue and weakness.
• Paleness (pallor).
• Shortness of breath.
• Heart palpitations or noticeably rapid heartbeat upon exertion.
• Sore, red, and glazed-looking tongue.
• Loss of appetite leading to weight loss.
• Abdominal swelling.
• Nausea and diarrhea.

• Certain blood disorders in which there is an increased demand for red cells (such as sickle cell anemia or thalassemia) can lead to depletion of body folate stores unless supplemental folic acid is provided.

PREVENTION
• Eat a balanced, sensible diet. The main sources of folic acid include fresh green leafy vegetables, raw fruit, mushrooms, lima and kidney beans, yeast, and organ meats such as liver and kidney.
• Avoid overcooking foods rich in folic acid (overcooking destroys their vitamin content).
• Consume alcohol only in moderation.

DIAGNOSIS
• A blood test that measures folic acid can determine whether the body's folate stores are adequate.

HOW TO TREAT IT
• Proper diet is frequently all that is required to correct the problem.
• Folic acid tablets can quickly correct the disorder. Depending on the cause of the deficiency, supplemental folic acid may be needed for a time; in rare instances, injections of folic acid are necessary.
• Elimination of causative factors (poor diet or excessive drinking, for example) is essential.
• Treatment of an underlying intestinal disorder causing folic acid deficiency may serve as a cure.

WHEN TO CALL A DOCTOR
• Make an appointment with your doctor if you have symptoms of anemia.
• If you're already being treated for folic acid deficiency and symptoms don't improve after two weeks, notify your doctor.
• All women who are considering pregnancy should discuss folic acid supplementation with their doctors. Such supplementation during the early weeks of pregnancy decreases the incidence of nerve (neural) defects in a developing child.

Anemia, Hemolytic

WHAT IS IT?

Hemolytic anemia occurs when circulating red blood cells are destroyed prematurely. Often the bone marrow cannot produce new red cells fast enough to compensate for the increased destruction (despite the fact that marrow is capable of producing red cells at up to six times the normal rate). The disorder is rarely life-threatening, but it may be difficult to treat.

WHAT CAUSES IT?

• Hemolytic anemia is either inherited or acquired. Inherited cases are due to a genetic abnormality in the red cells themselves, and anemia generally appears early in life. Hereditary forms include hemoglobinopathies such as sickle cell anemia, red cell membrane disorders like hereditary spherocytosis (a condition in which the red cells are spherical instead of the normal doughnut shape), and red cell enzyme disorders such as glucose-6-phosphate dehydrogenase deficiency (G6PD).

• In people with G6PD, red cell destruction (hemolysis) is usually provoked by exposure to certain substances. These include certain types of drugs such as sulfonamides and antimalarials, the medication nitrofurantoin, and the active ingredient in mothballs.

• Infection, fever, or disturbances of normal metabolism can also initiate hemolysis.

• Hemolytic anemia in one form of G6PD deficiency, common in the Greek isles, results from the ingestion of fava beans (or inhalation of pollen from the plant).

• Certain types of viral, bacterial, or parasitic infections can cause red cell destruction.

• For unknown reasons, the body occasionally produces antibodies to its own red cells. This is known as autoimmune hemolytic anemia and may occur alone or as a consequence of other diseases, such as lymphoma.

• Transfusion with incompatible blood will result in either immediate and severe or delayed hemolysis.

• Abnormalities in the lining of the blood vessels, artificial heart valves, or blood clots may cause mechanical damage that destroys red cells.

• Certain drugs, such as antibiotics, antihypertensives, and antiarrhythmics can cause hemolysis by either immune or nonimmune mechanisms.

PREVENTION

• When hemolytic anemia is provoked by specific substances, avoiding them can prevent recurrence.

DIAGNOSIS

• Blood tests, including a complete blood count, are necessary.

• A family history is conducted.

• Occasionally, when hemolysis is very mild and there is little evidence of anemia, a radioactive chromium test may be performed to assess red cell survival, which is always shortened.

• Other more specialized tests for abnormalities of the red cell membrane, enzymes, or hemoglobin may be necessary.

HOW TO TREAT IT

• Immunosuppressant drugs, such as corticosteroids (prednisone, for example), may be useful in cases caused by an autoimmune disorder.

• Anemia due to hereditary spherocytosis or autoimmune hemolysis can be greatly improved by removal of the spleen (splenectomy), as the spleen is the primary site of red cell destruction.

• Blood transfusions are sometimes required as emergency treatment.

• Folic acid supplementation should be provided.

WHEN TO CALL A DOCTOR

• Any symptoms of anemia warrant a call to your doctor.

SYMPTOMS

• Fatigue and weakness.
• Paleness (pallor).
• Shortness of breath.
• Palpitations or other heartbeat irregularities.
• Jaundice and dark urine (caused by excessive formation of the bile pigment bilirubin) as red cells are destroyed prematurely.

Anemia, Iron Deficiency

WHAT IS IT?

Iron deficiency anemia occurs when the body's usual stores of iron are so depleted that the bone marrow cannot produce enough hemoglobin, the iron-containing protein in red blood cells that carries oxygen in the bloodstream. Iron deficiency is the most common cause of anemia, is rarely serious, and is easily treated in most cases. In fact, in mild chronic cases, it often produces few or no symptoms and is generally discovered only when a doctor obtains a complete blood count (CBC). Of course, more severe anemia gradually leads to noticeable fatigue and other symptoms.

WHAT CAUSES IT?

• The most common cause of iron deficiency anemia is gradual, prolonged blood loss. For this reason, menstruating women are particularly prone to anemia. In men, the most common cause of iron deficiency is blood loss in the digestive tract, resulting from disorders such as peptic ulcer, inflammatory bowel disease, and stomach or colon cancer. Sometimes hemorrhoids bleed enough to result in anemia.
• Long-term use of aspirin (for heart attack prevention) or nonsteroidal anti-inflammatory drugs (such as ibuprofen and naproxen, used for pain relief) can irritate the lining of the stomach and cause bleeding, resulting in anemia.

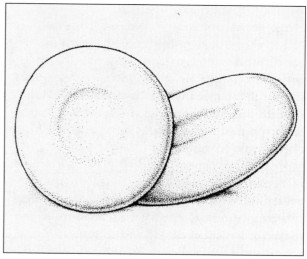

The shape of the red blood cell affords optimum surface area for the transport of oxygen molecules. All of the various types of anemia are characterized by a deficiency of healthy red blood cells.

• Pregnancy and breastfeeding increase the susceptibility of iron deficiency. Children with an inadequate diet may also be at risk.
• In chronically ill patients, repeated blood drawing for diagnostic testing can produce an iron deficiency.
• Poor absorption of iron may result from surgical removal of the stomach (gastrectomy), from intestinal disorders that cause chronic diarrhea, or from abnormal food habits such as the ingestion of clay (stemming from unusual cravings known as pica).
• Intestinal parasites such as hookworm can cause iron deficiency.

PREVENTION

• Eat a balanced, sensible diet.
• Pregnant and menstruating women should discuss iron supplementation with their doctors.
• If you must regularly take aspirin or nonsteroidal anti-inflammatory drugs, take them with food or an antacid (one containing magnesium and aluminum hydroxide is best).

DIAGNOSIS

• A blood test for the protein ferritin can usually determine whether there is an iron deficiency.
• A gastrointestinal endoscopy (the insertion of a lighted scope through the mouth and into the

---

SYMPTOMS

• Fatigue and weakness.
• Pallor (may be especially noticeable in the gums, eyelids, and nail beds).
• Heart palpitations, rapid heartbeat, or breathing difficulty, especially upon exertion.
• Irritability.
• Inability to concentrate.
• Smooth, sore tongue or tiny cracks at the corners of the mouth.
• Brittle nails.
• Black, tarry (or even bloody) stools (when anemia is due to substantial blood loss in the gastrointestinal tract).
• Unusual craving (called pica) for clay, dirt, or ice.

Anemia, Iron Deficiency   *continued*

esophagus) may be necessary to locate the source of gastrointestinal iron loss.

HOW TO TREAT IT

• First, it is essential for a doctor to determine the underlying cause of an iron deficiency, and each case is treated based on the doctor's conclusions. Do not attempt to treat iron deficiency anemia yourself.

• Iron supplementation may be required—but only under a doctor's supervision. Taking too much iron unnecessarily can lead to excessive storage of iron and serious health problems, including heart and liver damage. Also, if you are losing blood due to a disease such as colon cancer, supplements might mask the problem and delay the diagnosis.

• If iron supplements are prescribed, be sure to take them for the full term recommended by your doctor, even if you begin to feel well again. After the anemia is cured, your body needs to replenish its reserve stores of iron, which may take three months or more.

• Note that iron absorption is decreased by milk and antacids.

• Iron may be given by intravenous injection in patients who cannot tolerate oral iron therapy.

• In very rare and severe cases, iron deficiency anemia may be severe enough to require a transfusion of packed red cells.

WHEN TO CALL A DOCTOR

• Call your doctor if you experience the symptoms of anemia. Sometimes iron deficiency anemia is an indication of a more serious underlying disorder, such as peptic ulcer or colon cancer. Certain tests may be needed to confirm or rule out these possibilities.

• Women who are pregnant or menstruate heavily should contact their doctors to discuss iron supplementation.

• People on rapid weight loss programs should discuss their dietary needs for iron and other nutrients with a doctor or a qualified nutritionist. ▲

Anemia, Pernicious

WHAT IS IT?

Pernicious anemia is a rare type of anemia (an inadequate number of red blood cells) that results from an insufficiency of vitamin B_{12} (cobalamin), an essential component in the manufacture of red cells. A dietary deficiency of B_{12} is very rare; rather, this disorder usually occurs because the body cannot properly absorb the vitamin. Pernicious anemia, which develops and progresses subtly, may at first produce the characteristic symptoms of all types of anemia: weakness, fatigue, and paleness (pallor). Untreated, the disease may cause disturbances in the gastrointestinal and cardiovascular systems and especially the nervous system, because B_{12} is essential for proper nerve function. With treatment, prognosis is excellent, although severe neurologic damage is usually permanent. Pernicious anemia can occur at any age; among younger individuals it is most common in African American women.

WHAT CAUSES IT?

• Pernicious anemia almost always results from an impaired ability to absorb vitamin B_{12}. This can occur when cells in the stomach lining atrophy and fail to produce normal amounts of digestive acids as well as a substance called intrinsic factor, which is essential for the absorption of B_{12}. It may also result from an abnormality in the small intestine, where vitamin B_{12} is absorbed.

SYMPTOMS

• Fatigue and weakness.
• Heart palpitations; lightheadedness or dizziness.
• Pallor (may be especially noticeable in the lips, gums, eyelids, and nail beds).
• Shortness of breath or chest pain on exertion.
• Sore, red, and glazed-looking tongue.
• Irritability or inability to concentrate.
• Mild jaundice of the eyes or skin.
• Loss of appetite leading to weight loss.
• Nausea and diarrhea.
• Neurologic symptoms: numbness and tingling in the extremities, poor coordination, and loss of fine touch.

• The incidence of pernicious anemia is higher in those with a family history of pernicious anemia or other apparent autoimmune disorders, such as Graves' disease, hypothyroidism, or vitiligo.
• Partial or total surgical resection of the stomach or damage to the lining of the stomach may prevent secretion of intrinsic factor and hamper B_{12} absorption.
• Disorders of the small intestine can interfere with B_{12} absorption.
• Rarely, a dietary lack of B_{12} causes the disorder.

PREVENTION

• There is no way to prevent pernicious anemia, except in the rare cases caused by a dietary B_{12} deficiency, which may affect strict vegetarians who avoid meat and dairy products entirely. Such people should take vitamin supplements.

DIAGNOSIS

• Patient history and physical examination.
• A blood test to measure levels of B_{12} and red cell folate (the blood abnormalities of vitamin B_{12} and folate deficiency are identical).
• A Schilling test (using radioactive vitamin B_{12} to accurately measure the amount being absorbed into the bloodstream).

HOW TO TREAT IT

• Lifelong intramuscular injections of vitamin B_{12} (usually self-administered once a month) are necessary. Because the problem lies in the body's inability to absorb the vitamin, oral B_{12} is generally not used. However, massive oral doses of B_{12} are effective when injections are not feasible.
• Rarely, those with very severe anemia may need an initial blood transfusion.
• Pernicious anemia is associated with an increased risk of stomach cancer, so lifelong cancer screening is recommended.

WHEN TO CALL A DOCTOR

• Consult your doctor if you experience persistent fatigue, weakness, or pallor. Avoid self-medication with folic acid, which can mask the anemia of vitamin B_{12} deficiency and make the neurologic abnormalities worse. ⬛

Ankylosing Spondylitis

WHAT IS IT?

Ankylosing spondylitis (AS) is an uncommon type of inflammatory arthritis that primarily affects the joints of the spinal column. Typically, AS originates in the sacroiliac joints, where the vertebrae of the spine meet the pelvis. The disease tends to progress from the lower back up to the vertebrae in the neck. (Peripheral joints are also involved in as many as 25 percent of cases, especially among women.) Cartilage and other tissue between the joints gradually deteriorate and are replaced by hard, fibrous tissue. Eventually the bones fuse together and joint flexibility is lost. Symptoms—primarily lower back pain and stiffness—often first appear in late adolescence or early adulthood; onset after age 45 is very rare. Early onset of the disease is associated with a worse prognosis.

The most serious complication is spinal fracture that can result in quadriplegia; however, most patients suffer no serious disability despite the pain and are able to continue working. The disease may get progressively worse, stabilize, or go into remission at any point. About 25 to 30 percent of AS patients are affected by inflammation and scarring of structures within the eye (see Uveitis and Iritis), and a few patients may develop an abnormality of the aortic valve in the heart or scarring of lung tissue. Ankylosing spondylitis is more common among Caucasians than other races and is three times more prevalent in men than women.

WHAT CAUSES IT?

• The cause of AS is unknown, though hereditary factors appear to play a role. There is also evidence suggesting a link between intestinal bacteria or inflammation and the autoimmune activity (in which the body's defenses against disease attack healthy tissue) involved in the mechanism of joint deterioration.

PREVENTION

• There is no known way to prevent AS.

DIAGNOSIS

• No definitive laboratory tests exist to distinguish AS from similar inflammatory diseases. Diagnosis is primarily based on patient history, physical examination, and x-ray findings.
• Blood tests may detect a specific antigen (HLA-B27) that is present in 90 percent of patients with AS. The presence of this antigen does not confirm the diagnosis (it is also seen in 6 to 8 percent of normal Caucasians), but does suggest a genetic predisposition to the disease.
• X-rays may reveal signs of joint deterioration in the spine, pelvis, or hips.

HOW TO TREAT IT

• There is no specific way to treat AS; therapy is aimed at relieving discomfort and maintaining joint function.
• Nonsteroidal anti-inflammatory drugs (NSAIDs), especially indomethacin, are commonly prescribed to ease pain and inflammation.
• Strength-training exercises and other forms of physical therapy may help to maintain or improve flexibility.
• Braces and supports are not helpful and are not advised.
• Occasionally, direct injections of corticosteroids may be beneficial in patients unresponsive to NSAIDs.
• Severe arthritis in the hips may warrant total hip replacement surgery (arthroplasty).
• If uveitis occurs, it can be treated with corticosteroids and medicated eyedrops.

WHEN TO CALL A DOCTOR

• Make an appointment with a doctor for any persistent back pain.

SYMPTOMS

• Lower back pain that may be intermittent or persistent. Pain may be worse at night.
• Morning stiffness in the back or hips that improves with activity.
• Limited chest capacity due to pain and stiffness in the ribs.
• Neck or chest pain.
• Eye pain, blurred vision, watery eyes, and aversion to light (due to associated uveitis).
• Pain in the peripheral joints.

Anxiety States

WHAT IS IT?

Anxiety can be a natural, beneficial reaction to stress or danger. However, a state of anxiety is unhealthy when it becomes excessive or unreasonable, persists in the absence of obvious stress, interferes with normal daily functioning, or causes emotional discomfort. Anxiety states may occur episodically, as in panic disorder, which is marked by repeated episodes of sudden, intense, and unwarranted bouts of terror. Panic attacks are accompanied by dread and fear of dying; symptoms can be mistaken for a heart attack. People with recurrent panic attacks often develop a fear of being alone in a public place (agoraphobia).

Anxiety states can also be chronic and persistent. These include generalized anxiety disorder (GAD) and others. In GAD, a person experiences excessive anxiety and worry not linked to any one event or activity. Posttraumatic stress disorder is characterized by long-term psychological distress following a traumatic event, such as a natural catastrophe, warfare, rape, child abuse, or a car crash. Obsessive-compulsive disorder is marked by repetitive, nonsensical thoughts (such as constantly thinking of a particular word or of harming a family member) or by irrational behaviors and rituals (such as constant handwashing or checking to see if a door is locked). Phobias are unreasonable fears, such as of being in a confined space (claustrophobia) or driving across a bridge.

Anxiety states are exceedingly common. They have a higher prevalence in women and are among the most successfully treatable of all mental disorders. But untreated anxiety disorders increase the risk of hypertension, drug and alcohol abuse, and suicide.

WHAT CAUSES IT?

• The causes of anxiety states are generally unknown. A genetic or biochemical predisposition appears to be part of the explanation, but early childhood experiences and pivotal life events play a role.
• Various drugs or chemical substances can trigger anxiety; these include caffeine, nonprescription decongestants and cold remedies, thyroid hormone, and inhaled asthma drugs. Anxiety also accompanies withdrawal from caffeine, alcohol, tobacco, sedatives, narcotics, and other addictive drugs.

PREVENTION

• Those who have suffered anxiety states in the past may prevent future ones by receiving treatment.

DIAGNOSIS

• A thorough patient history establishes the diagnosis.
• Certain tests, such as blood tests and CT (computed tomography) scans may be done to rule out an underlying cause of anxiety, such as hyperthyroidism.

HOW TO TREAT IT

• Cognitive-behavioral psychotherapy, sometimes combined with drug therapy.
• Relaxation techniques, such as biofeedback, meditation, and yoga.
• Antidepressant drugs, often combined with psychotherapy, are effective for GAD, panic, posttraumatic stress, and obsessive-compulsive disorders.
• Short-term therapy with benzodiazepine tranquilizers is occasionally recommended. Long-term use can lead to dependence.

WHEN TO CALL A DOCTOR

• Consult a doctor if chest pain, shortness of breath, or panic attacks interfere with your quality of life. ▲

SYMPTOMS

• Heightened self-awareness and alertness to surroundings (hypervigilance).
• Intense worry and feelings of dread.
• Impaired concentration; fleeting attention span.
• Restlessness and irritability; insomnia.
• Profuse sweating; hot flashes.
• Muscle tension and trembling.
• Rapid, shallow breathing (hyperventilation) or breathlessness.
• Palpitations or chest pains.
• Dilated pupils.
• Dry mouth; a feeling of a lump in the throat.
• Excessive fatigue or weakness.
• Repetitive, unwanted thoughts or behaviors (obsessive-compulsive disorder).
• Nightmares and upsetting flashbacks (posttraumatic stress disorder).

Aortic Aneurysm

WHAT IS IT?

An aortic aneurysm is a weak spot in the wall of the aorta, the primary artery that carries blood from the heart to the head and extremities. There are three common types of aortic aneurysm. Saccular and fusiform aneurysms are balloonlike swellings of the arterial wall that can occur in the portion of the aorta within the chest or just below the kidney in the abdomen. A dissecting aneurysm is a longitudinal, blood-filled split in the lining of the artery, usually occurring in the aortic arch near the heart. As blood is pumped through the aorta, the weak spot in the elastic arterial wall bulges outward.

The risk is that an aneurysm will eventually rupture, with great bleeding internally and complete collapse of circulation. Sudden severe pain, shock, and loss of consciousness usually occur within seconds, and death is imminent in more than 50 percent of cases, even with emergency surgery. Thus, the goal is to detect and treat an aortic aneurysm before it ruptures. Aortic aneurysms generally affect people over 60 and are more common among men.

PREVENTION

• Eat a diet low in cholesterol and saturated fats to reduce the risk of atherosclerosis.

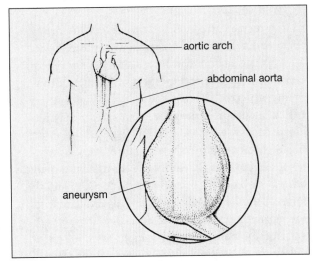

Just above the heart, the aorta branches upward to carry blood to the head and also arches downward to supply the lower extremities. An aneurysm may balloon outward anywhere along the aortic wall, but they are more common in the abdominal aorta.

• Take steps to prevent, detect, and treat high blood pressure.

WHAT CAUSES IT?

• Approximately 95 percent of aortic aneurysms are caused by atherosclerosis, the narrowing of an artery due to the buildup of fatty plaque.
• The muscular middle layer of the artery may be congenitally weak and thus prone to a dissecting aneurysm.
• High blood pressure (hypertension) intensifies the force of blood on the walls of the arteries and contributes to the development of dissecting aneurysms.
• Syphilis may cause a saccular or fusiform aneurysm near the heart (now rare).
• The arterial wall may be weakened as a result of trauma or complication of other diseases, possibly leading to saccular or fusiform aneurysms.

DIAGNOSIS

• Physical examination of your abdomen by the doctor may reveal a pulsing aneurysm.
• X-rays, CT scans, or ultrasound imaging may confirm the presence of an aneurysm.
• Angiography (an injection of an opaque dye into an artery to produce a clear x-ray image of the aorta) may be performed.

SYMPTOMS

• In the majority of cases there are no warning symptoms. More likely, an aortic aneurysm is detected with an x-ray or during a routine physical examination.
• Hoarseness, difficulty in swallowing, or persistent cough may indicate a saccular or fusiform aneurysm in the chest area.
• A throbbing lump in the abdominal area, severe backache, leg pain or a feeling of coldness in the leg (due to an embolus from a clot formed in an abdominal aneurysm), or severe abdominal pain (due to the rupture of an abdominal aneurysm) may indicate a saccular or fusiform aneurysm in the abdominal area.
• Severe chest pain that may be mistaken for a heart attack may signal a dissecting aneurysm.

Aortic Aneurysm *continued*

HOW TO TREAT IT

• Have regular physical exams to detect an aortic aneurysm before it has a chance to rupture. Your doctor may recommend x-rays and angiography to determine the size and location of an aneurysm if one is suspected.

• If an aneurysm is detected, your doctor may recommend watching and waiting (especially if it is small), since aneurysms tend to grow very slowly.

• Your doctor may prescribe a beta-blocking medication. Beta-blockers decrease blood pressure and the force of the heart's contraction, thus reducing pressure against the walls of the aorta.

• Periodic ultrasound examinations are used to follow the expansion of an aneurysm over time.

• Certain aneurysms require immediate treatment, often involving surgical removal of the affected portion of the artery and replacement with a synthetic arterial graft. Surgery may also be required if an aneurysm is causing pain, is larger than six centimeters, or is rapidly expanding. Surgery on an unruptured aneurysm has an 80 to 90 percent success rate.

WHEN TO CALL A DOCTOR

• Call a doctor if you experience symptoms of an aortic aneurysm.

• See your doctor regularly if you suffer from high blood pressure or high cholesterol, each a major risk factor for the different types of aneurysm. ⚠

Appendicitis, Acute

WHAT IS IT?

Acute appendicitis is inflammation of the appendix, the narrow, finger-shaped organ that branches off the first part of the large intestine on the right side of the abdomen. Although the appendix is a vestigial organ with no known function, it can become diseased. In fact, acute appendicitis is the most common reason for abdominal surgery in the world. If it is not treated promptly, there is the chance that the inflamed appendix will burst, spilling fecal material into the abdominal cavity. The usual result is a potentially life-threatening infection (peritonitis), but the infection may become sealed off and form an abscess. Appendicitis is uncommon among older people, and symptoms are generally mild, so that

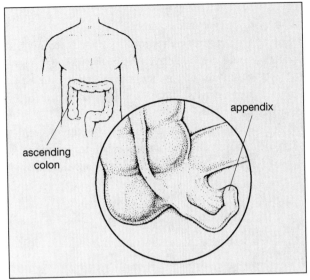

The appendix, about 3.5 inches long, extends from the bottom of the first or ascending portion of the colon. It serves no known function.

diagnosis of the acute episode is often not made. Members of this age group are thus at greater risk for rupture with peritonitis or abscess formation.

WHAT CAUSES IT?

- Appendicitis is usually caused by a bacterial infection, although the reason the appendix becomes infected is unknown.
- The appendix may become obstructed by a lump of feces or tumors, leading to inflammation and infection.

PREVENTION

- There are no specific preventive measures. Contrary to popular belief, swallowing seeds from fruit does not precipitate appendicitis.

DIAGNOSIS

- Physical examination is necessary to rule out other disorders that produce symptoms similar to those of appendicitis.
- A rectal examination may be performed.
- Blood and urine samples will be taken for analysis.
- An abdominal x-ray may be necessary.
- Viewing the appendix through a small incision in the abdomen or with a special instrument (laparoscope) may be needed to confirm the diagnosis.

SYMPTOMS

- In very young children or people over age 65, symptoms may be deceptively mild. Otherwise, symptoms can vary widely and may include the following:
- Vague discomfort near the navel (early in an attack), migrating to the right lower quadrant of the abdomen.
- Sharp, localized, persistent pain within a few hours.
- Pain that worsens with movement, deep breathing, coughing, sneezing, walking or being touched.
- Constipation and inability to pass gas, possibly alternating with diarrhea.
- Low fever (below 102°F). A high fever (possibly accompanied by chills) may indicate an abscessed appendix.
- Rapid heartbeat.
- Abdominal swelling (in late stages).
- Abrupt cessation of abdominal pain after other symptoms occur, indicating the appendix has burst—an emergency.
- Nausea and vomiting (in some cases).
- Loss of appetite.
- Coated tongue and bad breath.
- Painful urination.
- Blood in the urine.

Appendicitis, Acute *continued*

HOW TO TREAT IT

• Call your doctor immediately.

• The appendix must be removed (appendectomy). Surgery should not be delayed more than a few hours.

• If you are unsure of your symptoms, take your temperature every two hours and keep a record for your doctor.

• If you suspect appendicitis, avoid laxatives and enemas (they can cause an inflamed appendix to burst), and pain relievers (they may hinder an accurate diagnosis). Avoid eating or drinking (take small sips of water if you are thirsty), since anesthesia is safer on an empty stomach. Rest in a chair or bed.

• If an abscess has formed, your doctor may drain it and prescribe large doses of antibiotics. Appendectomy may be scheduled for a later date.

WHEN TO CALL A DOCTOR

• Call a doctor immediately if you experience symptoms that may indicate appendicitis. ▲

Asthma

WHAT IS IT?

Bronchial asthma is a condition caused by chronically hyperreactive and inflamed airways, punctuated by acute episodes of reversible obstruction of the airways. For reasons not fully understood, those suffering from asthma are hyperresponsive to irritants such as dust, cold air, and viral infections. Such irritants may periodically cause bronchospasm—contraction of the muscles within the bronchi (the airways between the trachea and the air sacs of the lungs)—and provoke increased mucus production. These two reactions further narrow the already inflamed airways and make it very difficult for the asthma sufferer to breathe. Attacks may be mild or severe and may last anywhere from a few minutes to days. Asthma may develop at any age, although 50 percent of children with asthma outgrow the condition as they get older and the bronchial passages widen.

WHAT CAUSES IT?

• While asthma is generally caused by allergy to some foreign substance (allergen) or irritant, no extrinsic trigger can be found in some types of asthma. Allergens include (but are not limited to) pollen, dust mites, feathers, animal dander, molds, some drugs such as aspirin, other allergic conditions such as eczema or hay fever, and rarely, foods. Irritants may include cold or dry air, smoke, air pollu-

tion, bronchitis and other lung infections, vigorous exercise, emotional excitement, or stress.
• A predisposition to asthma may be hereditary.

PREVENTION

• Try to identify allergens in home and work environments, and eliminate them if possible.
• Don't smoke; try to avoid secondary smoke.
• Reduce the amount of dust in your home: vacuum regularly, encase mattresses with plastic to discourage dust-mite infestation, and eliminate carpets that are difficult to clean.
• Avoid foods (such as milk, nuts, chocolate, fish) and medicines (such as aspirin or ibuprofen) that have triggered asthma attacks in the past.
• Drink at least eight glasses of liquid a day to keep mucus secretions loose.
• Each morning, practice deep breathing by inhaling fully, bending over with arms crossed over abdomen, and coughing to loosen accumulated lung secretions.
• Take preventive medications as prescribed.
• There is no need to avoid exercise; however, your doctor may advise you to take preventive medicines before exercising.

DIAGNOSIS

• Your doctor will conduct a physical examination.
• Allergy skin tests will be performed. A small amount of a suspected allergen will be injected just under the skin. If the area turns red or itchy, or a lump appears, you may be allergic to that substance.
• Chest x-rays will be required.
• Blood samples may be taken.
• Pulmonary-function tests that measure the strength and efficiency of your lungs will be performed.
• Keep a diary of the occurrence and severity of asthma attacks.

HOW TO TREAT IT

• A bronchodilator inhaler should be kept on hand in the event it is needed to relieve a severe attack. However, it is not recommended for regular use as overreliance on it may be harmful.
• If attacks are frequent, oral bronchodilator drugs (such as long-acting theophylline) or an antileukotriene agent (such as zafirlukast) may be used to help

---

SYMPTOMS

• Typical symptoms include: sudden breathing difficulty, wheezing, rapid, shallow breathing eased by sitting up, and a sense of suffocation; painless tightness in the chest; coughing, possibly with production of a thick, clear, or yellow sputum (symptoms in young children may in fact mimic those of a viral infection).
• More severe symptoms include: inability to speak more than a few words without gasping for breath; clenched or constricted neck muscles; rapid pulse; sweating; severe anxiety.
• Emergency symptoms: bluish tinge in the face or lips; extremely labored breathing; mental confusion; profound feeling of exhaustion.

Asthma *continued*

reduce frequency. Inhaled long-acting bronchodilators are sometimes used as well.

• Regular use of inhaled prescription corticosteroids
(anti-inflammatory drugs) helps control the underlying inflammation.

• When possible, inhalers should be used with a
spacer to help ensure that medicine reaches the
lungs, rather than just being absorbed in the back of
the throat.

• Your doctor may advise you to use a peak flow
meter (a small, handheld device that measures airflow). Your peak airflow will go down hours, and
sometimes even a day or two, before an attack, so
the meter can serve as an early warning system.

• Corticosteroid pills may be prescribed briefly
during severe attacks, which at times may require
an emergency room visit or hospitalization.

• Your doctor may give you desensitizing injections
to known allergy-causing agents.

WHEN TO CALL A DOCTOR

• **EMERGENCY** Call an ambulance if an attack does
not respond after two doses of prescribed inhalant.

• Call a doctor if you notice that the frequency of
attacks has increased significantly or if you need to
use a bronchodilator more than six times a day. ▟

Basal Cell Skin Cancer

WHAT IS IT?

Basal cell skin cancer is by far the most common form of skin cancer in the United States. It is believed to occur when excess ultraviolet radiation (usually sunlight) damages the genetic material of the basal cells located in the thin, top layer of the skin (epidermis). Basal cell skin cancer causes a local change in the skin, usually a pearly, whitish bump. As the bump grows, it may ulcerate and appear as an open sore.

The most common site for basal cell skin cancer is the face (typically the nose or ears), although it may appear anywhere. It is a painless, slow-growing cancer and very rarely, if ever, spreads to other parts of the body. Left untreated, however, it can slowly invade and even destroy the entire nose or an ear. Fortunately, with early detection and treatment, basal cell carcinoma is cured in 95 percent of cases, with only 5 percent of cases showing local recurrence.

WHAT CAUSES IT?

• Skin cells are damaged by cumulative exposure to ultraviolet radiation from the sun or from artificial sources (such as sunlamps). Although the risk of skin cancer increases steadily with age, even teenagers with excess sun exposure can develop skin cancers.
• People who sunburn easily, especially those with fair skin, blue eyes, or red or blond hair are most at risk, because they have relatively little natural pigment protection (melanin).
• Risk is greater in sunny climates and in locales near the equator, where the sun's radiation is most intense.

SYMPTOMS

• A small, flat, waxy or pearly bump, most common on the face, ears, back, or the "V" where the neck meets the chest.
• A skin blemish that grows steadily over a period of weeks and does not spontaneously disappear within a month. It may develop into a shallow ulcer with raised edges and a moist center. The ulcer may seem to heal or disappear, only to recur later.

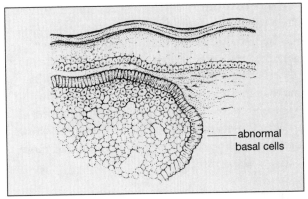

Ultraviolet radiation can damage basal cells in the epidermis. These cells may surface and produce a growth characteristic of skin cancer.

PREVENTION

• As much as possible, avoid exposure to direct sunlight between 10 a.m. and 2 p.m.
• Block the sun's rays with protective clothing such as hats and long sleeves.
• Before going outside, apply (and reapply often) a waterproof sunscreen lotion with a sun protection factor (SPF) of at least 15.
• Avoid sunlamps and tanning booths.
• Perform regular skin self-examinations, looking for any new growths or changes in existing lesions.
• People who have had one basal cell skin cancer have an approximately 50 percent chance of having a second nonmelanoma (basal or squamous cell) skin cancer within five years. For this reason, preventive measures are especially important after initial diagnosis.

DIAGNOSIS

• A biopsy (removal of a tissue sample for microscopic examination) will be performed.

HOW TO TREAT IT

• To remove cancerous cells, surgery or radiation therapy may be used.

WHEN TO CALL A DOCTOR

• Make an appointment with your doctor when you notice any change in the appearance of your skin. Just about everyone has some skin growths; most are harmless. Nonetheless, a biopsy may be needed.
• Schedule a skin examination at least once a year following an episode of basal cell skin cancer.

Bell's Palsy

WHAT IS IT?

Bell's palsy is paralysis of the muscles on one side of the face. It results from inflammation of the facial nerve, which runs through a tiny hole in the bone between the ear and the jaw. Inflammation of this nerve compresses it inside its bony channel, thus paralyzing the muscles between the forehead and mouth. Onset is usually sudden, typically occurring upon awakening, and most commonly strikes those between the ages of 30 and 60.

WHAT CAUSES IT?

• The cause is unknown in most cases.
• Viral infection (including herpes zoster, the same virus that causes chicken pox and shingles), physical trauma, and heredity have been proposed as potential causative factors.

PREVENTION

There is no way to prevent Bell's palsy at present.

DIAGNOSIS

• Physical examination is necessary. Other disorders, such as a stroke, will have to be ruled out.
• Electrical tests of the facial nerves (electromyography) may be performed to determine the extent of nerve damage.

HOW TO TREAT IT

• Spontaneous recovery occurs in 80 to 90 percent of cases (often beginning within three weeks), so many physicians believe treatment is unnecessary or

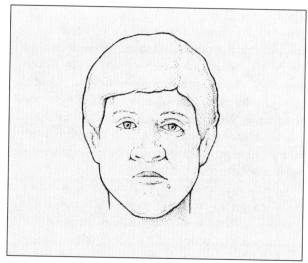

Bell's palsy is characterized by paralysis of the muscles on one side of the face, causing the affected brow, cheek, and side of the mouth to droop and making it difficult to close the eye.

ineffective. Outlook is most favorable when paralysis is incomplete and improvement begins soon after onset. Treatment is thus aimed at easing symptoms and preventing damage to the eye.
• Wearing goggles during the day and applying an eye patch at night to hold the eyelid shut may help protect the eye if the eyelid cannot close. An artificial tear solution may also be recommended.
• Nonprescription pain relievers and using a heating pad on the painful area for 15 minutes at a time eases mild to moderate pain.
• For more severe pain or for cases that fail to improve over time, corticosteroids (such as prednisone) may be prescribed—although the effectiveness of such therapy for Bell's palsy is a point of debate.
• As muscle strength returns, exercising the weak facial muscles is recommended.
• Plastic surgery may improve appearance and muscle function in the rare cases where facial paralysis persists.

WHEN TO CALL A DOCTOR

• Facial paralysis always warrants a doctor's attention. Although Bell's palsy is the most common cause and is not a medical emergency, more serious problems such as a stroke or tumor should be ruled out.

SYMPTOMS

• Drooping muscles and weakness on one side of the face, resulting in a distorted smile or an expressionless look.
• Drooping brow, inability to close the eyelids, and tearing on the affected side.
• Possible pain in the ear and on the affected side of the face.
• Drooling from one corner of the mouth.
• Possible changes in taste and increased sensitivity to noise.

Benign Paroxysmal Positional Vertigo BPPV

WHAT IS IT?

Benign paroxysmal positional vertigo is dizziness that arises abruptly upon changing the position of the head (for instance, while tilting the head to look upward, sitting up, or turning over in bed). Symptoms generally last less than a minute, but they can be extremely disconcerting and may be accompanied by loss of balance, nausea, and vomiting. Such episodes may recur several times a day. Contrary to popular belief, recurrent or chronic dizziness indicates a brain tumor less than 1 percent of the time.

WHAT CAUSES IT?

• Balance is maintained by otoliths, tiny calcium stones that press on hairlike fibers deep in the canals of the inner ear. When bent, these fibers send signals to the brain so it can calculate the head's position. As people age, minuscule amounts of debris may slough off and press on these fibers. This interferes with the sense of balance by sending false signals to the brain, resulting in BPPV.

• A prior head injury or viral infection of the inner ear may contribute to BPPV development.

PREVENTION

• Until you receive successful treatment, try to avoid the positions that induce dizziness.

• Avoid sudden, rapid head movements.

DIAGNOSIS

• Your doctor may order various tests to determine the exact cause of vertigo and to rule out a more serious underlying disorder.

HOW TO TREAT IT

• Lie down until dizziness and other symptoms go away.

SYMPTOMS

• Sudden, acute dizziness or a spinning sensation that occurs after changing the position of the head.

• Loss of balance.

• Nausea and vomiting.

• Certain medications—such as antihistamines (which can have an antinausea effect) and scopolamine (a motion-sickness drug)—may be prescribed to ease dizziness.

• In one treatment technique, a doctor will induce dizziness by moving the patient's head rapidly or slowly to one side, holding the position for a few minutes, then repeat the procedure for the opposite side. Afterward, the patient sits up and must keep the head upright for 48 hours (even while sleeping). This treatment produces complete remission in 60 percent of BPPV cases and improvement in another 30 percent.

• The patient is instructed to move his or her head in a way that induces dizziness. He or she then performs this technique several times a day for a few weeks. This treatment has been shown to be effective in the vast majority of patients.

WHEN TO CALL A DOCTOR

• Make an appointment with your doctor if you experience episodes of severe dizziness. ▲

Bipolar Disorder

WHAT IS IT?

Bipolar disorder is a condition characterized by episodes of low mood (depression) or elated mood (mania), separated by periods of normal mood and functioning. Mania is marked by inflated self-esteem; an elated, euphoric, or grandiose mood; increased activity; and a decreased need for sleep. Episodes of mania or depression can last from a few weeks to several months and are frequently severe enough to affect day-to-day functioning at work and at home. Men tend to have more bouts of mania; women have more episodes of depression (see Depression for more information). Bipolar disorder has also been called manic-depressive illness.

Affecting about 1 percent of the general population, bipolar disorder typically begins between ages 20 and 30, though it can start at any age. For most patients, the condition is recurring. The rate of this "cycling" varies among individuals. Fortunately, although bipolar disorder can be a lifelong condition, treatment helps the majority of patients to have less frequent and less severe episodes.

WHAT CAUSES IT?

• Genetics play a primary role in the development of bipolar disorder. If you have a family history of bipolar disorder, there is a greater chance that you will be vulnerable to it.
• Recurrent manic episodes may be caused by sleep deprivation or antidepressant drug therapy.
• The more episodes a patient has had, the more likely he or she is to have another.

PREVENTION

• There is no way to prevent bipolar disorder, but medications such as lithium, carbamazepine, and divalproex sodium may prevent recurrences.

DIAGNOSIS

• Physical examination and patient history by a mental health professional are necessary. Because symptoms of a single manic episode occasionally mimic those of schizophrenia (see Schizophrenia for more information), patients may need several exams before getting an accurate diagnosis.
• Laboratory tests should be done to rule out an underlying medical illness (such as hyperthyroidism), an adverse drug reaction, another medical or psychiatric condition, or the effects of alcohol or illicit drugs.

HOW TO TREAT IT

• Lithium and divalproex sodium are the treatments of choice for mania. Carbamazepine is also effective. Beneficial effects appear in two to six weeks.
• Because of the slow therapeutic response to these medications, antipsychotic medications may be administered for treatment of severe mania.
• Severe manic episodes may need to be treated in the hospital.
• Depressive episodes are typically treated with antidepressant drugs, psychotherapy, or both.

WHEN TO CALL A DOCTOR

• Call a doctor if you or someone you know shows significant signs of bipolar disorder.

SYMPTOMS

Depression: See Depression.
Mania:
• Elated mood.
• Feelings of irritability, grandeur, and inflated self-esteem.
• Diminished need for sleep.
• Being extremely talkative.
• Sensing that thoughts and ideas are racing.
• Being easily distracted.
• Increased productivity and/or activity at work, at school, or in social situations.
• Excessive involvement in high-risk activities that are likely to have painful consequences (such as extramarital affairs or unsound business deals).
• Increased sex drive.

Bladder Cancer

WHAT IS IT?

Bladder cancer is the growth of malignant cells in the lining of the bladder. Often, more than one tumor is present at a time, and the cancer may spread into and through the wall of the bladder. The most frequent symptom of bladder cancer is painless hematuria (blood in the urine), although commonly there are no symptoms at all. Therefore, when symptoms of a bladder disorder do arise, they are most often due to other, less serious, conditions such as infections, benign prostate enlargement, or bladder stones. Bladder cancer is rare before the age of 40 and is more common among men.

WHAT CAUSES IT?

• Smoking is associated with an increased incidence of bladder cancer.
• Exposure to toxic chemicals (such as those used in the rubber industry as well as industrial dyes and solvents) is a potential risk factor.
• A family history of bladder cancer is associated with an increased risk.

PREVENTION

• Don't smoke cigarettes.
• Exercise caution if you work with industrial dyes or in the rubber industry.
• If you have a family history of the disease, get regular checkups.
• See your doctor regularly if you have had bladder cancer to screen for recurrences.

DIAGNOSIS

• Patient history and physical exam help to establish the presence of a bladder disorder.
• Cystoscopy (the use of a thin, lighted tube that allows a surgeon to see the bladder directly) and biopsy (removal and analysis of tissue samples) are required for a definitive diagnosis.
• Urinalysis may be used to detect cancer cells and blood in the urine.
• CT (computed tomography) scans provide a view of the bladder and surrounding tissues to reveal any structural abnormalities.

HOW TO TREAT IT

• Tumors in the early stages may be removed surgically through the cystoscope. Such tumors may recur, thus requiring repeated cystoscopy every three months for one to two years, then every six months for one to two more years, and then yearly for life.
• Recurrences may also be treated with chemotherapeutic agents instilled directly into the bladder with a catheter.
• Chemotherapy given intravenously is used if evidence indicates that the cancer has spread.
• If the cancer is advanced, removal of the entire bladder is required. Radiation and chemotherapy may also be used.

WHEN TO CALL A DOCTOR

• Call a doctor if you have blood in the urine or you experience other symptoms of bladder cancer. ▲

SYMPTOMS

• Blood in the urine.
• Difficult, frequent, or painful urination.
• Pain in the pelvic region.
• Feeling of pressure in the back.
• Persistent fever.

Bladder Infection Cystitis

WHAT IS IT?

Bladder infection, also known as cystitis, occurs when bacteria, generally from outside the body, enter the urinary tract and infect the urethra and the bladder. It is most common in women.

WHAT CAUSES IT?

• About 80 percent of urinary tract infections are caused by bacteria that normally inhabit the anal area with no ill effect; however, if these bacteria enter the urinary tract, infection may ensue. The relatively short urethra of women, as compared to that of men, provides less of a barrier to bacteria.
• Use of a urinary catheter may introduce bacteria to the bladder.
• Sexual activity may bruise the urethra in women, promoting infection.
• Obstruction of urine flow by a bladder tumor or, in men, an enlarged prostate may lead to bladder infection.
• Women with recurrent disease may be genetically predisposed.

PREVENTION

• Obtain prompt treatment of bacterial infections elsewhere in the body, especially kidney infections.
• The use of spermicides and diaphragms may predispose women to urinary tract infections by altering vaginal bacteria, which may spread to the urethra.
• Urinate when you feel the urge (retaining a full bladder promotes infection).
• Women with serious or recurrent bladder infections associated with intercourse should ask their doctor about taking preventive antibacterial medications.

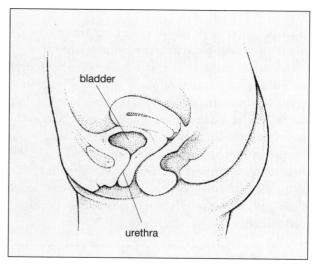

Bacteria may ascend the urethra to infect the bladder. Women are more prone to such infections, as the female urethra is relatively short.

• Research has not shown douching, the direction of wiping after toilet use, or urination after intercourse to have any clear association with urinary tract infections.

DIAGNOSIS

• Diagnosis is based upon a culture of a urine sample for bacteria.

HOW TO TREAT IT

• Your doctor may prescribe antibiotics to fight the infection. Take them for the full term prescribed.
• You may also be given antispasmodics and analgesics to relieve the pain.
• Drink cranberry juice to increase the acidity of the urine, as some medicines are more effective with acidic urine.

WHEN TO CALL A DOCTOR

• Call your doctor if you experience symptoms of a bladder infection, especially if they are accompanied by a high fever or if symptoms recur or persist despite treatment.
• Call your doctor if you develop pain in the lower back, which may indicate a kidney infection. Bacteria from the bladder infection may have migrated to the kidney. ▲

SYMPTOMS
• Burning sensation during urination.
• Frequent urination with only small amounts of urine passed on each occasion.
• Urgent need to urinate; lack of urinary control.
• Blood in the urine.
• Pain in the lower abdomen.
• Low-grade fever (under 102°F).
• Painful sexual intercourse.

Bladder Stones

WHAT IS IT?

Bladder stones form when substances (such as calcium oxalate) in the urine concentrate and coalesce into hard, solid lumps that lodge in the bladder. Often, several stones form at once. Normally, they are fairly small and are excreted in the urine without complications, but sometimes stones become trapped in the neck of the bladder and—as residues in the urine continue to accumulate—grow large enough to cause pain, urinary blockage, or infections, thus requiring surgical intervention. Bladder stones almost exclusively affect middle-aged and older men, but, for unknown reasons, are becoming increasingly rare.

WHAT CAUSES IT?

• Most commonly, stones become problematic when the neck of the bladder is obstructed due to prostate enlargement, a benign growth (adenoma) within the prostate, or abnormal contraction or stricture of the bladder neck. Stones often originate elsewhere in the urinary tract (such as the kidneys), or in the bladder itself. Hereditary factors may be involved.
• Other causes include the long-term use of a urinary catheter, chronic urinary tract infections, or a nerve injury that impairs bladder function.
• Mild, chronic dehydration concentrates the urine, which may promote stone formation.
• A diet high in oxalic acid (found in rhubarb, leafy vegetables, and coffee) may lead to stones.

PREVENTION

• Drink at least eight glasses of water a day.
• Get prompt treatment for urinary tract infections.

SYMPTOMS
• Interruption of the urine stream, inability to urinate except in certain positions, frequent urge to urinate but with only small amounts of urine passed.
• Blood in the urine, often only apparent in the last few drops.
• Pain—sometimes severe—in the pelvic region, genitals, lower abdomen, or lower back.
• Low-grade fever (under 102°F).

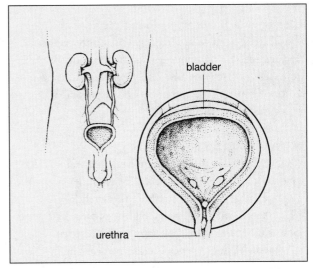

Bladder stones may grow large enough to lodge in the neck of the bladder and obstruct the outflow of urine through the urethra.

DIAGNOSIS

• A thorough medical history and physical exam (including a rectal exam) are necessary.
• Urine samples are taken and analyzed.
• Stones can be located with x-rays or ultrasound.
• Cystoscopy (inspection of the inside of the bladder using a scope) confirms the diagnosis.

HOW TO TREAT IT

• Your doctor may prescribe narcotic analgesics to relieve pain and antibiotics to treat an infection.
• Smaller stones can be removed through a cystoscope, a tube inserted through the urethra that allows the doctor to view the stones. The scope can also be outfitted with a device that crushes the stones, after which the fragments are washed away.
• Larger stones can be treated with extracorporeal shock-wave lithotripsy, which aims concentrated bursts of sound waves that pulverize the stones.
• On rare occasions, very large stones may require surgical removal (suprapubic lithotomy).
• The underlying problem (such as prostate enlargement) causing stones to be trapped in the bladder must be identified and treated to prevent recurrence.

WHEN TO CALL A DOCTOR

• Call a doctor for symptoms of bladder stones.

Blepharitis

WHAT IS IT?

Blepharitis is an inflammation of the edges of the eyelids, resulting in a persistent, unsightly redness and scaliness. The condition tends to recur, but it is generally not serious and rarely poses any threat to vision. Blepharitis often affects both eyes at once and is common among children.

WHAT CAUSES IT?

• Seborrheic dermatitis (seborrhea)—characterized by greasy, red, scaly, itchy patches of skin—may migrate from the scalp to affect the eyelids.
• Blepharitis may be associated with rosacea or acne (See Rosacea or Acne for more information).
• A bacterial infection can cause or complicate blepharitis due to seborrhea.
• Lice infestation of the eyelashes can cause the condition.
• Mascara or eye shadow may result in contact dermatitis of the eyelids (see Eczema).

PREVENTION

• Avoid locations where lice might be prevalent.
• Control seborrhea of the scalp with medicated shampoos.

DIAGNOSIS

• Patient history and physical examination are necessary. The doctor may culture material from an ulcer on the eyelid for bacteria.

HOW TO TREAT IT

• Apply warm-water compresses on eyelids for about 15 minutes to loosen scales. Then scrub scales away with a solution of water and sodium bicarbonate (baking soda) or water and baby shampoo.
• Your doctor may prescribe topical corticosteroid medications or antibiotics if a bacterial infection is present.
• For lice infestation, nits will be removed with forceps. An insecticide ointment may be prescribed for daily use.

WHEN TO CALL A DOCTOR

• If the condition does not respond to cleansing treatments within two weeks, call your doctor.
• Call your doctor if ulcers form on the eyelids. This suggests a bacterial infection.
• If you notice nits, make an appointment to see your doctor right away.

SYMPTOMS

• Red, sticky, and crusty eyelid edges.
• Thickened eyelids with prominent, visible blood vessels.
• Itching, burning, continual blinking, and a sensation that something is in the eyes.
• A crust that requires the eyelids to be pried apart in the morning.
• Greasy scales (from seborrhea), dry scales (from a bacterial infection), or flakes of skin appearing on the eyelid edges. (Scales or flakes may fall into the eye and cause conjunctivitis.)
• Small ulcerations on the eyelid (severe cases).
• Loss of eyelashes.
• Acne.
• Visible nits on the lashes, when blepharitis is caused by lice infestation.

Bone Cancer

WHAT IS IT?

Bone cancer is the growth of malignant cells that gradually replace normal bone cells, leading to weakness and pain in the affected bone. Primary bone cancer, which arises directly in the bone (usually in the leg), is relatively rare and generally strikes people under the age of 20. Much more common is metastatic or secondary bone cancer, which originates in another organ and then spreads to the bone. Cancer may also develop in associated bone structures, including the marrow and the connective tissues. Some types of bone cancer may spread to other organs. With modern therapies, the outlook for many patients (especially those with primary bone cancer) has improved significantly.

WHAT CAUSES IT?

• The cause of primary bone cancer is unknown, but hereditary factors, environmental factors, trauma, or excessive radiation therapy (to treat other types of cancer) may be involved.

• Metastatic bone cancer most often stems from cancer of the breast, lung, prostate, thyroid, or kidney. Multiple myeloma (a cancer of the bone marrow) may also affect the bones.

• The incidence of bone cancer is higher in patients with Paget's disease, a degenerative bone disease that primarily affects older people (see Paget's Disease for more information).

PREVENTION

• Get regular checkups to detect cancers elsewhere in the body before they have a chance to spread.

SYMPTOMS

• Pain and tenderness in the affected bones. The pain is usually dull and localized and is often worse at night.
• Swelling or a noticeable tumor or mass around the site of a primary tumor. (Swelling generally does not occur with metastatic tumors.)
• Greater susceptibility to bone fractures (as healthy bone cells are replaced by malignant ones).

DIAGNOSIS

• X-rays are taken.

• Diagnostic imaging techniques such as CT (computed tomography) scans or MRI (magnetic resonance imaging) are used to detect tumors and metastatic areas.

• A biopsy of the affected bone may be taken to confirm the presence of cancer (especially in the case of primary tumors, since cancer has usually already been diagnosed in the case of metastatic tumors).

• Blood tests may be performed.

HOW TO TREAT IT

• The bone or bones affected by primary tumors may need to be surgically removed. This may involve amputation, although in some cases only the tumor is removed and the remaining bone is reinforced with a metal prosthesis.

• Chemotherapy and radiation therapy may be required.

• Orthopedic surgery may be necessary to repair bone fractures.

WHEN TO CALL A DOCTOR

• Call a doctor if you feel persistent pain in one or more bones, if you develop weakness or paralysis in the limbs, or if you begin to limp unexpectedly. ▲

Botulism

WHAT IS IT?

Botulism is a life-threatening form of bacterial food poisoning that, unlike common forms of food poisoning, affects the central nervous system. Symptoms usually appear approximately 18 to 36 hours after eating contaminated food, and currently the disease is fatal in about 10 percent of cases, most often because of respiratory failure. Patients who exhibit symptoms in less than 24 hours of infection tend to experience the most severe course of the disease and have the highest mortality rate; those that survive the first few days can usually expect full recovery. The most common form of the disease involves infants younger than six months old. Both the incidence of botulism and its mortality rate are declining.

WHAT CAUSES IT?

• Botulism is caused by consumption of food contaminated with the bacterium *Clostridium botulinum,* which can produce the deadly toxin (botulin) that interferes with the transmission of signals across neural synapses. Undercooked foods or those with a low acid content are most likely to transmit botulism.
• The disease may rarely occur when spores of the bacterium infect an open wound.

PREVENTION

• Never eat even a minuscule amount of food from a can that is bulging (a sign of bacterial activity), leaking, or has an unusual odor or color.
• Do not feed honey to children less than a year old. Contaminated honey is a common cause of infant botulism, but does not appear to pose a problem for children or adults.

SYMPTOMS

• Dry mouth and sore throat.
• Blurred and double vision.
• Fixed, dilated pupils.
• Breathing and swallowing difficulty.
• Slurred speech.
• Abdominal cramps, diarrhea, nausea, and vomiting.
• Weakness in arms and legs, leading to paralysis.

• Be cautious with the following foods, which are most likely to be contaminated: home-canned fruits and vegetables (green beans in particular), fish, undercooked sausage and other pork products, smoked meats, red meat, and milk products.
• Keep foods at room temperature for no more than one hour before or after cooking. Refrigerate any leftovers promptly (divide large amounts of food into smaller batches before refrigerating).

DIAGNOSIS

• Patient history and physical examination are needed.
• Blood, stool, or stomach contents as well as the suspected food may be tested for the presence of botulin toxin and the bacterium, but the ultimate diagnosis rests on the presentation of symptoms.
• An electromyogram (EMG), which tests the conduction of electrical impulses along the nerves, may be done to rule out other disorders.

HOW TO TREAT IT

• Call an ambulance immediately; emergency care and hospitalization are necessary.
• If only a few hours have passed since eating contaminated food, induce vomiting.
• If possible, try to refrigerate some of the suspected contaminated food for analysis.
• Doctors will administer a botulism antitoxin, which can be lifesaving but can have pronounced unpleasant side effects. When botulism is strongly suspected, the antitoxin is given before laboratory confirmation of the diagnosis.
• Penicillin is also frequently given, but this is controversial as the actual bacteria is not the primary problem.
• Enemas and drugs that induce bowel evacuation may be given to help rid the body of the toxin.
• Mechanical respiration may be needed in the case of severe breathing difficulty.

WHEN TO CALL A DOCTOR

• **EMERGENCY** Get immediate medical help if you develop any of the symptoms of botulism. ⚠

Brain Abscess

WHAT IS IT?

A brain abscess is an accumulation of pus (due to infection) inside the brain. These abscesses produce symptoms by raising pressure inside the rigid skull or by destroying or irritating surrounding brain tissue. Brain abscesses are most common in the frontal and temporal lobes of the cerebrum—the portion of the brain that controls higher functions, including speech and thinking.

Prompt medical treatment usually ensures full recovery; however, approximately 10 percent of cases are fatal, while others result in some permanent neurological disorder such as epilepsy. Brain abscesses are becoming increasingly rare due to the widespread use of antibiotics to treat underlying infections before they can cause such complications.

WHAT CAUSES IT?

• Blood-borne infections may spread to the brain and result in an abscess or multiple abscesses. Patients with bacterial endocarditis (an infection of a heart valve) or immune deficiencies (such as AIDS) are prone to brain abscesses from infectious organisms carried in the blood.
• Brain abscesses may also result from the spread of an infection from another (typically adjacent) part of the body to the brain.
• A head wound that penetrates the skull can lead to brain infection and thus an abscess.

PREVENTION

• Receive prompt medical treatment for any infec-tions elsewhere in the body—especially those occur-ring in the middle ear or the sinuses.
• Wear protective headgear when engaging in any activity where risk of head injury is possible.

DIAGNOSIS

• Diagnosis is strongly suspected from CT (com-puted tomography) or MRI (magnetic resonance imaging) brain scans.
• A culture of organisms taken from the pus con-firms the diagnosis and is required to select appropri-ate antibiotic treatment.

HOW TO TREAT IT

• Large doses of antibiotics are given to attack the underlying infection.
• Some type of surgical procedure is often necessary as well. Frequently, a hole is drilled into the skull so that the abscess can be drained or completely removed. This procedure also allows doctors to iden-tify the precise underlying organism in order to determine the appropriate antibiotic treatment. After such surgery, antibiotics will usually be prescribed for one or two months.
• Anticonvulsant drugs may be prescribed if the abscess has caused epileptic seizures.

WHEN TO CALL A DOCTOR

• **EMERGENCY** See a doctor immediately if you have any signs of serious infection or symptoms such as speech difficulty, seizures, or partial paralysis. △

SYMPTOMS

• Headaches (often severe).
• Nausea and vomiting.
• Drowsiness.
• Partial paralysis, weakness, or loss of sensation on one side of the body or in the legs; or, progressive speech difficulty (depending on the location of the abscess).
• Epileptic seizures.
• Fever.
• Discharge of pus from the nose or ear.

Brain Hemorrhage Intracranial Bleeds

WHAT IS IT?

A brain hemorrhage, one of the two main types of strokes (see Stroke for more information), results when a ruptured artery causes bleeding into the brain (intracerebral bleed) or into the space between the membranes surrounding the brain (subarachnoid hemorrhage). Damage occurs two ways. First, blood supply is cut off to the parts of the brain beyond the site of the rupture in the artery. Second—and more dangerous—the escaped blood forms a mass that increases pressure on the surrounding brain tissue. Blood continues to flow until it coagulates or until it simply has no place left to go. Intracerebral bleeds usually occur in the cerebrum, the part of the brain that controls higher functions such as speaking and reasoning. Subarachnoid hemorrhages usually occur at the base of the brain. Massive hemorrhages are usually fatal; indeed, only about 25 percent of patients survive.

WHAT CAUSES IT?

• High blood pressure is the main cause.
• Atherosclerosis (the buildup of fatty plaque in the arteries) weakens arterial walls, further increasing the risk of bleeds due to hypertension.
• Bleeding disorders (such as hemophilia and leukemia) or the use of anticoagulant or thrombolytic drugs increase the risk of intracerebral bleeding.
• Aneurysms (weak spots in the wall of an artery that may burst) are a major cause of subarachnoid hemorrhage. They are often due to congenital defects.
• Blood vessel abnormalities such as arteriovenous malformation (AVM) may result in a stroke.

• A head injury may rupture arteries in the brain.
• Brain tumors may lead to intracerebral bleeding.

PREVENTION

• Keep blood pressure and weight under control.
• People with undiagnosed aneurysms often will have severe, sudden, unusual headaches initially. If the cause of these can be identified, arteriography (diagnostic imaging of the arteries) may reveal a surgically treatable aneurysm.

DIAGNOSIS

• Arteriography may be used to detect cerebral aneurysms before they rupture.
• A lumbar puncture (spinal tap) may be used to test for blood in the cerebrospinal fluid and to check for increased pressure within the skull.
• CT (computed tomography) scans of the head may be taken to identify and assess the amount of blood spillage in the brain.
• MRI (magnetic resonance imaging) can detect abnormal blood vessels, underlying tumors, and some aneurysms.

HOW TO TREAT IT

• Call an ambulance immediately.
• After careful evaluation, physicians may take emergency measures to reduce blood pressure in order to minimize flow of blood from the ruptured artery.
• Life support may be necessary.
• Surgical repair, if attempted at all, is usually delayed for one to two weeks after the incident, although another approach calls for more rapid surgical intervention in some cases.

WHEN TO CALL A DOCTOR

• **EMERGENCY** Call an ambulance immediately. ⚠

SYMPTOMS
• Stiff neck.
• Sudden, excruciating headache.
• Nausea and vomiting.
• Mental confusion.
• Sudden loss of consciousness without warning.
• Paralysis on one side of the face or body.
• Speech difficulty or loss of ability to speak.
• Blurred or double vision, dilated pupils, crossed eyes, or inability to move the eyes.

Brain Tumors

WHAT IS IT?

A brain tumor is an abnormal growth of cells in the brain or the membranes surrounding the brain (a tumor known as a meningioma). The tumor increases pressure inside the skull and so exerts pressure on the entire brain: this phenomenon is responsible for many of the symptoms of brain tumors regardless of whether they are benign or malignant. Primary brain tumors originate in the brain but are much less common than secondary, or metastatic, tumors, which spread to the brain from cancers elsewhere in the body. Symptoms tend to appear gradually and vary according to the area of the brain affected. Primary malignant brain tumors are rare, accounting for less than 2 percent of all cancers.

WHAT CAUSES IT?

• The cause of primary brain tumors is unknown.
• Metastatic tumors may spread from cancers of the lungs, liver, intestines, breast, skin, or other parts of the body.

PREVENTION

• Get regular checkups to detect cancers elsewhere in the body before they have a chance to spread.

DIAGNOSIS

• A thorough patient history and physical examination are necessary.

SYMPTOMS

• Frequent headaches that are more painful when lying down.
• Vomiting, with or without nausea.
• Blurred or double vision.
• Seizures.
• Impaired thinking, mental confusion, or even coma.
• Other symptoms depend on the location of the tumor within the brain and may include weakness or unsteadiness, paralysis on one side of the body, dizziness, speech difficulty, memory loss, loss of the sense of smell or hearing, or personality change.

• CT (computed tomography) scans or an MRI (magnetic resonance imaging) may be necessary to locate the tumor.
• A spinal tap or lumbar puncture (the use of a needle to remove and analyze a sample from the cerebrospinal fluid surrounding the spinal cord) is often performed. (However, spinal taps should not be performed if other diagnostic imaging techniques reveal evidence of a mass. Under such circumstances a spinal tap is dangerous.)
• A biopsy of the tumor will most likely be necessary to confirm the diagnosis.
• Electroencephalography may be used to measure and assess electrical activity in the brain.
• Cerebral arteriography may be used in preparation for surgery to outline the arteries supplying blood to the tumor.

HOW TO TREAT IT

• Tumors near the surface of the brain may be surgically removed. In many cases, however, it is only possible to remove a portion of a tumor, since taking it all out would cause unacceptable amounts of brain damage. Still, removing even part of it may afford a period of improvement by relieving pressure within the cranium.
• Tumors deep within the brain may be treated with microsurgery, laser surgery, or radiation therapy.
• For malignant primary tumors, surgery may be followed with radiation or chemotherapy. Surgery may also be preceded by radiation.
• Your doctor may prescribe corticosteroids to reduce swelling of brain tissue, anticonvulsant drugs to control seizures, and pain relievers.

WHEN TO CALL A DOCTOR

• Call a doctor if you ever have a seizure.
• Consult your doctor if you experience a severe, persistent headache, especially one that is worse in the mornings or when lying down.
• Call a doctor if you experience double vision or if you notice weakness, numbness, or loss of sensation in the limbs.

Breast Cancer

WHAT IS IT?

Breast cancer, the growth of malignant cells in the breast, is the most common cancer among women. It is rare but does occur in men. Breast cancer usually originates in the milk-carrying ducts, although it may arise in the milk-producing lobes or, more rarely, in the dense connective tissue of the breast. A breast tumor is not in itself life-threatening, but there is a high risk that the cancer will spread to other organs via the lymph nodes or the bloodstream, so early detection is imperative. In 90 percent of cases, only one breast is affected, although those who have had cancer in one breast are at increased risk of eventually developing it in the other. In all cases, early detection and treatment improve the outlook significantly.

WHAT CAUSES IT?

The precise cause is unknown, but the following factors correlate with a higher incidence of breast cancer:
• Age. The risk of breast cancer increases progressively after age 50.
• Family history. Women whose immediate or near-immediate family members have had breast cancer are at greater risk, especially if the cancer occurred at an early age.
• Having had children late in life or not at all. Women who have no children, have their first child

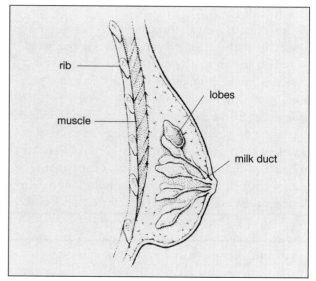

The breast contains 15 to 20 lobes, each containing dozens of milk-producing glands. Breast cancer originates in these glands.

in their 30s, or have never breastfed may be more susceptible to breast cancer.
• Early onset of menstruation (that is before age 11).
• Late menopause (that is not having reached menopause by one's early 50s).
• Nonmalignant cysts and tumors in the breasts.
• A diet high in animal fat.
• Possibly, environmental toxins.

PREVENTION

• Mammograms can detect tumors too small to feel. Women over 50 should have annual mammograms, and those between ages 40 and 50 should discuss their individual risk factors with their doctors to determine when to begin mammography. The exam should be performed by a radiologist specializing in mammography or by a mammography center accredited by the American College of Radiology. A list of accredited centers is available from the National Cancer Institute at 1-800-4-CANCER.
• Women should have a yearly breast exam performed by a doctor or other trained specialist.
• Women should perform monthly breast exams (the best time is two or three days after menstruation ends). Breast tissue is normally somewhat lumpy and uneven, so it is important to become familiar with the normal contour and texture of the breasts.

SYMPTOMS

• A lump or swelling, usually painless, anywhere in the breast or underarm area (but most commonly in the upper and outer region of the breast).
• Changes in the appearance of the breast's skin, including flattening, indentation, dimpling, creasing, redness, or scaliness.
• Changes in the nipple, including indentation, an itching or burning sensation, or dark or bloody discharge.
• Changes in the size or symmetry of the breasts.
• Discomfort or pain in the breast in advanced cases.

Breast Cancer *continued*

Changes in texture and appearance will then become more easily detectable. Follow these steps:
• Stand before a mirror and check both breasts for anything unusual. Look for puckering, dimpling, or scaling of the skin or a discharge from the nipples.
• Changes in position may reveal unusual lumps or indentations. Clasp your hands behind your head and press your hands forward. Look for any changes in the breasts' appearance.
• Next, press your hands firmly on your hips and bow slightly toward the mirror, pulling your shoulders and elbows forward (again, checking for anything unusual).
• Raise your left arm. Moving in tiny, gentle, circular motions with three or four fingers of your right hand, feel all around the left breast. Start at the outer part of the breast and work gradually toward the nipple in concentric circles. Pay special attention to the underarm area. Feel for any unusual lump or mass beneath the skin. Gently squeeze the nipple and look for any discharge.
• Repeat the previous step for the right breast.
• Repeat the last two steps while lying flat on your back, with a small pillow or folded towel placed under your shoulder.

DIAGNOSIS

• Breast examination or mammography may reveal the presence of a lump in the breast.
• A biopsy of the lump is necessary to determine whether cancerous cells are present. Tissue or fluid may be drawn out of the lump with a needle, or a sample of tissue may be removed during minor surgery.
• Ultrasound, thermography, or CT (computed tomography) scans may be recommended.

HOW TO TREAT IT

• Surgery is necessary to remove the tumor. The patient will be given the choice of having any necessary surgery performed at the time of the biopsy or in a subsequent operation. Depending upon how far the cancer has spread, surgery may involve removing only the mass or lump (lumpectomy) or the entire breast (mastectomy), either of which may include removal of the neighboring lymph nodes. If a tumor has invaded the muscle tissue under the breast, the removal of the breast and the underlying muscle tissue (radical mastectomy) may be advised.
• Radiation therapy may be required after surgery to prevent further spread of the cancer, especially if the lymph nodes were affected.
• Chemotherapy may be required before and after surgery to prevent further spread of the cancer. Such treatment generally lasts from six months to a year.
• Hormone therapy may be prescribed after surgery for estrogen-receptor-positive tumors. The estrogen-blocking drug tamoxifen may be continued indefinitely.
• Reconstructive plastic surgery is available for women who have had part or all of the breast removed. Women may have reconstructive surgery at the same time as surgery to remove the tumor or at a later date.

WHEN TO CALL A DOCTOR

• Make an appointment with a doctor if you notice a lump anywhere in the breast or under the arm. Most lumps are not cancerous, but a biopsy is necessary to diagnose breast cancer with certainty.
• Make an appointment with a doctor if you notice any change in the size, shape, or appearance of the breast or if you experience any discharge from the nipple. ▲

Bronchiectasis

WHAT IS IT?

Bronchiectasis is a rare chronic lung condition resulting from recurrent or persistent inflammation that ultimately damages the walls of the bronchial tubes. The ability to expel mucus is impaired, which leads to further infection and inflammation. Eventually (usually over a period of years), the affected air passages may be completely destroyed. Inflammation of the bronchial walls may be isolated to one area or may be distributed throughout the lungs. Bronchiectasis in childhood is now rare, thanks to vaccines to prevent whooping cough and antibiotics to control bacterial infections.

WHAT CAUSES IT?

• Currently, cystic fibrosis causes one-half of all cases of bronchiectasis.
• Other diseases that affect the lungs (such as pneumonia, chronic bronchitis, emphysema, measles, or tuberculosis) may result in bronchiectasis.
• A congenital bronchial defect may distort or weaken the walls of the bronchial tubes.
• Inhalation of foreign objects (such as a peanut) or aspiration of gastric contents may irritate and inflame bronchial walls, thus initiating a cycle of infection that may lead to bronchiectasis.
• Lung cancer or a lung abscess may cause bronchiectasis.

PREVENTION

• Be sure children have been properly vaccinated against childhood diseases.

DIAGNOSIS

• Patient history and physical examination are needed.
• Sputum samples will be analyzed.
• Chest x-rays or a CT (computed tomography) scan are often used to confirm the diagnosis.

HOW TO TREAT IT

• Don't smoke; avoid dust- and smoke-filled rooms.
• Drink plenty of fluids to dilute and loosen mucus secretions in the lungs.
• Your doctor may prescribe antibiotics to treat an infection. Take antibiotics for the full term prescribed.
• Your doctor may instruct you in how to expel mucus from your lungs by assuming various positions that lower your head below your torso (a technique known as postural drainage).
• Surgery may be required in advanced cases to remove affected portions of the lungs.

WHEN TO CALL A DOCTOR

• Call a doctor if you have a persistent cough, especially one that yields heavy sputum or mucus, or if you have recurrent respiratory infections. ▲

SYMPTOMS

• A persistent cough that produces large amounts of thick, foul-smelling gray-green sputum, possibly flecked with blood.
• Shortness of breath.
• Bad breath.
• Fits of coughing brought on by a change in posture, such as lying down.
• Frequent respiratory infections.
• Appetite loss, weight loss, clubbed fingers, fever, and anemia in more advanced cases.

Bronchitis, Acute

WHAT IS IT?

Acute bronchitis occurs when an irritant or infection causes inflammation and swelling of the lining of the bronchial tubes, which narrows the air passages. When the cells lining the airways are irritated beyond a certain point, the tiny cilia (hairs) that normally trap and eliminate foreign matter stop working properly. The buildup of irritants leads to the production of excess mucus, which clogs air passages further and produces the characteristic heavy cough of bronchitis. Although attacks of acute bronchitis are common and not usually a major health threat, the elderly and the very young are vulnerable to severe consequences. Attacks may also be a major threat to people with chronic lung diseases like emphysema and asthma. Generally, though, symptoms disappear spontaneously within a few days.

WHAT CAUSES IT?

• Viral infections (including the common cold and flu) and bacterial infections may lead to bronchitis.
• Irritants including chemical fumes, dust, smoke, or other air pollutants may provoke an attack.
• Smoking, asthma, poor nutrition, cold weather, congestive heart failure, and chronic pulmonary disorders may increase the risk of an acute attack.

PREVENTION

• Don't smoke; try to avoid second-hand smoke.
• People at increased risk should avoid exposure to potentially irritating airborne particles, such as dust, and avoid exercise on poor air-quality days.

DIAGNOSIS

• Patient history and physical examination are needed.
• Chest x-rays, sputum samples, or blood tests may be taken to rule out other lung disorders.

SYMPTOMS

• Deep, persistent cough that may produce gray, green, or yellowish sputum.
• Shortness of breath and wheezing.
• Fever.
• Chest pain, exacerbated by cough.

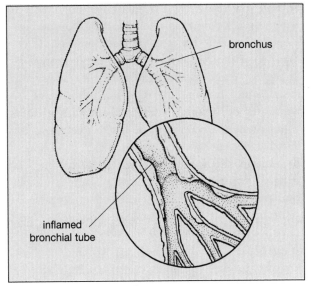

Inflammation of the bronchi and bronchial tubes results in swelling and narrowing of the air passages, and stimulates excess mucus production.

HOW TO TREAT IT

• Take aspirin or ibuprofen to reduce fever and pain.
• Take an over-the-counter cough suppressant containing dextromethorphan if you have a persistent dry cough that disrupts your sleep or normal activities. However, if you are coughing up sputum, suppressing the cough may encourage mucus accumulation in the lungs, potentially leading to serious complications.
• Stay in a warm room. Inhale steam, use a humidifier, or take frequent hot showers to loosen phlegm.
• Drink at least eight glasses of water a day to help thin mucus and make it easier to expel.
• Antibiotics may be prescribed if bacterial infection is suspected.
• Smokers should abstain from cigarettes.

WHEN TO CALL A DOCTOR

• Call a doctor if symptoms do not ease within 36 to 48 hours, or if episodes of acute bronchitis recur.
• Call a doctor if you suffer from a lung disease or congestive heart failure and are experiencing symptoms of acute bronchitis.
• Call a doctor if during an attack of bronchitis you cough up blood, become short of breath, or have a fever above 102°F.

Bunions

WHAT IS IT?

A bunion is a deformity of the first joint of the big toe. The bones in the joint protrude outward, forcing the toe to point inward toward the other toes. Shoes may exert pressure against the protruding joint, leading to painful bursitis (inflammation of a bursa, one of the small, fluid-filled sacs that produces a lubricating fluid to minimize friction between muscles and tendons and between muscles and bones). In addition, the skin over a bunion may become irritated owing to constant rubbing against the shoe. Bunions are common and, while not serious, may be painful and limit the toe's range of motion.

WHAT CAUSES IT?

• Wearing shoes with pointed toes and high heels is the most common cause of painful bunions.
• Rheumatoid arthritis and osteoarthritis may lead to joint deformity and the development of bunions.
• A hereditary trait known as hallux valgus may cause weakness in the joints of the toes and lead to the formation of bunions.

PREVENTION

• Avoid high-heeled shoes whenever possible. Choose shoes with low heels and plenty of room for the toes.

DIAGNOSIS

• Physical examination and x-rays of the affected toe confirm the diagnosis.

HOW TO TREAT IT

• Avoid wearing high-heeled shoes, especially those

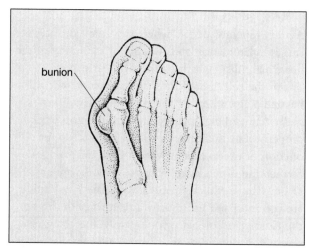

bunion

Inflammation of the joint at the base of the big toe may be further aggravated as shoes rub against the protruding bunion.

with pointed toes. Stretching your shoes may provide extra room and offer some relief.
• Commercially available felt pads or cushions may ease pressure from the shoe on the bunion and the other toes. Around the house it may be helpful to wear an old shoe with a hole cut out above the bunion.
• Arch supports, or an orthotic shoe insert prescribed by your doctor, may help to redistribute weight on the foot.
• Surgery to realign the joint and remove the bunion may be recommended in severe cases.

WHEN TO CALL A DOCTOR

• Make an appointment if you experience continuing pain due to a bunion or if the bunion is interfering with walking or other activities. 🔺

SYMPTOMS
• A painful, bony lump at the side of the base of the big toe.
• A big toe that points inward and possibly overlaps one or two toes.
• Foot pain and stiffness that may interfere with walking and other activities.
• Redness and swelling around the base of the big toe.

Bursitis

WHAT IS IT?

Bursitis is inflammation of a bursa—one of the small, fluid-filled sacs located near joints and bony prominences throughout the body. The bursae act as cushions between muscles and tendons and between muscles and bones. They produce a lubricating fluid to minimize friction at these sites, thus facilitating joint movement. Irritation, overuse, infection, or injury can inflame a bursa, resulting in painful bursitis. The shoulders, elbows, hips, knees, heels, and the base of the big toe are among the sites most often affected. Bursitis is so common that it has acquired a number of familiar names, including student's elbow and housemaid's knee. Bursitis is not serious and usually subsides on its own within one or two weeks if the aggravating activity is altered or stopped; however it has a tendency to recur.

WHAT CAUSES IT?

• Activities that put constant pressure on a bursa (such as resting the elbow on a desk or kneeling).
• Repetitive and vigorous joint movement.
• A blow or other injury to a bursa.
• Inflammatory arthritis, gout, and certain infections.
• Calcium deposits in, or degeneration of, a nearby tendon is sometimes associated with bursitis.

PREVENTION

• Wear protective gear when playing sports. Check with a coach, trainer, or professional to be sure that you are using proper techniques.
• Avoid overly strenuous or repetitive physical activities if possible.
• If you must work in a kneeling position, use knee pads or cushions, change positions often, and take frequent breaks.

• To prevent bursitis in the feet, wear high heels only when you must; buy new running shoes when old ones wear out; wear shoes with a properly fitting heel.

DIAGNOSIS

• Patient history and physical examination are needed.
• X-rays of the affected area may be necessary to rule out other disorders.

HOW TO TREAT IT

• Rest and avoid putting pressure on the affected area. Your doctor may prescribe splints, braces, or slings to keep the joint still.
• Take an over-the-counter pain reliever as needed.
• Use ice packs for the first 48 hours to relieve pain and swelling. Then, if desired, switch to heat packs, which stimulate blood flow and ease pain.
• To reduce swelling, your doctor may draw excess fluid from the bursa with a syringe and then tightly bandage the joint.
• Your doctor may administer injections of corticosteroids and a local anesthetic to reduce swelling and ease pain.
• Gradually resume using the affected joint to prevent stiffening and muscle atrophy, although naturally you should temporarily avoid any activities that aggravate the condition.
• Surgery to remove the bursa may be necessary in severe, persistent cases.

WHEN TO CALL A DOCTOR

• Make an appointment with a doctor if joint pain or swelling persists for more than two weeks despite treatment. 🔺

SYMPTOMS

• Pain and swelling around a joint.
• Restricted and painful movement of the affected joint.
• Pain spreading into the neck or arms due to bursitis in the shoulder.
• Fever (when associated with an infection).

Candidiasis

WHAT IS IT?

Candidiasis (also known as moniliasis) is a fungal infection that may affect the mouth, vagina, gastro-intestinal tract, skin, nails, or mucous membranes throughout the body. The infection can spread from the genitals or mouth to other moist regions of the body. Normally, the body harbors a small amount of the fungus *Candida albicans*, in addition to some harmless bacteria that compete with this fungus and thus keep it under control. If the number of such bacteria diminish for any reason (with the use of antibiotics, for example), the fungus may grow without restriction and begin to cause symptoms.

Candidiasis occurring in the vagina—better known as a yeast infection—is very common and tends to recur, but it is not serious. However, among drug addicts and immunosuppressed or other seriously ill people, the Candida fungus may enter the bloodstream and invade the kidneys, lungs, or brain, although this is rare.

WHAT CAUSES IT?

• The use of antibiotics may kill the bacteria that normally keep the fungus in check.
• Oral contraceptives or pregnancy may disrupt the normal acidity and moisture of the vagina, thus promoting a yeast infection.

SYMPTOMS

• Vaginal itching, discomfort, and redness, in addition to a thick, white, odorless discharge. Vaginal infections may also cause discomfort during urination and sexual intercourse.
• Oral infections (thrush) produce a cream-colored or bluish-white discharge on the tongue or mouth, with sore, creamy yellow, raised patches in the mouth.
• Skin infections produce an itchy, red rash with flaky white patches. In infants, skin infections may accompany diaper rash.
• Male genital infections produce inflammation of the head of the penis (balanitis).
• Serious, widespread infections may produce chills, fever, and severe malaise.

• Patients with diabetes mellitus are at greater risk of Candida infections.
• A weakened immune system may encourage the growth of the fungus. Those taking immunosuppressant drugs or undergoing chemotherapy and people with AIDS or other immune disorders are especially susceptible.

PREVENTION

• Women should wear cotton undergarments. Nylon fibers, which do not "breathe," create a warm, moist environment that may encourage fungal growth.
• Douche or use feminine hygiene sprays only when so advised by your doctor.
• Avoid sexual intercourse with a partner infected with *C. albicans* until the infection is cured.
• Women prone to candidiasis and using oral contraceptives should consider another birth control method.
• Pregnant women in the third trimester should be examined for candidiasis to avoid spreading an infection to the baby.
• Those prone to Candida infections of the skin should keep their skin as dry as possible.

DIAGNOSIS

• Analysis of skin scrapings, vaginal discharge, pus, or sputum is necessary to confirm the diagnosis.
• Blood or tissue cultures may be required.

HOW TO TREAT IT

• For candidiasis of the vagina, penis, mouth, or throat, your doctor may prescribe antifungal creams, suppositories, or tablets. Preparations for vaginal yeast infections are also available over the counter but should not be used without seeing a doctor initially.
• Your doctor may advise using a gentle mouthwash to loosen hardened secretions in the mouth.
• Intravenous antifungal drugs may be prescribed in severe cases of candidiasis of the mouth, throat, and digestive system.

WHEN TO CALL A DOCTOR

• Call a doctor if you experience any symptoms of candidiasis. ⚠

Canker Sores

WHAT IS IT?

Canker sores (also called aphthous ulcers) are small, painful, craterlike ulcers in the lining of the mouth. They often occur two or three at a time, but it's not unusual for 15 or more to appear at once. Canker sores may sometimes be contagious. They are very common, occurring predominantly among those between the ages of 10 and 40, especially women. Canker sores usually heal within two weeks, but they may recur. Although they pose no serious health threat, severe canker sores can make eating and talking unpleasant.

WHAT CAUSES IT?

While the precise cause of canker sores is unknown, there are several things that may trigger them:
• Injuries due to rough dentures, toothbrushes, chipped or jagged teeth, dental work, or burns from hot food or liquids may lead to mouth ulcers.
• Canker sores are more likely to appear during periods of emotional stress or physical exhaustion.
• Viral or bacterial infections may induce canker sores; thus, close contact (including sharing utensils) with others who have canker sores may increase risk.
• Irritation from certain foods, including citrus fruits, pineapple, vinegar, or highly salted foods, may cause mouth ulcers.
• Food allergies, allergic rhinitis, and certain vitamin deficiencies are associated with canker sores.
• Often canker sores occur spontaneously.

DIAGNOSIS

• In severe or persistent cases, a biopsy of the ulcers may be taken to rule out oral ulcers occurring in association with other disorders including cancer and erosive lichen planus (a chronic, itching skin disease of unknown cause).
• A blood sample may also be required.

SYMPTOMS
• Small, painful, white or gray, craterlike, red-rimmed ulcers located anywhere inside the mouth, including the gums, tongue, and lips. Ulcers may appear singly or in groups.

PREVENTION

• Brush and floss your teeth regularly.
• Try to determine if certain foods seem to trigger canker sores and then avoid those foods.
• Because canker sores may be contagious, avoid intimate contact with someone who has them.

HOW TO TREAT IT

• Apply an ice cube to the sore area to relieve pain.
• Rinse the mouth several times a day with warm salt water.
• Avoid spicy or acidic foods that irritate the ulcers.
• For recurrent or more severe ulcers, a doctor may recommend using an antiseptic mouthwash. In addition, a doctor may prescribe topical anesthetics, antihistamines, or corticosteroids to speed healing.
• A waterproof ointment may be used to cover the ulcer as it heals.

WHEN TO CALL A DOCTOR

• Call your doctor if, in addition to canker sores, you develop a high fever or swollen glands.
• Consult your doctor if you experience severe pain from the ulcers.
• Call your doctor if the ulcers persist for longer than two weeks despite treatment.

Carcinoid Tumors and Carcinoid Syndrome

WHAT IS IT?

A carcinoid tumor is a growth composed of cells with properties of both endocrine and nerve tissues. By far the most common site for carcinoid tumors is the wall of the intestines, but they may occur in other organs, such as the lungs or pancreas. This rare type of tumor can be benign or malignant. Even when malignant, the tumor grows very slowly and thus may never produce any symptoms or affect general health in any way. Occasionally a tumor may cause abdominal pain or intestinal bleeding or grow large enough to cause intestinal obstruction.

In about 10 percent of cases, however, the cells of a malignant carcinoid tumor get into the bloodstream, spread to other organs (especially the liver), and multiply. Carcinoid tumors secrete a number of powerful substances (serotonin, histamine, prostaglandins, and several hormones). Consequently, tumors that have spread to the liver produce unpleasant symptoms that characterize what is called carcinoid syndrome. Although carcinoid tumors can be life-threatening, the tumors grow so slowly that the patient may live 10 or 20 years after initial diagnosis. If they are detected before spreading, surgical treatment may allow for full recovery.

SYMPTOMS

- Carcinoid tumors may cause no symptoms, but they can possibly cause abdominal pain, gastrointestinal bleeding, or intestinal obstruction. Carcinoid syndrome, however, may produce a number of the following symptoms:
- Flushing or redness of the face and neck lasting up to several hours owing to the secretion of excess hormones and other substances. Such symptoms may be triggered by exercise, alcohol consumption, stress, or certain foods.
- Gas and profuse diarrhea with possible abdominal cramping and vomiting.
- Wheezing or breathlessness.
- Watery, swollen eyes.
- Palpitations or symptoms of congestive heart failure (CHF), as the abundance of serotonin may damage heart valves.

WHAT CAUSES IT?

- The cause of carcinoid tumors is unknown.
- Risk factors may include obesity, smoking, and excessive alcohol consumption.

PREVENTION

- There is currently no known way to prevent carcinoid tumors.

DIAGNOSIS

- A urine sample is analyzed for the presence of a byproduct of the breakdown of serotonin, the major substance secreted by carcinoid tumors.
- Abdominal x-rays and possibly a CT (computed tomography) scan of the abdomen will be done.
- An octreotide (hormone) scan may be performed.
- Endoscopy or sigmoidoscopy (examination of the bowel using a small, flexible, illuminated scope) is often performed. A biopsy of any suspicious tissue in the colon may be taken during these procedures.
- Carcinoid tumors may be detected during abdominal surgery for another, unrelated disorder.

HOW TO TREAT IT

- If carcinoid tumors are detected before they have spread or in the early stages after spreading, surgery will be performed in an attempt to remove them.
- Chemotherapy may be used to slow the progress of the carcinoid tumor.
- If the carcinoid tumor has invaded the liver, treatment is aimed at relieving the symptoms of carcinoid syndrome. Medical treatments may include serotonin-blocking drugs and bronchodilators (to relieve wheezing and shortness of breath).
- Niacin supplements may be given because the chemical activity of the tumors results in a niacin deficiency that, in fact, causes a number of the symptoms associated with carcinoid syndrome.
- Injections of octreotide (a synthetic hormone) may be used to decrease the body's secretion of hormonal substances.

WHEN TO CALL A DOCTOR

- The symptoms of carcinoid syndrome warrant a doctor's attention.

Cardiac Arrhythmias

WHAT IS IT?

Cardiac arrhythmias are disturbances in the normal rhythm of the heartbeat. An occasional palpitation or fluttering is usually not serious, but a persistent arrhythmia may be life-threatening.

There are many different types of cardiac arrhythmias. The heart may beat too rapidly (tachycardia) or too slowly (bradycardia), or it may beat irregularly. Atrial fibrillation and atrial flutter are common cardiac arrhythmias, which lead to an irregular and sometimes rapid heart rate. These atrial arrhythmias may interfere with the heart's ability to pump blood properly from its upper chambers (atria). The atria may not always empty completely, and blood remaining there too long may stagnate and potentially clot. Such clots may travel to other parts of the body, where they may cause blockages in the blood supply to the limbs, brain, or heart.

In ventricular fibrillation, the lower chambers of the heart (ventricles) quiver feebly instead of contracting powerfully. This is the most severe type of arrhythmia, causing death in minutes unless medical assistance is obtained immediately.

WHAT CAUSES IT?

• Disorders that damage the heart or its valves, such as endocarditis, myocarditis, and rheumatic fever.
• Disorders of the thyroid gland.
• Chest- or heart-surgery patients may develop an arrhythmia soon after an operation.
• Dehydration or depletion of potassium or other electrolytes may trigger an arrhythmia.
• Some drugs, including digitalis, stimulants, and diuretics, as well as overdoses of cocaine, marijuana, or antidepressants may provoke an arrhythmia.

SYMPTOMS
• Palpitations or irregular-feeling heartbeats.
• Shortness of breath.
• Chest pain.
• Dizziness, lightheadedness, and fainting spells.
• Mental confusion.
• Loss of consciousness.
• In some cases there may be no symptoms.

• Injury to the heart due to a heart attack.
• Risk increases with smoking, excess consumption of caffeine or alcohol, advancing age, high blood pressure, kidney disease, and stress.

PREVENTION

• Engage in regular aerobic exercise. Avoid cigarettes, illegal drugs, and excessive amounts of alcohol and caffeine. Try to reduce emotional stress.
• Carefully follow instructions for prescription drugs.

DIAGNOSIS

• Electrocardiography (ECG), to monitor the electrical impulses that control heartbeat; may require Holter monitoring (portable ECG) for a brief period (usually 24 hours).
• Blood pressure and blood tests.
• Exercise (treadmill) stress test.
• Chest x-rays and angiography (injection of a contrast material into an artery to produce a clear x-ray image of the blood vessels).
• Echocardiogram (use of ultrasound to map the heart's movements and structure).
• An electrophysiologic study (a sophisticated electrical test of the heart involving electrical monitoring and stimulation inside the heart) may be performed.

HOW TO TREAT IT

• Antiarrhythmic drugs (such as a beta-blockers, calcium channel blockers, amiodarone, or procainamide) may be prescribed.
• Anticoagulants (such as aspirin or warfarin) may be prescribed to prevent the formation of blood clots, particularly for atrial arrhythmias.
• Digitalis (a drug that slows ventricular response to the rapid impulses coming from the atrium) may be prescribed for those with atrial arrhythmias.
• Defibrillation—a jolt of electricity applied to the chest by an emergency medical team—may restore normal heart rhythm if administered within a few minutes of the onset of ventricular fibrillation. An electric shock (cardioversion) may also be administered under nonemergency conditions to correct atrial arrhythmias.
• A pacemaker may be implanted in the chest if the heart rate is dangerously slow.

Cardiac Arrhythmias *continued*

• An ablation procedure (removal of damaged heart tissue) may be recommended to interrupt an abnormal electrical pathway. This can often be performed during an electrophysiologic study.

• Surgery may be done to interrupt an abnormal electrical pathway in the heart, replace a damaged heart valve, or bypass blocked coronary arteries.

WHEN TO CALL A DOCTOR

• **EMERGENCY** Call an ambulance if you experience severe chest pain, shortness of breath, or prolonged palpitations.

• **EMERGENCY** Call an ambulance if someone loses consciousness. If heartbeat or breathing has stopped, perform cardiopulmonary resuscitation (CPR).

Cardiomyopathy

WHAT IS IT?

Cardiomyopathy is the term for any disease of the heart muscle that interferes with the heart's ability to pump blood with sufficient force. There are several forms of it: Dilated (or congestive) cardiomyopathy is weakness in the walls of the heart that causes them to balloon out, compromising the heart's efficiency and increasing the risk of congestive heart failure, arrhythmias, and the formation of blood clots (which may cause heart attacks or strokes). Hypertrophic cardiomyopathy, overgrowth or thickening of heart muscle, may compromise blood flow through the heart. Restrictive cardiomyopathy involves loss of elasticity of the heart walls that prevents the heart from adequately filling with blood prior to contracting. Except when caused by viral infections, cardiomyopathy develops slowly and may produce no symptoms until the later stages. The disorder is relatively rare, accounting for only 1 percent of heart disease fatalities in the United States, although it is one of the more common causes of serious heart disease in younger people.

WHAT CAUSES IT?

• In many cases of cardiomyopathy, the cause is unknown.
• Hypertrophic cardiomyopathy appears to run in families.

SYMPTOMS

• Often there are no symptoms until the disease's very advanced stages. These may include the following:
• Shortness of breath, especially during exertion.
• Swelling of the feet, ankles, or hands (edema).
• Fatigue.
• Palpitations.
• Dizziness or fainting.
• Wheezing and a dry cough, or a cough producing foamy, bloody phlegm.
• Chest pain (may be mild).
• Stroke or painful and cold extremity due to a blood clot blocking a blood vessel.

• Viral infections of the heart cause inflammation of the heart muscle (myocarditis) and may result in permanent damage to the muscle.
• Excess consumption of alcohol may be toxic to the heart muscle over time.
• Nutritional deficiencies (such as lack of vitamin B_1 or potassium) and hormone imbalances may damage and weaken the heart muscle.
• Amyloidosis, a disorder in which the walls of the heart are infiltrated by a waxy substance, may cause restrictive cardiomyopathy (see Amyloidosis for more information).
• The risk of developing cardiomyopathy increases with smoking, obesity, or chronic diarrhea.
• Advanced coronary artery disease may be a cause.

PREVENTION

• To reduce the risk of heart disease in general, eat a well-balanced low-fat diet, exercise regularly, and lose weight if you are overweight. Limit yourself to no more than two alcoholic beverages each day, and don't smoke.

DIAGNOSIS

• An electrocardiogram (ECG) monitors the electrical impulses that control the heartbeat. You may be asked to wear a portable electrocardiogram device, known as a Holter monitor, for 24 hours.
• Chest x-rays may be taken.
• Your doctor may perform an echocardiogram, which uses ultrasonic waves to image the structure and the movements of the heart.
• A biopsy of heart muscle may be taken.

HOW TO TREAT IT

• Your doctor may prescribe medications to reduce heart muscle exertion, improve the heart's pumping ability, regulate the heartbeat, and ease symptoms.
• Avoid strenuous physical activity.
• Abstinence from alcohol may be necessary.
• A heart transplant may be advised if the heart muscle has been badly damaged.

WHEN TO CALL A DOCTOR

• Symptoms of cardiomyopathy indicate late-stage disease, warranting prompt attention from a doctor. ▲

Carpal Tunnel Syndrome

WHAT IS IT?

Carpal tunnel syndrome results when the median nerve, which passes through a narrow tunnel of wrist bones (carpals) and a ligament at the base of the hand, is compressed by surrounding tissue or excess fluid. Symptoms, including numbness, tingling, and pain in the hand, wrist, or arm, may appear suddenly or gradually and often affect both hands. The disorder occurs most often among women between the ages of 30 and 60.

WHAT CAUSES IT?

• Activities that require prolonged bending of the wrist or constant repeated hand motions may lead to carpal tunnel syndrome. Such activities include typing, assembly-line work, knitting, sewing, tennis, and canoeing.
• Injury to the wrist may damage the median nerve.
• Hormonal changes due to pregnancy or birth control pills may cause fluid accumulation in the carpal tunnel.
• Diseases such as rheumatoid arthritis, diabetes mellitus, hypothyroidism, and acromegaly may promote carpal tunnel syndrome.

PREVENTION

• Take frequent breaks when engaged in strenuous work or activities requiring repetitive hand motions,

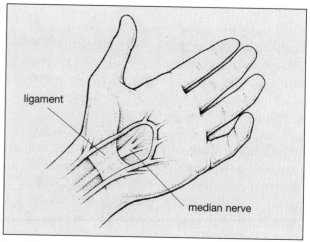

Repetitive hand motion can narrow the carpal tunnel, which may exert pressure on the median nerve and cause pain, numbness, or tingling.

and try to vary activities so that wrists are not constantly bent.
• Use a wrist-support pad while typing.

DIAGNOSIS

• Physical examination and patient history are needed.
• The hands and wrists may be x-rayed.
• A nerve conduction velocity study may be used to monitor the electrical impulses along the median nerve to determine if it is compressed.

HOW TO TREAT IT

• Over-the-counter analgesics can be used for pain.
• A wrist splint may be prescribed, especially for nighttime use.
• Diuretics may be prescribed to reduce fluid accumulation in swollen tissue.
• Corticosteroids may be injected in more severe cases to reduce inflammation.
• If symptoms persist despite treatment, surgery may be recommended to relieve pressure on the median nerve.

WHEN TO CALL A DOCTOR

• Call a doctor if symptoms of carpal tunnel syndrome become sufficiently troublesome or begin to interfere with normal daily activity. ◣

SYMPTOMS

• Numbness, tingling, and eventually pain in the first three fingers, and perhaps half of the fourth finger.
• Pain, often worse at night, possibly severe enough to awaken you.
• Possible pain in the entire hand, forearm, and occasionally above the elbow.
• Weakness in the hands and fingers that may make it difficult to pick up or hold onto objects.
• A sensation of swelling in the fingers (without any visible swelling).
• Atrophy of the muscles at the base of the thumb.

Cataracts

WHAT IS IT?

A cataract is a loss of transparency in the normally clear lens of the eye. At first, a small, hazy spot may appear in the field of vision. Gradually (often over a period of years), as the lens grows more opaque, vision becomes more blurry, especially at night or in very bright light. In the United States about 75 percent of all people over age 60 show some signs of cataracts. Advanced cases are easily treated with surgery (although most patients can postpone surgery for years).

WHAT CAUSES IT?

• Aging is the single greatest risk factor for cataracts, as cumulative exposure to the sun's ultraviolet rays over a lifetime appears to be a primary cause.
• Exposure to radiation, including x-rays and microwaves, may promote cataracts.
• Physical injury to or inflammation of the eye (for example, uveitis or iritis) may lead to cataracts.
• The long-term use of corticosteroid drugs, hereditary factors, and birth defects may be contributing factors.
• Cataracts may occur at a younger age in people with diabetes mellitus.

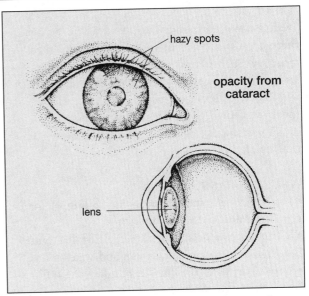

The eye's lens is normally perfectly clear, but when a cataract forms light is absorbed and diffused by the opacity, resulting in blurred vision.

SYMPTOMS

• Gradual, painless, increasingly blurred or double vision.
• Halos or blurriness around lights. Vision may actually be better in dim light, since bright light causes the pupil to constrict, restricting the passage of light to the part of the lens most affected by a cataract.
• Increased sensitivity to light and glare.
• Dulled color perception.
• Temporary improvement in near vision (patient may no longer need reading glasses for a brief period).
• Frequent changes in eyeglass or contact lens prescriptions.
• Difficulty driving at night or in bright light.
• Yellowish or milky white appearance of the lens in advanced cases.

PREVENTION

• Wear sunglasses marked "general purpose" or "special purpose," or those that indicate they block at least 95 percent of ultraviolet-B (UVB) rays.

DIAGNOSIS

• Eye examination by an ophthalmologist.

HOW TO TREAT IT

• To minimize glare outdoors, wear a wide-brimmed hat and amber-tinted sunglasses.
• Indoors, use floor or desk lamps with incandescent bulbs instead of ceiling or fluorescent lights. Avoid pinpoint halogen lights, which cause the pupils to constrict. Installing dimmer controls is advised.
• When reading, try large-print books and newspapers.
• Surgery (successful in 95 percent of cases) is the only cure for cataracts. It can often be postponed indefinitely but is advised when cataracts interfere with normal activities. During the operation the lens is removed and replaced with a plastic intraocular lens implant. (Special contact lenses or eyeglasses may be used when an implant is ruled out.)

WHEN TO CALL A DOCTOR

• See an ophthalmologist for any vision problems.

Cervical Acceleration/Deceleration Injuries Whiplash

WHAT IS IT?

Whiplash is a neck injury sustained when the head is thrown backward and then forward (or vice versa) violently. Such trauma may damage the muscles, ligaments, tendons, and cartilaginous disks in the neck and may even result in fractures of the cervical (neck) vertebrae. Typically, pain and stiffness are much worse a day or two following the injury; fortunately, full recovery is likely.

WHAT CAUSES IT?

• Car accidents (especially rear-end collisions) are the most common cause of whiplash.
• Whiplash may occur during recreational activities like high-impact sports, dancing, and waterskiing.
• Osteoarthritis of the spine may stiffen the spine and increase vulnerability to neck injuries.

PREVENTION

• Use properly adjusted headrests in the car and always use lap and shoulder belts.

DIAGNOSIS

• X-rays of the neck and spine may be taken.
• Your doctor will perform a physical examination to detect changes in motor ability and sensation.

HOW TO TREAT IT

• Apply ice packs for the first 24 hours after the injury to reduce pain and swelling.
• Take nonprescription pain relievers.
• Sleep without a pillow. Instead, place a rolled towel (less than two inches in diameter) behind your neck, or sleep wearing a neck brace.

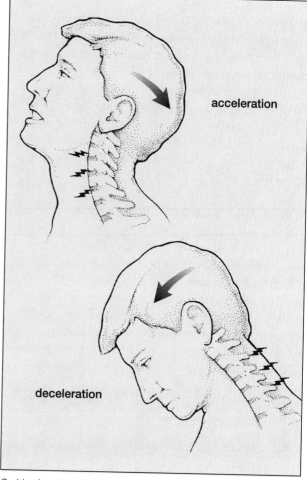

Sudden forward acceleration causes the head to be thrown back; the head is then thrown forward as the force of rear impact is absorbed.

• After 24 hours, use either heat or ice packs as desired. Try hot showers or warm compresses.
• Your doctor may recommend a padded neck brace or collar to immobilize the injured region for several days or weeks as pain subsides. In more severe cases, short-term traction may be recommended.
• Muscle relaxants or narcotics may be prescribed in more severe cases. (Avoid alcohol with such drugs.)
• During recuperation, don't lift heavy objects, and be especially cautious when driving.

WHEN TO CALL A DOCTOR

• Call a doctor if you suffer a painful neck injury or if you develop severe pain, numbness, or weakness in the arm or face. ▲

SYMPTOMS

• Neck pain or stiffness, appearing within 24 hours of an injury. Often, pain in the front of the neck diminishes over several days, while pain in the back of the neck intensifies.
• Dizziness and headache.
• Nausea and vomiting.
• Numbness or stiffness in the arms.
• Gait instability.

Cervical Cancer

WHAT IS IT?

Cervical cancer is the growth of malignant cells in the cervix, the narrow opening of the uterus. Cervical cancer develops slowly from a distinct precancerous stage (dysplasia). Cancer confined to the surface of the cervix is classified as preinvasive, while cancer that has spread into deeper layers or to other organs is termed invasive. Symptoms may not appear until the cancer reaches the more dangerous invasive phase; however, with early diagnosis and treatment, long-term prognosis is extremely favorable.

WHAT CAUSES IT?

• The cause is unknown, but risk factors include sexual activity at an early age, multiple sexual partners, multiple pregnancies, a history of herpes or other venereal infections, and smoking.
• Infection with certain varieties of the human papillomavirus, which cause genital warts, has a strong association with cervical cancer.
• Women whose mothers took the synthetic hormone DES during pregnancy may be at greater risk.

PREVENTION

• Women who are sexually active, over age 18, or whose mothers took the drug DES during pregnancy should have a Pap smear (microscopic examination of a small sample of cells scraped from the cervix and upper vagina) at least once a year.

DIAGNOSIS

• A Pap smear to detect cancerous cells or dysplasia.
• Colposcopy (inspection of the vagina and cervix with a lighted instrument) to identify suspicious

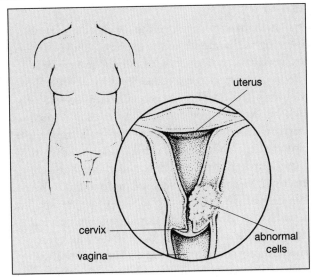

The cervix, located at the end of the vaginal canal, marks the entrance to the uterus. It is the most common site of gynecological cancer.

growths; biopsy of suspicious lesions on the cervix.
• Conization (a biopsy of a cone-shaped section of the cervix) to detect and remove abnormal cells in patients whose Pap smear suggests preinvasive cancer.
• Dilatation and curettage (D&C), in which the cervix is dilated to obtain tissue samples for analysis.
• Blood and urine samples.

HOW TO TREAT IT

• Preinvasive cervical cancer may be treated by cauterization (use of heat to burn away cancerous cells), cryosurgery (use of liquid nitrogen to freeze and destroy cancerous cells), or laser surgery. Preinvasive cancers may also be totally removed during conization or, rarely, with hysterectomy (removal of the cervix and uterus).
• Surgery for invasive cervical cancer is usually treated by radical hysterectomy (removal of all of the internal reproductive organs and neighboring lymph nodes); very severe cases may also require removal of the bladder and rectum (very rare).
• Radiation and chemotherapy may be used if cancer has spread throughout the uterus or to other organs.

WHEN TO CALL A DOCTOR

• Schedule regular Pap smears. Call your doctor if you note any symptoms of cervical cancer. 🔺

SYMPTOMS

• No symptoms during early stages.
• Abnormal vaginal bleeding between periods, after intercourse, or after menopause; heavier and lengthier monthly periods (in later stages).
• Persistent, unusual vaginal discharge.
• Back and abdominal pain.
• General malaise and loss of weight and appetite after cancer has spread.

Cervical Disorders, Nonmalignant

WHAT IS IT?

Nonmalignant disorders of the cervix (the narrow opening at the mouth of the uterus) include cervicitis, cervical eversion, cervical polyps, and cervical dysplasia. Cervicitis is a broad term for an inflammation or infection of the cervix. Cervical eversion, also known as ectropion (often mistakenly termed cervical erosion), is the migration of cells from the lining of the endocervical canal (endocervix) to the outer portion of the cervix (ectocervix). The cells from the endocervical canal are more delicate than the cells of the ectocervix and thus more susceptible to infection. Actual erosion or abrasion of cervical tissue is quite rare but may occur following certain medical procedures, sexual intercourse, or the use of an intrauterine birth control device (IUD).

Cervical polyps are grapelike growths from the surface cells lining the cervix. They may occur singly or in groups, and in some women, large polyps may interfere with conception by creating a barrier to sperm. In very rare cases, polyps are an early precursor of cervical cancer. Cervical dysplasia is the presence of abnormal cells on the surface of the cervix and may be classified as mild, moderate, or severe, depending upon the extent of the cellular abnormality. Although dysplasia (at any stage) is not cancerous and milder degrees may go away spontaneously, it may be the first step in the eventual development of cervical cancer and thus warrants prompt attention.

WHAT CAUSES IT?

• Cervicitis may be caused by vaginal infections, sexually transmitted diseases, and pelvic inflammatory disease. Tears or lacerations in the cervix occurring during childbirth or abortion may lead to cervicitis.
• The cause of cervical eversion is not known. The condition is normal in early puberty, and some women are born with it. Pregnancy and long-term use of oral contraceptives may increase risk.
• The growth of cervical polyps may be triggered by injury to the cervix, vaginal infections, or hormonal changes. They tend to recur after removal, but are almost always benign.
• The cause of cervical dysplasia is not known, although it may be linked to cervical eversion and sexually transmitted diseases, especially those associated with the human papillomavirus. Women who have had many sexual partners are at greater risk (see Cervical Cancer for more information).

PREVENTION

• Women should have regular Pap smears for early detection of any irregularities in the cervix.
• Prompt treatment should be obtained for any vaginal infection or sexually transmitted disease.
• Women should wear cotton undergarments. Nylon fibers, which cannot "breathe," create a warm, moist environment that may encourage infections.

DIAGNOSIS

• A Pap smear (microscopic examination of a small sample of cells scraped from the cervix and upper vagina) is necessary.
• A sample of vaginal discharge, if any is present, may be taken for analysis (including culture or microscopic examination).
• Colposcopy (inspection of the vagina and cervix with a special scope) can identify abnormalities.
• A biopsy of cervical tissue may be performed.

SYMPTOMS

• Cervicitis: clear, gray, or yellow vaginal discharge; vaginal bleeding after intercourse or between periods; burning and itching of external genitalia. (Simultaneously occurring infections of adjacent organs may produce additional symptoms of frequent and urgent need to urinate, painful urination, and lower abdominal or back pain.)
• Cervical eversion: white or slightly bloody vaginal discharge, often appearing one week prior to a period; vaginal bleeding after intercourse or between periods.
• Cervical polyps: heavy, watery, and bloody vaginal discharge; vaginal bleeding after intercourse, between periods, or after a bowel movement; heavy bleeding during periods; pelvic cramps.
• Cervical dysplasia: no symptoms. A Pap smear is necessary to detect it.

Cervical Disorders, Nonmalignant *continued*

HOW TO TREAT IT

• Cervicitis: Your doctor may prescribe antibiotics, or antifungal or antiviral agents. If symptoms persist, the affected area of the cervix may be painlessly destroyed by heat (cauterization), the use of liquid nitrogen (cryosurgery), or laser surgery. If the infection has penetrated deeply into the cervical tissue, the affected tissue may be surgically removed in a conical section (conization).

• Cervical eversion: The affected tissues may be destroyed by cauterization, cryosurgery, or laser surgery. Treatment is unnecessary if the condition produces no symptoms.

• Cervical polyps: Polyps are removed surgically. Single growths may be removed under a local anesthetic in the doctor's office. Removal of groups of larger polyps may require brief hospitalization.

• Cervical dysplasia: Mild cervical dysplasia may disappear without treatment. Surgery for persistent cervical dysplasia may include laser surgery, cryosurgery, cauterization, or conization. In severe cases, which border on cervical cancer, a hysterectomy may be advised (see Cervical Cancer for more information).

WHEN TO CALL A DOCTOR

• Make an appointment with a gynecologist if you experience symptoms of any cervical disorders.

• See your gynecologist for regularly scheduled Pap smears. ⚗

Chiggers

WHAT IS IT?

Chiggers are the larvae of the harvest mite or red bug. The tiny larvae, measuring only about a third of a millimeter in length, inhabit grasses, weeds, shrubs, and brush, primarily in the southern United States (although they may be found as far north as Canada). They most often attach themselves to human hosts at the ankles and legs, since these are the parts of the body most commonly exposed to the low-lying vegetation where chiggers dwell. However, chiggers generally prefer warm, moist places and so may lodge in the groin area, the armpits, the crook of the elbow, beneath the waistband of clothing, or any region where clothing is tight. Chiggers release an enzyme that dissolves the skin; then they insert a feeding tube into their victim's bloodstream. They feast on their host's blood for up to four days, until they become engorged and drop off. Skin at the site of the chigger bite may react in a variety of ways. An allergic reaction is common, producing extremely itchy red patches. Blisters and swelling may also appear.

While serious diseases due to chigger bites are not a threat in the United States, minor secondary infections may ensue, especially if the sufferer scratches itchy skin until it bleeds. Although itching and discomfort may persist for weeks, chigger bites cause no permanent ill effects.

WHAT CAUSES IT?

• Spending time in the woods or fields during the summer increases the risk of chigger bites.

PREVENTION

• Use an insect repellent during outdoor summer activities.

• When walking in the woods or fields, cover your legs completely by wearing long pants and tucking them into your socks or boots.

DIAGNOSIS

• Diagnosis is determined by visual observation and generally does not require a doctor.

HOW TO TREAT IT

• Try not to scratch chigger bites (scratching increases the risk of infection).
• Calamine lotion may soothe itching.
• Take an antihistamine such as pseudoephedrine or diphenhydramine to relieve allergic reaction and itching.
• Over-the-counter corticosteroid creams (hydrocortisone) may alleviate itching. More potent hydrocortisone creams are available by prescription.
• Your doctor may prescribe antibiotics to treat a secondary infection. Antibiotics should be taken for the full term prescribed.

WHEN TO CALL A DOCTOR

• Call a doctor if you suffer an allergic reaction (such as hives) to chigger bites or if over-the-counter treatments fail to relieve severe itching. ⚠

SYMPTOMS
• Extremely itchy, red bumps about one-half inch in diameter. Chiggers may be visible in the center of unscratched bumps. Itching may persist for weeks.
• Hives, blisters, swelling, or large red patches at the site of the bite(s).

Chlamydia

WHAT IS IT?

Chlamydia is any of a group of highly contagious microorganisms that can infect various sites in the body, including the genitals, eyes, lymph nodes, and respiratory tract. In developed countries, it most commonly appears as a sexually transmitted genital infection, marked by inflammation of the urethra (urethritis) in men and cervical infection in women.

Diagnosis of genital chlamydia may be difficult, especially in women, because the infection may cause no symptoms. In women, untreated infection may involve the fallopian tubes (salpingitis), creating disorders also known as pelvic inflammatory disease. These may lead to sterility and/or an increased risk of ectopic (tubal) pregnancy. In men, untreated infection may lead to epididymitis, a painful inflammation of the structure that connects the testes to the urethra. Prompt diagnosis and treatment with antibiotics improves prognosis. In underdeveloped countries, chlamydia infection of the eyes (trachoma) is the leading cause of blindness. Chlamydia has also been identified as a potential cause of coronary artery disease, but these organisms are of a different subtype than those that cause genital infection.

SYMPTOMS

- Painful or burning urination; possible redness and itching in and around the urethra.
- Watery mucus discharge from the penis or vagina.
- Painful swelling of the scrotum; inflamed, painful lymph nodes in the groin area.
- Lower abdominal pain.
- When the eyes are affected, inflammation of the lining of the eyelids and the membrane covering the whites of the eyes (conjunctivitis), leading to blindness if untreated.
- In newborns, difficulty in breathing and a staccato cough, indicating a respiratory chlamydial infection.
- High fever (103°F to 106°F), a symptom of psittacosis pneumonia. Other symptoms range from those of a mild flu to those of severe pneumonia.

WHAT CAUSES IT?

- Chlamydial infections may be transmitted by vaginal or anal intercourse and by oral-genital contact.
- Infection of the cervix in pregnant women may cause eye and respiratory infections in newborns.
- Touching the eyes with contaminated hands may transfer the infection to the eyes.
- A respiratory chlamydial infection *(Chlamydiaceae pneumoniae)* is a common cause of community-acquired pneumonia.
- *C. psittaci,* spread to people via infected birds, may lead to a rare form of pneumonia (psittacosis).

PREVENTION

- Avoid intimate contact with infected people until the infection is cured.
- A monogamous sexual relationship or complete abstinence will protect against genital infection; otherwise, use condoms, other barrier methods, and spermicides to help reduce risk.
- To prevent psittacosis, make sure that any imported or exotic pet bird has been quarantined for 30 days, and that birds of the parrot family have been treated with necessary antibiotics, before buying them.

DIAGNOSIS

- A culture of urethral or cervical discharge is taken.
- Traces of chlamydia DNA can be detected in the urine using a new test.
- Persons at risk—especially those under age 25 who are sexually active—should be screened every six to 12 months, whether or not symptoms are present.

HOW TO TREAT IT

- To treat all chlamydial infections, your doctor will prescribe antibiotics such as azithromycin or doxycycline, which should be taken for the full term. Antibiotics will be administered to both sexual partners for genital chlamydia. Only one partner may exhibit symptoms, but both must be treated.

WHEN TO CALL A DOCTOR

- Make an appointment with a doctor if you or your partner experience symptoms of genital chlamydia, if your inner eyelids become inflamed, or if you develop a high fever (over 102°F).

Cholesteatoma

WHAT IS IT?

A cholesteatoma is a benign, cystlike tumor in the eardrum or middle ear. Most commonly, a cholesteatoma develops when the eustachian tube (the passage between the ear and nose) is blocked for a prolonged period. Gradually, the air trapped in the middle ear is absorbed by surrounding tissue, resulting in greater air pressure outside the eardrum than inside. This pressure imbalance pushes the weakest part of the eardrum inward, creating a pocket. Old skin cells normally shed by the eardrum collect into a ball inside this pocket and form a cyst. If the eardrum is perforated, a cyst may form directly in the middle ear.

Cholesteatomas have the capacity to destroy bone and nerve tissue that lie in its path of growth. The most common problem associated with these tumors is permanent, mild-to-moderate hearing loss due to damage to the delicate bones in the middle ear. If left untreated, the cyst may also eventually begin to erode the eardrum, the facial nerve, the bones lining the ear canal, or even the skull. In such advanced cases, complications can include epidural abscess and meningitis, two types of potentially life-threatening infections of the tissues surrounding the brain.

WHAT CAUSES IT?

• Repeated middle ear infections resulting from blockage of the eustachian tube, creating the conditions conducive to the development of a cholesteatoma.
• A congenital defect may prevent the eustachian tube from opening as it normally should during infancy.
• Risk of cholesteatoma is higher among those with a childhood history of ear infections.

SYMPTOMS
• Hearing loss, ranging from mild to severe.
• Pus leaking from the ear.
• Headaches and earaches.
• Weakness of facial muscles.
• Dizziness.

PREVENTION

• Judicious use of antibiotics and myringotomy tubes (placed in the eardrums) can help an otitis-prone child avoid the later development of cholesteatoma.
• If your child has frequent ear infections, he or she should not be subjected to second-hand cigarette smoke, which can lead to even more frequent ear infections.
• Ongoing followup is required for otitis-prone children.

DIAGNOSIS

• Patient history and physical examination are necessary. Your doctor will examine your ear with an otoscope, a device that permits a clear view of the entire ear canal.
• If your doctor suspects a cholesteatoma, a thorough examination by an otolaryngologist (ear, nose, and throat specialist) will be required.
• MRI (magnetic resonance imaging) may be used to confirm the diagnosis.

HOW TO TREAT IT

• Surgery is the sole cure for cholesteatoma. Cyst removal usually requires opening the middle ear and, possibly, the mastoid process (a honeycomb-like bone behind the ear). This is often performed on an outpatient basis. To minimize the risk of recurrence, great care must be taken during the procedure to remove all traces of the cholesteatoma.
• In more advanced cases, several operations may be necessary to rebuild the bones of the ear. Additional operations may be required to remove cysts that have grown back.
• If the cyst extends to the mastoid process and cannot be cured by antibiotics, a mastoidectomy (removal of the mastoid process) may be necessary.
• A hearing aid may be prescribed if normal hearing cannot be restored.

WHEN TO CALL A DOCTOR

• Call a doctor if you experience hearing loss or any of the symptoms of cholesteatoma. ▲

Chronic Fatigue Syndrome

WHAT IS IT?

The term chronic fatigue syndrome is used to designate a group of symptoms that includes, among other things, extreme and persistent weakness and exhaustion. Several criteria must be met to establish a diagnosis of chronic fatigue syndrome. For one, symptoms such as fatigue and malaise after exercise must interfere with the patient's ability to work and function normally for a period of at least six months. Other medical and psychiatric disorders must be ruled out as well.

The causes of chronic fatigue are extremely elusive, and thus the disorder is fertile ground for unproven theories and quack remedies. No true cure exists; however, in most cases, symptoms are at their worst early on and gradually diminish on their own.

WHAT CAUSES IT?

• The cause of chronic fatigue is unknown. For a time, it was believed that the Epstein-Barr virus was the cause, since tests showed that most chronic fatigue sufferers had been exposed to it. However, almost 90 percent of healthy people have also been exposed to the virus with no ill effects, and not everyone with chronic fatigue symptoms has been exposed. Thus there is no evidence that chronic fatigue is caused by any virus or that it is contagious.
• Another proposed theory is that chronic fatigue is an autoimmune disorder, meaning that the immune system overcompensates in response to a perceived threat (such as a virus) and ultimately attacks otherwise healthy body tissues.
• A new (and as yet unconfirmed) theory suggests that people with chronic fatigue symptoms have lower levels of specific hormones (cortisol and corticotropin-releasing hormone) involved with mood and energy levels.
• Psychological and lifestyle factors appear to play contributory roles.

PREVENTION

• Chronic fatigue syndrome cannot be prevented. Contrary to popular opinion, you cannot "catch it" from someone else.

DIAGNOSIS

• Patient history and physical examination are needed.
• The patient must exhibit all of the aforementioned symptoms. Tests need to be conducted to rule out anemia, infection, diabetes, heart disease, thyroid disease, and other ailments that may produce persistent weakness and exhaustion.

HOW TO TREAT IT

• Over-the-counter pain relievers may be used for muscle and joint pain and headaches.
• Exercising vigorously may exacerbate symptoms. Instead, maintain moderate levels of activity and slowly increase your tolerance for exercise.
• Getting plenty of rest and eating a healthy, balanced diet is recommended.
• Low-dose antidepressants may improve sleep disturbances and decrease fatigue and muscle pain.
• Psychological counseling may be helpful—not because chronic fatigue is a psychosomatic disorder but because it is often accompanied by depression (see Depression for more information). Treating the depression may make the overall illness less debilitating.

WHEN TO CALL A DOCTOR

• Make an appointment with your doctor if you have symptoms of chronic fatigue syndrome. 🔺

SYMPTOMS

• Severe, debilitating fatigue, usually made worse by exercise.
• Recurrent flu-like symptoms, including a chronic sore throat.
• Aches and pains in the muscles and joints.
• Painful lymph nodes in the armpits and neck.
• Headaches.
• Low-grade fever (99.5°F to 100.5° F) and chills.
• Depression.
• Mental confusion, irritability, and loss of memory.
• Sleep difficulties.

Chronic Obstructive Pulmonary Disease COPD

WHAT IS IT?

Chronic obstructive pulmonary disease (COPD) is an umbrella term for conditions that obstruct the air passages (bronchi) or damage the small air sacs (alveoli) in the lungs, resulting in progressively impaired breathing. Two primary disorders that constitute COPD are emphysema and chronic bronchitis; many patients with COPD exhibit a combination of both.

Chronic bronchitis is a persistent inflammation of the bronchial tubes in the lungs, producing a recurrent cough with large amounts of mucus. When the cells lining the airways are irritated beyond a certain point, the tiny cilia (hairs) that normally trap and eliminate foreign matter cease to function properly. The buildup of irritants leads to the production of excess mucus, which clogs air passages and produces the characteristic heavy cough of bronchitis. Bronchitis is classified as chronic when the patient coughs up sputum most of the days of a three-month period, two consecutive years in a row.

Emphysema is progressive damage to the lungs, resulting from loss of elasticity in the alveoli, where oxygen enters and carbon dioxide exits the bloodstream. If the lungs are damaged by the chemicals in cigarette smoke or by the persistent inflammation and coughing of chronic bronchitis, the delicate walls of the alveoli may become progressively enlarged, inelastic, and far less functional. The loss of elasticity, often combined with narrowing of the small airways in the lungs (sometimes to the point of

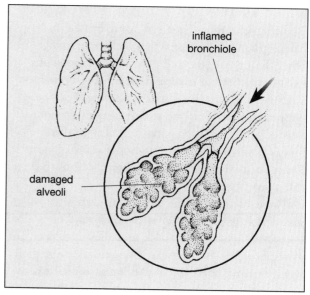

As the alveoli (the tiny air sacs at the ends of the bronchial trees) are damaged by emphysema, the lungs are able to transfer less and less oxygen to the bloodstream, causing shortness of breath. Also, chronic inflammation of the airways may inhibit the entry of air into the alveoli.

collapse), traps stale air instead of allowing it to be exhaled. The affected air sacs are thus unable to deliver oxygen to the bloodstream or to remove carbon dioxide—producing the characteristic shortness of breath of emphysema. Lung damage may progress until breathing is severely impaired, at which time the condition is potentially life-threatening. Low blood-oxygen levels may cause the pressure in the pulmonary arteries to become elevated (pulmonary hypertension), which in turn may prevent the right side of the heart from adequately pumping blood.

Onset of COPD is usually very gradual. It develops over a number of years, and symptoms may not appear until the disease has already progressed quite far. Lung damage is permanent, but it is preventable in many cases by avoiding smoking. COPD is two to three times more common in men than in women.

WHAT CAUSES IT?

- Smoking is the most common cause of COPD.
- Air pollution may be a contributing factor.
- Industrial or chemical fumes can damage the airways.
- Repeated viral or bacterial lung infections may thicken the lining of the bronchial walls, narrow the

SYMPTOMS

- Shortness of breath and wheezing.
- A persistent, mucus-producing cough, especially in the morning (a symptom of chronic bronchitis).
- A chronic dry cough (a symptom of emphysema).
- In severe cases, symptoms of COPD may include coughing up blood, chest pain, and blue-purple complexion.
- Swollen legs and ankles from right-sided heart failure (cor pulmonale).
- Difficulty in exhaling.

Chronic Obstructive Pulmonary Disease COPD *continued*

airways, and stimulate excessive mucus production in the lungs.

• A hereditary deficiency of the enzyme alpha-1-antitrypsin may cause the walls of the alveoli to break down.

• People with occupations that require constant exposure to dust, chemicals, or other lung irritants or that require heavy use of the lungs, such as glass-blowing or playing a wind musical instrument, may be more susceptible to emphysema.

• The labored breathing resulting from the narrowed airways of chronic bronchitis may strain the alveoli and lead to emphysema.

• Asthma or recurrent respiratory allergies are associated with greater risk of COPD.

• Young children living with heavy smokers are more susceptible to chronic respiratory inflammation.

PREVENTION

• Don't smoke (smoking is the primary cause of COPD).

• Avoid spending long periods outside on days when the air quality is poor.

DIAGNOSIS

• Patient history and physical examination are needed.

• A sputum sample may be taken for analysis.

• Blood samples will be taken from both an artery and a vein (to measure oxygen and carbon dioxide levels).

• A chest x-ray will be performed.

• Spirometry and various other pulmonary-function tests that measure breathing capacity and efficiency will be done.

• Tests that measure the strength and efficiency of the heart muscle may be ordered.

HOW TO TREAT IT

• Don't smoke; avoid smoke-filled rooms.

• Drink plenty of fluids to loosen mucus secretions. Avoid caffeine and alcohol, however, since they have a diuretic effect and may lead to dehydration.

• When indoors, moisten the air with a cool-mist humidifier.

• Try to avoid going outside on cold days or days when the air quality is poor, and avoid exposure to cold, wet weather. If bronchitis is advanced and unrelenting, you may want to consider moving to a warmer and drier climate.

• Don't use cough suppressants. Coughing is necessary to clear accumulated mucus from the lungs, and suppressing it may potentially lead to serious complications.

• A cold virus may trigger a flare-up in those suffering from COPD; decrease the risk of catching one by minimizing contact with people suffering from respiratory infections and washing your hands often. Get vaccinated for influenza (annually) and pneumonia (a one-time inoculation).

• A bronchodilator may be prescribed to widen the bronchial passages. Oxygen may be administered in more severe cases.

• Your doctor may prescribe antibiotics to treat or to prevent bacterial lung infections, since patients with COPD are more susceptible to these. Antibiotics should be taken for the full term prescribed.

• Your doctor may instruct you on how to drain mucus from your lungs by assuming various positions that lower your head below your torso (a technique known as postural drainage).

• Breathing exercises (as instructed by your doctor) may prove beneficial.

• In very severe cases of emphysema with extensive lung damage, a lung transplant may be advised (heart-and-lung transplants are advised if progressive lung disease has weakened the heart).

WHEN TO CALL A DOCTOR

• **EMERGENCY** Get medical assistance immediately if your complexion turns bluish or purplish.

• Call a doctor if symptoms become more severe; for example, if shortness of breath or chest pain becomes more intense, your cough worsens or you cough up blood, you develop a fever, you begin to vomit, or your legs and ankles swell more than usual.

• Make an appointment with a doctor if you have experienced a recurrent, persistent, mucus-producing cough for parts of the last two years, or if you experience persistent shortness of breath. ▲

Cirrhosis

WHAT IS IT?

Cirrhosis is characterized by progressive destruction of liver cells and the formation of fibrous scar tissue. The loss of liver cells interferes with the organ's ability to process nutrients, hormones, and drugs and slows the production of proteins and other important substances manufactured in the liver. Eventually liver failure may result. The scar tissue interferes with blood flow from the intestine through the liver via the portal vein. Pressure in the portal vein increases (portal hypertension), the spleen becomes enlarged, and blood is shunted around the liver through enlarged, fragile veins (varices) in the stomach and esophagus. Toxic substances formed in the intestine, and normally cleared in the liver, bypass the liver and are carried to the brain, where they can interfere with its function (hepatic encephalopathy). People with cirrhosis may exhibit no symptoms until the damage—which is irreversible—is quite extensive. Cirrhosis is twice as common among men as women, and some forms of it are associated with an increased risk of liver cancer.

WHAT CAUSES IT?

• Alcoholism is the primary cause of cirrhosis, owing to a combination of the alcoholic's poor diet and the

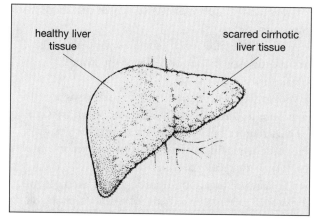

In the cirrhotic liver, healthy cells die and are replaced by scar tissue. Initially, the liver enlarges; in end-stage cirrhosis, the organ shrivels.

direct toxic effects of alcohol. Many alcoholics are also infected with hepatitis C.
• Chronic viral hepatitis (types B, C, and D) or chronic autoimmune hepatitis may lead to cirrhosis.
• Some hereditary diseases, such as cystic fibrosis, hemochromatosis (iron accumulation), and Wilson's disease (deposition of copper), may injure the liver.
• Bile ducts, through which bile is released to the intestines to aid in digestion, may become blocked, inflamed, or scarred, resulting in a type of cirrhosis called biliary cirrhosis. Bile ducts may also be injured during gallbladder surgery.
• Prolonged exposure to certain medications, or to toxic chemicals like insecticides, herbicides, cleaning solvents, and engine exhaust, may harm the liver.
• Congestive heart failure may lead to cirrhosis.

PREVENTION

• Consume no more than two drinks a day. If you suspect that you may have a drinking problem, seek help immediately. You will need to avoid alcohol completely in order to halt the progress of cirrhosis, and a doctor or support group can help you achieve this goal.
• Eat a healthy, balanced diet.

DIAGNOSIS

• In late stages of cirrhosis, diagnosis is very often evident from the history and findings on physical examination. Other tests mentioned are confirmatory in late stages but essential in early stages.

SYMPTOMS

• No symptoms in early stages.
• Loss of appetite; weight loss; nausea; diarrhea.
• Fatigue, weakness, and exhaustion.
• Jaundice; small, red, spidery veins (spider nevi) appearing on the skin, along with a tendency to bruise or bleed easily; severe itching.
• Swelling in the legs and ankles (edema) or abdomen (ascites).
• Darkened urine.
• Impotence, testicular atrophy, and enlarged breasts in men; cessation of menstruation (amenorrhea) in women.
• Black or bloody stools; vomiting of blood.
• Inability to concentrate, impaired memory, and irritability; mental confusion.
• Trembling hands.

Cirrhosis *continued*

• Blood tests are conducted to measure the synthesis of certain proteins by the liver and any increased release of certain enzymes that indicate inflammation. Blood tests are also done to detect the presence of hepatitis B or C.

• A liver biopsy or scan may be done.

• In some cases, the liver may be examined with a viewing instrument (laparoscope) inserted through a small incision in the abdomen.

HOW TO TREAT IT

• Stop drinking alcohol completely. Even if cirrhosis is not alcohol–induced, the liver may be further damaged by alcohol.

• If swelling in the legs, ankles, or abdomen is present, eat a low-salt diet to reduce fluid retention. (Diuretics may be prescribed for this purpose as well.)

• Antibiotics may be prescribed if excess fluid retained in the abdomen has become infected.

• Cholestyramine may be prescribed to relieve severe itching by binding bile salts in the small intestine.

• Antihypertensive drugs such as beta–blockers may be prescribed to lower pressure within the portal vein and thus reduce the risk of bleeding from esophageal varices.

• Endoscopic procedures to close off esophageal varices may be warranted.

• Restriction of dietary protein may ease or prevent neurological changes (hepatic encephalopathy).

• Laxatives (such as lactulose) may be used to speed the passage of toxins through the intestine.

• In advanced cases, a liver transplant may be recommended.

WHEN TO CALL A DOCTOR

• **EMERGENCY** If you begin to vomit blood, call an ambulance.

• Make an appointment with a doctor if you develop symptoms of cirrhosis.

• Seek help from a health professional or a support group if you are worried that you or someone close to you has a drinking problem. ▲

Colitis, Ulcerative

WHAT IS IT?

Ulcerative colitis is a persistent inflammation of the lining of the colon; small ulcers form and eventually develop into abscesses. Episodes of painful, bloody diarrhea and other symptoms may vary in intensity and alternate with symptomless periods of normal bowel function. The condition may develop gradually over a period of years or appear without warning in a sudden, severe attack. In very severe episodes, the patient is at risk for potentially life-threatening blood poisoning (due to toxins found in infected abscesses) and excessive blood loss (due to bloody diarrhea). Other serious complications include massive dilatation of the colon (toxic mega-colon) and perforation of the colon wall, allowing intestinal contents to infect the abdominal cavity (peritonitis). Those who have had ulcerative colitis for 10 years or more are at increased risk of colorectal cancer. The disorder most often affects young adults.

WHAT CAUSES IT?

• The precise cause of ulcerative colitis is unknown, though it appears to be an autoimmune disorder (the body's immune system is overstimulated and attacks its own tissues; in this case, the colon).
• Hereditary factors may play a role.
• Stress, anxiety, or depression may result from suffering from this chronic, often debilitating illness. Though not a cause, emotional factors may intensify symptoms in those with ulcerative colitis.

SYMPTOMS

• Recurrent episodes of bloody, pus- and mucus-filled diarrhea.
• Pain on the left side of the abdomen that lessens after a bowel movement.
• Painful bowel movements; feeling of incomplete evacuation; rectal urgency, pain, cramps.
• Weight loss.
• Symptoms in remote sites of the body, including arthritis and inflammation of the eyes.
• Severe attack: nausea, vomiting, dehydration, profuse sweating, appetite loss, bloating, high fever (104°F), heart palpitations.

• Certain foods may exacerbate symptoms in people sensitive to them (such as milk in those with lactose intolerance).

PREVENTION

• Ulcerative colitis cannot be prevented at present.

DIAGNOSIS

• Blood and stool samples are taken.
• Sigmoidoscopy or colonoscopy (use of a lighted viewing tube) is used to inspect the large intestine.
• A biopsy of the colon lining is usually taken during the sigmoidoscopy or colonoscopy.
• A barium enema with x-ray may be performed.
• Periodic screening for early colon cancer (with colonoscopy) is recommended for those who have had ulcerative colitis for more than 10 years.

HOW TO TREAT IT

• A hot water bottle or a heating pad may be applied to the abdomen to relieve cramps.
• Guard against irritating the colon during a flare-up by avoiding milk and milk products if sensitive.
• Bed rest may be necessary during severe attacks.
• Anti-inflammatory drugs such as sulfasalazine are often prescribed for mild attacks and to prevent recurrence.
• Corticosteroids are the most effective treatment for more severe attacks.
• Enemas containing corticosteroids or aspirin-like drugs may be used to treat internal inflammation.
• Nutritional supplements may be recommended if there is malnutrition or anemia.
• When diarrhea is severe, patients may be hospitalized and fed intravenously.
• Surgical removal of part or all of the colon may be required if the inflammation does not respond to medication. Results of such surgery are often very favorable. Some physicians recommend removal of the colon to prevent colon cancer in those who have had active ulcerative colitis for 10 to 20 years.

WHEN TO CALL A DOCTOR

• Call a doctor if you experience diarrhea that contains blood or mucus or if abdominal pain becomes severe, especially with a high fever.

Colon Polyps

WHAT IS IT?
Colon polyps are nodular growths on the lining of the colon. Generally, they produce no symptoms and are only discovered when a colonoscopy (use of a flexible, lighted tube called a colonoscope to examine the colon) is performed. Polyps are common; two out of every three people over age 60 have them. However, 90 percent of colorectal cancers arise from initially benign polyps, and the larger the polyp, the more likely it is to become cancerous. Thus, early detection and treatment are imperative (see Colorectal Cancer for recommendations on early detection screening procedures).

WHAT CAUSES IT?
• The cause of most colon polyps is unknown.
• Chronic inflammation of the colon due to ulcerative colitis may lead to the development of polyps.
• A diet high in fat (especially from red meat) and low in fiber may contribute to polyp formation.
• Hereditary factors may be involved. One disorder, known as familial colonic polyposis, is characterized by the growth of a large number of polyps (as many as 1,000 or more) in the colon. Gardner's syndrome, another hereditary disorder, produces multiple colonic and intestinal polyps as well as nonmalignant tumors in the bones and skin.
• People who have had colon polyps in the past or have a family history of them are at increased risk of future polyps.

PREVENTION
• Eat a diet low in animal fat and red meat, but high in fiber.
• Get regular checkups if you have had colon polyps, if members of your family have had colon cancer or polyps, or if you are over age 50. The checkup may include testing of a stool sample for bleeding.

SYMPTOMS
• Rectal bleeding.
• Blood and mucus in the stool.
• Change in bowel movements.
• Abdominal pain.

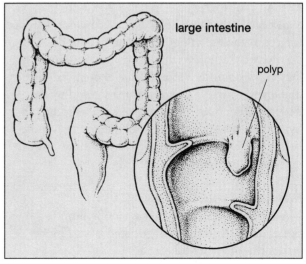

large intestine

polyp

Polyps may form anywhere along the wall of the large intestine. Most are benign, although almost all colon cancers originate as polyps.

DIAGNOSIS
• A small, lighted viewing tube will be passed through the anus to the lower large intestine (sigmoidoscopy) or to the entire large intestine (colonoscopy) to examine the colon.
• A barium enema may be necessary (barium provides an outline of the colon on x-ray). This procedure is not as sensitive in detecting polyps—nor can it differentiate between benign and malignant polyps or remove polyps—as the tube can.
• Blood and stool samples may be taken. Stool samples are examined for hidden (occult) blood.

HOW TO TREAT IT
• Generally, polyps are removed upon detection during the diagnostic colonoscopy. In a few cases, a small incision (laparotomy) may be made in the abdomen to gain access to a portion of the colon. Surgery may involve removing the polyp and possibly a section of the colon and nearby lymph nodes.

WHEN TO CALL A DOCTOR
• Make an appointment with a doctor if you experience symptoms of colon polyps.
• Children in families with a hereditary predisposition toward colon polyps should be screened for colon disorders by age 12. ◣

Colorectal Cancer

WHAT IS IT?

Colorectal cancer, one of the most common types of cancer, is the growth of malignant cells in the colon or rectum. Tumors in the colon are slow-growing, but may eventually become large enough to obstruct the digestive tract. The cancer may spread to the liver, lymph nodes, or other parts of the body, and symptoms may not appear until the cancer is quite advanced. However, if detected and treated early, the outlook is optimistic.

WHAT CAUSES IT?

• A diet high in animal fats (especially from red meat) and low in fiber is associated with a higher incidence of colorectal cancer.
• A personal or family history of colon polyps or ulcerative colitis increases the likelihood of colorectal cancer. A family history of colorectal, breast, or endometrial cancer is also a risk factor.
• The risk of colorectal cancer increases after age 40.

PREVENTION

• Eat a diet low in animal fat and high in fiber.
• Get regular checkups if you have a personal or family history of colon or digestive tract disease.
• The American Cancer Society recommends that people over 40 have an annual digital rectal exam (half of all colorectal cancers occur in the rectum).

SYMPTOMS

• Often there are no symptoms in early stages.
• Change in bowel habits (constipation, diarrhea, or extremely narrow stools) lasting for more than 10 days.
• Bloody or black, tarry stools.
• Pain or tenderness in the lower abdomen.
• Bloating, cramps, gas pains, and a protracted feeling of fullness.
• Loss of appetite and loss of weight.
• Fatigue, paleness (pallor), and heart palpitations due to anemia that often occurs in conjunction with colorectal cancer.
• Inability to pass stools (a sign of intestinal obstruction, an emergency situation).

• People over 50 also should have an annual stool sample test for hidden bleeding and a sigmoidoscopy (in which a lighted viewing tube is used to examine the colon) every three to five years, provided that two successive examinations have proved negative.

DIAGNOSIS

• Blood and stool samples are taken.
• A digital rectal exam (in which the doctor examines the rectum with a gloved finger) is performed.
• Sigmoidoscopy or colonoscopy is used to view the bowel, during which a biopsy may be taken to determine whether the tumor is benign or malignant.
• A barium enema may be necessary. The barium creates a sharp image of the colon during x-ray.
• Colon cancer should always be suspected (and proper tests conducted) in older men and in postmenopausal women with iron deficiency anemia.

HOW TO TREAT IT

• Surgery is necessary to remove the tumor. If the cancer is detected early, the surgery may be limited to a bowel resection, in which the cancerous part of the colon is removed and the healthy parts are rejoined. Nearby lymph nodes are also removed.
• If the tumor is blocking the colon, the cancerous part of the colon is removed, and the end of the remaining upper portion of the colon is brought through an opening created in the abdominal wall for waste to pass through, into a bag. This procedure (colostomy) may be temporary, to allow the colon to heal after the operation, or permanent, when cancer is extensive (about 15 percent of cases).
• Radiation therapy may be used before surgery to reduce the size of the tumor or after surgery to destroy remaining cancer cells; chemotherapy may be used to halt the spread of the cancer.

WHEN TO CALL A DOCTOR

• Call a doctor if you experience rectal bleeding or if you have changes in your bowel movements that persist for three weeks or more.
• Make an appointment with a doctor if you have a personal or family history of colon disease.
• **EMERGENCY** Get immediate medical attention if you experience a total inability to pass stools.

Common Cold

WHAT IS IT?

The common cold is a general term for a group of minor, highly contagious viral infections that cause inflammation of the mucous linings of the nose and throat. Symptoms generally develop one to two days after exposure to the virus, and the cold is contagious for the first two to three days of symptoms. No cure exists, but spontaneous recovery generally occurs within a week to 10 days. Colds tend to be more frequent in the winter than in the summer and more common among children than adults, since immunity to many cold viruses develops with age. Colds may, however, cause serious complications in patients suffering from chronic respiratory disorders.

WHAT CAUSES IT?

• Over 200 different strains of viruses (predominantly rhinoviruses and coronaviruses) cause colds.
• Infected persons may spread cold viruses by direct contact, such as shaking hands or kissing, or through the air, by coughing or sneezing. The virus may also spread via contaminated objects, such as drinking glasses or playing cards.
• Contrary to popular belief, colds are not caused by fatigue, cold air, wet hair, or wet clothes.

PREVENTION

• Wash hands frequently with soap and warm water, especially after visiting public places.

SYMPTOMS

• Nasal and sinus congestion.
• Nasal discharge and watering eyes.
• Sneezing.
• Dry cough, or a cough that produces little sputum.
• Sore throat.
• Headache.
• Mild fever (under 102°F) with chills.
• Fatigue.
• Cold sores on the mouth (due to the cold virus reactivating a dormant herpes simplex infection).
• General muscle and joint aches.

• Avoid touching the face with unwashed hands.
• Don't share towels or drinking glasses.
• Try to limit exposure to people with colds.
• Contrary to popular belief, taking large doses of vitamin C has not been shown to prevent colds.

DIAGNOSIS

• Diagnosis is made by observation of symptoms and does not require a doctor.

HOW TO TREAT IT

• Take aspirin or acetaminophen to relieve headaches and muscle aches and to reduce fever. Acetaminophen is recommended for children under 12.
• Use cold medications sparingly. Avoid "shotgun" remedies that claim to treat all cold symptoms—they are often ineffectual. Nasal decongestant sprays and drops should not be used for more than a few days, as they may actually aggravate congestion with extended use. If you are coughing up mucus, avoid cough suppressants, since they will permit mucus to accumulate in the lungs.
• Drink plenty of fluids to help loosen mucus secretions in the lungs.
• Gargle with warm, salty water several times a day to soothe a sore throat. Sucking on hard candy will help keep the throat lubricated.
• Rest at home (in bed if you feel like it) for the first day or two to aid recovery and to prevent spreading the cold to others.
• Antibiotics do not help treat a cold, but they may be prescribed if you develop a secondary bacterial infection.
• Zinc lozenges have been reported in some studies to shorten the duration of the common cold, but other investigations have found no difference with their use.

WHEN TO CALL A DOCTOR

• Call a doctor if cold symptoms persist for more than two weeks, especially if they increase in severity.
• Call a doctor if you suffer from a chronic respiratory disorder and you catch a cold. ▲

Concussion

WHAT IS IT?

A concussion is characterized by a brief loss of consciousness following an injury or blow to the head. The blow is forceful enough to cause the brain to bump against the skull and temporarily disturb the normal electrical activity in the brain, but it is not traumatic enough to result in more severe injuries such as cerebral lacerations or bruises. Indeed, concussion is the mildest form of brain-skull impact, and full recovery generally occurs within 24 to 48 hours; however, repeated concussions may eventually cause permanent brain damage.

WHAT CAUSES IT?

• Automobile crashes, industrial accidents, and falls are the most common causes of head injury.
• Blows to the head sustained due to boxing, sports injuries, or physical assault may cause a concussion.

PREVENTION

• Wear lap and shoulder belts in the car. Wear a helmet if you ride a motorcycle or bicycle.
• Wear protective headgear when playing sports.

DIAGNOSIS

• Your doctor will request a thorough description of the accident or event that resulted in the concussion.

• An observation period of 24 to 48 hours will be recommended to monitor your mental state, level of alertness, and any symptoms.
• X-rays of the neck and CT (computed tomography) scans of the brain may be necessary.

HOW TO TREAT IT

• Call a doctor immediately after any loss of consciousness following a head injury. The doctor will recommend 24 hours of bed rest under observation.
• Avoid driving a car until the doctor has ruled out any complications.
• Acetaminophen or ibuprofen may be recommended to relieve pain. However, avoid aspirin, because it may provoke internal bleeding.

WHEN TO CALL A DOCTOR

• See a doctor immediately if you or someone you know has sustained a concussion. The doctor will run tests to determine whether more severe head injuries have occurred in addition to the concussion.
• Call a doctor if the initial symptoms do not diminish within a few days after the first examination.
• **EMERGENCY** After the preliminary examination, call the doctor back immediately if any of the following symptoms occur: the patient cannot awaken or is incoherent upon awakening; convulsions; severe headaches; repeated vomiting; visual disturbances; persistent drowsiness; shortness of breath; speech difficulty; or a staggering gait. ▲

SYMPTOMS

• Brief loss of consciousness.
• Headache, dizziness, and blurred vision.
• Occasional nausea and vomiting.
• Inability to remember events immediately prior to the injury.
• Drowsiness; mental confusion.
• Persistent insomnia, headaches, dizziness, irritability, moodiness, and depression. This combination of symptoms is known as post-concussive syndrome and may continue for several weeks.
• Slow thinking, impaired concentration, and slurred speech—known as punch-drunk syndrome—as a result of repeated concussions (an occupational hazard for boxers).

Congestive Heart Failure

WHAT IS IT?

Congestive heart failure (CHF) is a serious condition marked by the inability of the heart to pump enough blood to meet the body's oxygen demands. Heart failure can result from either a reduced ability of the heart muscle to contract or from a mechanical problem that limits the ability of the heart's chambers to fill with blood. When weakened, the heart is unable to keep up with the demands placed upon it; blood returns to the heart faster than it can be pumped out so that it gets backed up or congested—hence the name of the disorder.

The heart attempts to compensate in a number of ways. It beats faster and expands somewhat more than usual as it fills with blood, so that when it contracts, more blood is forced out to the body. In addition, the decreased volume of blood reaching the kidneys causes them to stimulate a hormonal cascade (renin–angiotensin system), which results in the retention of sodium and water. These efforts help meet the body's demands in the short term, but they ultimately have deleterious long-term effects. Faster beating allows less time for the heart to refill after contraction, so that less blood ends up being circulated. Also, the extra effort increases the heart muscle's demand for oxygen; if this need is not met adequately, heart rhythm can become dangerously erratic (see Cardiac Arrhythmias for more information) and ultimately fatal.

Failure of the left side of the heart (left-sided failure) is more common. It leads to increased pressure in the pulmonary veins in the lungs, which forces fluid into the surrounding microscopic air sacs, or alveoli, that transfer oxygen to the bloodstream. As the alveoli fill with fluid, they no longer function properly, which limits the amount of oxygen available to the body (see Pulmonary Edema for more information) and produces the most characteristic symptoms of congestive heart failure: fatigue and shortness of breath. In right-sided failure, the increased pressure in the veins returning blood from the rest of the body combined with the compensatory retention of sodium and water leads to fluid accumulation and swelling in the abdomen, liver, and legs. Often, both left- and right-sided heart failure occur together.

Congestive heart failure should not be confused with a heart attack, which involves sudden tissue death of the heart muscle. Although heart failure may occur suddenly in some cases, gradual loss of function is more common. Fatigue, shortness of breath on exertion, and increased frequency of nighttime urination develop and worsen over time. Shortness of breath is often worse when lying down—a condition known as orthopnea—as fluid from the legs pools in the lungs. Elevating the head with pillows eases chest congestion, but in advanced stages the patient may be unable to recline at all without severe breathlessness, and may need to sleep upright in a chair.

CHF occurs most frequently in those over age 60 and is the leading cause of hospitalization and death in that age group. In over 50 percent of cases, sudden death occurs due to a cardiac arrhythmia, or

---

SYMPTOMS

- Severe fatigue and weakness.
- Irregular or rapid heartbeat.
- Shortness of breath and wheezing after limited physical exertion. In advanced cases shortness of breath occurs even at rest, and attacks of severe breathlessness disturb sleep (left-sided failure).
- Dry cough or cough that produces frothy or bloody sputum (left-sided failure).
- Frequent urination during the night (right-sided failure).
- Swelling of the ankles and feet, or swelling in the lower back if the patient is bedridden (right-sided failure).
- Rapid weight gain due to fluid retention (right-sided failure).
- Abdominal pain and a feeling of fullness (right-sided failure).
- Swollen neck veins (right-sided failure).
- Loss of appetite (anorexia); nausea and/or vomiting.
- General feeling of poor health.
- Anxiety; in severe cases irritability, restlessness, and mental confusion may occur.

Congestive Heart Failure *continued*

irregular heartbeat. Unfortunately, antiarrhythmic medications may not be effective in controlling arrhythmias caused by CHF.

There is no cure for heart failure, although measures are taken to treat the underlying cause, if possible. Restricted salt intake, and medication are used to ease the strain on the heart and to relieve symptoms. CHF is a serious health risk; for many patients the outlook is uncertain and depends on the extent of the disease and the patient's response to therapy. However, with proper treatment it is possible for many patients to live with CHF and to manage many symptoms effectively. It is important that patients adhere to prescribed treatment regimens; noncompliance with a doctor's recommendations regarding diet or medication increase the risk that the disease will worsen.

WHAT CAUSES IT?

• Coronary artery disease (obstruction of the coronary arteries by atherosclerotic plaque so that heart tissue is starved of oxygen) often leads to a heart attack, which damages the heart muscle and causes CHF (see Coronary Artery Disease and Myocardial Infarction for more information).
• Heart muscle injury due to viral infections (see Myocarditis) or long-term drug or alcohol use (see Cardiomyopathy) may result in CHF.
• Conditions that overwork the heart may lead to CHF. Such conditions include: heart valve defects, high blood pressure, increased levels of thyroid hormones (thyrotoxicosis), and anemia.
• Infiltration of the heart muscle by other tissue, as occurs with amyloidosis (accumulation of a waxy substance), may cause CHF.
• Triggers for CHF to develop in a weakened heart include pulmonary embolism, severe bacterial or viral infections, pregnancy or childbirth, and physical overexertion.
• Right-sided heart failure commonly results from left-sided heart failure.
• CHF may result from restricted entry of blood into the heart due to thickening of the tissue surrounding the heart (pericardium), or to accumulation of excessive fibrous tissue in the heart muscle.

PREVENTION

• Don't smoke.
• Consume no more than two alcoholic beverages a day.
• Eat a healthy, balanced diet low in salt and fat, exercise regularly, and lose weight if you are overweight.
• Adhere to a prescribed treatment program for other forms of heart disease.

DIAGNOSIS

• Patient history and physical examination.
• Chest x-rays.
• Blood and urine tests.
• An electrocardiogram (ECG) may be performed to measure the electrical activity of the heart. ECG abnormalities can indicate rhythm disturbances, heart muscle damage, inadequate blood flow to segments of the heart, and enlargement of the heart muscle. You may be given a portable ECG device, known as a Holter monitor, to measure the heart's electrical activity over a 24-hour period.
• Exercise stress testing, in which blood pressure, heart rate, ECG, and oxygen consumption rates are measured while you walk on a treadmill.
• An echocardiogram, which uses sound waves to produce images of the heart, may be performed.
• A coronary angiography may be performed to evaluate narrowings of the coronary arteries. In this procedure a tiny catheter is inserted into an artery in a leg or arm and threaded up to the coronary arteries. A contrast material is then injected, which provides a clear image of the blood vessels on x-ray.

HOW TO TREAT IT

• Your doctor will advise you to reduce your salt intake (salt contributes to fluid retention and swelling) and to eat smaller, more frequent meals (less effort is required to digest smaller portions).
• Caffeine, which may exacerbate heartbeat irregularities, should be avoided.
• Vasodilators, such as hydralazine or ACE inhibitors (for example, captopril and enalapril), may be prescribed to dilate blood vessels, thus reducing blood pressure and easing blood flow.
• Various types of diuretics, such as hydrochloro-

Congestive Heart Failure *continued*

thiazide, metolazone, furosemide, or bumetanide, will be prescribed to help eliminate excess fluid from body tissues.

• Digitalis glycosides may be prescribed to strengthen contractions of the heart muscle (in the United States digoxin is the most commonly prescribed type of digitalis).

• Other medications, including anticoagulants such as warfarin, beta-blockers such as carvedilol, calcium channel blockers such as amlodipine, and tranquilizers such as diazepam, may be prescribed to improve blood flow, ease breathing, and relieve anxiety.

• Special elastic support stockings that reduce swelling in the legs may be prescribed.

• In severe cases it may be necessary to administer oxygen through a nasal tube. Mechanical devices for administration of oxygen are available for home use after the condition has stabilized in the hospital.

• Surgery may be required to repair or replace heart valves or bypass blocked coronary arteries.

• Percutaneous transluminal angioplasty (insertion and then inflation of a small balloon in an obstructed coronary artery via a catheter) may be performed to widen the artery and improve blood flow.

• A heart transplant may be advised if the heart muscle has been badly damaged. The survival rate for this surgery is 80 percent after one year and over 60 percent after four years.

WHEN TO CALL A DOCTOR

• **EMERGENCY** Call an ambulance immediately if you experience severe breathlessness.

• **EMERGENCY** Call an ambulance if you experience crushing chest pain, with or without nausea, vomiting, profuse sweating, breathlessness, weakness, or intense feelings of dread. Such symptoms may indicate a heart attack.

• Make an appointment with a doctor if you regularly experience fatigue and shortness of breath after mild physical activity.

• Call a doctor if you experience any of the following during treatment for congestive heart failure: fever, rapid or irregular heartbeat, wheezing, severe shortness of breath, or any worsening of the other symptoms of congestive heart failure. ▲

Conjunctivitis

WHAT IS IT?

Conjunctivitis is an inflammation of the mucous membranes (conjunctiva) that line the inner surface of the eyelids and the whites of the eyes. It may be triggered either by an infection or an allergic reaction. Known as pinkeye because the blood vessels in the whites of the eyes dilate and redden, conjunctivitis is highly contagious when caused by an infection. It is usually not serious, although it should be treated promptly to prevent possible complications and transmission to others. With proper treatment, conjunctivitis generally disappears within two or three weeks.

WHAT CAUSES IT?

• Bacterial or viral infections are the most common causes of conjunctivitis.
• Allergies (to such things as pollen, cosmetics, and contact lens cleaning solution) are a possible cause.
• Air pollution or chemical irritants may lead to conjunctivitis.
• Cervical infections (chlamydia, genital herpes, or gonorrhea) in a pregnant woman may result in potentially blinding conjunctivitis in the baby.
• A partially blocked tear duct is a possible cause.

PREVENTION

• Try never to touch the eyes when, for example, handling contact lenses.
• Wash your hands often with soap and warm water.
• Change towels and pillowcases often.
• Do not share towels.
• Do not share eye makeup; replace cosmetics every four to six months.
• Avoid substances that trigger eye irritation.

SYMPTOMS

• Redness of the white of the eye.
• Itching and a gritty sensation in the eye.
• Oozing discharge from the eyes.
• Excessive tearing.
• Dried crusts that form during sleep, which may bind the eyelids together.
• Swollen eyelids.
• Aversion to bright lights (photophobia).

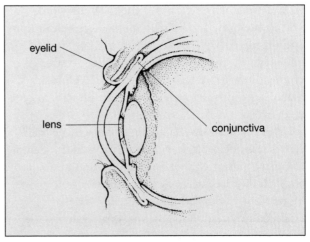

Inflammation of the conjunctiva produces characteristic redness and irritation in the eyes but seldom affects vision.

DIAGNOSIS

• The diagnosis can generally be made by the typical findings on physical examination.
• Swab samples may be taken and cultured to identify the type of bacterial infection involved.

HOW TO TREAT IT

• First, consult a doctor or ophthalmologist to confirm the diagnosis. It is important to determine whether infectious conjunctivitis is bacterial or viral in origin. Bacterial conjunctivitis is the more serious of the two and requires treatment; viral conjunctivitis typically resolves on its own, without complication.
• Your doctor may prescribe antibiotic or steroid eyedrops or ointments. Use as directed and be careful not to allow the tip of the eyedrop bottle to touch the eyes.
• For infectious conjunctivitis, soak a clean cloth in warm water, wring it dry, and apply it to the eye.
• For allergic conjunctivitis, apply cool compresses to the eye. Antihistamines may be recommended.

WHEN TO CALL A DOCTOR

• Call a doctor if conjunctivitis symptoms do not improve after three or four days of treatment, especially if fever, increased pain, or changes in vision develop. In the case of bacterial conjunctivitis, prompt treatment will avert complications. ▲

Constipation

WHAT IS IT?

Constipation is characterized by infrequent bowel movements with stools that are often hard and sometimes painful to pass. In constipation, intestinal contractions slow down, allowing more time for the bowels to remove water from food wastes. This results in hard stools that are difficult to pass. However, it should be noted that normal frequency of bowel movements varies greatly from person to person. It is perfectly normal for some people to have three bowel movements a day, while others have as few as three a week; true constipation involves the passage of hard stools less than three times in a week and is usually accompanied by bloating and discomfort. (Any change in a person's usual frequency of bowel movements, however, may be a sign of a more serious underlying disorder.)

WHAT CAUSES IT?

- Lack of fiber in the diet or inadequate fluid intake.
- Prolonged inactivity or severe depression.
- Irregular or abnormal contractions of the bowel muscles owing to lack of exercise or to disorders such as irritable bowel syndrome, diabetes mellitus, hypercalcemia, hypothyroidism, or colorectal cancer.
- Failure to go to the bathroom when the urge strikes may lead to the formation of hard, impacted stools.
- Overuse of laxatives, aspirin, or aluminum- or calcium-based antacids may impair normal bowel function.
- Constipation may occur as a side effect of certain medications, including antihypertensive drugs (calcium channel blockers and beta-blockers), tricyclic antidepressants, narcotics, and atropine.

SYMPTOMS

- Infrequent, difficult, and possibly painful bowel movements.
- Straining during bowel movements.
- Continued sensation of fullness after bowel movements.
- Hard, dry stool.
- Abdominal swelling.

PREVENTION

- Eat high-fiber, low-fat foods. Try to get at least five servings a day of fiber-rich foods, including raw fruits and vegetables, whole-grain breads and cereals, bran, dried peas and beans, and potato skins.
- Drink at least eight glasses of water a day.
- Exercise regularly.
- Go to the bathroom as soon as the urge strikes.

DIAGNOSIS

- Evaluation will include medical history (with emphasis on bowel habits) and a physical exam.
- Blood and stool samples may be obtained.
- A sigmoidoscopy (use of a flexible, lighted scope to view the lower large intestine) may be performed.
- A barium enema may be necessary. The barium creates a sharp image of the colon on x-ray.

HOW TO TREAT IT

- Follow the prevention tips above.
- Drink a cup of hot liquid (such as coffee or tea), especially first thing in the morning, since it may activate what is known as the gastrocolic reflex, which induces a bowel movement by stimulating the colon.
- Use laxatives only as a last resort, on your doctor's advice. Bulk-forming agents, including bran, psyllium (Metamucil, Konsyl), and methyl cellulose (Citrucel, Cologel), are usually the best choice. Never use mineral oil as a laxative.
- Do not use enemas unless otherwise instructed by your doctor.

WHEN TO CALL A DOCTOR

- Make an appointment with a doctor if constipation persists for two weeks or more, and increased fiber intake and exercise have failed to help.
- Consult a doctor if fever or severe abdominal pain occurs with constipation, if abdominal bloating, cramping, or other discomfort disrupts your routine, or if you notice blood in the stool.
- Call a doctor if you experience constipation shortly after beginning a new medication. The prescription may need to be adjusted.
- Call your doctor if you notice any major change in normal bowel habits.

Corneal Ulcers

WHAT IS IT?

A corneal ulcer is an open sore on the eye's cornea, the tough, transparent membrane that covers and protects the pupil and iris (colored portion). Corneal ulcers are typically very painful, especially when caused by a bacterial infection, and feel as if something is intractably lodged in the eye even if no foreign object is visible upon close inspection. A simple abrasion on the surface of the cornea produces the same sort of pain, but this usually subsides within 48 hours. If pain persists longer, chances are great that some type of infection has set in, causing an ulceration, which requires immediate treatment. If neglected, corneal ulcers may scar the cornea, resulting in permanent vision impairment. In rare cases the infection may penetrate the cornea to involve other structures of the eye, requiring emergency surgery.

WHAT CAUSES IT?

• Corneal ulcers most often originate as a corneal abrasion (due to a scratch from an insect or a tiny fleck of steel, glass, dirt, or dust) that then becomes infected with bacteria, viruses, fungus, or protozoans like amoebae. Viral corneal ulcers are most often due to infection with the herpes simplex virus.
• Contact lens wearers and chronically ill or debilitated patients are more prone to corneal ulcers.
• Eye surgery or preexisting corneal disease may increase the likelihood of corneal ulceration.
• Chemical irritation may be a cause.
• Hyperthyroidism (Graves' disease) often causes the eyelids to retract, preventing the eyes from being bathed in tears, thus promoting corneal ulcers.

PREVENTION

• If you wear contact lenses, remove and clean them daily (or as recommended by the manufacturer or your ophthalmologist). Do not clean them with saliva or tap water.
• Avoid smoke and other airborne irritants.
• Wear protective goggles when warranted (at a workbench, for example); wear sunglasses outdoors on windy days.
• Wash hands frequently and keep your fingers away from your eyes if you have cold sores.

DIAGNOSIS

• Physical examination by an ophthalmologist is usually all that is required to diagnose a corneal ulcer. A special dye (fluorescein) that provides a clear view of the corneal surface when blue light is shined upon it may be used to aid in diagnosis.
• A swab culture of the ulcer or, if necessary, a biopsy (tissue sample) will be obtained to identify the infectious organism.

HOW TO TREAT IT

• Corneal ulcers caused by bacterial infections are treated with antibiotic eyedrops or ointments, and sometimes oral antibiotics. In severe cases antibiotics may be injected near the eye for faster absorption.
• Viral ulcers may be treated with antiviral drops or pills. Further ulcers may occur, however, in cases where the infection is persistent, such as those caused by the herpes simplex virus.
• Fungal or amoebic corneal ulcers are treated with an appropriate drug.
• Topical corticosteroid drops may be prescribed in some cases to reduce inflammation.
• Severe cases that result in corneal scarring may warrant corneal transplant.
• Any underlying eye disorder is also treated.

WHEN TO CALL A DOCTOR

• See an ophthalmologist right away for any eye pain that persists for more than several hours. If you are wearing contact lenses, remove them at once.

SYMPTOMS

• Severe eye pain; feeling that something is lodged in the eye.
• Redness in or discharge from the eyes.
• Heightened sensitivity to light; aversion to bright light.
• Excessive tearing.
• Blurred vision.
• Eyelid spasms.
• Visible white, gray, or yellow ulceration on the cornea.

Corns and Calluses

WHAT IS IT?

A callus is a patch of rough, thickened skin that forms on the feet, hands, or other sites where constant pressure or irritation provokes the skin cells in the affected area to grow at an accelerated rate. The callus itself is generally painless (and in fact, forms to protect the skin below), although the underlying skin may be tender. A corn is a small, round callus on the surface that extends into the skin like a cone, with the point within the foot, hence the pain when pressed. They are found on or between the toes. Corns and calluses are common, minor problems that usually respond promptly to treatment. However, corns and calluses put people with diabetes mellitus at greater risk of foot infection and other complications.

WHAT CAUSES IT?

• Constant pressure from ill-fitting shoes is the most common cause of corns and calluses on the feet.
• Activities such as tennis, carpentry, dancing, writing, or playing the violin or guitar may cause calluses by putting repeated pressure and friction on the hands, fingers, or other parts of the body.

PREVENTION

• Wear comfortable shoes that fit well.
• Wear work gloves when performing manual labor.

DIAGNOSIS

• Diagnosis is based on visual examination of the affected area and does not require a doctor.

HOW TO TREAT IT

• Some calluses, such as those formed by dancing or playing the guitar, protect the skin from abrasion and need not be treated.

> ### SYMPTOMS
> • For calluses: a thickened, hard, rough, sometimes yellowish patch of skin.
> • For corns: a small bump of thickened skin on the side or top of a toe joint or between the toes. Pressure on the corn causes pain.

• Corns and calluses on the feet often disappear on their own if ill-fitting shoes are replaced with good, comfortable footwear.
• Doughnut-shaped felt pads or moleskin (available in drugstores) may ease pressure from shoes around the corn or callus.
• Soak the affected area in warm water daily for at least five minutes, then use a pumice stone or callus file to rub away the upper layers of the thickened skin. (However, abrading a callus in this manner is not recommended for those with diabetes or poor circulation.)
• The doctor may use surgery or chemical peels to remove a corn or callus that is resistant to treatment.

WHEN TO CALL A DOCTOR

• Because sensation and circulation may be diminished, people with diabetes mellitus should see a doctor if corns or calluses develop on the feet. They should be instructed by a doctor or nurse on how to conduct daily self-examinations of the feet.
• Make an appointment with a doctor or podiatrist if the corn or callus persists despite treatment and it is interfering with your normal daily activities.
• See a doctor or a podiatrist as soon as possible if the area around the corn or callus becomes red, painful, swollen, hot, or ulcerated; these are signs of inflammation, possibly due to infection.

Coronary Artery Disease

WHAT IS IT?

Coronary artery disease (CAD), the leading cause of death in the United States, is a narrowing of the coronary arteries, the vessels that supply blood to the heart muscle. Physical activity increases the oxygen needs of the body, and the heart responds to the greater demand by pumping blood more vigorously, which in turn increases the oxygen needs of the heart muscle.

In CAD, narrowed coronary arteries limit the supply of blood to the heart muscle. If narrowing is not extensive, difficulties may occur only during physical exertion, when the narrowed arteries are unable to meet the increased oxygen requirements of the heart. However, as the disease worsens, the narrowed arteries may starve the heart muscle of oxygen during periods of normal activity, or even at rest.

Coronary artery disease is generally due to the buildup of plaques in the arterial walls, a process known as atherosclerosis. Plaques are composed of cholesterol-rich fatty deposits, collagen, other proteins, and excess smooth muscle cells. Atherosclerosis, which usually progresses very gradually over a

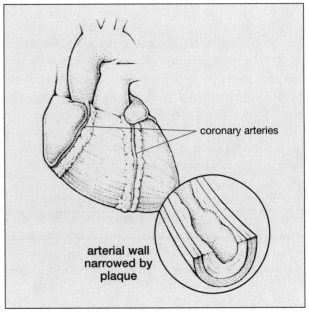

coronary arteries

arterial wall narrowed by plaque

The coronary arteries supply the heart muscle with freshly oxygenated blood. A buildup of atherosclerotic plaque in these arteries may deprive the heart of a sufficient amount of oxygen (causing chest pain) and, if the artery becomes totally blocked, result in a heart attack.

lifetime, thickens and narrows the arterial walls, impeding the flow of blood. Blood clots form more easily on arterial walls roughened by plaque deposits. The clots may block the narrowed coronary artery completely and cause a heart attack (see Myocardial Infarction for more information). Arteries may also narrow suddenly as a result of an arterial spasm. (Spasms are most commonly triggered by smoking.)

Symptoms of coronary artery disease usually develop insidiously. In the early stages of the disease, there are generally no symptoms. As the disease progresses, chest pain (angina pectoris) may develop during periods of physical activity or emotional stress, because the narrowed arteries cannot supply the heart with the increased amount of blood and oxygen necessary at those times. Angina usually subsides quickly with rest, but over time, symptoms arise with less exertion, and CAD may eventually lead to a heart attack. However, in a third of CAD cases, angina never develops, and a heart attack can occur suddenly with no prior warning.

Although CAD can be a life-threatening condition, the outcome of the disease is in many ways up

SYMPTOMS

- No symptoms in the early stages of coronary artery disease.
- Chest pain (angina), or milder pressure, tightness, squeezing, burning, aching, or heaviness in the chest, lasting from 30 seconds to five minutes. The pain or discomfort is usually located in the center of the chest just under the breastbone, and may radiate down the arm (usually the left), up into the neck, or along the jaw line. The pain is generally brought on by exertion or stress and stops with rest. The amount of exertion required to produce angina is reproducible and predictable.
- Shortness of breath, dizziness, or a choking sensation, accompanying chest pain.
- A sudden increase in the severity of angina, or angina at rest, is a sign of unstable angina that requires immediate medical attention because a heart attack may shortly occur.

Coronary Artery Disease *continued*

to the patient. Damage to the arteries can be slowed or halted with lifestyle changes, including smoking cessation, dietary modifications, and regular exercise, or by medications to lower blood pressure and cholesterol levels. Additional goals of treatment, which may involve medication and sometimes surgery, are to relieve symptoms, ease circulation, and prolong life.

WHAT CAUSES IT?

• Smoking promotes the development of plaque in the arteries. Also, by increasing the amount of carbon monoxide in the bloodstream and decreasing the amount of oxygen available to the heart, smoking increases the likelihood of angina.

• High blood cholesterol levels lead to coronary artery disease. LDL (low-density lipoprotein) enters the lining of the arterial walls where, after being chemically altered, its cholesterol can be incorporated into plaque (see Hypercholesterolemia for more information).

• High blood pressure predisposes one to CAD.

• People with diabetes mellitus are at greater risk for atherosclerosis.

• Obesity may promote atherosclerosis.

• Lack of exercise (a sedentary lifestyle) may encourage atherosclerosis.

• Men are at greater risk than women for coronary artery disease, although the risk for postmenopausal women approaches that of men as estrogen production decreases with menopause. Ongoing studies will determine whether this risk may be partly offset by estrogen replacement therapy.

• Women over age 35 who take oral contraceptives and smoke cigarettes have a higher risk of atherosclerosis.

• A family history of premature heart attacks is associated with greater CAD risk.

• A spasm of the muscular layer of the arterial walls may cause an artery to contract and produce angina. Spasms may be induced by smoking, extreme emotional stress, or exposure to cold air.

PREVENTION

• Don't smoke.

• Eat a diet low in saturated fat, cholesterol, and salt.

• Pursue a program of moderate, aerobic exercise for at least 30 minutes, three days a week. People over age 50 who have led a sedentary lifestyle should check with a doctor before beginning an exercise program.

• Lose weight if you are overweight.

• See your doctor regularly to have your blood pressure and cholesterol measured.

• Your doctor may advise you to take a low dose of aspirin every day if you are at high risk for CAD. Aspirin reduces the tendency for the blood to clot, thereby decreasing the risk of heart attack. However, such a regimen should only be initiated under a doctor's recommendation.

• Women at or approaching menopause may want to discuss the possible cardioprotective benefits of postmenopausal estrogen replacement therapy with their doctors.

DIAGNOSIS

• Patient history and physical examination. If you suffer a heart attack, diagnosis will often be made immediately upon examination by a doctor or emergency medical technician.

• An electrocardiogram (ECG) may be performed to measure changes in the electrical activity of the heart resulting from abnormalities in the flow of blood or a prior heart attack. In some cases your doctor may provide you with a portable ECG device, known as a Holter monitor, in order to record the electrical activity of the heart over a 24-hour period.

• Chest x-rays.

• Blood tests.

• Stress testing. Blood pressure, heartbeat, and breathing rates are measured by ECG while you walk on a treadmill. If you cannot exercise adequately, a medication may be injected instead.

• An injection of a radioisotope such as thallium may be given after an exercise test to gauge blood flow to the heart.

• An echocardiogram, which uses ultrasound waves to create moving images of the heart, may be performed.

• A coronary angiography is performed to determine the presence of narrowings of the coronary arteries. In this procedure a tiny catheter is inserted into an artery of a leg or arm and threaded up into the

Coronary Artery Disease *continued*

coronary arteries. A contrast material is then injected from the end of the catheter into the coronary arteries, and x-rays are taken.

HOW TO TREAT IT

• Emergency treatment and immediate hospitalization is necessary if a heart attack occurs—commonly signaled by crushing, persistent chest pain (see Myocardial Infarction for more information).

• Follow prevention tips for a heart-healthy lifestyle, including a low-fat diet and regular physical exercise. Avoid excessive alcohol consumption, nasal decongestants, and diet pills, all of which may raise blood pressure.

• Rapidly acting nitrates, such as nitroglycerin, or longer-acting nitrates like isosorbide dinitrate may be prescribed to dilate blood vessels and relieve or prevent symptoms of angina. A nitroglycerin tablet placed under the tongue (sublingually) at the onset of an angina attack usually relieves the pain within minutes. Sublingual nitroglycerin may also be taken just prior to activities that commonly provoke angina. However, for any given angina attack, you should not take more than three nitroglycerin tablets at five-minute intervals—pain lasting longer than this may signal a heart attack. Intravenous nitrates may be administered in patients with unstable angina. Nitrates may also be prescribed in the form of patches or ointments for continuous protection.

• Beta-blockers such as propranolol or metoprolol are prescribed to reduce the heart's oxygen demand by slowing the heart rate and lowering blood pressure.

• ACE inhibitors such as enalapril may be prescribed to reduce blood pressure and dilate blood vessels.

• Calcium channel blockers such as verapamil, diltiazem, or nifedipine may be prescribed to reduce the heart's oxygen demands and to increase coronary blood flow.

• Anticoagulants such as heparin or warfarin will be administered to reduce the risk of blood clots in patients with unstable angina.

• Vasodilators such as captopril, enalapril, or hydralazine may be prescribed to expand blood vessels, thus reducing blood pressure and facilitating blood flow.

• An obstructed coronary artery may be opened with percutaneous transluminal coronary angioplasty (PTCA). In this procedure a small balloon is inserted into the circulatory system via a catheter and guided to the site of an arterial blockage. The balloon is then inflated, compressing the plaque, widening the passageway, and improving blood flow. PTCA usually requires a hospital stay of only a few days.

• Coronary bypass surgery may be performed to improve blood flow to the heart. A mammary artery or a vein taken from the leg is grafted onto the damaged coronary artery to circumvent a narrowed or blocked portion.

• A heart transplant may be advised in severe cases in which the heart muscle has been badly damaged. The survival rate for heart transplant is 80 percent after one year and 63 percent after four years.

WHEN TO CALL A DOCTOR

• **EMERGENCY** Call an ambulance if you experience crushing chest pain, with or without nausea, vomiting, profuse sweating, shortness of breath, weakness, or intense feelings of dread.

• **EMERGENCY** Call an ambulance if chest pain from previously diagnosed angina does not subside after 10 to 15 minutes.

• **EMERGENCY** Call an ambulance the first time you experience intense chest pain.

• See your doctor if attacks of previously diagnosed angina become more frequent or more severe or occur at rest.

Costochondritis

WHAT IS IT?

Costochondritis is an inflammation of the cartilage of the rib cage. It usually involves the upper ribs near the top of the breastbone. It is most common in women and in those over age 40. Tietze's syndrome (after the German physician who identified it) is a similar condition that generally affects young adults and occurs in both sexes with equal frequency. The symptoms of chest pain and tenderness, which can come on gradually or suddenly, vary from mild to intense. The pain is often aggravated by body movement and may radiate to the shoulder or arm. Even though costochondritis is not a serious disorder, it may cause great anxiety, since the intense chest pain can be mistaken for that of a heart attack. The condition may last for a week, or up to several years. While some patients experience recurrent episodes, spontaneous and permanent remission is the norm.

WHAT CAUSES IT?

• The cause of costochondritis is unknown in the majority of cases.

• Costochondritis may result from an injury or blow to the chest or even from an episode of especially vigorous coughing.

• Costochondritis may be one feature of polyarthritis (widespread inflammation of cartilage).

PREVENTION

• Wear protective gear when playing sports.

DIAGNOSIS

• Physical examination and patient history are needed.

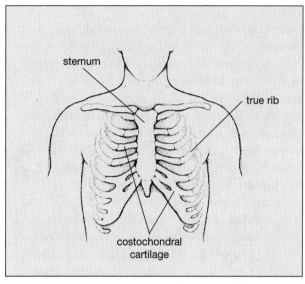

The rib cage is not comprised entirely of bone; a significant portion of it is cartilage that connects the true ribs to the sternum (breastbone).

• A chest x-ray, an electrocardiogram (a test to monitor the heart's electrical activity), and blood tests may be performed to rule out more serious underlying disorders, including heart and lung diseases.

HOW TO TREAT IT

• Rest and avoid exercises or movements that aggravate the inflammation and cause pain; symptoms generally disappear on their own over time.

• Take aspirin, acetaminophen, or nonsteroidal anti-inflammatory drugs (NSAIDs) such as ibuprofen to relieve pain.

• Applying heat (for example, with a heating pad) may provide relief.

• Corticosteroid injections may be used to reduce pain and swelling in more severe cases.

WHEN TO CALL A DOCTOR

• The pain of costochondritis is not serious. However, any intense chest pain warrants immediate emergency medical evaluation, since it may be a sign of a more serious problem, such as a heart attack. ⚠

SYMPTOMS

• Chest pain, usually in the front of the rib cage. The pain is exacerbated by movements that change the position of the ribs or by the direct application of pressure on the affected region.

• Swelling of the tissues around the breastbone may occur.

• Anxiety and hyperventilation during acute episodes of pain occur rarely.

Crohn's Disease

WHAT IS IT?

Crohn's disease, also known as regional ileitis, is a chronic inflammation of the intestinal wall, most commonly in the final portion of the small intestine or the colon. Less often, the upper digestive tract may also be affected. The inflammation involves deep layers of the intestinal wall, where ulcers and abscesses may form. The ulcers may erode the wall completely, creating abnormal passages (fistulas) to other parts of the intestine, to other organs such as the bladder, or to the skin. Deep cracks (fissures) may also develop in and around the anus (see Anal Fissures). Inflammation may thicken the intestinal wall until the passageway becomes blocked. Symptoms of Crohn's disease appear during flare-ups, which alternate with periods of remission. Some people suffer only one or two attacks before entering into permanent remission; others experience recurrent attacks over a lifetime. Crohn's disease is relatively rare, but the incidence among the general population has been increasing in recent decades.

WHAT CAUSES IT?

• The cause of Crohn's disease is unknown.
• Hereditary factors seem to play some role in the development of this disorder.
• Various theories suggest these possible causes: viral or bacterial infections, autoimmune disorders, food allergies, or lymphatic obstruction.

SYMPTOMS

• Spasms of abdominal pain or cramps, often located near the navel or in the lower right abdomen.
• Persistent watery diarrhea.
• Rectal bleeding or blood in the stool.
• Anal fissures.
• Nausea.
• Fever.
• Fatigue.
• Loss of appetite and weight.
• Systemic complications such as joint pain from arthritis, inflammation of the eyes, and skin lesions.

PREVENTION

• At present there is no known way to prevent Crohn's disease.

DIAGNOSIS

• Patient history and physical exam are necessary.
• Blood tests may be taken.
• Upper gastrointestinal (GI) series of x-rays are taken to view the small intestine.
• A barium enema may be performed. The barium creates a sharp image of the colon on x-ray.
• Sigmoidoscopy (to inspect the lower large intestine) or colonoscopy (to view the entire large intestine) may be performed.
• A biopsy of the colon lining is generally taken during the sigmoidoscopy or colonoscopy to distinguish Crohn's disease from ulcerative colitis.

HOW TO TREAT IT

• For mild attacks, over-the-counter antidiarrheal medications and pain relievers may be taken.
• Anti-inflammatory medications, such as sulfasalazine or corticosteroids, may be recommended.
• Antibiotics may be prescribed to suppress secondary infections.
• Enemas containing corticosteroids or aspirin-like drugs may be used to treat internal inflammation.
• Immunosuppressive drugs may be prescribed on a long-term basis to quell autoimmune activity.
• Dietary changes, vitamin or mineral supplements, or vitamin B_{12} injections, to replace nutrients lost from poor bowel absorption, may be advised.
• In some cases of extremely severe attacks, periods of intravenous feeding may be necessary to allow the bowel to rest.
• Surgery may be required to repair blockages, fistulas, or abscesses in the rectum or intestine.
• In advanced, long-standing cases of Crohn's disease, the damaged portion of the bowel may be removed.

WHEN TO CALL A DOCTOR

• Call a doctor if you experience symptoms of Crohn's disease (especially lower-right abdominal pain, which may signal appendicitis).
• Call a doctor if you experience black or bloody stools, a swollen abdomen, or a fever over 101°F.

Croup

WHAT IS IT?

Croup is a condition marked by obstruction of breathing due to inflammation and narrowing of the air passages. It develops from a respiratory infection, such as a cold or the flu, peaks in severity between three and five days, and resolves by the sixth day. Symptoms include noisy breathing, stridor (a high-pitched whistling sound when inhaling), and a tight, barking cough (like a seal). These may fluctuate from mild to severe, but are usually worse at night. Croup generally affects children up to the age of five. It is more common in boys than girls and is more likely to occur in the winter. Older children and adults are not at risk for croup because their airways are wider and thus resistant to collapse.

WHAT CAUSES IT?

• Viral infections—including flu, measles, and colds—are the most common cause of croup.
• Bacterial infections sometimes lead to croup.

PREVENTION

• Wash hands frequently with warm water and soap to prevent spreading the infection to other children.

DIAGNOSIS

• Physical examination and patient history are needed.

SYMPTOMS

• Loud, barking cough.
• Breathing difficulty, which manifests itself as wheezing or a high-pitched whistling sound when inhaling (stridor).
• Nasal flaring; retractions (ribs appearing more prominent during breaths).
• Hoarseness; chest discomfort.
• Emergency symptoms indicate life-threatening obstruction of the airways and include the following: great difficulty in swallowing; drooling; inability to bend the neck forward; a bluish tinge to the lips; increased breathing difficulty; worsened coughing; extremely rapid heartbeat; high-pitched wheezing noises upon inhaling; loss of consciousness.

• A neck x-ray or laryngoscopy (using a lighted scope to view the inside of the throat) may be performed to locate specific sites of airway obstruction.

HOW TO TREAT IT

• Have the child inhale moist air from a bowl of steaming water, cool-mist humidifier, or hot shower, to help relieve congestion during an attack. Having the child breathe cool night air may also help open the airways.
• Sitting up straight makes breathing easier. Infants may be placed in a child seat.
• Acetaminophen may be administered to reduce fever. (Do not give aspirin to children.)
• Be calm and reassure the child; anxiety and crying aggravate symptoms.
• The use of corticosteroids (injected or taken orally) may improve stridor.
• Antibiotics may be prescribed if there is thought to be an additional bacterial infection; they should be taken for the full term prescribed.
• Hospitalization may be necessary for severe attacks. The child may be placed in a humidified oxygen tent and given the drug epinephrine, which helps to decrease the swelling of the airway.
• In very serious cases, the doctor may insert a breathing tube down the child's throat through the mouth or through a small incision in the neck (tracheostomy). The tube can usually be removed within 24 hours.

WHEN TO CALL A DOCTOR

• **EMERGENCY** Call an ambulance immediately if your child experiences serious breathing difficulty or develops other emergency symptoms of severe lung obstruction.
• Call a doctor if your child develops noisy, rapid breathing.
• Be alert for signs of ear infections and pneumonia, potential complications of croup that may arise a few days after an attack subsides. ▲

Cushing's Syndrome

WHAT IS IT?

Cushing's syndrome—an uncommon disorder named for the twentieth-century American surgeon who identified it—is caused by elevated blood levels of cortisol (an essential corticosteroid hormone). Cortisol is produced by the cortex of the adrenal glands, grape-size organs located above each kidney that form part of the body's endocrine system. Cortisol secretion is stimulated by the release of adrenocorticotropic hormone, or ACTH, from the pituitary gland. Cushing's syndrome is due to overproduction of cortisol by the adrenals or administration of excessive amounts of cortisone in the treatment of a number of diseases. The disorder is known as Cushing's disease when symptoms are due to increased production of ACTH by a tumor in the pituitary gland. Common complications are hypertension, diabetes mellitus, osteoporosis, and muscle weakness. Both Cushing's syndrome and Cushing's disease respond well to treatment.

WHAT CAUSES IT?

• Large or long-term doses of oral corticosteroid medications—prescribed to treat disorders such as

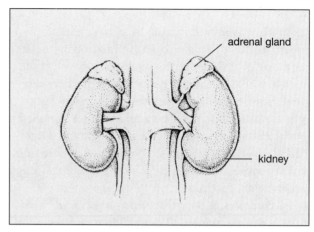

The adrenal glands, located on the top of each kidney, secrete several hormones, including the steroid cortisol, made in the adrenal cortex.

rheumatoid arthritis, inflammatory bowel disease, or asthma—are now the most common cause of Cushing's syndrome.

• An adrenal tumor or overgrowth (hyperplasia) of adrenal cortex cells may cause Cushing's syndrome.

• A pituitary tumor that secretes excess ACTH overstimulates cortisol production by the adrenal glands and causes Cushing's disease.

• Occasionally, tumors elsewhere in the body, such as in the lungs, may produce excess ACTH (ectopic ACTH-producing tumor).

PREVENTION

• If you are taking corticosteroids on a long-term basis, ask your doctor about taking the lowest possible doses of these medications.

DIAGNOSIS

• Blood and urine tests to measure levels of adrenal hormones.

• CT (computed tomography) scans or MRI (magnetic resonance imaging) of the abdomen or skull (to image the pituitary gland).

HOW TO TREAT IT

• If Cushing's syndrome is caused by long-term treatment with corticosteroid medications, your doctor may gradually reduce the dosage and switch you to another form of treatment, if possible. Never stop taking corticosteroids on your own, because serious

---

SYMPTOMS

• A round or "moon-shaped" face.
• Fat accumulation on the torso and between the shoulder blades.
• Thin legs and arms.
• Fatigue and muscle weakness.
• Skin changes, including easy bruising; acne; purple stretch marks on the abdomen, thighs, and breasts; thin skin; a reddish appearance of the face.
• Insomnia.
• Changes in mental state, such as mood swings, depression, paranoia, or euphoria.
• In men: growth of breasts (gynecomastia); impotence.
• In women: growth of hair (hirsutism); the cessation of menstruation (amenorrhea).
• Back or hip pain from bone fractures due to osteoporosis.

Cushing's Syndrome   *continued*

side effects may occur; slow withdrawal should be planned and supervised by a doctor.

• A pituitary or adrenal tumor can be surgically removed.

• Radiation therapy, either alone or in conjunction with surgery, may be used to treat tumors.

• Medications that inhibit the secretion of cortisol, such as ketoconazole, aminoglutethimide, metyrapone, or mitotane, may be prescribed when surgery is impossible or unsuccessful, or when the tumor is malignant.

• Hormone replacement therapy (temporary or life-long) may be necessary to supplement or replace adrenal and thyroid hormone following surgery or radiation treatment to the pituitary.

WHEN TO CALL A DOCTOR

• Call a doctor if you develop excess fat on your face and torso, accompanied by any of the other symptoms of Cushing's syndrome. ▲

Depression

WHAT IS IT?

Depression is a mood disorder characterized by a persistent sad or empty feeling, irritability, and a loss of interest in everyday activities. The condition is twice as common in women as in men and is usually episodic. But unlike normal sadness or grieving, most bouts of depression last for weeks, months, or even years. Some people with depression have a chronic, low-grade form of the condition called dysthymia. A smaller number suffer from bipolar disorder—bouts of depression interspersed with periods of elevated (manic) mood (see Bipolar Disorder).

Although depression is usually not considered life-threatening, it can lead to thoughts of and attempts at suicide. As many as 70 percent of suicides in the United States are related to depression, and about 15 percent of severely depressed people commit suicide. Fortunately, the overwhelming majority of people with depression can be helped by counseling (psychotherapy), antidepressant drugs, or other therapies, thus lowering the suicide risk.

WHAT CAUSES IT?

• Although the cause of most cases of depression is unknown, it is thought to be associated with a combination of medical, genetic, and environmental factors.

• Imbalances of chemicals that transmit nerve signals (neurotransmitters) in the brain may play a role.

• The condition appears to run in families, although no specific genes have been identified.

• Initial episodes may be connected to a major life event, such as the death of a loved one or loss of a job. Recurrent episodes, however, appear unrelated to such events.

• In about 15 percent of cases, depression develops in response to a medical illness (especially heart disease, cancer, or a neurologic disorder such as Parkinson's disease or stroke) or from long-term use of some medications, including beta-blockers for high blood pressure and corticosteroids for arthritis. Other causes of this "secondary depression" include alcoholism, an underactive thyroid gland (see Hypothyroidism for more information), vitamin deficiencies, and schizophrenia (see Schizophrenia).

PREVENTION

• Although the initial onset of depression cannot be prevented, recurrent episodes may be controlled or avoided altogether with ongoing psychotherapy and/or drug therapy. The longer a person stays in treatment, the less likely he or she is to experience a relapse.

DIAGNOSIS

• Because there are no reliable laboratory tests to diagnose depression, physical examination and psychological evaluation are essential.

• Expression of either of the first two symptoms of depression (see Symptoms box), in conjunction with other symptoms, for a period of two or more consecutive weeks.

• A positive family history of depression or a prior depressive episode helps establish the diagnosis.

HOW TO TREAT IT

• Psychotherapy is as effective as drug treatment in mild cases. Psychotherapy may also be used in conjunction with drug therapy.

• Antidepressant medications, such as selective serotonin reuptake inhibitors (SSRIs), tricyclics, and monoamine oxidase (MAO) inhibitors, are mainstays of treatment.

SYMPTOMS

• Persistent feelings of sadness, apathy, or hopelessness lasting more than two weeks.

• Diminished interest in most daily activities, particularly pleasurable ones.

• Decreased appetite and subsequent weight loss; increased appetite and weight gain.

• Lack of sleep (insomnia), frequent awakening throughout the night, or conversely, an increased need for sleep.

• Anxiety; diminished ability to think or concentrate.

• Older people may initially focus on physical or cognitive complaints brought on by their depression. Insomnia and agitation are also more common in older patients.

Depression *continued*

• Electroconvulsive therapy (using an electric current to cause a brief convulsion) is sometimes used in severe cases.

• Exposure to bright light, known as light therapy, may be effective, particularly when depression is related to seasonal changes (seasonal affective disorder).

• In secondary depression, the underlying cause is addressed, although antidepressant therapy may also be prescribed.

WHEN TO CALL A DOCTOR

• Anyone with symptoms of depression should see a doctor for an evaluation and possible referral to a mental health professional.

• **EMERGENCY** Anyone who has persistent thoughts of suicide should get immediate psychological or medical treatment. 🔺

Dermatomyositis

WHAT IS IT?

Dermatomyositis is a rare connective tissue disease characterized by inflammation of the muscles and skin. As dermatomyositis progresses, muscle tissue is wasted and gradually replaced by useless scar tissue. Muscle weakness is the primary symptom. Typically affected are the large skeletal muscles (those in the arms, shoulders, pelvis, and thighs), but the heart and the involuntary muscles that control swallowing and breathing may also be involved. Some people develop polymyositis alone, which results in these muscle problems exclusively; in others, the skin (dermis) is involved too, hence the name dermatomyositis. Onset of symptoms may be sudden or gradual. Dermatomyositis is potentially life-threatening when vital organs are affected, but the survival rate has improved in recent years (currently about 75 percent of patients survive beyond six or seven years of diagnosis), and the majority of patients improve with treatment. Two-thirds of those afflicted with dermatomyositis are women.

WHAT CAUSES IT?

• The cause of dermatomyositis is unknown.
• Dermatomyositis or polymyositis can occur alone (idiopathic) or may be associated with another rheumatic disease, such as systemic lupus erythematosus or Sjögren's syndrome.

PREVENTION

• Dermatomyositis cannot be prevented.

DIAGNOSIS

• Physical examination and patient history are needed.
• Blood tests are taken to look for enzymatic evidence of muscle inflammation.
• Electromyography (which measures electrical activity in the muscles) may be performed.
• A biopsy may be performed to remove a sample of affected muscle tissue for examination under a microscope.

HOW TO TREAT IT

• Corticosteroid drugs such as prednisone are usually prescribed (often in high doses) to reduce inflammation.
• Immunosuppressant drugs may be used if corticosteroids are not effective in relieving inflammation.
• Physical therapy may be advised to minimize shrinkage of the muscles.

WHEN TO CALL A DOCTOR

• Call a doctor if you develop symptoms of dermatomyositis.

SYMPTOMS

• Weakness, stiffness, and pain in the muscles, especially the muscles of the shoulder and hip. It may even be difficult to perform such simple actions as brushing hair.
• Red, sometimes itchy rash on the face, neck, upper torso, and upper arms and legs. A rash may form on the knees, knuckles, elbows, or other joints or bony prominences.
• Purple discoloration and swelling of the eyelids, especially apparent upon awakening.
• Skin that feels thicker than normal (over affected areas).
• Hands and feet unusually sensitive to cold (Raynaud's phenomenon).
• Difficulty speaking or swallowing.
• Weight loss.

Diabetes Insipidus

WHAT IS IT?

Diabetes insipidus, not to be confused with the more common diabetes mellitus, is a relatively rare disorder resulting from a failure to produce sufficient amounts of vasopressin, also known as antidiuretic hormone (ADH). Vasopressin, secreted by the posterior pituitary gland, helps the kidneys to reabsorb water and maintain proper fluid balance. If the pituitary fails to produce enough ADH, water is not conserved but simply passed through the kidneys and excreted, typically in very large quantities. More rarely, the kidneys fail to respond properly to ADH; this is known as nephrogenic diabetes insipidus. Dehydration is the primary health risk associated with either form. Diabetes insipidus affects both sexes equally. With proper treatment, overall prognosis is good (except in cases caused by cancer).

WHAT CAUSES IT?

• In approximately half of all cases, the cause of diabetes insipidus is unknown.
• Hereditary factors may play a role in some cases.
• Damage to the pituitary gland from a head injury, a pituitary tumor, radiation therapy, or surgery may lead to diabetes insipidus.

PREVENTION

• There is no known way to prevent diabetes insipidus.

DIAGNOSIS

• Physical examination and patient history are needed. Diagnosis of diabetes insipidus is suspected when a patient reports unusually large and frequent urine output.
• A urinalysis is done to discover dilute urine (low specific gravity).
• A water deprivation test may be conducted. The patient consumes no fluids for eight hours while urine output and specific gravity are monitored. Patients with diabetes insipidus continue to produce large amounts of urine despite dehydration. An injection of vasopressin reduces urine volume and produces a concentrated urine in those with pituitary diabetes insipidus (but not nephrogenic diabetes insipidus).
• Blood tests may be taken to assess water and salt balance.

HOW TO TREAT IT

• Vasopressin (synthetic ADH) may be administered (either in a nasal spray or by injection) to replace or supplement the body's ADH production. Such hormone therapy is usually necessary for a lifetime, although if diabetes insipidus is caused by a head injury or surgery, it may be possible to discontinue treatment after a year or so.
• To treat nephrogenic diabetes insipidus, your doctor may advise a low-salt diet to reduce thirst and slow the excretion of water. Certain diuretics may also be prescribed. (Nephrogenic diabetes insipidus does not respond to ADH treatment.)
• Drink plenty of fluids to prevent dehydration.
• Consume plenty of high-fiber foods and fruit juices to prevent or treat constipation.

WHEN TO CALL A DOCTOR

• See a doctor immediately if you develop symptoms of diabetes insipidus.
• **EMERGENCY** Call an ambulance if you observe someone lose consciousness. ⚠

SYMPTOMS

• Frequent and excessive urination. Output may be as high as 25 to 35 quarts within 24 hours and may be as frequent as every 30 minutes, even at night.
• Extreme thirst.
• Dry skin.
• Constipation.
• Emergency symptoms of dehydration, including dizziness, weakness, and unconsciousness.

Diabetes Mellitus

WHAT IS IT?

Diabetes mellitus is a metabolic disorder with abnormally high blood glucose levels (hyperglycemia) as its most prominent feature. During intestinal digestion, carbohydrates and proteins are broken down into simple sugars and amino acids, respectively. The liver converts all of the sugars and some of the amino acids into glucose, a simple sugar that is used for energy by every cell in the body. Glucose passes from the bloodstream into the cells with the help of insulin, a hormone produced by the pancreas (a pear-shaped organ located just below the stomach). By attaching to receptor sites on the surface membrane of a cell, insulin promotes the movement of glucose-transport proteins from the interior of the cell to its surface, where they bind with glucose and carry it into the cell. In diabetes mellitus, several problems may interfere with this process: pancreatic insulin production may be partially or completely impaired, or body cells may become unable to use normal amounts of insulin efficiently.

These underlying problems in fact distinguish the two main types of the diabetes. In type 1, or insulin-dependent diabetes mellitus (IDDM), also known as juvenile diabetes, the pancreas produces little or no insulin. Type 1 diabetes develops suddenly and most commonly affects those under age 30; the average age of onset is between 12 and 14. However, IDDM accounts for only 7 to 10 percent of cases of diabetes mellitus. In the much more common type 2, or non-insulin-dependent diabetes mellitus (NIDDM), also known as adult-onset diabetes, insulin production by the pancreas is normal or only slightly reduced, but cells are unable to respond efficiently to insulin—a condition referred to as insulin resistance. The onset of type 2 diabetes is usually gradual and tends to affect people over age 40, particularly those who are overweight. Infrequently, an adult may develop type 1 diabetes.

In both type 1 and type 2 diabetes, the hyperglycemia leads to excretion of glucose in the urine and an accompanying increase in urine production. If inadequate amounts of insulin are administered to patients with type 1 diabetes, unrestrained release of fatty acids from adipose (fat) tissue leads to the overproduction of ketone bodies in the liver. Accumulation of ketone bodies can cause a life-threatening condition known as diabetic ketoacidosis (DKA). DKA may occasionally affect those with type 2 diabetes in periods when the body is highly stressed, for example, during a severe infection.

People with type 2 diabetes are susceptible to another life-threatening condition known as a hyperosmolar nonketotic state, characterized by extremely high blood sugar levels. This condition usually occurs in elderly persons with some other serious underlying illness. An episode of either DKA or the hyperosmolar state may be the first indication that someone has diabetes.

People with diabetes may also suffer from low blood sugar (hypoglycemia) if too much insulin or oral hypoglycemic agent is given for treatment (see Hypoglycemia for more information).

After 10 to 20 years of diabetes, patients are likely to develop complications, such as vision disorders, kidney damage, and peripheral nerve degeneration (neuropathy). Strict control of blood glucose can delay or prevent these complications. Loss of sensation in the feet may allow injuries to go unchecked

---

SYMPTOMS

- Excessive and frequent urination (as often as every hour or so). Nighttime awakening to urinate is common.
- Increased thirst.
- Increased appetite.
- Unintentional weight loss.
- Blurred vision.
- Fatigue and weakness.
- Recurring or persistent infections of the bladder, skin, or gums.
- Numbness and tingling in feet and hands.
- Symptoms of hypoglycemia (see Hypoglycemia for more information).
- Emergency symptoms of hyperosmolar nonketotic states: extreme thirst, lethargy, weakness, mental confusion, coma.
- Emergency symptoms of diabetic ketoacidosis: nausea and vomiting, labored breathing, mental confusion, coma.

Diabetes Mellitus *continued*

and become infected. In addition, people with diabetes are at increased risk for developing narrowing of the coronary arteries (see Coronary Artery Disease for more information) as well as narrowing of arteries supplying the brain and legs. The combination of foot infections and decreased blood supply can lead to gangrene (tissue death), which may require amputation. Diabetes mellitus (and its complications) is the fourth leading cause of death in the United States.

Treatment of type 1 diabetes requires between one and four daily injections of insulin. (Insulin cannot be taken orally, since digestive juices would destroy it.) In addition, diet and exercise must be carefully planned to ensure that blood glucose levels are neither too high nor too low. Type 2 diabetes may be controlled with a combination of diet, exercise, and weight loss, although medications (including insulin) are often necessary. Treatment is largely a process of self-management. Although there is no cure, almost all people with diabetes are able to control their symptoms and lead full, productive lives.

WHAT CAUSES IT?
• Type 1 diabetes is an autoimmune disorder, resulting from a mistaken attack by the immune system on insulin-producing cells in the pancreas.
• Genetic factors are important in type 2 diabetes.
• Obesity predisposes individuals to the development of type 2 diabetes.
• Certain drugs, such as corticosteroids or thiazide diuretics, may increase the risk of type 2 diabetes.
• Other disorders, such as hemochromatosis, chronic pancreatitis, Cushing's syndrome, or acromegaly, may lead to diabetes. Surgical removal of the pancreas may also lead to diabetes.
• Pregnant women may develop diabetes mellitus (gestational diabetes), which may disappear after childbirth; there is an increased risk that these women will subsequently develop type 2 diabetes.
• Contrary to popular belief, eating lots of foods rich in sugar does not promote diabetes.

PREVENTION
• To prevent the development of type 2 diabetes, lose weight if you are more than 20 percent over-

weight, and maintain weight within healthy limits.
• Exercise regularly.
• There is no known way to prevent type 1 diabetes.
• People with diabetes should get regular eye examinations to aid in early detection and treatment of diabetes-related vision disorders (diabetic retinopathy).

DIAGNOSIS
• Patient history and physical examination are needed.
• Diagnosis is made when fasting blood tests show high glucose levels (126 mg/dL or greater).
• When test results are ambiguous, a glucose tolerance test may be done. A drink containing 75 grams of glucose is swallowed and blood glucose levels are measured every 30 minutes over a two-hour period.
• Urine samples may be analyzed for protein content.
• Blood glycohemoglobin is calculated as the average of blood glucose level readings over the preceding two months.

HOW TO TREAT IT
For type 1 diabetes:
• Daily injections of insulin are necessary. One to four daily injections are required to control blood glucose levels. Long-acting and rapid-acting insulin preparations are available; a combination of the two kinds is often prescribed.
• A strict diet and schedule of meals are necessary to control blood glucose levels. Your doctor may recommend a diet low in fat, salt, and cholesterol, and may advise you to see a nutritionist for dietary planning.
• Because both exercise and insulin lower glucose levels, exercise and insulin injections must be timed so that they do not combine to cause a dangerous drop in blood sugar (hypoglycemia).
• Strict adherence to the timetable of injections, meals, and exercise is necessary for proper management of the disease.
For type 2 diabetes:
• A diet low in fat and other calories, in addition to regular exercise, is necessary to control weight.
• Oral hypoglycemic drugs, such as tolbutamide, chlorpropamide, glyburide, glipizide, or repaglinide may be prescribed to increase insulin production by the pancreas, if exercise and diet do not lower glucose levels sufficiently.

Diabetes Mellitus *continued*

• Other oral agents can reduce insulin resistance (metformin and troglitazone) or slow the absorption of sugars from the intestine (acarbose).

• Insulin injections may be necessary in more severe cases of type 2 diabetes, or if a patient with type 2 diabetes contracts an additional illness.

For both types of diabetes:

• Blood tests to measure glucose levels should be performed as your doctor recommends, one to four times a day. Your doctor will recommend a blood monitoring device to use at home.

• Careful attention must be paid to the risk factors for atherosclerosis because of its increased occurrence with diabetes. Those suffering from diabetes should not smoke, should reduce dietary saturated fat, cholesterol, and salt, and should take any medications prescribed for high blood pressure or high cholesterol levels.

• People with diabetes should drink generous amounts of water when stricken with another illness such as the flu. This replaces lost fluid and prevents diabetic coma. When ill, people with type 1 diabetes should test their urine for ketones every four to six hours.

• People with diabetes should practice good foot care and check their feet every day. Nerve damage from diabetes mellitus reduces sensation in the feet, and small foot problems may turn into major infections.

• Laser photocoagulation to prevent the rupture of tiny blood vessels in the eye may be used to prevent or treat vision problems due to diabetes mellitus (diabetic retinopathy). Most patients with diabetes need an eye examination by an ophthalmologist at least once a year to detect the earliest manifestations of retinopathy.

• Dialysis, an artificial blood-filtering process, may be necessary to treat kidney failure. In advanced cases a kidney transplant may be advised (see Renal Failure, Chronic, for more information).

• Amitriptyline or desipramine, medications usually used to treat depression, may be prescribed to relieve the pain in the limbs (see Peripheral Neuropathy for more information).

• Excellent control of blood glucose levels delays or prevents late complications affecting the eyes, kidneys, and nerves.

• Kidney damage can be slowed by controlling blood pressure and using ACE inhibitors.

• The American Diabetes Association can provide information about support groups in your area.

WHEN TO CALL A DOCTOR

• Call a doctor if you notice a sudden or gradual increase in hunger, thirst, and urine output.

• Call a doctor if you have been diagnosed with diabetes mellitus and an additional illness such as a cold or the flu causes blood sugar levels to go out of control. Do not take over-the-counter medications without first consulting your doctor.

• **EMERGENCY** Call an ambulance if a person with diabetes loses consciousness. Inform the doctor or the rescue worker that the person has diabetes.

• **EMERGENCY** (in type 2 diabetes) Call an ambulance immediately if you develop symptoms of a hyperosmolar nonketotic state; these include extreme thirst, lethargy, weakness, and mental confusion.

• **EMERGENCY** (in type 1 diabetes) Call an ambulance immediately if you develop symptoms of diabetic ketoacidosis; these include dry mouth, dry and flushed skin, sweet or fruity-smelling breath, labored breathing, vomiting, and abdominal pain, with or without excessive urination and extreme thirst.

• **EMERGENCY** (in type 1 diabetes) Call your doctor right away if urine tests detect the presence of ketones and the steps given by your doctor fail to control the problem. 🛆

Diarrhea, Acute

WHAT IS IT?

Acute diarrhea, the passage of frequent, loose, or watery stools, is not a disease itself but rather a symptom of an underlying disorder. As food passes through the digestive system, water is normally reabsorbed through the wall of the large intestine. Diarrhea—and, at times, dehydration—results when fluid is not reabsorbed but remains in and is expelled with the fecal matter. Although diarrhea usually subsides without treatment within two or three days, any resulting dehydration is serious (particularly among infants and the elderly) and needs quick treatment.

WHAT CAUSES IT?

- Food poisoning from various causes, including viruses or bacteria.
- Non-food-related viral infections.
- A reaction to certain foods (such as citrus fruits or beans) in some people.
- Large amounts of artificial sweeteners, such as sorbitol, xylitol, and mannitol, which are found in diet foods, chewing gum, and other products.
- Alcoholic beverages.
- Some drugs including antihypertensives, drugs to combat heart disease, over-the-counter antacids containing magnesium, and certain antibiotics.
- Infectious diseases such as traveler's diarrhea, typhoid fever, amoebic dysentery, and bacillary dysentery (shigellosis).
- Emotional stress and anxiety.

PREVENTION

- Do not eat food that you suspect has spoiled.
- Avoid foods to which you are sensitive.
- When traveling abroad, drink only bottled or boiled water or other bottled beverages. Eat cooked foods and fruit you can peel yourself. Local water or raw foods may contain bacteria that can cause diarrhea.
- Learn ways of coping with emotional stress, and try to avoid stressful situations.

DIAGNOSIS

- Diarrhea may be self-diagnosed by the observation of characteristic symptoms.
- Laboratory stool analysis may be warranted in cases of persistent diarrhea.

HOW TO TREAT IT

- Prevent dehydration (especially important for the elderly and young children) by drinking a solution of one teaspoon of salt and four teaspoons of sugar in one quart of water. Measure accurately: Too much salt may worsen dehydration. Drink one pint of solution each hour while diarrhea lasts.
- Do not take over-the-counter antidiarrheal medications for the first few hours (the diarrhea may be ridding your body of infectious agents or irritants). If work or other obligations necessitate the use of an antidiarrheal medication, use one containing loperamide (such as Imodium A-D) or bismuth subsalicylate (such as Pepto-Bismol).
- Limit (or avoid) milk products, alcohol, and foods rich in fiber during recovery.
- For infants: While diarrhea persists, do not feed them milk. Instead, feed them an electrolyte solution available from a pharmacist. If diarrhea clears up within two days, reintroduce milk gradually over a 24-hour period. Feed the infant a solution of one part milk and three parts water at first, gradually increasing the amount of milk over the next three feedings. Use a solution of half-milk/half-water for the second feeding; three-quarters milk for the third feeding; undiluted milk for the fourth.

WHEN TO CALL A DOCTOR

- Call a doctor if diarrhea persists for more than 48 hours or is accompanied by lightheadedness, severe cramping, fever over 101°F, or blood in the stool.
- Call a doctor if diarrhea recurs frequently.
- **EMERGENCY** Call a doctor promptly if an infant or an elderly person shows symptoms of dehydration.

SYMPTOMS

- Loose, watery stools.
- Increased frequency of bowel movements.
- Abdominal cramping and pain.
- Emergency symptoms of dehydration in infants: drowsiness; unresponsiveness; slackness of the skin; glazed eyes; a dry, sticky mouth and tongue; persistent crying.

Dislocations and Subluxations

WHAT IS IT?

A dislocation is a complete loss of contact between the bone surfaces in a joint that normally meet; a subluxation is a partial loss of contact. Within a normal joint, ligaments hold the bones together so that their surfaces are in close contact, and the entire joint is encased in a membrane (joint capsule). When the bones become dislocated or subluxated (usually because of a violent physical trauma), damage to the ligaments and joint capsule occurs, resulting in severe pain and loss of mobility. Commonly affected joints include those of the shoulders, fingers, knees, hips, ankles, and feet.

Dislocations and subluxations usually respond well to treatment, and normal joint movement is usually restored within two months of the injury. However, in some cases the ligaments may remain slightly stretched after healing and recurrent subluxation or dislocation may occur. In more severe cases a dislocation may involve nerve damage and result in some degree of paralysis.

SYMPTOMS

- Deformity of the affected joint. The joint may be bent at an awkward angle or look misshapen.
- Difficulty moving the affected joint.
- Pain (often severe) or tenderness in the joint.
- Swelling and stiffness within 30 minutes of a physical trauma.

WHAT CAUSES IT?

- Injury is the most common cause of dislocations.
- Certain joints, such as the hip, are congenitally prone to dislocations in some people.
- Previous injuries of a joint may so weaken surrounding tissues that subsequent subluxation or dislocation may occur with little provocation.

PREVENTION

- Because most are due to injury, dislocations and subluxations cannot be prevented.

DIAGNOSIS

- Physical examination and patient history.
- X-rays rule out or confirm the condition.

HOW TO TREAT IT

- Get immediate professional medical care; prompt treatment can prevent additional tissue, nerve, and blood vessel damage. Do not try to reposition the joint yourself. On the contrary, the joint should be immobilized with a splint or sling if possible.
- Apply ice to the affected area to reduce swelling while awaiting professional care.
- Do not eat or drink (a full stomach interferes with the anesthesia that may be necessary during the repositioning of the joint).
- A doctor or other medical personnel will reposition the joint. Local or general anesthesia may be used to reduce pain during the procedure.
- Surgery may be required to reposition the joint in more severe dislocations. Wire may be used to keep the bones in place.
- A splint, cast, or traction may be required to immobilize the joint after repositioning, to allow damaged ligaments to heal.
- A program of physical therapy may be prescribed to build strength and mobility after the affected joint has healed.

WHEN TO CALL A DOCTOR

- Call a doctor immediately if you think you have dislocated a joint, because it becomes increasingly difficult to reposition the joint properly as the surrounding tissues swell.
- **EMERGENCY** Call an ambulance or get to a doctor immediately if you experience paralysis, lack of a pulse, or extreme pain near a dislocated joint. This may indicate that the blood supply to the area has been blocked by the injury. ▲

Disseminated Intravascular Coagulation

WHAT IS IT?

Disseminated intravascular coagulation (DIC), also known as defibrinogenation syndrome, is a rare disorder marked by excessive blood coagulation, which paradoxically results in simultaneous uncontrolled bleeding. Normally, clotting factors cause blood platelets to coagulate into a solid plug at the site of an injury, preventing blood loss from an open vein or artery. In DIC, however, clotting occurs in small blood vessels throughout the body, even where no injury is apparent. This decreases the available quantity of clotting factors and platelets, thereby increasing the risk of severe bleeding. Furthermore, the body steps up its anticoagulation system to dissolve the numerous clots, which only compounds the likelihood of uncontrolled bleeding. In addition, blockage of blood vessels by clots may damage the kidneys and extremities, and sometimes even the brain, lungs, pituitary and adrenal glands, and the gastrointestinal lining. DIC occurs as a complication of a variety of severe disorders and injuries. Effective treatment requires proper diagnosis and treatment of the underlying disorder.

WHAT CAUSES IT?

• Blood infection (bacterial sepsis) may cause widespread coagulation and subsequent bleeding.
• Leukemia or other systemic cancers may cause disruption of the clotting mechanisms in the blood.
• Extensive, serious burns destroy body tissues and may disturb the normal balance of clotting factors.

SYMPTOMS

• Abnormal bleeding from anywhere in the body, possibly at several sites at once.
• Tiny, red, pinpointlike dots (petechiae).
• Vomiting of blood.
• Bloody or black stools.
• Blood in the urine.
• Vaginal bleeding.
• Unexplained bruises.
• Severe abdominal or back pain.
• Seizures or loss of consciousness in advanced cases (rare).

• Heatstroke or shock (for example, due to massive blood loss) may lead to DIC.
• Other serious disorders, such as cirrhosis of the liver or cardiac arrest, may cause DIC.
• Complications during pregnancy and childbirth may disrupt the blood's clotting mechanisms.
• Some kinds of surgery, such as cardiopulmonary bypass surgery, may induce DIC.
• A poisonous snakebite may cause excessive coagulation and bleeding.
• Transfusion of an incompatible blood type may lead to DIC.

PREVENTION

• Disorders that could result in DIC require prompt treatment.

DIAGNOSIS

• Blood tests are performed.
• A thorough physical examination and other tests and procedures are required to identify an underlying cause of DIC.

HOW TO TREAT IT

• Hospitalization is necessary to properly treat and monitor DIC.
• Treatment of the underlying disorder is of prime importance.
• A transfusion of whole blood, plasma, platelets, or packed red blood cells may be necessary after the underlying cause is treated.
• Anticoagulants may be used to prevent excessive clotting.

WHEN TO CALL A DOCTOR

• **EMERGENCY** Call an ambulance if you develop symptoms of DIC.

Diverticular Disorders

WHAT IS IT?

Diverticulosis is a condition marked by the formation of diverticula—small pouchlike herniations along the wall of the gastrointestinal tract. Most commonly, diverticula appear in the left side of the colon; rarely, they also develop as far up as the throat (pharynx). As many as half of all Americans over the age of 50 have diverticulosis, although few ever have any noticeable symptoms. Diverticulosis only requires treatment if it causes discomfort (painful diverticular disease) or complications.

In some cases the diverticula become inflamed or infected—a painful condition known as diverticulitis. In severe cases, an inflamed diverticulum may perforate or burst, resulting in abscesses or peritonitis (inflammation of the lining of the abdominal cavity, which may be fatal unless treated immediately). Diverticula may also cause rectal bleeding. Diverticular disorders are not related to colon cancer.

WHAT CAUSES IT?

• Diverticulosis is usually caused by chronically increased pressure and strain on the colon wall.
• A low-fiber diet (common in industrialized Western countries) is correlated with diverticular disease. The disorder is almost unheard of in rural Asian and African societies, where a high-fiber diet is the norm.

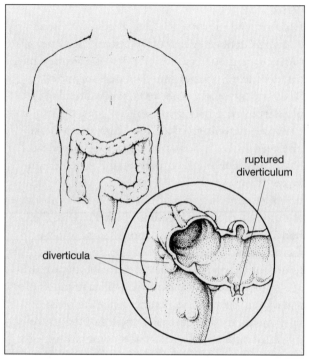

In diverticulosis, small pouches (diverticula) form in weakened spots on the colon wall. If they become inflamed (diverticulitis), they may rupture or bleed.

• Hereditary factors may play a small role in the development of diverticulosis.
• Increased pressure on the colon resulting from straining during bowel movements or from chronic constipation or laxatives may lead to the formation of diverticula.

PREVENTION

• Eat a high-fiber, low-fat diet. Foods high in fiber include fruits, vegetables, and whole-grain breads and cereals.
• Drink plenty of fluids (at least eight full glasses of water a day) to help soften stools.
• Exercise regularly to help maintain regularity.

DIAGNOSIS

• A barium enema may be performed. The barium creates a sharp image on x-ray of the digestive tract.
• Colonoscopy (use of a thin, lighted scope to view the colon) may be performed.
• A CT (computed tomography) scan may be performed to help diagnose acute diverticulitis.

SYMPTOMS

• Diverticulosis usually causes no symptoms. However, some patients do develop mild complaints, including bloating, gas, nausea, constipation alternating with diarrhea, and tenderness or pain, most often in the lower left abdomen.
• Symptoms are pronounced when a diverticulum becomes inflamed or perforated (diverticulitis). Severe abdominal cramping, usually on the lower left side, is most prominent. Pain may be immediately severe or start off gradually and increase in severity over several days. Other symptoms may include tenderness over the abdomen, fever, nausea, blood in the stool, and impaired bowel function.

Diverticular Disorders *continued*

HOW TO TREAT IT

• Following prevention tips for diet (especially incorporating fiber) and exercise is important.

• Your doctor may recommend a bulking laxative containing the fiber psyllium or an artificial fiber like calcium polycarbophil. However, do not take laxatives without consulting your doctor and never use enemas—these may only further aggravate a diverticular disorder.

• For diverticulitis, your doctor may prescribe antibiotics and bed rest, often in the hospital.

• Injections of painkillers may be warranted in severe cases of diverticulitis.

• Antispasmodic drugs may be prescribed to relax the muscles around the digestive tract.

• You may need to have your stomach kept empty (with a tube passed through the mouth into the stomach) and to be fed intravenously to allow inflamed diverticula to heal. You should be able to eat and drink normally when symptoms have subsided (generally in a few days).

• Surgery may be necessary to drain an abscess.

• In severe or recurrent cases, surgery may be necessary to remove the affected part of the colon. In a few cases, a temporary colostomy may be required, with later operations to reconnect the colon.

WHEN TO CALL A DOCTOR

• Call a doctor immediately if you experience severe abdominal pain, with or without fever or abdominal bloating.

• Call a doctor if you notice a change in your bowel habits that lasts longer than two weeks, especially if you also experience rectal bleeding.

• Call a doctor if minor symptoms of diverticulosis (nausea, bloating, constipation, and others) develop and persist. ▣

Dry Mouth Xerostomia

WHAT IS IT?

Dry mouth, also known as xerostomia, is abnormal dryness of the mucous membranes in the mouth, due to a reduction of the flow or change in the composition of saliva. It can occur as a symptom of many possible underlying disorders or as a side effect of certain medications. Dry mouth is not a serious medical problem in itself, but it may contribute to poor nutrition, psychological discomfort, mouth infections, and tooth decay if left untreated. Medical care is aimed at relieving symptoms and treating the underlying disorder.

WHAT CAUSES IT?

• Dry mouth may occur as a side effect of many medications, including antihypertensive drugs, anti-depressants, painkillers, tranquilizers, diuretics, and antihistamines.
• Radiation therapy for tumors in or near the mouth can cause severe dry mouth.
• A bone marrow transplant may produce dry mouth.
• Sjögren's syndrome, an autoimmune disorder in which the body's own natural defenses against disease inappropriately begin to attack healthy tissue (see Sjögren's Syndrome for more information), may lead to dry mouth as well as dry eyes.
• Injury to the head or neck may damage nerve endings and thus interfere with the function of the salivary glands.
• Dry mouth may be associated with neurological changes that occur with brain-centered disorders like a stroke or Alzheimer's disease (see Stroke and Alzheimer's Disease for more information).
• Nutritional deficiencies may be a cause.
• Fear, stress, anxiety, and depression may lead to dry mouth.
• Some people report the sensation of chronic dry mouth, even though their salivary glands are normal.

PREVENTION

• Eat a healthy, balanced diet.
• Drink plenty of fluids.
• Be aware of the side effects of medications.

DIAGNOSIS

• Chronic dry mouth can be self-diagnosed by observation of symptoms. However, your doctor or dentist should be notified.

HOW TO TREAT IT

• Sip water frequently, especially when speaking or eating. Avoid beverages that contain caffeine or sugar, which may aggravate dryness.
• Chew sugarless gum or suck on sugarless hard candies to stimulate saliva production, or try sucking on a peach pit or a small piece of lemon.
• Avoid tobacco, alcohol, and foods that are salty, spicy, or highly acidic.
• At night, use a humidifier, and keep a glass of water by your bed in case you awaken with dry mouth.
• Use lip balm to prevent the lips from cracking.
• The use of prescription topical fluoride may be necessary to reduce the risk of tooth decay.
• An artificial saliva solution can help moisten the mouth's mucous membranes.
• Your doctor may prescribe the medication pilo-carpine for dry mouth induced by radiation therapy or Sjögren's syndrome.

WHEN TO CALL A DOCTOR

• Make an appointment with your doctor or dentist if you develop dry mouth. ▲

SYMPTOMS

• Dry or burning sensation in the mouth.
• Difficulty in chewing, swallowing, tasting, and speaking.
• In advanced cases, cracked lips, changes in the tongue's surface, widespread tooth decay, and mouth ulcers.
• Oral fungal infection (thrush) is common and may be subtle (such as intolerance of spicy foods, occasional cracks at the corner of the mouth).

Dupuytren's Contracture

WHAT IS IT?

Dupuytren's contracture, named after the nineteenth-century French surgeon who first described it, is a painless and usually progressive disorder characterized by the hardening of a band of tissue just beneath the skin on the palm of the hand (palmar fascia). For unknown reasons, the tissue hardens and shrinks into a fibrous, scarlike mass. It initially appears as a puckering on the palm of the hand, just below the fingers. As the condition progresses, the contracted tissue pulls one or more of the fingers inward, so that it becomes increasingly difficult, if not impossible, to straighten out the affected digits.

Ordinarily, the ring and little fingers are affected, but the middle and index fingers and even the thumbs are sometimes involved. (Although Dupuytren's contracture typically affects the hands—usually both of them—the feet and toes also are sometimes affected.) In most cases, the condition is nothing to worry about; it is rarely painful, and it causes few limitations. But should it begin to interfere with normal activities, minor surgery can correct the problem.

WHAT CAUSES IT?

• The cause of Dupuytren's contracture is unknown.
• Age, gender, and hereditary factors play a role in the development of Dupuytren's contracture. Older men—particularly those of northern European descent—are most likely to be affected. In fact, one in five Caucasian men over the age of 65 has some signs of the condition.
• Diabetes, lung disease, epilepsy, and alcoholism have been associated with Dupuytren's contracture.
• People whose occupations require the use of hand-held tools (especially tools that vibrate, such as jack-hammers, electric drills, and chainsaws) may have an increased risk of developing the condition.

PREVENTION

• There is no known way to prevent Dupuytren's contracture.

DIAGNOSIS

• Physical examination and patient history are usually all that is required to make a diagnosis.
• A useful test for the disease is to try to lay the hand flat, palm side down, on a table. If this cannot be done because the fingers stay bent, the disease is likely present.

HOW TO TREAT IT

• No treatment is needed unless the contracture interferes with the use of the hand. Splints are of no benefit.
• Physical therapy and corticosteroid injections may ease symptoms.
• If the use of the hand is impaired, surgery can be performed to correct the problem. Sometimes a skin graft is necessary.
• Following surgery, physical therapy may restore mobility and strength in the affected area. However, the ability to perform precision work, such as playing a musical instrument, may not be fully regained. Some numbness may result after surgery if the contracture involved any nearby nerves.

WHEN TO CALL A DOCTOR

• Make an appointment with a doctor if the inability to straighten your fingers interferes with normal activities. ▲

SYMPTOMS

• A thickened lump of tissue in the palm of the hand at the base of a finger.
• Puckering of the skin above the lump.
• Weakness in the grasp.
• Inability to fully straighten one or more fingers, most commonly the ring and little fingers.

Dysentery, Bacillary Shigellosis

WHAT IS IT?

Bacillary dysentery, also known as shigellosis, is a potentially dangerous and extremely contagious bacterial infection of the colon. Symptoms develop after an incubation period of one to four days and generally subside within 10 days. (Severe cases may last as long as six weeks, but most cases are mild). Shigellosis is most prevalent in children between the ages of one and four. Common in overpopulated areas with poor sanitation, shigellosis often occurs in epidemics; isolation or quarantine of affected people is often practiced to curb the spread of the disease. Shigellosis is uncommon in the United States; most citizens who contract it do so while traveling abroad.

WHAT CAUSES IT?

• The shigella bacillus, a bacterium that invades the lining of the colon, is one of several infections that can cause dysentery.
• Other causes of dysentery include the parasite amoeba and the bacteria *E. coli, Yersinia,* and others.
• The shigella bacillus is typically spread via contact with the fecal matter of an infected person.
• Failure to wash the hands thoroughly after a bowel movement may help to transmit shigellosis.
• Flies may spread the bacteria from feces (more common in areas with poor sanitation.)
• Contaminated food or water may spread infection.

PREVENTION

• To prevent the spread of infection, wash your hands frequently with warm water and soap, especially after a bowel movement or before handling food. (Because dysentery has an incubation period of up to four days, you may be carrying the disease without realizing it.)
• When traveling abroad or in areas with poor sanitation, drink only bottled or boiled water or other bottled beverages, and eat only cooked foods and fruit you can peel yourself.
• Avoid contact with infected persons if possible.

DIAGNOSIS

• Dysentery is distinguished from more routine causes of infectious diarrhea by the presence of blood.
• Physical examination and patient history are needed.
• Stool samples are taken for examination under a microscope and for a laboratory culture to confirm the presence of the shigella bacillus.
• Blood tests may be taken to look for electrolyte (essential mineral salt) abnormalities or anemia.

HOW TO TREAT IT

• A solution of electrolytes (such as sodium and potassium) and fluids may be administered to treat dehydration, although water or other beverages are usually sufficient. In severe cases, fluids must be replaced intravenously.
• While waiting to see a doctor, prevent dehydration by drinking sports drinks, like Gatorade, or a solution of one teaspoon salt and four teaspoons sugar in one quart of water. It is important to measure accurately: Too much salt may worsen dehydration. Drink one pint each hour while diarrhea persists.
• Do not take over-the-counter antidiarrheal medications unless otherwise instructed by your doctor. Diarrhea helps rid the body of infectious organisms.
• Although the infection often clears on its own, antibiotics are often given to limit its transmission. These must be taken for the full term prescribed.
• Isolation from others is required to prevent spread of the disease.

WHEN TO CALL A DOCTOR

• Call a doctor as soon as you notice symptoms of dysentery. The disease is dangerous and extremely contagious, and should be treated quickly. ▲

SYMPTOMS
• Watery diarrhea initially. It may evolve to contain mucus and blood.
• Straining during bowel movements, with accompanying rectal pain.
• Abdominal pain; body aches.
• Nausea and vomiting.
• Fever.
• Rapid dehydration and weight loss. (The very young and the elderly are especially susceptible to dehydration.).

Dyspareunia Painful Intercourse

WHAT IS IT?

Dyspareunia is pain that occurs only (or primarily) during sexual intercourse. It is not a disease but rather a symptom of an underlying physical or psychological disorder. The pain, which can be mild or severe, may occur in the genitals, the pelvic region, or the lower back. The condition is much more common among women than among men. Treatment for dyspareunia is aimed at identifying and properly treating the underlying disorder.

WHAT CAUSES IT?

• For women, causes include vaginismus (a condition characterized by involuntary spasms of the vaginal muscles); insufficient vaginal lubrication; scars from an episiotomy (an incision made to facilitate childbirth); thinning and dryness of the vaginal wall due to estrogen deficiencies accompanying menopause or breastfeeding; and inadequate foreplay.
• Disorders that may cause pain upon deep vaginal penetration include pelvic inflammatory disease; ovarian cysts; endometriosis; varicose veins in the pelvis; and ectopic pregnancy.
• Other causes include infections, such as sexually transmitted diseases, which may irritate the vaginal walls or the skin of the penis; bladder or other urinary tract disorders such as cystitis or urethritis; cancer in the sex organs or the pelvic region; arthritis, especially in the lower back; and allergies to spermicides or to the latex in condoms and diaphragms.
• For men, dyspareunia can result from such disorders as irritation of the skin of the penis due to an allergic rash; physical abnormalities of the penis, such as a tight foreskin or a bowed penis with erection (chordee); and infections of the prostate gland or testes.

SYMPTOMS

• Any type of pain that occurs during intercourse—from burning sensations in the genitals caused by infection to lower back pain due to arthritis—qualifies as dyspareunia. The pain may be mild or severe, and it may last throughout sexual activity or occur only under certain circumstances.

PREVENTION

• Practice safe sex techniques to reduce the possibility of infection. Use condoms during intercourse.
• Use water-based lubricants during intercourse.
• Experiment with different coital positions to determine which ones minimize discomfort.

DIAGNOSIS

• Detailed history (including sexual) and physical examination.
• Various laboratory tests may be performed to determine the underlying cause.
• The diagnosis of vaginismus is made only after exclusion of other potential causes.

HOW TO TREAT IT

• Medications are prescribed to treat infections.
• If you suspect an allergy to latex, consult your doctor for alternative methods of birth control and disease prevention.
• If your spermicide is causing discomfort, try a different brand or consider using an alternative method of birth control.
• A water-based lubricant may help ease discomfort and friction. However, avoid oil-based lubricants, such as petroleum jelly, since they dissolve the latex in condoms and may actually promote infection.
• Insertion of a graduated set of dilators into the vagina may be used to treat vaginismus.
• Pain during intercourse due to an episiotomy generally subsides over time.
• Psychological evaluation may be advised if no underlying physical anomalies can be identified.

WHEN TO CALL A DOCTOR

• Make an appointment with a doctor if you or your partner is experiencing pain during intercourse.
• Call a doctor if pain worsens or if symptoms do not abate with treatment. ▲

Ear Infection, Middle Otitis Media

WHAT IS IT?

Otitis media is an infection of the middle ear, the cavity between the eardrum and the delicate structures of the inner ear. Typically, it occurs when viruses causing an upper respiratory tract infection (such as a cold) or bacteria migrate along the eustachian tube, the passageway between the nasal passages and the middle ear. Infection often causes the tube to become blocked, producing a vacuum-like effect and preventing the mucus, pus, and other fluids produced during an infection from draining out of the middle ear. This causes pain as these fluids exert pressure on the eardrum, possibly rupturing it. Otitis media is very common in children (because the eustachian tube is smaller), and it tends to recur, especially in winter. With prompt treatment, the chances of full recovery are excellent. Persistent forms of the disorder, chronic otitis media, produce milder symptoms. Left untreated, however, chronic otitis media may eventually cause severe structural damage in the ear and skull, resulting in irreversible hearing loss or facial nerve weakness.

WHAT CAUSES IT?

• A viral or bacterial infection of the upper respiratory tract is the most common underlying cause.
• Nasal allergies or childhood adenoids may cause blockage of the eustachian tube.
• A ruptured eardrum facilitates the entrance of infectious agents into the middle ear.

SYMPTOMS

• Sensation of fullness in the ear, eventually leading to severe pain.
• Some temporary hearing loss in affected ear.
• Fever.
• Dizziness.
• Nausea and vomiting.
• Clicking or popping sounds in the ear when moving the jaw.
• Pain when pulling on the earlobe.
• Persistent pus seepage and mild hearing loss, often without earache (the primary symptoms of chronic otitis media).

• Children with congenital problems of the facial skeleton (such as cleft lip) and those with Down syndrome are at greater risk of middle ear infection.
• Certain groups of people (such as the Navajo) have a hereditary predisposition to ear infections.
• Second-hand exposure to cigarette smoke raises the risk of middle ear infection in children.
• Recurrent bacterial ear infections may result in chronic otitis media.

PREVENTION

• Wash bed linens, towels, and heating pads regularly to prevent reinfection from pus residues. Discard cotton balls and swabs after use.
• Wash hands frequently with soap and warm water to prevent the spread of infection, particularly in school and day-care settings.

DIAGNOSIS

• The doctor will examine the ear canal with an otoscope, a small, lighted viewing instrument.
• A culture of the fluid discharge may be taken.

HOW TO TREAT IT

• Antibiotics (to be taken for the full term prescribed) may be needed to treat a bacterial infection.
• Take aspirin or acetaminophen to ease pain and fever. Children should be given acetaminophen only.
• Your doctor may recommend decongestants or antihistamines to treat symptoms.
• A small incision (myringotomy) may be made in the eardrum to allow pus to drain. This incision heals by itself in two to three weeks. A tube may be placed within the myringotomy to aerate the middle ear when fluid repeatedly accumulates.
• Enlarged adenoids may require surgical removal.
• Rarely, the mastoid process, a bone just behind the ear, becomes infected and must be surgically removed (mastoidectomy).

WHEN TO CALL A DOCTOR

• Call a doctor if you or your child develops an earache that persists despite treatment, especially if symptoms worsen or are accompanied by swelling around the ear, facial twitches, or severe ear pain that suddenly ceases (indicating eardrum rupture). ▲

Ear Infection, Outer Otitis Externa

WHAT IS IT?

Otitis externa, also known as swimmer's ear, is inflammation (often due to infection) of the skin of the outer ear, which includes not only the visible ear but also the portion of the ear canal that leads up to the eardrum. In some cases, the inflammation may be localized, producing a boil. Although it can be painful and unpleasant, otitis externa is generally not serious and responds well to treatment. However, people with diabetes, the elderly, and those with weakened immune systems are susceptible to malignant otitis externa, a rare, noncancerous (despite its name) form of this disorder. Malignant otitis externa may spread to surrounding bones and soft tissues and can be fatal if not treated.

WHAT CAUSES IT?

• Moisture in the ear fosters fungal and certain kinds of bacterial infections. Swimming, especially in contaminated water, thus increases the risk of otitis externa. Showering, washing your hair, or getting caught in the rain is less likely to raise risk.
• Skin disorders, such as eczema or seborrheic dermatitis, may cause inflammation.
• Objects inserted into the ear, like cotton swabs, may irritate the skin or cause small cuts that are vulnerable to infection.
• Inadequate production of earwax renders the ear more vulnerable to infection.

SYMPTOMS

• Itching in the ear canal in the early stages.
• Ear pain that may become intense. The ear is tender to the touch and pain worsens when pulling the ear.
• Discharge of fluid or pus from the ear canal.
• Redness and swelling of the skin of the ear canal (and occasionally of the external ear).
• A small, painful lump or boil in the ear canal.
• Eczema (dandruff-like patches of flaky, itchy, red, oozing skin) around the ear opening.
• Temporary hearing loss due to pus accumulation in the ear canal.
• Fever.

• Over-the-counter earwax removers, hair dyes, shampoos, hairsprays, or chlorinated water may irritate skin in the ear canal.

PREVENTION

• Do not insert objects, even cotton swabs, into the ear canal, and do not clean the ear with alcohol or over-the-counter solutions. (Your doctor can remove earwax safely.)
• If you experience frequent itching of the ear canal, consult a doctor. Control of an underlying skin condition can prevent secondary infection.
• Avoid swimming in waters that may be polluted.

DIAGNOSIS

• The doctor will examine the ear canal through an otoscope, a small, lighted viewing instrument.
• A culture of fluid discharge may be taken.

HOW TO TREAT IT

• Over-the-counter pain relievers may be taken. (Children should take acetaminophen, not aspirin.)
• Your doctor may use a small suction device to remove excess fluid and pus from the ear canal.
• Topical antibiotics or antifungal ear drops may be prescribed to treat infection, in addition to corticosteroid drops to reduce inflammation. A spongelike wick may be inserted into the ear to allow medication to travel deeply into the ear canal.
• Oral antibiotics may be given for severe infection.
• Surgical removal of dead tissue may be required to treat malignant otitis externa.
• Codeine or narcotics may be prescribed to relieve severe pain.
• After symptoms disappear, avoid getting water into the ear canal for up to three weeks. During this period, protect your ears when showering or washing your hair; avoid swimming.
• In the event of recurrence, keep a supply of the prescription ear drops on hand to ease symptoms.

WHEN TO CALL A DOCTOR

• Call a doctor if otitis externa symptoms persist for longer than a week despite treatment.
• People with diabetes should notify a doctor when they develop an ear infection.

Eardrum, Perforated

WHAT IS IT?

A perforated eardrum is a tear or a hole in the membrane (eardrum) that divides the outer ear canal and the middle ear. This translucent membrane receives sound vibrations and transmits them to the tiny bones (ossicles) in the middle ear, the initial step in the process of converting sound waves to nerve impulses. Consequently, when the eardrum is perforated or ruptured, hearing is temporarily compromised. Additionally, a ruptured eardrum provides greater opportunity for bacteria to enter and infect the middle ear. With prompt medical treatment, small perforations generally heal on their own within a month or two. Larger punctures and those that do not heal within three months may require microsurgery to repair or rebuild the eardrum. Once an eardrum is healed, there is usually little or no residual hearing loss provided that the ossicles have not been damaged.

SYMPTOMS
- Earache or sudden pain in the ear.
- Partial hearing loss.
- Slight bleeding or discharge from the ear. Pain associated with infection may ease as built-up fluid is released.
- Ringing or buzzing in the ear (tinnitus).

WHAT CAUSES IT?

- A severe middle ear infection (otitis media) may erode the eardrum or cause it to burst.
- Inserting an object (a cotton swab, paper clip, etc.) into the ear may perforate the eardrum.
- A sudden increase or decrease in the air pressure in the outer ear canal relative to that of the middle ear may cause the eardrum to rupture (barotrauma). Changes in pressure strong enough to rupture the eardrum may be caused by a nearby explosion or a blow to the ear (such as a slap to the head or direct force from water contact such as occurs during diving or water skiing). Scuba diving or flying may also cause a pressure change strong enough to injure the eardrum.

PREVENTION

- Do not insert objects, even cotton swabs, into the ear canal, and you should not attempt to clean the ear with alcohol or over-the-counter solutions. If impacted earwax interferes with hearing or causes discomfort, allow your doctor to remove it safely.
- Do not swim in polluted waters, which can cause ear infections.
- Get prompt treatment for ear infections.
- Avoid scuba diving (and flying if possible) when you have an allergy, cold, or throat infection.

DIAGNOSIS

- The doctor will examine the eardrum through an otoscope, a small, lighted viewing instrument.

HOW TO TREAT IT

- If you suspect a ruptured eardrum, see a doctor. In the meantime, cover the affected ear with a clean, dry pad to discourage infection. Take an over-the-counter pain reliever if necessary. Acetaminophen should be given to children instead of aspirin.
- Your doctor may prescribe antibiotics to treat or prevent infection in the middle ear.
- A warm heating pad or towel may be placed over the ear to relieve pain.
- Keep the eardrum dry as it heals. Protect the ear in the shower and when washing your hair; avoid swimming. An ear patch may be recommended for daytime use.
- If the eardrum fails to heal on its own, it may be surgically repaired with a tissue graft (myringoplasty or tympanoplasty).

WHEN TO CALL A DOCTOR

- Call a doctor if you experience symptoms of a ruptured eardrum.
- Consult an otolaryngologist (ear, nose, and throat specialist) if normal hearing is not restored within a month following a ruptured eardrum. ▲

Eczema Dermatitis

WHAT IS IT?

Eczema or dermatitis is a common inflammatory skin condition. Red raised lesions, oozing, and crusting may be seen in the acute phase; the chronic stage, often brought on by rubbing or scratching, is characterized by scaly, red, darkened, thickened patches of skin. The various types of eczema are grouped by cause or appearance, but all types are very itchy and red, and may worsen and spread if scratched. Occasionally, a secondary bacterial infection develops at the irritated site. Eczema is generally not a serious health risk, and in many cases, symptoms may be eased with over-the-counter creams and ointments.

WHAT CAUSES IT?

• Eczema may be associated with a personal or family history of allergies to foods, pollen, and animal dander, among others (atopic eczema).
• Eczema may be caused by contact with a variety of substances, including plants such as poison ivy; metals, especially nickel (used in rings and watchbands); rubber or latex; dyes; cosmetics; fragrances; leathers; topical medications; and dishwashing liquid, cleaning agents, and solvents (contact dermatitis).
• Some drugs, such as penicillin, may cause eczema when taken internally by people allergic to them.
• Poor circulation in the legs may lead to eczema (stasis dermatitis).
• In some cases, the cause of eczema is unknown.

PREVENTION

• Avoid direct contact with poison ivy, sumac, or oak.
• Stay away from substances to which you know you are allergic.

SYMPTOMS

• Itchy patches of dry, swollen, scaly, rough, cracked, or reddened skin.
• Oozing and crusting in the affected areas.
• Coin- or disk-shaped scaly patches of skin (nummular eczema).
• Swollen legs (stasis dermatitis).
• Thick, dry patches of skin in chronic cases.

• Use a cool-mist humidifier to moisten indoor air.
• Apply unscented moisturizer to dry skin as needed.
• For baths or showers, use cool or lukewarm (not hot) water. Avoid soaps with perfumes or deodorants. Apply moisturizer liberally while the skin is still wet. Gently pat the skin dry; do not rub.
• Wear cotton gloves under rubber gloves to prevent irritation when washing dishes or handling substances containing chemical irritants.
• Do not dress an infant in so many layers that he or she becomes overheated (heat may worsen eczema).

DIAGNOSIS

• Diagnosis may be made upon visual inspection and usually does not require a doctor.
• Allergy patch tests, blood tests, or a skin biopsy may be taken.

HOW TO TREAT IT

• Scratching the affected area should be avoided. Scratching makes eczema worse and can spread the irritation. Covering the affected area with a sterile bandage may help prevent scratching.
• If you come in contact with poison ivy, sumac, or oak, immediately washing the affected area with soap and water can remove the irritating plant chemicals.
• Over-the-counter corticosteroid creams (hydrocortisone) may be used to soothe skin. Oral antihistamines may also help to relieve itching.
• Your doctor may prescribe stronger corticosteroid ointments or ointments containing coal tar to soothe inflammation.
• Oral corticosteroid medications may be prescribed for extensive or severe cases that do not respond to topical treatments.
• Special support stockings may improve circulation in the legs to treat stasis dermatitis.
• Wearing cotton clothes next to the skin can be beneficial. Cotton is less irritating than wool, silk, or synthetics.
• Antibiotics may be needed to treat a secondary bacterial infection.

WHEN TO CALL A DOCTOR

• Call a doctor if eczema does not respond to self-treatment, is widespread, infected, or recurrent.

Empyema

WHAT IS IT?

Empyema is an accumulation of pus (which forms as a result of infection) in any body cavity, although the term is generally used to refer to the buildup of pus between the lungs and the ribcage (the pleural space). Normally, a small amount of sterile fluid is present inside this space, serving as a lubricant. But if this fluid becomes infected, pus may build up to quantities of a pint or more, exerting pressure on the lungs, which can cause pain and shortness of breath. This disorder has become uncommon since the development of antibiotics. Empyema occurring in other organs results in different symptoms. For example, when it affects the gallbladder, abdominal pain and jaundice may occur.

WHAT CAUSES IT?

• Pleural empyema (within the chest cavity) occurs as a complication of chest surgery, a serious chest injury, or an infection in the lungs (such as pneumonia or tuberculosis) or pleural space.
• Infection elsewhere in the body may spread to the chest cavity and cause pleural empyema. For example, an infection of the kidney may spread upward, through the diaphragm, and form an empyema in the chest.

PREVENTION

• Prompt treatment for infections, especially of the lungs, helps prevent empyema.

DIAGNOSIS

• A chest x-ray is taken, which shows fluid surrounding part of the lung.
• Diagnosis is confirmed by microscopic examination

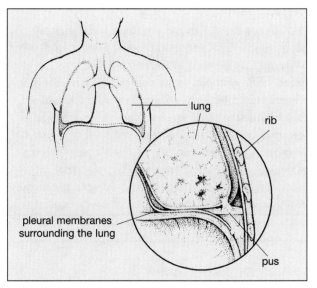

In pleural empyema, the space between the lung and the pleural membranes becomes infected, resulting in a buildup of pus.

of pus and by culturing it (allowing the infectious agent to grow in the laboratory so that it may be identified).

HOW TO TREAT IT

• Pain relievers, such as aspirin, acetaminophen, or narcotics, are recommended.
• Antibiotics are administered (often intravenously in a hospital) to combat bacterial infection.
• Pus is removed by thoracentesis, a procedure that involves withdrawing fluid into a syringe after inserting a needle through the chest wall into the pleural cavity. Repeated procedures may be necessary.
• Surgery may be required in severe cases or when the fluid is too thick to be removed by thoracentesis. A drainage tube may be implanted through a small incision in the chest wall into the pleural space (thoracostomy). In some cases a large incision that opens the chest cavity (thoracotomy) may be needed.

WHEN TO CALL A DOCTOR

• Call a doctor if you experience the symptoms of empyema or any persistent symptoms of infection. ⬛

SYMPTOMS

• Chest pain, especially when breathing deeply.
• Shortness of breath.
• Dry cough.
• Fever and chills.
• Profuse sweating, including night sweats.
• Exhaustion.
• Weight loss.

Encephalitis

WHAT IS IT?

Encephalitis, a rare disorder, is inflammation of the brain, almost always due to a viral infection. In most cases a virus attacks the brain directly after it is contracted from the bite of an infected mosquito or, less often, a tick. Encephalitis may occur as an isolated case or in epidemics. Most cases occur during the summer and early fall, although infection is possible year-round in warm regions. Depending on the specific virus involved, the onset of symptoms may be sudden or may take over a week to develop. In some cases a flu-like illness with symptoms of fever, headache, muscle aches, and fatigue may be present for several days before more severe symptoms of vomiting, stiff neck, extreme drowsiness, or seizures develop; in other cases severe symptoms may appear immediately. In addition, symptoms may vary among different age groups. In infants, a swelling in the soft spot of the skull (fontanel) and a stiff neck may be pronounced; children may complain of a headache and exhibit a sensitivity to light; in adults, neurological disturbances—both physical and mental—may be prominent. Although most cases of encephalitis are mild and may be mistaken for a cold or flu, in some cases (especially among the very young and very old) encephalitis is life-threatening. The outlook is good for those who survive the first two weeks of the infection; however, neurological symptoms may take many months to subside fully. Severe attacks bear the risk of permanent brain damage or epilepsy. Chemotherapy is available only for infections with the herpes simplex virus. In other cases treatment is aimed at relieving the severity and duration of symptoms.

WHAT CAUSES IT?

• Viral infection causes encephalitis. Most commonly, mosquitoes or ticks acquire an arbovirus from infected domestic animals (especially horses) or wild or domestic birds and may then transfer the virus to humans.
• Occasionally, infections with herpes simplex virus may spread to the brain.
• Human immunodeficiency virus (HIV) infection, measles, chicken pox, and infectious mononucleosis may cause an autoimmune encephalitis.
• Rarely, an adverse reaction to a vaccine may lead to encephalitis.

PREVENTION

• Prevent insect bites by using insect repellent containing DEET (diethyltoluamide) during outdoor summer activities. Apply repellent to clothing; use sparingly on skin.
• Cover exposed skin when in grassy, wooded, or swampy areas where mosquitoes and ticks may be present. Tuck long pants into socks, wear shoes instead of sandals, and wear long-sleeved shirts. Light-colored clothing makes ticks more visible.
• During a more widespread encephalitis outbreak, limit outdoor exposure during times of greatest mosquito activity: early morning, late afternoon, and early evening.
• Use fine-tipped, curved tweezers to remove a tick attached to your skin (see Lyme Disease for more information about tick removal). Do not use petroleum jelly, kerosene, or a lit cigarette to remove a tick; contrary to popular belief, these removal methods are ineffective and may increase the likelihood of infection.
• If possible, avoid areas where there is an outbreak of encephalitis.

SYMPTOMS
• Headache.
• Fever.
• Nausea and vomiting.
• Fatigue and loss of appetite.
• Double vision, or pupils of different size.
• Speech impairment, loss of hearing.
• Stiff neck and back, due to an associated infection of the meninges—the three layers of tissue covering the brain (see Meningitis for more information).
• Extreme sensitivity to light,
• Mental confusion, irritability, memory loss, personality changes, and hallucinations.
• Seizures.
• Paralysis of one side of the body.
• Drowsiness, gradual loss of consciousness, and coma. Coma may persist for days or weeks.

Encephalitis   *continued*

DIAGNOSIS

• Lumbar puncture (spinal tap).
• Blood tests.
• Electroencephalogram (EEG).
• CT (computed tomography) scans or MRI (magnetic resonance imaging).
• In severe cases a brain biopsy may be required to determine the underlying cause and thus guide further treatment. Under general anesthetic, a tiny hole is drilled in the skull, and a needle is used to extract a sample of the affected brain tissue.

HOW TO TREAT IT

• The antiviral drug acyclovir may be administered intravenously to treat encephalitis due to the herpes simplex type 1 or type 2 viruses.
• Oral corticosteroid drugs, such as dexamethasone, may be administered to reduce any inflammation of the brain.
• Anticonvulsant drugs, such as phenytoin, may be given to prevent seizures.
• Sedatives may be recommended to calm the patient.
• Pain relievers like aspirin, acetaminophen, ibupro-fen, or naproxen may be administered to reduce pain and fever. Aspirin should not be given to children with viral infections, owing to the risk of side effects (see Reye's Syndrome for more information).
• Fluids and electrolytes (such as sodium and potassium) may be administered intravenously to prevent dehydration during treatment, and liquid nutrients may be given through a tube placed in the stomach via the nose.
• A mechanical respirator may be required to aid breathing.
• Antibiotics may be administered to treat an associated bacterial infection.
• Speech, physical, and occupational therapy may be necessary during recovery in cases where a patient has suffered lasting brain damage.

WHEN TO CALL A DOCTOR

• Call a doctor immediately if you or your child develops nausea, severe headache, and a stiff neck, with or without a preceding flu-like illness.
• **EMERGENCY** Call an ambulance immediately if someone loses consciousness.

Endometrial Hyperplasia

WHAT IS IT?

Endometrial hyperplasia is the abnormal thickening of the lining of the uterus due to an increase in the number of endometrial glands. This disorder most often affects young women who are just beginning to menstruate and older women approaching menopause. In most cases endometrial hyperplasia is not a serious health risk. In some women, microscopic examination of endometrial tissue may reveal abnormalities in cellular nuclei, a precancerous disorder sometimes referred to as adenomatous hyperplasia, which may lead to endometrial (uterine) cancer. However, most cases of endometrial hyperplasia are benign and respond well to treatment with hormones or minor surgery. Symptoms of abnormal vaginal bleeding may cease with menopause.

WHAT CAUSES IT?

• An overproduction of estrogen causes endometrial hyperplasia in young women.
• Unopposed estrogen replacement therapy (taking estrogen without progesterone) in postmenopausal women is associated with a higher incidence of endometrial hyperplasia.
• Young women who have just begun to menstruate, and women who have (or who have had) irregular menstrual cycles, are at greater risk for endometrial hyperplasia when taking estrogen after menopause.

PREVENTION

• Although endometrial hyperplasia cannot be prevented, women should have regular pelvic examinations once they reach age 18 or become sexually active, to aid in early detection and treatment of any abnormalities.
• Postmenopausal estrogen replacement should be accompanied by a progestational agent or frequent endometrial biopsies.

DIAGNOSIS

• Although a Pap smear is performed (a small sample of cells is scraped from the cervix and examined under the microscope), it is done mostly to rule out other abnormalities. The Pap smear has a low detection rate for endometrial abnormalities.
• A biopsy of endometrial tissue may be taken during a pelvic examination.
• A dilatation and curettage (D&C) may be performed. In this procedure the cervix is widened, and tissue samples are obtained from the uterine lining.
• Blood levels of estrogen are measured.

HOW TO TREAT IT

• In most cases removal of excessive uterine tissue during the diagnostic D&C is all that is needed.
• Postmenopausal women on unopposed estrogen therapy who have recurrent endometrial hyperplasia should discuss with a gynecologist the options of either stopping the therapy or supplementing it with a progestational agent.
• In premenopausal women who have recurrent endometrial hyperplasia, oral contraceptives or a progestational agent such as Depo-Provera may be prescribed for a few months to thin the endometrial lining.
• A hysterectomy, the surgical removal of the uterus (and perhaps other reproductive organs), may be advised for postmenopausal women (or premenopausal women who no longer wish to have children) to reduce the risk of cancer when adenomatous hyperplasia does not respond to progestational agents.

WHEN TO CALL A DOCTOR

• Call a doctor if you develop heavy vaginal bleeding or if you experience vaginal bleeding between periods or after menopause. 🔺

SYMPTOMS
• Vaginal bleeding between menstrual periods or after menopause.
• Heavy menstrual bleeding.
• Periods that last longer than usual.

Endometrial Polyps

WHAT IS IT?

Endometrial polyps are small, spherical or cylindrical growths on the endometrium, the lining of the uterus. The exact cause of endometrial polyps is not known, but they tend to accompany other conditions involving overgrowth of uterine cells, such as endometrial hyperplasia or uterine fibroids (see Endometrial Hyperplasia or Fibroids, Uterine for more information). Polyps may appear singly or in clusters and are most common between the ages of 30 and 60, particularly among women over age 50. Although they are usually not a health risk, polyps occasionally contain cancerous cells.

Polyps generally cause no symptoms and, indeed, often go undetected. In some instances, however, endometrial polyps may cause heavy menstrual bleeding, bleeding between periods, or postmenopausal bleeding. Occasionally polyps may protrude into the vagina through the cervix, where they may bleed and cause pain. Cylindrical polyps attached to the uterine wall by a stalk may become twisted, which cuts off their blood supply and leads to infection. Polyps can grow large enough to fill or even stretch the uterus and therefore interfere with conception. Endometrial polyps can usually be removed with minor surgery.

WHAT CAUSES IT?

• The cause of endometrial polyps is unknown.

PREVENTION

• While endometrial polyps cannot be prevented, women should have regular pelvic examinations and Pap smears once they reach age 18 or become sexually active, to aid in early detection and treatment of any abnormalities.

DIAGNOSIS

• A pelvic examination may reveal the presence of endometrial polyps that protrude through the cervix.
• An abnormal Pap smear may reflect an underlying endometrial polyp.
• A hysterosalpingogram (HSG; injection of a contrasting dye into the uterus), ultrasound, or hysteroscopy (viewing the uterine lining with a camera) may be used to detect polyps inside the uterus.
• Dilatation and curettage (D&C) may be performed. In this procedure the cervix is widened so that the uterine lining can be scraped to obtain a tissue sample.

HOW TO TREAT IT

• Endometrial polyps may be scraped and removed from the uterine lining during the D&C procedure used for diagnosis. The D&C is generally performed at a hospital on an outpatient basis and requires local anesthesia.

WHEN TO CALL A DOCTOR

• Call a doctor if you develop bleeding between periods, if your periods are heavier or lengthier than normal, or if you have postmenopausal bleeding. ▲

SYMPTOMS
• No symptoms in many cases.
• Light bleeding or spotting between periods, especially after sexual intercourse.
• Heavy bleeding during menstrual periods.
• Periods that last longer than usual.
• Pelvic cramps.
• Foul-smelling vaginal discharge (if infection occurs).
• Postmenopausal bleeding or spotting.

Endometriosis

WHAT IS IT?

Endometriosis is a benign disorder characterized by the presence of endometrial tissue (the tissue that lines the uterus) outside the uterine cavity where it becomes attached to reproductive or abdominal organs. The patches of endometrial tissue swell with blood during menstruation as if they were still in the uterus. Because this blood is trapped within the tissue and cannot be shed through the vagina, blood blisters form, and they may develop further into cysts, scar tissue, or adhesions (fibrous bands that link together other tissues that are normally separated). Cysts may range from the size of a pinhead to the size of a grapefruit; cysts, scars, and adhesions may all lead to infertility.

Endometriosis is a common disorder, most prevalent between the ages of 25 and 40. Symptoms vary and are not strictly correlated with the severity of the disease; they may worsen with time, but tend to diminish during pregnancy and cease with menopause. Many women have no symptoms at all. Treatment depends on the severity of symptoms, the age of the woman, and whether she wishes to have children.

WHAT CAUSES IT?

• The cause of endometriosis is unknown. Hereditary factors may be involved.

SYMPTOMS

• Pain in the vagina, lower abdomen, and lower back. Pain often begins just prior to monthly periods, continues during menses, and worsens just after the cessation of blood flow.
• Abnormal or heavy menstrual bleeding.
• Vaginal pain during sexual intercourse (see Dyspareunia for more information).
• Diarrhea, constipation, or pain during bowel movements.
• Bleeding from the rectum or blood in the urine during menses.
• Nausea and vomiting just prior to monthly periods.
• Infertility. (Endometriosis is one of the most common causes of infertility.)

• Hormonal changes or recent pelvic surgery may promote endometriosis.

PREVENTION

• While endometriosis cannot be prevented, women should have regular pelvic examinations once they reach age 18 or become sexually active, to aid in early detection and treatment of any reproductive system abnormalities.

DIAGNOSIS

• A pelvic examination may reveal a suspicion of endometriosis. The doctor presses upon the uterus and ovaries to feel for any abnormalities.
• A definitive diagnosis requires direct visualization and biopsy or sampling of the extrauterine endometrial tissue. This is usually done by laparoscopy (the insertion of a thin, lighted viewing instrument into the abdomen through a small incision).

HOW TO TREAT IT

• Young women with endometriosis who wish to bear children may be advised to have children sooner rather than later.
• Over-the-counter pain relievers may be taken for mild menstrual pain.
• Danazol, progestins, or Gn-RH (gonadotropin-releasing hormone) agonists may be administered to halt menstruation for three to six months in an effort to shrink endometrial tissue.
• Surgical removal of the tissue may be required to relieve severe symptoms or to allow impregnation. Tissue may be destroyed by heat (electrocautery) or removed with lasers during laparoscopy (usually done on an outpatient basis under local anesthesia).
• A hysterectomy, the surgical removal of the uterus (and sometimes other reproductive organs), may be advised in severe cases. Hormone replacement is required if both ovaries are removed.

WHEN TO CALL A DOCTOR

• Call a doctor if you experience severe pain and heavy bleeding during menstruation, with or without additional symptoms of endometriosis. ⓐ

Epididymitis

WHAT IS IT?

Epididymitis is an infection of the epididymis, a tightly coiled, tubular structure located along the side of each testicle. Newly manufactured sperm cells mature as they slowly pass through the epididymis. The epididymic infection, which almost always affects only one epididymis, is common, easily treated, and not associated with permanent damage; however, epididymitis that affects both sides may lead to sterility if left untreated. Epididymitis does not occur prior to puberty.

WHAT CAUSES IT?

• A bacterial infection is the most common cause of epididymitis. The infection may be sexually transmitted or may spread from a bacterial infection in the bladder, urethra, or prostate.
• Straining upon urination may force urine into the reproductive tract and cause chemical irritation of the epididymis.
• Genital injury is sometimes a cause.
• Urinary tract instrumentation (such as a catheter) or prostate surgery can lead to epididymitis.

PREVENTION

• Use a condom to help prevent sexually transmitted disease.
• Obtain prompt treatment for urinary tract infections (see Bladder Infection for more information).

DIAGNOSIS

• Physical examination. A digital rectal examination may be performed by inserting a gloved, lubricated finger into the rectum to feel for abnormalities.
• Samples of urine and prostate gland secretions may be taken.

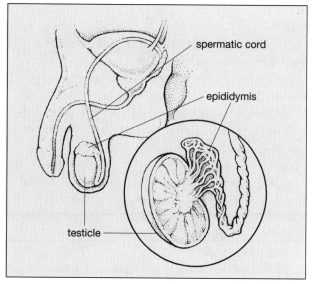

Sperm cells newly produced by the testicles mature during their journey through the long, coiled tubules of the epididymis.

HOW TO TREAT IT

• Antibiotics are prescribed to treat a bacterial infection. Sexual partners may need to be treated as well.
• Over-the-counter analgesics may be used to ease pain and inflammation.
• Bed rest may be advised until symptoms subside. When resting, it is advised to support the scrotum on a rolled bath towel.
• An ice pack may be used to relieve swelling. (Heat should not be used, because it may damage sperm-producing cells.)
• Sexual activity should be avoided for as long as symptoms persist.
• An athletic supporter may ease discomfort during recuperation. Full recovery may take several weeks or longer.
• Surgical removal of the epididymis may be necessary for very severe or recurrent cases that do not respond to antibiotic therapy.

WHEN TO CALL A DOCTOR

• Call a doctor for any severe or persistent testicular pain or swelling. ▲

SYMPTOMS

• Rapid onset of pain, heat, and swelling along the side of one testicle (and sometimes both), followed by swelling and hardening of the scrotum.
• Fever.
• Burning on urination.

Epiglottitis

WHAT IS IT?

Epiglottitis, a medical emergency, is a rare infection of the epiglottis—the small flap of cartilage in the throat that closes upon swallowing to prevent food and liquids from entering the windpipe. When infected, the epiglottis becomes inflamed and swollen, causing rapidly progressive breathing difficulty, especially in children. In an attempt to ease breathing, a person with epiglottitis commonly assumes a characteristic posture of leaning forward in a sitting position with the neck extended. Swelling of the epiglottis may lead to complete blockage of the airway within 12 hours of onset, so immediate treatment is necessary. Hospitalization is necessary so that breathing may be aided by tubes or emergency surgery in the event of complete obstruction of the airway. However, once treatment is initiated, symptoms generally subside within 36 to 48 hours, leaving no permanent damage. Epiglottitis most commonly affects children between the ages of two and eight, but it can occur in adolescents and adults.

WHAT CAUSES IT?

• Bacterial infection causes epiglottitis. The most common cause in children is *Hemophilus influenzae* which is highly infectious and may dictate antibiotic treatment of other family members. Streptococcal infection can also cause epiglottitis in both children and adults.

• Adults who have a weakened immune system due to leukemia, Hodgkin's disease, AIDS, or chemotherapy treatment for cancer are at higher risk for epiglottitis.

SYMPTOMS

• Sore throat.
• Fever.
• Increasing difficulty or pain upon swallowing.
• Drooling.
• Increasingly muffled speech; hoarseness.
• Irritability and restlessness.
• Emergency symptoms: breathing difficulty, a bluish tinge to the skin (cyanosis), loss of consciousness.

PREVENTION

• As much as possible, try to limit exposure to people with contagious respiratory illnesses.

DIAGNOSIS

• Examination of the throat using a tongue depressor or laryngoscope (a special lighted scope). Because there is a danger that this may cause an inflamed epiglottis to completely block the airway, such an examination should not be attempted at home.

• Neck x-ray.

• Blood and throat cultures.

HOW TO TREAT IT

• Hospitalization is necessary to treat epiglottitis. Symptoms may quickly become life-threatening.

• Oxygen may be administered to aid breathing.

• Obstruction of the airway may make it necessary to pass a tube down the throat, through the nose or mouth, to permit breathing.

• A temporary surgical opening in the throat, known as a tracheotomy, may be performed in some cases. In this procedure a small tube is surgically inserted into the throat, allowing the patient to breathe. The tube is removed after symptoms and epiglottal inflammation subside.

• Antibiotics (usually a cephalosporin) are administered intravenously to treat the underlying bacterial infection.

• Fluids may be administered intravenously to prevent dehydration.

• Corticosteroid medications may be given to reduce inflammation of the epiglottis.

WHEN TO CALL A DOCTOR

• **EMERGENCY** Call an ambulance or get to a hospital immediately if you or your child begins to experience swallowing or breathing difficulty, or if your child turns blue or loses consciousness. 🔺

Erectile Dysfunction Impotence

WHAT IS IT?

Erectile dysfunction, commonly known as impotence, is the inability to achieve or maintain an erection adequate for satisfactory sexual performance. It may occur at any age but becomes increasingly frequent as men grow older. The mechanisms for erection are fairly complex: A sensory stimulus triggers the brain to send nerve impulses down through the spinal cord. These signals trigger the release of a chemical messenger that causes the vessels supplying blood to the penis to dilate. The rod-shaped spongy tissues (corpora cavernosa) in the penis then fill with blood and expand, pressing against the veins that normally allow blood to drain from the penis, thus producing an erection. Interference with any part of this process—whether psychological or physiological—may cause erectile dysfunction. Although an occasional inability to maintain an erection is common and not a sign of a chronic problem, a doctor should be consulted if impotence persists. Treatment depends upon the underlying cause.

WHAT CAUSES IT?

• Emotional and psychological difficulties such as guilt or anxiety (especially performance anxiety, in which fear of not having an erection becomes so distracting that it becomes a self-fulfilling prophecy).
• Conditions that affect the brain and decrease the libido (sex drive), including depression or schizophrenia; use of drugs that act on the central nervous system (sedatives, antidepressants, some antihypertensives, antipsychotics, and alcohol); and chronic illnesses such as heart, lung, kidney, or liver disease, and certain types of cancer.
• Hormonal disturbances that decrease the libido, including diminished testosterone levels, elevated prolactin (due to a pituitary tumor; see Hyperprolactinemia), and hyper- or hypothyroidism.
• Brain disorders (that do not affect libido but have neurological consequences that affect sexual functioning), including brain tumor and stroke.
• Spinal cord disorders, such as multiple sclerosis or spinal cord trauma.
• Damage to the peripheral nerves due to diabetes mellitus or pelvic surgery for disorders such as prostate cancer or rectal cancer.
• Medications that can sometimes cause sexual dysfunction, including anticholinergics, antihistamines, beta-blockers (and other kinds of antihypertensives), and long-term use of nicotine.
• Peripheral vascular disease (impaired blood flow to the extremities and the penis).
• Fatigue.
• Advancing age.

PREVENTION

• Have no more than two alcoholic beverages a day.
• Don't smoke.
• Talk to a therapist about improving communication with your sexual partner.

DIAGNOSIS

• Patient history and physical examination are required.
• Blood may be taken to measure testosterone, prolactin, and thyroid hormones.
• Psychological causes may be identified by ruling out a physiological cause. A band of stamps or perforated tape is placed around the penis before sleep. An erection during the night will break the perforations, demonstrating that there is no organic cause for the erectile dysfunction.
• The drug alprostadil may be injected into the penis to test for vascular problems.

HOW TO TREAT IT

• Avoid nicotine, alcohol, and other drugs.
• Your doctor may change your prescriptions if a medication has caused impotence.
• Psychological counseling may be recommended.
• Testosterone injections or skin patches are given if blood testosterone levels are low.
• Hyperthyroidism or hypothyroidism is treated if necessary.
• Bromocriptine therapy is given to correct elevated prolactin levels.

SYMPTOMS

• Inability to achieve or maintain an erection sufficient for satisfactory sexual performance.

Erectile Dysfunction Impotence *continued*

• The oral medication sildenafil citrate (Viagra) is effective in up to 80 percent of men with erectile dysfunction. The drug is taken one to two hours prior to sexual activity and requires sexual stimulation to work. Side effects include headache, flushing, and upset stomach. Men taking nitrate-containing medication (such as nitroglycerin) should not take sildenafil.

• A special vacuum device may be used to produce an erection. Air is pumped out of a plastic tube placed securely over the penis, and the resulting vacuum pulls blood into the corpora cavernosa within a few minutes. The device is removed and a rubber band is placed at the base of the penis to maintain the erection.

• Self-administered injections of alprostadil, a vasodilator drug, dilate the blood vessels in the penis to produce an erection. Your doctor will instruct you on the correct injection technique.

• Surgical implants for the penis are available. In one procedure an inflatable device with a small fluid reservoir is inserted. In another, flexible rods are implanted that can be either bent upward to produce an erection or tucked close to the body.

• Your doctor may rarely advise vascular surgery to improve blood flow to the penis.

WHEN TO CALL A DOCTOR

• Call a doctor if you experience a persistent inability to achieve or maintain an erection.

Esophageal Cancer

WHAT IS IT?

Esophageal cancer is the growth of malignant cells in the esophagus, the passageway from the throat to the stomach. An esophageal tumor blocks the passage of food to the stomach, erodes the esophageal lining, and contributes to the development of fistulas (abnormal channels between normally separate organs) between the esophagus and the trachea (the major airway to the lungs). Although uncommon, esophageal tumors worsen rapidly: by the time symptoms develop, the outlook is poor. In North America this cancer is more common among blacks than whites and affects men more frequently than women. It occurs most often in those over age 50. Although a cure may be attempted when the cancer is detected at an early stage, treatment is generally aimed at relieving symptoms and making the patient as comfortable as possible.

SYMPTOMS

- Progressive swallowing difficulty, first with solid foods, then liquids; painful swallowing.
- Chest pain.
- Weight loss.
- Regurgitation of bloody mucus.
- Vomiting or regurgitation of swallowed food.
- Repeated respiratory infections. Material may spill into the airway and lungs from frequent regurgitation or from an esophagotracheal fistula.

WHAT CAUSES IT?

- The cause of esophageal cancer is unknown.
- Smoking and excess consumption of alcohol are believed to be the greatest risk factors.
- Swallowing lye or other corrosive chemicals may lead to esophageal cancer.
- The habit of drinking extremely hot beverages may, over time, damage the esophagus and predispose it to cancer.
- Persistent gastric reflux is associated with a higher risk of esophageal cancer (see Gastroesophageal Reflux for more information).

PREVENTION

- Do not smoke.
- Have no more than two alcoholic beverages a day.

DIAGNOSIS

- X-ray after swallowing barium to create a clear image of the esophagus.
- Endoscopy (a small, lighted viewing tube inserted into the esophagus through the mouth under local anesthesia).
- A biopsy is performed during the endoscopy to remove a sample of esophageal tissue for examination under a microscope.

HOW TO TREAT IT

- Surgery may be performed in an attempt to remove the tumor.
- If the tumor cannot be completely removed, laser surgery may be used to reduce its size and open a passageway into the stomach.
- Radiation therapy may be used after or in conjunction with surgery to decrease tumor size and prevent its spread.
- Chemotherapy may be used to destroy remaining cancer cells instead of, or in addition to, surgery and radiation therapy.
- An esophageal dilator may be used to widen the stricture. Dilation is usually repeated periodically to maintain the opening.
- Patients who are unsuited for surgery may have a plastic tube inserted through the esophagus (intubation) to bypass the site of the tumor.
- An artificial opening in the stomach (gastrostoma) or small intestine (ileostoma) may be created surgically, so that food may bypass the entire esophagus.
- Painkillers and tranquilizers are prescribed to relieve pain and anxiety.

WHEN TO CALL A DOCTOR

- Call a doctor if you experience difficulty in swallowing.

Esophageal Rupture

WHAT IS IT?

An esophageal rupture is a tear in the esophagus, the passageway from the throat to the stomach. It is a medical emergency, requiring prompt diagnosis and treatment. The esophagus may be ruptured by forceful vomiting, chemical injury, trauma, or other disorders of the esophagus, such as esophageal cancer (see Esophageal Cancer for more information). Chest pain from a large tear in the esophagus may mimic symptoms of a heart attack (see Myocardial Infarction for symptom information). Leakage of esophageal contents such as saliva, food, or vomit into the neighboring chest cavity can cause chemical injury or a serious bacterial infection or abscess. Treatment usually involves surgery to repair the tear and remove esophageal contents from the chest cavity, combined with antibiotics to prevent or treat a bacterial infection. If the esophagus has been severely damaged, surgical removal of part or all of the esophagus may be necessary.

WHAT CAUSES IT?

- Forceful vomiting.
- Ingestion of a foreign object.
- Ingestion of lye or other corrosive chemicals (see Esophageal Stricture for more information).
- Infection, ulcer, or cancer of the esophagus.
- Trauma, such as an automobile accident.
- Accidental injury from insertion of tubes or instruments into the esophagus during medical procedures. (Approximately half of esophageal ruptures are caused this way.)

PREVENTION

- Keep small objects and household chemicals that may be swallowed away from young children.

SYMPTOMS

- Moderate or severe chest pain that may worsen upon breathing or swallowing following an episode of retching or vomiting.
- Fever.
- Rapid, shallow breathing.
- Excessive sweating.

- Obtain prompt treatment for disorders that cause severe nausea and vomiting.

DIAGNOSIS

- Chest x-ray. You may be required to swallow a contrast material during an x-ray, so that the site of rupture in the esophagus can be clearly identified.

HOW TO TREAT IT

- Surgical repair of the rupture is necessary for all but relatively small tears. In cases of severe esophageal damage, the affected portion of the esophagus may be removed surgically.
- Small tears can often be treated medically. In such cases, the patient will not be permitted to eat and oral suction may be used to keep the esophagus empty.
- Intravenous fluids and nutrients may be administered to maintain hydration and nutrition until the tear has healed.
- Intravenous antibiotics may be administered to treat or prevent an associated bacterial infection.

WHEN TO CALL A DOCTOR

- **EMERGENCY** Call an ambulance for any severe chest pain. Heart attack, esophageal tear, and other serious disorders will need to be ruled out. 🔺

Esophageal Stricture

WHAT IS IT?

An esophageal stricture is a narrowing of the esophagus, the passageway from the throat to the stomach. Stomach acid, esophageal cancer, accidentally swallowed harsh chemicals, and other irritants may injure the esophageal lining, causing inflammation (esophagitis) and the formation of scar tissue. This may gradually lead to obstruction of the esophagus, preventing food and fluids from reaching the stomach.

WHAT CAUSES IT?

• Persistent reflux of gastric acid into the esophagus (see Gastroesophageal Reflux for more information).
• Systemic sclerosis (scleroderma), which is often associated with severe reflux and esophageal stricture (see Scleroderma for more information).
• Swallowing lye or other corrosive chemicals.
• Pills lodged in the esophagus.
• Esophageal surgery or protracted use of a nasogastric tube (used in hospitals for feeding).
• Esophageal cancer may narrow the esophagus and produce the same symptoms.

PREVENTION

• Aggressive treatment of chronic gastroesophageal reflux is necessary.
• Store all corrosive chemicals where they will be inaccessible to children.
• Take all pills with a full glass of liquid.

DIAGNOSIS

• Barium x-ray studies. You may be required to swallow barium, which helps to create a sharp image of the esophagus on an x-ray.
• Endoscopy (insertion of an illuminated scope into

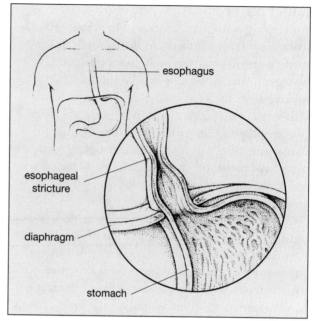

Injury to the lining of the esophagus, the narrowest portion of the digestive tract, may result in esophageal stricture.

the esophagus through the mouth under local anesthesia) may be performed.

HOW TO TREAT IT

• Your doctor may advise a diet of liquids or soft foods until food can be swallowed without difficulty.
• Mechanical dilation of the esophagus (esophageal bougienage) may be performed to widen the stricture.
• In severe cases the affected portion of the esophagus may be removed and replaced with a segment of the large intestine.
• In a few cases patients who are unsuited for surgery may have a feeding tube inserted through the stricture. Alternatively, such patients may have a small tube placed into the stomach (gastrostomy), so that food may bypass the esophagus completely.

WHEN TO CALL A DOCTOR

• **EMERGENCY** Call an ambulance if someone has swallowed a corrosive material.
• **EMERGENCY** Go to an emergency room if food becomes stuck in the esophagus and cannot be dislodged by drinking water or other maneuvers.
• Call a doctor if you experience progressive difficulty in swallowing. ⬛

SYMPTOMS

• Progressive swallowing difficulty, first with solid foods, then liquids; chest pain after meals; increased salivation.
• Regurgitation of foods and liquids. These may be aspirated into the lungs, causing cough, wheezing, and shortness of breath.
• Weight loss.

Essential Tremor

WHAT IS IT?

Essential tremor, also known as intention or familial tremor, is a rhythmic shaking movement caused by involuntary muscle contractions. This tremor, termed essential because it is not related to an underlying disorder, most frequently affects the hands and neck; it generally spares the muscles of the torso and lower limbs. Characteristically, essential tremor becomes more pronounced during activities such as writing or using a knife and fork, as distinguished from tremors in Parkinson's disease, which often diminish with movement (see Parkinson's Disease for more information). Essential tremor usually develops in middle age or later. Symptoms appear gradually. The most common of the so-called shaking disorders, essential tremor is not a serious health risk. It responds well to treatment and in fact seems to be an indicator of an unusually long life.

WHAT CAUSES IT?

• The cause of essential tremor is unknown.
• Genetic factors play a role in about half of all cases (familial tremor).

PREVENTION

• There is no known way to prevent essential tremor.

DIAGNOSIS

• Patient history and physical examination are needed.

SYMPTOMS

• Rhythmic shaking of the hands and fingers and, less frequently, the head, tongue, larynx, eyelids, or other parts of the body. The speed of the shaking movements may be rapid or moderate.
• Worsening of the tremor under the following conditions: with emotional or physical stress; when voluntarily moving the hands, head, and other muscles; when voluntarily trying to hold the head or hands still.
• Cessation of the tremor when at rest.
• Shaky handwriting.
• Quavering voice.

HOW TO TREAT IT

• Beta-blocking drugs (commonly used to treat high blood pressure) such as propranolol are generally the most effective medications for treating essential tremor.
• Other drugs, including anticonvulsants (such as primidone) and tranquilizers (such as clonazepam, lorazepam, or alprazolam), may be used to treat muscle tremors that do not respond to beta-blockers.
• Patients may be advised to drink one glass of wine or one ounce of 80-proof liquor a day, because alcohol has been shown to ease tremors in some cases. However, sometimes a rebound effect occurs, causing the tremor to worsen after the effect of the alcohol has worn off. In addition, some doctors fear the potential risk of alcohol abuse.
• Avoid the consumption of caffeine and other stimulants, which may exacerbate the tremor.
• In severe, disabling cases that do not respond satisfactorily to medications, controlled injections of botulinum toxin (which causes the muscle paralysis associated with botulism) into muscles of the forearm or neck may stop tremors.
• Surgical destruction of specific cells within the brain, or electrical stimulators implanted in certain regions of the brain, may provide relief from symptoms in severe cases that do not respond to other forms of treatment, but this is done only as a last resort.

WHEN TO CALL A DOCTOR

• Make an appointment with a doctor if involuntary trembling or shaking of the hands, head, or other muscles interferes with normal activities. ⚠

Eye Cancers

WHAT IS IT?

Eye cancer is the growth of malignant cells in the tissues of the eye. In adults, most eye cancers are secondary tumors that spread to the eye from other parts of the body (often the breast, although cancers of the lungs, kidneys, and prostate gland are sometimes involved). These cancers spread via the bloodstream or the lymphatic system.

Two primary tumors arise within the eyes: retinoblastomas and melanomas. Among children, retinoblastoma is the most common primary eye cancer; it affects children under age five. Malignant melanoma of the eye is found most frequently in adults (the average age at diagnosis is 60 to 65 years old). Most eye cancers affect only one eye, but retinoblastoma involves both eyes in about one-third of cases.

Symptoms may not be evident in the early stages of any form of eye cancer; growing tumors may increasingly cause pain and impair vision, however. Cancer of the eye may spread (metastasize) to the optic nerve, the brain, or the rest of the body, so early diagnosis and treatment are important. Treatment for eye cancer is aimed at destroying cancerous cells, relieving symptoms, and preserving sight as much as possible. Treatment for secondary eye tumors also involves treating the primary cancer elsewhere in the body.

SYMPTOMS

- Gradual distortion and loss of vision in the affected eye.
- Pain and redness in the affected eye.
- Different color irises in each eye.
- Bleeding in the eye.
- In retinoblastoma, an eye may turn in or out (crossed eyes). Later, visible whiteness in the pupil may be seen.
- Melanomas often produce no symptoms. Sometimes blurred vision or seeing flashing lights occurs. A black or brown spot on the iris or the white of the eye can develop.
- Bulging eyes (with a secondary tumor located behind the eyeball).

WHAT CAUSES IT?

- It is unknown why primary eye melanomas arise.
- The most common cause of metastatic eye cancer in adults is the spread of a tumor from another site in the body.
- Genetic factors play a role in retinoblastoma.

PREVENTION

- If retinoblastoma runs in your family, genetic counseling is advised before having children.
- Newborns and children in families with a history of retinoblastoma should have regular eye examinations.

DIAGNOSIS

- An ophthalmologist will conduct a complete eye examination, possibly using general anesthesia on children.
- An ultrasound examination and sometimes CT (computed tomography) scans of the head and eye may be performed. Ultrasound is the more useful and common.

HOW TO TREAT IT

- Laser surgery or cryosurgery (freezing the targeted tissue with liquid nitrogen) may be used to destroy small tumors.
- Radiation therapy may be used to kill cancerous cells, in conjunction with or in lieu of surgery.
- Chemotherapy may be used to halt or limit the spread of the cancer. Recently, new chemotherapeutic agents have been successful in treating retinoblastoma within the eye.
- Surgical removal of the eye may be necessary to prevent the cancer from spreading, or when an eye is completely blinded and painful.

WHEN TO CALL A DOCTOR

- Make an appointment with an ophthalmologist if you develop any of the symptoms of eye cancer.

Fibrocystic Breast Changes

WHAT IS IT?

Fibrocystic breast changes are characterized by the presence of noncancerous lumps, or cysts, in the breast. The cysts may vary in size, number, and composition; some may be filled with fluid, and others may be solid. Over 60 percent of women develop cysts in the breast, mainly between the ages of 25 and 50. Most experts now believe that the condition represents only a variety of common, natural states or changes in the breast and is not a disease at all. Symptoms of pain and tenderness tend to be more pronounced just prior to menstrual periods. Cysts are not cancerous; however, a biopsy is the only way to make a certain diagnosis of any lump found in the breast. Symptoms may disappear after menopause.

WHAT CAUSES IT?

• The cause of fibrocystic breast changes is unknown.
• Estrogen and other ovarian hormones may influence the development of cysts.

PREVENTION

• There is no way to prevent fibrocystic changes. For the purpose of early detection, women should perform monthly breast exams, have a yearly breast exam performed by a doctor or other trained specialist, and begin having mammograms after age 50 (see Breast Cancer for more information).

DIAGNOSIS

• Breast examination or mammography may reveal the presence of a lump in the breast.
• A biopsy of the lump, using a needle aspiration to

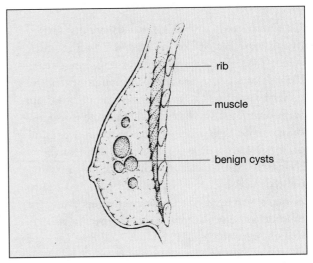

The lumps that characterize fibrocystic breast changes may alter in their size or feel in response to hormonal changes during the menstrual cycle.

extract fluid, or minor surgery to remove solid tissue is the only certain way to determine whether a breast lump or cyst is benign or malignant.

HOW TO TREAT IT

• Needle aspiration or biopsy may drain or remove the lump completely.
• A full-support bra (often worn both day and night) may help relieve minor breast discomfort.
• Over-the-counter pain relievers can reduce pain.
• A reduction in caffeine consumption may help relieve symptoms.
• Hormonal treatment (such as with oral contraceptives) may be prescribed to relieve symptoms, but this is not very effective and may be associated with undesirable side effects.

WHEN TO CALL A DOCTOR

• Make an appointment with a doctor if you notice the development of a new lump anywhere in the breast or under the arm, especially when no other lumps are present. Most lumps are not cancerous, but a biopsy is necessary for a definite diagnosis.
• Make an appointment with a doctor if you notice that a breast lump has become harder or more painful, changed in size, or if you experience discharge from the nipple. ▲

SYMPTOMS

• One or more lumps or swellings, often painless, anywhere in the breast.
• Discomfort or pain around the lump or in the breast, especially during the week before a menstrual period.
• Changes in the size or symmetry of the breasts.
• Symptoms are rare in postmenopausal women not taking hormone replacement therapy.

Fibroids, Uterine

WHAT IS IT?

Uterine fibroids are benign (noncancerous) growths of the muscular wall of the uterus. The growths, which may appear singly or in groups, range from the size of a pea to the size of a grapefruit, and may either be confined to the uterine wall or grow outward on thin stalks. Fibroids often cause no symptoms, unless they grow so large as to press painfully on other organs or even distort the shape of the abdomen. Also, a fibroid with a stalk may become twisted, which cuts off its blood supply and results in sharp, severe pain, requiring emergency surgery. Fibroids are quite common; they generally affect women between ages 30 and 45, and may shrink or disappear with the onset of menopause. The growths rarely become cancerous, although large fibroids may narrow the uterine cavity and lead to miscarriage or infertility.

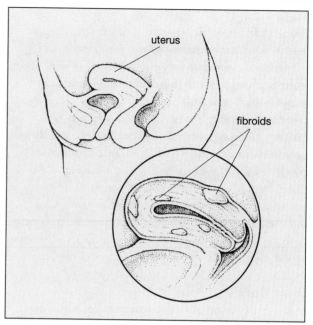

Small fibroids in the uterus wall may be unnoticeable; larger ones may cause pain, along with menstrual, urinary, or fertility problems.

WHAT CAUSES IT?

• The cause of uterine fibroids is unknown.
• Oral contraceptives or pregnancy may promote fibroid growth.

PREVENTION

• Women should have annual pelvic exams once they reach age 18 or become sexually active, to aid in early detection and treatment of any abnormalities.
• Women diagnosed with asymptomatic fibroids should have pelvic examinations once a year so that fibroid growth may be monitored.

DIAGNOSIS

• A pelvic examination, during which a doctor presses upon the uterus and ovaries to feel for any abnormalities, may reveal the presence of uterine fibroids.
• A pelvic ultrasound scan can confirm the diagnosis.

HOW TO TREAT IT

• Asymptomatic fibroids rarely require treatment.
• Iron supplements may be advised if a patient has heavy bleeding during menstrual periods.
• Surgical removal of the fibroids that leaves the uterus intact (myomectomy) is an option for some patients. Myomectomies usually have higher blood losses than hysterectomies, however, they preserve the chance for future pregnancies.
• Emergency surgery is necessary to remove a twisted fibroid.
• A hysterectomy, the surgical removal of the uterus (and perhaps of other reproductive organs), may be recommended for severe or recurrent cases.

WHEN TO CALL A DOCTOR

• Call a gynecologist if you develop symptoms of uterine fibroids.
• **EMERGENCY** Get immediate medical attention for sharp, sudden pain in the lower abdomen.

SYMPTOMS
• Heavier bleeding during menstrual periods.
• Abdominal discomfort, fullness, or pain.
• Lower back pain.
• Frequent urination; constipation.
• Emergency symptom: sharp, sudden pain in the lower abdomen (when a fibroid with a stalk becomes twisted).

Fibromyalgia

WHAT IS IT?

Fibromyalgia (previously called fibrositis) is a common, but poorly understood disorder characterized by chronic, widespread pain and stiffness in various muscles, tendons, and ligaments. Profound fatigue frequently accompanies the pain, and both are made worse by seemingly trivial physical activity. Diagnostic tests show no abnormalities of the joints and no muscle damage. Fibromyalgia is more common in women and increases in frequency with age. It often accompanies other illnesses, such as lupus or rheumatoid arthritis, but does not lead to joint or muscle damage. Treatment is aimed at the relief of symptoms.

WHAT CAUSES IT?

• The cause of fibromyalgia is unknown.
• Sleep disturbances or interruptions, especially of deep sleep (known as stage IV sleep), may provoke a flare-up of fibromyalgia.
• Underused muscles, poor fitness, and impaired blood circulation may contribute to fibromyalgia.
• Emotional stress and depression may worsen the illness.
• Sometimes an injury or infection will precede the onset of fibromyalgia; whether they cause the disease is unclear.

PREVENTION

• There is no known way to prevent fibromyalgia.
• Eating a healthy, well-balanced diet and getting regular exercise may help decrease the risk.

SYMPTOMS

• Widespread muscle aches, pains, and stiffness. Physical activity may relieve stiffness but worsen pain. Stiffness is usually worse upon awakening in the morning, but may be present all day.
• Chronic fatigue and unrefreshing sleep.
• Symptoms of irritable bowel syndrome, dysmenorrhea, migraine, or irritable bladder are sometimes present.

DIAGNOSIS

• Patient history and physical examination are needed.
• Although there are no specific tests for fibromyalgia, the diagnosis is strengthened when the physician applies pressure to 18 characteristically tender sites and the patient reports pain in at least 11 of them.
• Further tests to rule out rheumatoid arthritis and other diseases may be done. Indeed, a diagnosis of fibromyalgia is dependent upon the exclusion of other disorders.

HOW TO TREAT IT

• Over-the-counter pain relievers such as acetaminophen may be taken as necessary. Narcotic pain relievers should be avoided.
• A regular program of physical exercise may relieve pain and stiffness and improve circulation. Exercise may aggravate pain at first; therefore, in consultation with your doctor, start with low-impact activities such as walking, swimming, and bicycling, sustaining the activity for 20 to 30 minutes at a time. You may slowly work up to more vigorous exercises like jogging, racquetball, or aerobics.
• Medications such as amitriptyline, doxepin, or cyclobenzaprine may be prescribed to promote restful sleep and decrease pain.
• A hot bath, heating pad, or massage may provide temporary relief from muscle pain.
• Practice good posture during the day. A firm mattress may help prevent muscle pain at night.
• Psychological counseling may be beneficial and help to ease emotional stress that may trigger painful flare-ups. Relaxation techniques such as meditation or biofeedback may help reduce muscle tension and stress.
• Although the pain of fibromyalgia may be difficult to control, the disease is never life-threatening and does not lead to damage of the body or progressive disability.

WHEN TO CALL A DOCTOR

• Make an appointment with a doctor if you experience symptoms of fibromyalgia for more than three consecutive days, or if symptoms recur. ▲

Food Poisoning

WHAT IS IT?

Food poisoning refers to illness brought on by ingesting foods contaminated with living micro-organisms, toxins produced by microorganisms, poisonous chemicals, or poisonous fish, shellfish, or plants (such as mushrooms). The digestive tract is most commonly affected. However, botulism, a life-threatening form of food poisoning, primarily affects the nervous system and may cause respiratory failure (see Botulism for more information).

Food poisoning may result from improper storage and handling of food, such as inadequate refrigeration or touching food with soiled hands or machinery. Symptoms generally develop within one to 48 hours after eating. Some types of food poisoning (notably cholera and shigellosis) may take from three to five days to produce symptoms.

Food poisoning is suspected when sudden, acute gastrointestinal symptoms arise. It is difficult to prove that food poisoning is the cause of illness unless several people develop symptoms after sharing a meal or after eating in the same restaurant. The illness often subsides spontaneously after one to five days; however, severe or persistent symptoms require treatment and sometimes hospitalization.

SYMPTOMS
- Diarrhea.
- Abdominal pain and cramps.
- Nausea.
- Vomiting.
- Fever.
- Headaches.
- Bloody stool.

WHAT CAUSES IT?
- Preformed bacterial toxins produced by overgrowth of certain bacteria before food is eaten.
- Contamination with live microorganisms that proliferate in the intestine and may invade tissues or produce toxins.
- Poisonous metals.
- Poisons in fish, shellfish, and plants (mushrooms).

PREVENTION
- Wash your hands thoroughly with warm water and soap before preparing food.
- Make sure food is handled, cleaned, cooked, and refrigerated properly.
- Don't buy or use food in cans that are rusty, bulging, or leaking.
- Avoid tasting food to check for contamination.
- Don't eat mushrooms you have picked.
- Don't consume unpasteurized dairy products.
- Throw away any questionable leftovers.

DIAGNOSIS
- Vomit, feces, or blood may be cultured or tested.
- If available, samples of suspected foods are examined for contaminants.

HOW TO TREAT IT
- Drink plenty of fluids to prevent dehydration from diarrhea, and take antidiarrheal medications.
- An oral solution containing electrolytes and sugar may be needed to replace minerals lost with severe diarrhea.
- Intravenous fluids may be needed to treat severe dehydration.
- Medication to prevent vomiting (antiemetics) may be prescribed in severe cases, although vomiting may help rid the body of toxins.
- Antibiotics may be prescribed in some cases, depending upon the specific infectious agent involved.

WHEN TO CALL A DOCTOR
- The elderly, young children, and anyone with a weakened immune system (such as those diagnosed with AIDS or undergoing treatment for cancer) should be taken to a doctor immediately if they develop even mild symptoms of food poisoning. These people are at greater risk of life-threatening complications.
- Call a doctor if you develop any of the following: sudden, severe or bloody diarrhea; a fever over 102°F; severe abdominal pain.
- Call a doctor if food poisoning symptoms do not subside within a week.

Frostbite

WHAT IS IT?

Frostbite is the freezing of skin and damage to underlying blood vessels upon exposure to extreme cold. Blood flow halts in frostbitten skin, and the area must be thawed and rewarmed swiftly to prevent tissue death (gangrene) and infection. The ears, nose, hands, and feet are especially susceptible. Frostbite is sometimes accompanied by a life-threatening drop in internal body temperature, known as hypothermia, which must be treated first (see Hypothermia for more information). Less severe forms of frostbite are referred to as frostnip and chilblain.

WHAT CAUSES IT?

• Exposure to extremely cold temperatures (32°F or below) for prolonged periods of time causes frostbite. The risk becomes greater as the temperature drops and the wind increases.

• Wet clothing and skin increase the risk of frostbite.

• Certain conditions, such as diabetes mellitus, poor circulation, or previous frostbite predispose a person to frostbite.

• Fatigue and dehydration increase the risk of frostbite, as do alcohol and drugs.

PREVENTION

• Wear several layers of warm, protective clothing when you go out in cold weather. Clothing should be dry and should not be restrictive. Mittens are preferable to gloves and protection of the head and ears is important.

• Do not allow yourself to become overly tired, dehydrated, or hungry.

• Avoid smoking or drinking before venturing out into extreme cold. Tobacco decreases circulation by constricting blood vessels, and alcohol increases heat loss and impairs judgment.

DIAGNOSIS

• Presence of symptoms points toward frostbite.

• Mild frostbite (without blisters or numbness) may be treated at home. If there is any question as to the severity of frostbite, go immediately to an emergency room for evaluation.

HOW TO TREAT IT

• Go inside as soon as possible. Do not rub snow on the affected area.

• Remove clothing from frostbitten skin and cover the affected area with warm blankets. Do not rub or massage the affected area.

• Do not attempt to warm the area using hot air or an open flame.

• Warm, not hot, water (100°F to 108°F) may be used to thaw the affected area. It is important not to allow the affected area to refreeze.

• If the frostbite is severe, do not attempt to thaw the area. Go directly to an emergency room.

• Ibuprofen or other over-the-counter pain relievers should be taken immediately to ease pain during thawing.

• Aloe vera may be applied to the skin to ease pain and inflammation.

• Your doctor may prescribe painkillers to relieve severe pain, and antibiotics to prevent damaged tissue from becoming infected. A tetanus shot should also be given.

• In severe cases, surgery may be necessary to remove damaged tissue. It may take several weeks to determine the full extent of the damage. Rarely, amputation is necessary.

WHEN TO CALL A DOCTOR

• **EMERGENCY** Call an ambulance or go to an emergency room if you are concerned that frostbite may be severe. 🏥

SYMPTOMS

• In mild frostbite, a stinging or burning sensation is felt, accompanied by redness and swelling.

• As frostbite becomes more severe, the skin may appear bluish gray and feel numb.

• Blisters and bruising may appear upon rewarming.

Gallbladder Disorders

WHAT IS IT?

The gallbladder, a small, pear-shaped organ located just below the liver, concentrates and stores bile, a substance produced by the liver to aid in the digestion of fats. Bile is stored in the gallbladder and secreted into the duodenum (the portion of the small intestine joined to the stomach) during digestion. Gallstone formation—known as cholelithiasis—is the most common gallbladder disorder. It usually occurs when excessive amounts of cholesterol in the bile clump together into solid masses. People with hemolytic anemia (marked by rapid destruction of red blood cells) may develop gallstones composed of bilirubin, a bile pigment.

The quantity and size of gallstones may vary from one large stone to thousands of tiny ones. More common in women than in men, most gallstones are referred to as "silent gallstones," as they cause no symptoms and so require no treatment. Sometimes, however, gallstones produce acute symptoms by blocking the cystic duct (which leads from the gallbladder to the common bile duct) or the bile duct. Blockage of the cystic duct causes inflammation of the gallbladder, known as cholecystitis. A blocked bile duct is also prone to bacterial infection. In some cases an infected gallbladder may become filled with

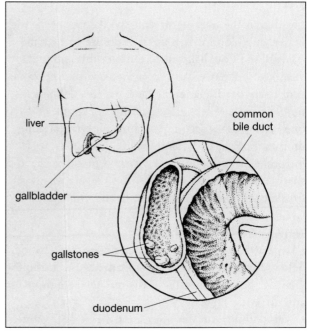

Gallstones may remain in the gallbladder or pass without incident through the bile duct into the duodenum. Symptoms arise when stones become trapped in the bile duct or the gallbladder is inflamed.

pus, a condition known as empyema that requires immediate surgery (see Empyema for more information). Rarely, the gallbladder may be the site of tumor formation. For reasons that are unclear, gallstones increase the risk of gallbladder cancer; although few people with gallstones develop cancer, the majority of those with gallbladder cancer also have gallstones. Cancer of the gallbladder, which normally strikes at age 70 or older, is inoperable upon diagnosis in 75 percent of cases, and the outlook is generally poor.

Treatment for most gallbladder disorders involves surgical removal of the gallbladder (cholecystectomy). Gallstones may be dissolved with chemical agents or sound waves, but tend to recur if the gallbladder is not removed. The absence of the gallbladder does not inhibit digestion; bile simply passes directly from the liver into the small intestine.

WHAT CAUSES IT?

• The exact cause of gallstones is unknown, but cholesterol stones are usually associated with an abnormal composition of the bile.

SYMPTOMS

• Moderate to severe pain in the upper-right abdomen, often spreading into the chest, right shoulder, and back. Pain due to gallstones may occur in separate episodes lasting from 30 minutes to four hours. Inflammation of the gallbladder causes pain that gradually increases in severity and may worsen upon deep breathing. Cancer of the gallbladder produces steady pain.
• Possible nausea and vomiting accompanying the attacks of pain.
• Fever and chills (gallbladder inflammation).
• Abdominal fullness or bloating.
• Severe belching, heartburn, and gas.
• Weight loss (cancer of the gallbladder).
• Jaundice.

Gallbladder Disorders *continued*

• Age, obesity, a high-calorie diet, very rapid weight loss, Crohn's disease, cirrhosis, hemolytic disorders, or intestinal surgery increase the risk of gallstones.

• Multiple pregnancies, oral contraceptives, or estrogen therapy may provoke the development of gallstones in women.

• Obstruction of the cystic duct (usually by gallstones), injury, or bacterial infection (usually in conjunction with bile duct obstruction) may lead to inflammation or abscess of the gallbladder.

• Gallstones are associated with a higher risk of gallbladder cancer.

• Hereditary factors may play a role; for example, among certain Native American tribes such as the Pima Indians of Arizona, nearly 70 percent of the women have gallstones by age 30.

PREVENTION

• Maintain ideal body weight.

• Check with your doctor before pursuing any diet for rapid weight loss.

DIAGNOSIS

• Physical examination is needed. The doctor may press on the upper abdomen to feel for an enlarged or tender gallbladder.

• Ultrasound scans may be performed.

• ERCP (endoscopic retrograde cholangiopancreatogram) may be done using a thin, lighted viewing tube (endoscope), which is passed down the throat into the small intestine. Contrast material is injected into the bile duct, and x-rays are taken.

HOW TO TREAT IT

• Cholecystectomy, or surgical removal of the gallbladder, is the treatment of choice for most gallbladder disorders and virtually prevents further attacks of gallstones by eliminating their source. Conventional abdominal surgery may be used, although increasingly, a newer procedure called laparoscopic cholecystectomy is preferred. With this method a scope is inserted through small abdominal incisions and then used to excise the gallbladder. The technique dramatically reduces postoperative pain and recovery time.

• Prior to surgery, meperidine or pentazocine is given to relieve pain. Intravenous feeding and fluids are also initiated, and antibiotics may be administered to prevent or treat an associated bacterial infection.

• In patients who have acute gallbladder inflammation but are too weak for cholecystectomy, a surgical opening in the gallbladder (cholecystostomy) may be created and a tube inserted to drain the gallbladder's contents. Complete removal of the gallbladder may be performed after the patient's condition has improved sufficiently.

• Oral ursodeoxycholic acid or chenodeoxycholic acid—bile acids that dissolve cholesterol gallstones over a period of months or years—may be prescribed. However, such therapy is effective only for small stones composed entirely of cholesterol. It is expensive and is successful less than 50 percent of the time. Even when it does work, there is a 30 to 50 percent chance that stones will recur.

• A long, thin needle may be used to infuse the solvent methyl tert-butyl ether (MTBE) directly into the gallbladder via a catheter. This method dissolves cholesterol gallstones within one or two days. Again, recurrence is a possibility.

• Sound wave therapy (extracorporeal shock-wave lithotripsy) has been used with limited success to shatter some types of gallstones and avoid surgery.

• Radiation or chemotherapy may be used to treat cancer of the gallbladder.

WHEN TO CALL A DOCTOR

• Call a doctor if you develop severe abdominal pain.

• **EMERGENCY** Call an ambulance if you experience upper-right abdominal pain and nausea accompanied by shortness of breath and sweating. Such symptoms may also signal a heart attack. 🔺

Ganglion

WHAT IS IT?

A ganglion is a round swelling or cyst that develops just under the skin near a joint or tendon. The back of the wrist is by far the most common site; however, ganglia may appear elsewhere, including the fingers, ankles, and feet. They vary from the size of a pea to, rarely, the size of a golf ball. They are usually painless or only somewhat bothersome. The thick, clear, jellylike fluid inside of a ganglion is believed to be composed of the same elements as the fluid that lubricates the joints and tendons. A buildup of this fluid within a tendon sheath or joint capsule causes these membranes to balloon outward. Because ganglia pose no health risk and are typically painless, they rarely require treatment, and they may disappear spontaneously without any medical intervention. Many patients seek treatment for cosmetic reasons.

WHAT CAUSES IT?

• The cause of ganglia is unknown, but may be related to trauma, repetitive use, or overuse.

PREVENTION

• There is no known way to prevent ganglia.

DIAGNOSIS

• Diagnosis is typically made upon visual inspection of clinical manifestations.
• In rare cases, x-rays or ultrasound may be used to confirm the diagnosis, and other tests may be performed to rule out a more serious disorder (such as a malignant growth) that might cause such a lump.

HOW TO TREAT IT

• Treatment is generally not necessary for a small, painless ganglion unless the patient desires it for cosmetic reasons.

SYMPTOMS
• An unusual lump under the skin (usually on the back of the wrist), which may feel soft and rubbery, or hard and solid.
• Pain or tenderness in the lump (although this is uncommon).

• Your doctor may use a large needle to puncture and drain the ganglion—a procedure known as needle aspiration. An anti-inflammatory corticosteroid medication may then be injected into the affected area. Needle aspiration may eventually need to be repeated, as ganglia treated in this manner have a tendency to recur.
• Surgery may be used to remove a ganglion that recurs or causes discomfort. After such surgery, recurrence is extremely unlikely.

WHEN TO CALL A DOCTOR

• Make an appointment with a doctor if you notice the development of a lump anywhere on your body. A ganglion is nothing to worry about; however, more serious disorders should be ruled out.
• Consult your doctor if a ganglion begins to cause discomfort, interferes with normal activities, or is cosmetically unacceptable to you. ▲

Gastroesophageal Reflux Heartburn

WHAT IS IT?

Gastroesophageal reflux, the most common cause of heartburn (which actually has nothing to do with the heart), is the regurgitation of the contents of the stomach and duodenum (the first portion of the small intestine) into the esophagus, the muscular tube through which food travels from the mouth to the stomach. Because the esophagus lacks the protective lining of the stomach, it is easily irritated by digestive juices; the irritation causes a "burning" sensation in the chest.

The lower esophageal sphincter (LES), a circular band of muscle located at the junction of the esophagus and stomach, is usually clenched but opens when a person swallows to permit food or liquid to enter the stomach. Reflux occurs when, for a variety of possible reasons, the LES allows stomach contents to pass upward into the esophagus. Severe, long-standing reflux can cause esophageal inflammation (esophagitis), which leads to scarring (stricture) that can cause considerable swallowing difficulty.

WHAT CAUSES IT?

• Weakness or inappropriate opening of the LES.
• Hormonal changes and increased abdominal pressure during pregnancy.
• Smoking.
• Overeating and obesity.
• Excessive consumption of alcohol.

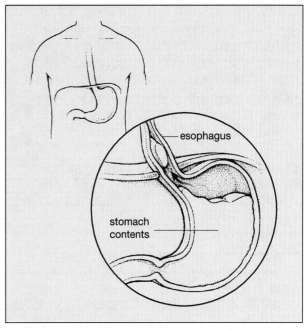

The stomach contains powerful acids and enzymes that are needed to break down proteins. Sometimes, especially following a large meal, stomach contents may be regurgitated into the esophagus (reflux). Because the esophagus is not protectively lined like the stomach, the acid causes a stinging sensation, commonly known as heartburn.

• Fatty, spicy, or acidic foods and drinks; chocolate; and mints (such as spearmint and peppermint).
• Excessive consumption of caffeinated beverages, which weaken the LES pressure and also stimulates acid secretion. For uncertain reasons, decaffeinated coffee also stimulates acid secretion and can increase the severity of reflux.

PREVENTION

• Avoid overeating or eating within two or three hours of going to bed, and avoid napping after a meal. Also don't exercise immediately after eating.
• Avoid tight pants, girdles, and belts.
• Lose weight if you are overweight.
• Avoid excessive consumption of alcohol.
• Don't smoke.
• Decrease your consumption of coffee and caffeinated beverages.

DIAGNOSIS

• Patient history usually indicates the diagnosis. Frequent episodes of a burning sensation in the chest or

SYMPTOMS

• Burning sensation (heartburn) in the chest behind the sternum, or breastbone. In rare cases, pain may radiate to the neck and arms, mimicking a heart attack.
• Difficulty swallowing liquids or foods.
• Regurgitation of food, usually tasting sour or bitter, when lying down or bending forward.
• Pain upon swallowing.
• Hoarseness or wheezing from regurgitation into the throat and lungs.
• Chest pain, thought to be due to an esophageal spasm set off by acid irritating the esophagus.

Gastroesophageal Reflux Heartburn *continued*

of sour or bitter liquid or food coming back to the mouth are hallmarks of gastroesophageal reflux.

• X-rays are taken after the patient swallows barium, which clearly outlines the esophagus and stomach and may demonstrate reflux.

• Monitoring of pH, in which a small acid-sensitive catheter is placed through the nose and into the esophagus to confirm and measure the severity of reflux.

• Endoscopy (the insertion of a lighted scope into the esophagus through the mouth) may be performed to look for evidence of esophagitis.

HOW TO TREAT IT

• Follow preventive measures.

• Elevate the head of the bed by six inches to reduce reflux at night.

• Take an over-the-counter (OTC) antacid that does not contain calcium or an OTC histamine (H2) blocker such as cimetidine, ranitidine, famotidine, or nizatidine on an as-needed basis, according to the label instructions. Frequent and long-term need for these drugs suggests severe reflux, so check with a doctor if you need more than occasional relief.

• Your doctor may prescribe medication to suppress the secretion of stomach acids or to speed the passage of food from the stomach to the small intestine. Medications include histamine (H2) blockers, proton pump inhibitors (such as omeprazole and lansoprazole), and prokinetic drugs (such as bethanechol, metoclopramide, and cisapride). These drugs are usually very effective and are the treatment of choice when simple self-care methods fail.

• In severe cases, surgery may be necessary to tighten the LES.

WHEN TO CALL A DOCTOR

• Call a doctor if symptoms of heartburn persist or recur frequently despite self-treatment.

• **EMERGENCY** Call an ambulance if you experience severe chest pain—this may signal a heart attack.

Genital Herpes

WHAT IS IT?

Genital herpes is a viral infection characterized by outbreaks of painful sores on the genitals. Most often it spreads through sexual contact. Once infected, a person carries the virus permanently in a latent form in the nerve cells; there is no cure. An initial attack and any recurrences generally last from one to three weeks, after which the infection may go into remission for months or years. Subsequent attacks tend to be less severe, and in about one-third of cases, permanent remission follows the initial outbreak.

Most people with genital herpes have no symptoms. Recent studies by the Centers for Disease Control and Prevention estimate that 40 million U.S. adults are infected. Genital herpes is highly contagious, and one partner may transmit it to another even when no visible sores or lesions are present. It is more easily transferred from men to women than vice versa; it may also be transferred to babies of infected mothers during childbirth, possibly causing blindness, retardation, or even death. Genital herpes is also a risk factor for HIV infection.

WHAT CAUSES IT?

• Herpes simplex virus type 2 (HSV-2) is the most common cause of genital herpes.
• Herpes simplex virus type 1 (HSV-1), the virus that commonly causes cold sores around the mouth, may also cause genital herpes.

SYMPTOMS

• Often no symptoms.
• Pain or itching in the genital area.
• Watery blisters in the genital area that break to form painful, shallow ulcers. The ulcers scab over and disappear spontaneously within three weeks. Occasionally, blisters and ulcers around the mouth may accompany genital sores.
• Painful urination in women.
• Fever, fatigue, loss of appetite, and enlarged lymph nodes in the groin (typically occurring only with the initial attack).
• Possibly headache (in those who develop viral meningitis).

• Recurrence in both sexes may be triggered by sexual intercourse, exposure to ultraviolet light, fatigue, injury, heat, cold, and stress. In women, recurrence may also be triggered by menstrual periods.
• People with weakened immune systems, such as those undergoing cancer treatment or those with AIDS, are more likely to have a severe case.

PREVENTION

• Avoid sexual contact if symptoms are present in either partner.
• Latex condoms during sexual intercourse reduce the risk of transmission, but they are not foolproof.
• To prevent ultraviolet light from triggering a recurrence of genital herpes, use sunscreen (SPF 15 or higher) before going outdoors.

DIAGNOSIS

• Patient history and physical examination.
• Culture of fluid from blisters or sores.
• Microscopic examination of lesion samples.

HOW TO TREAT IT

• Treatment is aimed at relieving symptoms. The antiviral drugs acyclovir, valacyclovir, and famciclovir may be prescribed to lessen the duration and severity of outbreaks. In people who have frequent recurrences (more than six a year), these drugs may be used long-term as suppressive therapy.
• Take aspirin, acetaminophen, or ibuprofen to relieve pain.
• Frequent warm baths may lessen discomfort during an outbreak.
• Women may urinate through a small tube, such as a toilet-paper roll, to prevent urine from irritating open sores on the vagina.
• A cesarean section may be necessary for pregnant women who have active genital herpes at time of delivery, in order to avoid transferring the infection to the infant during childbirth. The mother and infant may both be treated with acyclovir.

WHEN TO CALL A DOCTOR

• Call a doctor if you develop symptoms of genital herpes.

Genital Warts

WHAT IS IT?

Genital warts, also known as condylomata acuminata, are small growths in the genital area, commonly appearing around the vaginal opening or inside the vagina on the cervix, around the anus, on the penis, and on the perineum (the area between the genitals and anus). They are highly contagious, and are most commonly spread through sexual or other intimate body contact. It may take from three to 12 months after infection for a wart to appear. In addition, the virus may remain in skin tissues even after warts are removed, making recurrence common. Conditions producing excess vaginal moisture and discharge, such as yeast infections or pregnancy, may encourage wart growth in women.

Genital warts are linked to an increased risk of cervical and penile cancer. (Cervical cancer is detected in the early curable stages by Pap smear. All sexually active women should have a Pap smear at least every one to three years, so that if cancer develops, it may be detected early.) Other sexually transmitted diseases, such as syphilis or gonorrhea, may be transmitted at the same time as the genital wart virus.

WHAT CAUSES IT?

• The human papillomavirus (HPV) causes genital warts. Most of the more than 80 strains of the virus produce only harmless warts, but some have been associated with greater risk of cervical or penile cancer. Most persons with HPV infection are completely without symptoms.
• Genital warts may be spread by sexual intercourse.
• As with other sexually transmitted diseases, genital warts in children may be evidence of sexual abuse.

PREVENTION

• Use a latex condom during sexual intercourse to help prevent spreading or contracting the disease.

> ### SYMPTOMS
> • Small, red, rounded or flat, itchy bumps on or around the vagina, anus, penis, or perineum.
> • Several warts may grow together into a cauliflower-like configuration.

DIAGNOSIS

• Patient history and physical examination are needed. Women's pelvic examinations should include a Pap smear (a test in which a small sample of cells is scraped from the cervix); in addition, the doctor may examine the vagina with a colposcope (a magnifying instrument for viewing the inside of the vagina and the cervix).
• Blood samples may be taken to rule out other sexually transmitted diseases.
• A culture of vaginal or penile discharge may be taken to rule out gonorrhea or chlamydia.
• A biopsy (removal and analysis of tissue samples) may be performed to rule out cancer.

HOW TO TREAT IT

• A doctor may apply podophyllin, imiquimod, or trichloroacetic acid, chemical solutions that gradually destroy warts.
• Genital warts may be removed by applying liquid nitrogen, which freezes and thus destroys warts (cryosurgery). Warts may also be burned away with an electric probe (electrocauterization) or destroyed with laser surgery.
• The sexual partner(s) of the infected person should be examined as well. However, in many cases, they will have no symptoms.
• Do not attempt to remove genital warts using over-the-counter wart preparations. Such chemical solutions are too harsh for sensitive genital skin and may cause disfigurement.

WHEN TO CALL A DOCTOR

• Make an appointment with a doctor if you or your sexual partner display symptoms of genital warts.

Gingivitis

WHAT IS IT?

Gingivitis is an inflammation of the gums (gingiva), usually caused by the buildup of plaque at the base of the teeth. Bacteria within this sticky, colorless substance produce toxins that can inflame the gums, causing them to bleed. Without proper dental care, gingivitis may lead to more serious periodontitis (involving destruction of the bone that anchors the teeth in place) and eventual tooth loss.

WHAT CAUSES IT?

• Poor or improper oral hygiene is the most common cause.
• Poor nutrition, certain chronic diseases (such as diabetes), hormonal changes (such as those that occur during menopause), and some medications (including anticonvulsants) may promote gingivitis.

PREVENTION

• Brush your teeth at least twice a day using a soft nylon-bristle toothbrush. Scrub with a gentle circular motion, then whisk the brush up (on lower teeth) and down (on upper teeth), away from the gums. Brushing teeth too vigorously will only erode the gums. Be sure to clean the inside surfaces of the teeth (nearest to your tongue), because plaque deposits tend to be heavy there.
• Brush your tongue; it collects the same bacteria that stick to your teeth.
• Floss after brushing. With a gentle sawing motion, ease the floss between the teeth, forming a crescent against one side of a tooth. Using your thumbs and index fingers, gently scrape up and down, from just under the gum line to the top of the teeth.
• Consider using irrigation devices such as Waterpik or plaque removal devices such as Interplak—but check with your dentist first.
• See a dentist at least once a year. Professional

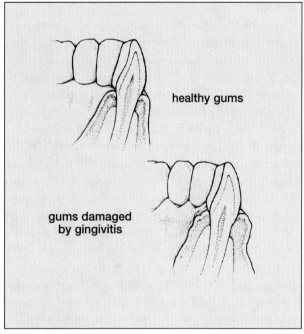

In gingivitis, plaque builds up on the teeth and irritates the gums. Eventually plaque wedges into pockets between the teeth and gums, damaging the gums and causing them to recede.

cleaning is required to remove deposits of hardened plaque (tartar).
• Limit your consumption of sugary drinks and sweet, starchy, or sticky foods, which stimulate the production of acid and lead to tooth and gum decay. Fruits and vegetables with high fiber content help to clean teeth and prevent gingivitis.

DIAGNOSIS

• An oral examination by a dentist is required to determine the extent of gum disease.

HOW TO TREAT IT

• Follow preventive tips for proper dental care.
• Your dentist or hygienist will scrape plaque and tartar off teeth and may prescribe an antibacterial mouthwash.
• Vitamin supplements may be recommended to treat a nutritional deficiency.

WHEN TO CALL A DOCTOR

• See a dentist at least once a year or if you develop symptoms of gingivitis. ▲

SYMPTOMS

• Red, shiny, swollen, tender gums that bleed easily (when brushing the teeth or while flossing, for example).
• Bad breath.

Glaucoma

WHAT IS IT?

Glaucoma is a sight-threatening disorder marked by an increase in intraocular pressure (IOP), that is, the pressure within the eyeball. It occurs as a result of an excess buildup of aqueous humor—the clear fluid inside the eyeball that provides nutrients to and carries waste products away from the lens and cornea of the eye, the only parts of the body with no blood supply. Each day, the eye produces about one teaspoon of aqueous humor. Normally, this fluid escapes from the eye, through a spongy mesh of connective tissue called the trabecular meshwork, at the same rate at which it is produced. In a common type of glaucoma, production of aqueous humor appears to exceed the rate of its escape and the pressure rises.

There are two forms of glaucoma: open angle and closed angle. Open-angle glaucoma, which accounts for 90 percent of all cases, is a slow, progressive disease that produces no symptoms in its early stages. By contrast, closed-angle glaucoma is relatively uncommon and is characterized by rapid and extreme elevations of IOP, often causing acute symptoms such as severe eye pain and rapid blurring of vision. Both types of glaucoma may lead to blindness by damaging the optic nerve; however, early detection and treatment can usually control IOP and prevent severe vision loss. Most prevalent among those over age 40, glaucoma is more common in African Americans or when there is a positive family history.

WHAT CAUSES IT?

• It is theorized that open-angle glaucoma occurs when, for reasons not completely understood, the trabecular meshwork becomes partially blocked.

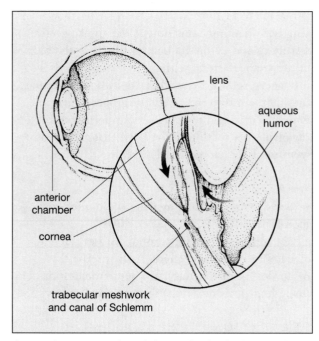

Aqueous humor passes through the anterior chamber between the lens and the cornea. It is then drained through the spongelike trabecular meshwork, and funnelled into the body's circulatory system through a passageway known as the canal of Schlemm. If the trabecular meshwork becomes clogged, drainage of the aqueous humor is impaired and pressure within the eye (intraocular pressure) increases.

IOP builds up as more aqueous humor is formed, but pressure doesn't rise high enough to cause any noticeable symptoms initially. When IOP remains elevated or continues to rise, however, fibers in the optic nerve are compressed and destroyed, leading to a gradual loss of vision over a period of years.
• Closed-angle glaucoma is caused by a sudden blockage near the iris that prevents aqueous humor from reaching the trabecular meshwork. The blockage results in the rapid onset of extremely high IOP that may cause severe, permanent vision loss within a day or two.
• A family history of visual-field loss due to glaucoma increases the risk of optic nerve damage. Evidence also suggests that cardiovascular disease, diabetes, and myopia (nearsightedness) increase the risk of nerve damage from glaucoma.

PREVENTION

• While there is no way to prevent glaucoma, early detection and treatment may prevent damage to the

---

SYMPTOMS

• Open-angle glaucoma: gradual loss of peripheral vision, marked by blind spots. Symptoms only develop at the later stages of the disease. Screening exams are advised.
• Closed-angle glaucoma: acute attacks involving severe eye pain, nausea and vomiting, blurred vision, and the appearance of rainbow-colored halos around lights.

Glaucoma   *continued*

optic nerve. See an ophthalmologist for a complete eye exam every two years after age 50. Those of African descent should start having such exams at age 40.

DIAGNOSIS

Glaucoma is diagnosed by an eye examination which emphasizes eye pressure measurement, viewing of the optic nerve, and assessment of optic nerve function:
• Tonometry (use of an instrument to apply slight pressure upon the eyeball to measure IOP).
• Ophthalmoscopy (in which the pupils are dilated with eye drops so that the optic nerve may be magnified and examined with an ophthalmoscope, a lighted viewing instrument).
• Perimetry (a visual-field test that determines the extent of peripheral vision).

HOW TO TREAT IT

• Glaucoma is a chronic disorder that cannot be cured. Open-angle glaucoma can often be treated safely and effectively by medical or surgical measures, though lifelong therapy is almost always necessary. Medications are nearly always used first. However, initial laser surgery is becoming a more common option.
• Eye drops are the most frequent medical treatment for glaucoma because they have fewer overall side effects than oral medications. Depending on which type, eye drops must be applied one to four times a day, regularly and on schedule, to maximize IOP control. Five types of eye drops are currently used: miotics (such as pilocarpine), beta-blockers (like timolol or levobunolol), adrenergic agonists (such as epinephrine or dipivefrin), topical prostaglandins (latanoprost), and carbonic anhydrase inhibitors (dorzolamide). Miotics (drugs that constrict the pupil) and adrenergic agonists increase the outflow of aqueous humor. Beta-blockers diminish the production of aqueous humor. Latanoprost, the newest type of glaucoma eyedrop, reduces IOP by increasing the outflow of aqueous humor. Because it works differently than other glaucoma drugs, it can be used along with a second medication to reduce IOP further. Dorzolamide drops, previously available only as tablets, decrease production of aqueous humor.

• Carbonic anhydrase inhibitor pills are generally used when optic nerve damage continues or seems highly likely despite maximal topical treatment. These oral medications initially lower IOP by 20 to 30 percent on average, but significant systemic side effects (such as numbness or tingling in the extremities, malaise, and loss of appetite) and occasional serious complications (such as kidney stones, depression, diarrhea, and blood abnormalities) can limit their use.
• Periodic ophthalmologic examinations are essential throughout medical therapy. These may initially be required daily or weekly for those with severe nerve damage or extreme elevations of IOP, or only every three to six months for patients with stable IOP and minimal optic nerve damage.
• Surgery is successful more often than medical treatment. However, it carries a greater risk of complications, including the development of cataracts, and repeat procedures may be required. About 10 percent of those with open-angle glaucoma require surgery, when drug therapy fails or when the patient has a medical condition (such as hypertension or severe heart or lung disease) that precludes maximal drug therapy. The two most common surgical procedures—laser trabecular surgery and filtration surgery—reduce ocular pressure by opening a passage for aqueous humor.
• Unless high IOP is relieved promptly during an acute attack of closed-angle glaucoma, blindness can occur within a day or two. Making a hole in the iris (iridotomy) creates a drainage path for the aqueous humor. Iridotomy in the other eye is generally recommended owing to the high likelihood that it will be involved in a future acute attack. The procedure can usually be performed with a laser.

WHEN TO CALL A DOCTOR

• Contact an ophthalmologist right away if you develop symptoms of acute closed-angle glaucoma.
• See an ophthalmologist for a complete eye exam every two years after age 50. (Those of African descent should start having such exams at age 40.) People with a family history of glaucoma should also have periodic exams. ▲

Glomerulonephritis, Acute

WHAT IS IT?

Acute glomerulonephritis is a term used to describe a number of underlying disorders that cause a sudden inflammation of the glomeruli, the tiny structures in the kidneys that filter waste products from the blood. Inflammation of the glomeruli impedes the filtering process, trapping waste products in the blood and allowing red blood cells and proteins to escape into the urine. Kidney malfunction may also lead to high blood pressure and fluid retention. Acute glomerulonephritis is most common among children, often occurring after a streptococcal infection of the throat or sometimes the skin. Although a few severe cases (about 5 percent) lead to kidney failure, most subside spontaneously within two weeks to several months.

WHAT CAUSES IT?

• The condition may occur as a complication of a bacterial infection. A throat or skin infection can trigger the formation of protein aggregates called immune complexes in the glomeruli, which cause inflammation that interferes with normal kidney function, usually within 14 days of the initial infection.
• Viral infections, such as mononucleosis, measles, and hepatitis B or C, and parasitic infections, such as malaria, are infrequent causes of the disorder.
• Autoimmune disorders, such as systemic lupus erythematosus or other causes of vasculitis (inflammation of small blood vessels) may produce glomerulonephritis and persistent kidney damage.

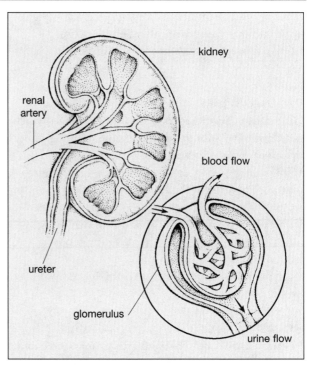

Blood enters the kidney through the renal artery; wastes are filtered out in the tiny glomeruli and excreted as urine through the ureter. Damaged glomeruli allow proteins and red blood cells to escape too.

PREVENTION

• There is no way to prevent acute glomerulonephritis.

DIAGNOSIS

• Patient history and physical examination.
• Blood and urine tests.
• A kidney biopsy (using a tissue sample taken with a needle) may be done if symptoms persist or if an underlying systemic disorder is suspected.

HOW TO TREAT IT

• High blood pressure is treated with antihypertensive drugs.
• Diuretics and a low-salt diet may be used to reduce excess fluid retention and increase urine output.
• If the disorder is the result of an underlying bacterial infection, antibiotics may be prescribed.
• Short-term kidney dialysis is sometimes needed.

WHEN TO CALL A DOCTOR

• Call a doctor if you or your child develop symptoms of acute glomerulonephritis. ▲

SYMPTOMS

• Abrupt onset of blood in the urine (color may range from light brown to bright red).
• Passing only small amounts of urine.
• Swelling of the ankles, the abdomen and scrotum, or the tissues around the eyes, due to fluid accumulation (edema).
• Shortness of breath, due to fluid accumulation in the lungs.
• In severe cases, symptoms of kidney failure, including fatigue, nausea and vomiting, loss of appetite, headache, back pain, fever, and impaired vision.

Glomerulonephritis, Chronic

WHAT IS IT?
Chronic glomerulonephritis is a kidney disorder caused by slow, cumulative damage and scarring to the tiny blood filters in the kidneys. These filters, known as glomeruli, remove waste products from the blood. In chronic glomerulonephritis, scarring of the glomeruli impedes the filtering process, trapping waste products in the blood while allowing red blood cells or proteins to escape into the urine, eventually producing the characteristic symptoms of high blood pressure and swelling in the legs and ankles. The disorder may first come to one's attention because of high blood pressure. Long-term inflammation and scarring (sclerosis) of the kidneys may lead to kidney failure in severe cases. Damage may progress without symptoms for months or years; by the time symptoms finally appear, the course of the disorder may be irreversible.

WHAT CAUSES IT?
• The specific cause of most cases of chronic glomerulonephritis is unknown.
• Viral infections, such as hepatitis B or C and acquired immunodeficiency syndrome (AIDS), may lead to chronic glomerulonephritis.
• Autoimmune disorders, such as systemic lupus erythematosus, or other causes of vasculitis (inflammation of small blood vessels) may cause chronic glomerulonephritis.
• Acute glomerulonephritis may, after a symptomless period of many years, reappear as chronic glomerulonephritis.

PREVENTION
• There is no known way to prevent chronic glomerulonephritis.

DIAGNOSIS
• Blood and urine tests.
• An ultrasound study of the kidneys may be performed to evaluate the size of the kidneys.
• A kidney biopsy may be performed. Under local anesthesia, the doctor inserts a needle into the kidney through the back to extract a small sample of tissue.

HOW TO TREAT IT
• Antihypertensive drugs may be prescribed to reduce high blood pressure.
• Diuretics may be prescribed to reduce excess fluid retention and increase urine production.
• Your doctor may advise you to eat a low-protein, low-salt diet and to take iron or vitamin supplements. (Do not take iron supplements without your doctor's approval.)
• In severe cases where kidney failure occurs, dialysis may be necessary. Dialysis performs the functions of the kidney by removing waste products and excess fluid from the blood when the kidney cannot (see Renal Failure, Chronic for more information).
• A kidney transplant is an alternative to dialysis in cases of kidney failure.

WHEN TO CALL A DOCTOR
• Call a doctor if you develop symptoms of chronic glomerulonephritis. ⚕

SYMPTOMS
• Blood or protein in the urine may be found on routine urinalysis.
• Swelling of the legs or ankles or other parts of the body, due to fluid accumulation (edema).
• Shortness of breath during exertion due to anemia.
• Headache or other symptoms of high blood pressure.
• In severe cases, symptoms of kidney failure, including fatigue; nausea and vomiting; loss of appetite; overall itching; headache; and impaired vision.

Goiter

WHAT IS IT?

A goiter is an enlargement or swelling of the thyroid, a gland in the throat that secretes a hormone which regulates body growth and metabolism. Goiters vary in size and, though sometimes unsightly, are generally painless. Rarely, a goiter may press against the trachea or esophagus, causing difficulty in breathing or swallowing. The disorder affects women four times more often than men.

WHAT CAUSES IT?

• A goiter is a common manifestation of Graves' disease (hyperthyroidism) and Hashimoto's thyroiditis, two serious thyroid disorders.
• Benign or malignant tumors of the thyroid gland may result in a goiter.
• Certain drugs designed to slow thyroid hormone production may cause goiters.
• Goiters may appear in women because of hormonal changes that occur with pregnancy.
• Goiters can be caused by insufficient amounts of iodine in the diet. This is now rare in the United States since the advent of iodized salt.

PREVENTION

• There is no known way to prevent goiter except in cases caused by a dietary insufficiency of iodine.

DIAGNOSIS

• Patient history and physical examination are needed.
• Blood tests, taken to evaluate the functional status of the thyroid gland, may also help to determine the underlying cause of the goiter.
• Thyroid scan with radioactive iodine or an ultrasound exam may be done.
• Fine-needle biopsy may be performed to rule out malignancy.

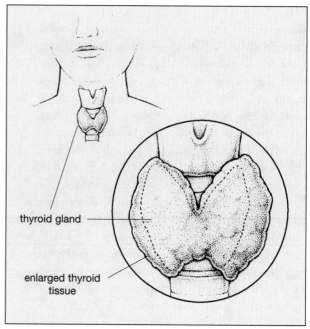

thyroid gland

enlarged thyroid tissue

Hyperthyroidism and other disorders affecting the butterfly-shaped thyroid in the neck can cause the gland to enlarge, resulting in a goiter.

HOW TO TREAT IT

• Thyroid-hormone-replacement therapy may ease the demand on the gland to produce thyroid hormone, which may cause it to decrease in size.
• Surgical removal of all or part of the thyroid may be necessary if the goiter is large, causes difficulty in breathing or swallowing, or is due to a malignant tumor.
• Your doctor may alter your prescription if the goiter is due to a medication.
• A diet that includes iodized salt and fish is advised in the unlikely event of iodine deficiency.

WHEN TO CALL A DOCTOR

• Call a doctor for any swelling in the neck. ▦

SYMPTOMS

• A swelling in the neck, ranging from a barely noticeable lump to a large growth.
• Difficulty in breathing or swallowing, or unexplained hoarseness (although these symptoms are rare).

Gonorrhea

WHAT IS IT?

Gonorrhea is a contagious bacterial infection, most commonly acquired through sexual contact with an infected partner. In men, the disease often infects the urethra (the conduit in the penis that carries urine and sperm) and may spread to other structures in the genitals or urinary tract. In women, gonorrhea usually infects the cervix but may eventually spread to other parts of the reproductive system (uterus and fallopian tubes), a condition known as pelvic inflammatory disease, which can lead to infertility. Less commonly, infections may occur in the throat, rectum, or eyes. Symptoms usually develop within two to 10 days after exposure, although many people, particularly women, experience no symptoms at all.

This disease generally strikes people between the ages of 18 and 30, particularly those who have had multiple sexual partners. Left untreated, the infection may spread via the bloodstream to the joints and tendons as well as to valves in the heart. Gonorrhea also increases the risk of HIV infection. With proper treatment, however, prognosis is excellent, although reinfection is common.

WHAT CAUSES IT?

• Gonorrhea is most often contracted via sexual contact, including anal, oral, and vaginal intercourse.
• An infected pregnant mother may transmit the disease to her baby during childbirth. This may cause blindness in the infant.
• Touching the eyes with contaminated hands can result in a gonococcal eye infection.

PREVENTION

• Abstinence or maintaining a monogamous sexual relationship are the only sure ways to prevent sexually transmitted gonorrhea.
• Men are advised to use a latex condom during sex.

DIAGNOSIS

• Diagnosis is confirmed by taking a culture or other diagnostic test of the discharge or infected tissue.

HOW TO TREAT IT

• A doctor will prescribe an antibiotic such as cefixime, ciprofloxacin, or ofloxacin. In addition, all people with gonorrhea should be treated for chlamydia, usually with azithromycin or doxycycline. Take antibiotics for the full term prescribed.
• Abstain from sexual activity until you are assured by your doctor that the infection is completely cured.
• Nonprescription pain relievers may be used to ease discomfort.
• Gonorrhea in the eye is treated with intravenous antibiotics as well as irrigation of the eye with an antibiotic solution.
• Sex partners should be referred for treatment.

WHEN TO CALL A DOCTOR

• See a doctor if you develop any of the symptoms of gonorrhea.
• If you discover that a sexual partner has gonorrhea, consult a doctor.

SYMPTOMS

• Pain during urination.
• Yellowish, puslike discharge from the penis or vagina.
• Rarely, pain during sexual intercourse.
• Redness or swelling at the infection site.
• Abnormal vaginal bleeding or lower abdominal pain in women (although these are rare).
• Sore throat (due to orally contracted infection); unusual rectal discharge or constant urge to move the bowels (anal infection).

Gout

WHAT IS IT?

Gout is a systemic disorder (that is, one potentially affecting the entire body), marked by elevated blood levels of uric acid, one of the body's waste products. This buildup in the blood can be caused by overproduction of uric acid, impaired excretion of it in the urine, or sometimes a combination of both. As it accumulates, uric acid may form crystals in the joints. Thus, gout is often first recognized by inflammation of a single joint. The immune system typically reacts to these crystals as if they were foreign invaders and releases substances that produce inflammation. The affected joint becomes swollen, red, warm, and severely painful. Often the first episode of gout affects the base of the big toe (this joint is eventually affected in 75 percent of patients).

Although symptoms gradually subside within a week, subsequent attacks are likely. These generally strike with no warning, occur with increasing frequency, and affect a number of joints, including the knees, elbows, wrists, and those of the hands and feet. Significantly elevated uric acid levels in the blood, if untreated, may result in kidney stones or deposition of uric acid in the kidneys, possibly causing kidney failure. About 90 percent of those affected with gout are adult men. In women, the disorder usually strikes after menopause.

WHAT CAUSES IT?

• Genetic factors are often involved; one in four gout sufferers has a family history of the disorder.
• A kidney malfunction may result in a buildup of uric acid and thus an attack of gout.
• Low doses of aspirin, certain antibiotics, diuretics, and alcohol may raise uric acid levels.
• Foods high in purines (like liver, anchovies, kidneys, and sweetbreads) may raise uric acid levels.

SYMPTOMS

• Sudden and severe pain in a joint, often the big toe.
• Swelling and redness around the affected joint.
• Fever (in some cases).
• Kidney stone symptoms.

• Obesity and high blood pressure are risk factors.
• Chemotherapy may raise uric acid levels as it rapidly destroys cells.

PREVENTION

• There is no way to prevent gout, but after the first attack, the risk of recurrences can be minimized.
• Daily doses of colchicine can reduce the frequency of episodes.
• Control your weight, but do not fast; fasting may raise uric acid levels.
• Avoid excessive alcohol consumption.
• If possible, medications that raise uric acid should be changed to others that do not.
• Several medications, including allopurinol (which blocks uric acid formation) and the drugs probenecid and sulfinpyrazone (which increase uric acid excretion in the urine), reduce uric acid levels.

DIAGNOSIS

• To confirm the diagnosis, fluid from the affected joint will be removed and analyzed for the presence of uric acid crystals and to rule out an infection.
• Blood samples will be taken and measured for uric acid levels.
• X-rays are taken to look for permanent joint damage in people with chronic gout.

HOW TO TREAT IT

• NSAIDs (nonsteroidal anti-inflammatory drugs) are the treatment of choice for gout.
• A doctor may prescribe colchicine to relieve pain and decrease swelling during an acute episode. The drug is taken hourly until symptoms subside or side effects (nausea, vomiting, cramps, diarrhea) begin.
• Your doctor may prescribe more powerful analgesics, including codeine or meperidine, for rapid relief of severe pain.
• Corticosteroids may be administered in pill form, intravenously, or by direct injections into the joint.
• Bed rest may be necessary. Make a small "tent" of the bedding to keep it from touching the affected area.

WHEN TO CALL A DOCTOR

• Call a doctor if you experience any of the symptoms of gout. ▲

Hammer Toe and Mallet Toe

WHAT IS IT?

A hammer toe is a deformity of the middle joint of a toe, producing a clenched, clawlike appearance in the affected digit. The tendons in the toe become abnormally contracted, causing the toe to bend downward, which, in turn, forces the joint to protrude upward. A mallet toe is a deformity in which the end joint of a toe becomes bent downward, so that the toe curls underneath itself. In either case the affected joints are stiff, and the toe cannot be straightened out. Constant rubbing against shoes may furthermore cause a painful corn (a round patch of rough, thickened, calloused skin) to develop over the joint or at the tip of the affected toe. Hammer and mallet toes may occur in any toe, although the second toe is the most common site. These deformities are often painful and limit the toe's range of motion—sometimes requiring surgery.

WHAT CAUSES IT?

• Wearing shoes that are too short or that have pointed toes may produce hammer toe.
• Long-term diabetes mellitus commonly causes nerve damage in the feet and so may lead to hammer toe.
• The cause of mallet toe is unknown.

PREVENTION

• Wear wide, comfortable shoes that have plenty of room for the toes.

DIAGNOSIS

• Examination of the affected toe is required.
• X-rays may be taken.

HOW TO TREAT IT

• Wear wide shoes with resilient soles. Avoid wearing shoes with pointed toes.
• Commercially available felt pads or cushions may ease pressure from the shoe on the toe. Toe caps (small, padded sleeves that fit around the tip of the toe) may relieve the pain of hammer toe.
• Arch supports or an orthotic shoe insert prescribed by your doctor or podiatrist may help to redistribute weight on the foot. These devices do not cure the problem but may ease the symptoms of either hammer toe or mallet toe.
• Surgery to realign the affected joint may be recommended if pain persists despite treatment.

WHEN TO CALL A DOCTOR

• Make an appointment with your doctor or a podiatrist if you experience continuing pain on account of a hammer toe or mallet toe, if the affected toe interferes with walking or other activities, or if the rubbing produces a sore or ulceration. ▲

SYMPTOMS

• A toe (usually the second digit, next to the big toe) bent at the middle joint and clenched into a painful, clawlike position (hammer toe). As the toe points downward, the middle joint may protrude upward.
• A toe with an end joint that curls under itself (mallet toe).
• Redness or a painful corn on top of the bent joint or at the tip of the affected toe, because of persistent rubbing against shoes.
• Pain in the toes that interferes with walking, jogging, dancing, and other normal activities, possibly leading to gait changes.

Headache, Cluster

WHAT IS IT?

Cluster headaches are characterized by sudden, intensely painful headaches occurring on one side of the head, centering around one eye. They tend to occur repeatedly, night after night, in periods or "clusters" of several weeks or months at a time. Pain usually appears one to three hours after falling asleep, during rapid eye movement (REM) sleep, and lasts for about an hour or more.

Clusters may be separated by symptom-free months or years. Rarely, cluster headaches may be chronic, lasting for several years. This disorder is four times more common in men than women and most commonly strikes between the ages of 20 and 40. Although cluster headaches may produce severe pain, they do not cause permanent harm (such as brain damage) and do not lead to other disorders.

SYMPTOMS

- Steady, intense pain around one eye, lasting from 30 minutes to two hours. Pain may spread to affect one entire side of the head.
- Nasal blockage on the affected side, later followed by profuse watery nasal discharge.
- Bloodshot, watery eye. Pupil may be constricted and eyelid may droop.
- Swollen cheek.
- Flushed face.

WHAT CAUSES IT?

- The cause of cluster headaches is unknown.
- Substances that may trigger headaches include alcohol, nicotine, and nitroglycerin (used in the treatment of angina).
- Certain foods have been implicated, specifically those containing tyramine. Such foods include pepperoni, red wine, chicken livers, active yeast preparations, and Camembert, cheddar, and other aged cheeses.
- Heavy smokers and drinkers are at greater risk for cluster headaches.
- Stress, overwork, or emotional duress may promote cluster headaches.

PREVENTION

- Avoid substances that appear to trigger headaches. Keep a detailed headache diary to help identify possible culprits. Keep a daily record of food and drink intake, activities, and the duration and severity of headaches.
- Avoid cigarettes and excessive alcohol consumption.

DIAGNOSIS

- Patient history and physical examination are needed.
- Tests may be performed to rule out sinusitis, glaucoma, cerebral aneurysm, or other disorders that may produce symptoms similar to those of cluster headaches.

HOW TO TREAT IT

- Do not lie down during an episode—this often worsens the pain.
- Standard over-the-counter pain relievers often work too slowly to relieve the pain of a cluster headache.
- Your doctor may prescribe inhalation of 100 percent oxygen for five to 15 minutes at the beginning of an episode to relieve pain.
- Your doctor may prescribe ergotamine tartrate, which may relieve pain at the first sign of a headache. A more effective approach is to prevent headaches by taking one of a number of different medications (steroids, anti-inflammatories, antidepressants, and antihypertensive drugs) throughout the duration of a cluster.
- Surgery to sever certain nerves near the site of the headaches may be recommended in severe cases that do not respond to other therapy. Surgery provides relief about two-thirds of the time but may have serious side effects, including muscle weakness and loss of sensation in some areas of the face.

WHEN TO CALL A DOCTOR

- Call a doctor immediately if you have never had a cluster headache, and you develop a sudden, intense headache centered on one eye. Other, more severe disorders may produce similar symptoms.
- Make an appointment with a doctor if your headaches are not responding to treatment.

Headache, Migraine

WHAT IS IT?

A migraine is a throbbing, intensely painful headache, usually beginning on one side of the head. It is sometimes preceded by distinct early warning symptoms, collectively called an aura. Incapacitating pain may last for up to two days, and the frequency of episodes may vary from several times a week to once every few years. Migraines afflict about 10 percent of the population, usually first appearing during childhood or adolescence, and are more common among women than men. The pain of a migraine usually moderates with age, but auras often continue to occur and may be confused with transient ischemic attack (TIA) or stroke (see TIA or Stroke for more information). There is no cure, but symptoms can be prevented or controlled with proper treatment.

WHAT CAUSES IT?

• The precise cause of migraines is unknown. One theory holds that abnormal constriction followed by dilation of arteries supplying the brain and scalp may be involved.
• Hereditary factors may play a role.
• Factors that may trigger migraines include: stress and overwork; relaxing periods following stressful ones (weekends, vacations); caffeine withdrawal; menstrual periods; oral contraceptives; vasodilating drugs; and exposure to bright lights or viewing certain visual patterns.
• Nitrites (such as are found in bacon and cured meats) and, possibly, foods containing the chemical tyramine (pepperoni, red wine, chicken livers, active yeast preparations, and cheddar and other aged cheeses) may trigger an attack.

PREVENTION

• Reduce stress and allow time for relaxation and recreation.
• Keep a daily record of food and drink intake to help identify possible triggers, and then avoid suspected items.
• Avoid oversleeping, which may lead to a migraine.

DIAGNOSIS

• Patient history and physical examination.
• Brain imaging (CT scan or MRI) is not necessary unless apparent migraine coexists with seizures, stroke, or vision problems upon neurological exam.

HOW TO TREAT IT

• Over-the-counter analgesics may be effective for mild attacks.
• Lying down in a dark, quiet room while symptoms last and using an ice pack on the forehead may be soothing.
• Medications, including ergotamine tartrate, dihydroergotamine, or sumatriptan and related drugs, may abort symptoms of a severe migraine if taken at the onset of the headache.
• Verapamil, propranolol or other beta-blockers, amitriptyline, and divalproex may prevent frequent recurrences.
• Relaxation training or biofeedback may be advised if stress is a trigger.

WHEN TO CALL A DOCTOR

• Call a doctor if headaches are severe, frequent, or persist for more than 24 hours, if there is a change in the pattern of your headaches, or if you experience speech difficulty.

SYMPTOMS

• Severe, throbbing pain, usually beginning on one side of the head, lasting up to two days.
• Nausea and vomiting.
• Sensitivity or aversion to light.
• Early warning symptoms (aura): temporary blind spots or blindness and other visual disturbances (such as seeing patterns of flashing lights); dizziness; numbness on one side of the face; weakness of an arm or leg; fatigue and listlessness.

Headache, Tension

WHAT IS IT?

Tension headaches, or stress headaches, are the most common type of headache in adults. They were so named because it was once theorized that tensing and stretching of the scalp and neck muscles caused the pain. However, it is now known that muscle tension itself does not cause such headaches (although it may exacerbate them). Such headaches are presumed to be the body's response to stress in a person's life, although the stress cannot always be identified. Precipitating stress is a factor in tension headache as well as in migraine (a severe form of headache). Tension headache symptoms may overlap with migraine, and in fact, people may suffer simultaneously from both tension headaches and migraines because both are so common (see Headache, Migraine, for more information). Pain and pressure from tension headaches may occur intermittently and last for hours at a time. Tension headaches most commonly affect people of middle age and older. Treatment is aimed at relieving symptoms.

WHAT CAUSES IT?

• The cause of tension headaches is unknown. However, certain conditions seem to be associated with the onset or worsening of a tension headache, including stress and fatigue; depression or anxiety; too little or too much sleep; a noisy environment; physically exhausting work; and eyestrain.
• Contrary to popular belief, mental concentration in itself does not cause headaches; eyestrain and poor posture from hunching over a desk are more likely culprits in such cases.
• Whether depression and anxiety are the cause or the result of chronic, unremitting tension headaches is controversial.

PREVENTION

• Get plenty of rest.
• Reduce stress; allow time in your schedule for regular exercise and relaxation.

DIAGNOSIS

• Patient history and the presence of symptoms suggest positive diagnosis.
• In severe or persistent cases, a doctor may perform vision tests or sinus x-ray. MRI or CT scan is not necessary unless a neurological exam is abnormal. Although brain tumor is often feared by patients, the chance that tension headache alone would be caused by a tumor is less than one in 10,000.

HOW TO TREAT IT

• Over-the-counter pain relievers (such as aspirin, ibuprofen, naproxen, or acetaminophen) may be taken as needed, according to label instructions.
• Massaging the muscles of the scalp and neck may help reduce pain.
• A hot bath may help relax muscles and ease the headache.
• A brief nap or even a rest in a dark, quiet room may be helpful.
• Relaxation training may be advised.
• Biofeedback—a technique in which the patient learns voluntary control over certain of the body's activities—may be used to treat tension headaches.
• Patients with continuous daily headaches over months or years usually have depression or anxiety. Antidepressant medications or tranquilizers may be prescribed.

WHEN TO CALL A DOCTOR

• Call a doctor if headache is severe, persists more than 24 hours, or is accompanied by other symptoms, such as fever, drowsiness, nausea and vomiting, blurred or double vision, or weakness. 🔺

SYMPTOMS

• Steady pain or pressure in the scalp, temples, or back of the head. Pain may be dull, intense, sharp, or diffuse, and persist for hours at a time.
• Pain or pressure that may feel like a constricting band encircling the head.
• Unlike migraines, which typically begin on only one side of the head, the pain of a tension headache involves both sides.
• Also unlike migraines, tension headaches do not cause nausea and vomiting or sensitivity to light (photophobia).

Heatstroke

WHAT IS IT?

Heatstroke is a medical emergency that occurs when overexposure to heat overwhelms the body's internal temperature-regulating mechanisms. Consequently, the protective sweating reflex ceases to function, even though evaporation of sweat on the skin's surface is one of the primary means for the dissipation of excess heat. Body temperature subsequently soars to dangerous heights (104°F or above—in some cases as high as 107°F). Unless emergency medical assistance is obtained promptly, shock, coma, brain damage, kidney failure, or even death may result. Infants and the elderly are at the greatest risk of severe consequences, but heatstroke may occur even in highly trained athletes.

WHAT CAUSES IT?

• Prolonged exposure to hot climates and high humidity.
• Dehydration or insufficient fluid intake.
• Electrolyte disturbances (imbalances in mineral salts, such as potassium, calcium, and magnesium).
• Impaired sweat gland function, which may be present at birth (congenital).
• Strenuous work, exercise, or sports participation in hot climates.
• Alcohol consumption and overeating increase risk.
• Risk is greater among older people (as internal temperature-regulating mechanisms become less responsive with age) and overweight people (as extra layers of body fat tend to retain heat).
• Certain medications, including diuretics and antihistamines, may increase risk of heatstroke.
• Heart disease and diabetes are risk factors.
• A recent dehydrating illness (one that involved excessive vomiting or diarrhea) increases susceptibility.

PREVENTION

• In hot, humid weather, increase fluid intake, wear light clothing, take frequent cool baths, try to remain in a cool (preferably air-conditioned) environment, and avoid alcohol and strenuous activity. These recommendations are especially important for the elderly, the chronically ill, or the very young.
• The body gradually adjusts to hotter climates over a period of one to three weeks. When the weather changes or you travel to warmer environs, spend increasingly longer amounts of time in the heat, followed by periods of rest in cool conditions to promote full acclimatization.

DIAGNOSIS

• Suspect heatstroke when confusion or altered behavior develops after exposure to a hot environment, especially after exertion.
• Urine and blood tests may be performed to determine a heatstroke victim's degree of dehydration.

HOW TO TREAT IT

• Heatstroke is an emergency: summon professional medical assistance at once.
• While waiting for emergency help to arrive, move the patient into a shady area or, ideally, a room with air conditioning. Elevate his or her feet. Loosen or remove clothing. Sponge the person with cold water or place in a cool bath. Offer cool liquids only if the person is awake and can drink normally.
• Professional treatment involves controlled, gradual cooling of the patient, fluid and electrolyte replacement (via oral or intravenous delivery), and tranquilizers to control seizures.

WHEN TO CALL A DOCTOR

• **EMERGENCY** Call an ambulance if signs of heatstroke develop.

SYMPTOMS

• Body temperature of over 104°F.
• Headaches, dizziness.
• Hot, dry, red skin; appears gray in later stages.
• Conspicuous absence of sweating, despite high body temperature. (Profuse sweating may occur initially, then cease as the body's temperature-regulating mechanisms break down.)
• Rapid heartbeat.
• Shallow and rapid breathing.
• Dilated pupils.
• Muscle cramps.
• Confusion, delirium, or stupor, progressing to seizures or loss of consciousness.

Hemochromatosis

WHAT IS IT?

Hemochromatosis, or iron overload, is a disorder resulting from an excessive accumulation of iron in the liver, pancreas, heart, testes, and other organs. It is usually caused by a genetic abnormality found in one of every 200 to 300 people, but may also be brought on by excessive iron intake, either in the diet or through blood transfusions. Symptoms often do not appear until late middle age, but by the time they do appear, the disease may be very advanced.

Excess iron in the pancreas may lead to diabetes mellitus, while excess iron in the liver may lead to cirrhosis of the liver, liver cancer, and liver failure. Untreated hemochromatosis may also lead to congestive heart failure. The gene for the disease is recessive, meaning that both parents must carry it for a child to have a chance of developing it. Men from high-risk families are 10 times more likely to develop the disease than women because men have a greater iron intake (they consume more food), and because women lose iron through menstruation. Boys from high-risk families should be tested at the onset of puberty, and girls before age 20.

WHAT CAUSES IT?

• Most cases are caused by a genetic abnormality resulting in excess iron absorption.
• The use of iron supplements or iron cookware does not lead to iron overload, except in those who are genetically predisposed.
• Excessive alcohol intake can worsen the liver damage caused by hemochromatosis.
• Patients with certain types of anemia may accumulate excessive iron from repeated blood transfusions (secondary hemochromatosis).

PREVENTION

• Early detection and treatment are essential for staving off symptoms and complications.
• If you are at risk for hemochromatosis, limit your intake of foods high in iron, such as liver, red meats, and iron-enriched breads and cereals, and do not take iron supplements unless advised by your doctor.

DIAGNOSIS

• Tests measuring the blood levels of iron can suggest the diagnosis.
• A family history of the disorder is often present.
• CT (computer tomography) scans or MRI (magnetic resonance imaging) may reveal organ abnormalities, which help determine the disorder's severity.
• A liver biopsy (removal of a tissue sample for microscopic examination) is the most definitive test.

HOW TO TREAT IT

• Periodic withdrawal of blood (phlebotomy) is necessary to rid the body of excess iron. This may be needed weekly for several years in severe cases; when iron stores have been reduced to normal, phlebotomy is required only three or four times a year.
• Testosterone therapy may be administered to men to correct loss of sexual desire and changes in secondary sexual traits.
• A diet low in iron-rich foods may be advised, although a completely iron-free diet is not necessary.
• Administration of the medication deferoxamine is required to remove iron in patients with secondary hemochromatosis.

WHEN TO CALL A DOCTOR

• Call a doctor if you develop symptoms of hemochromatosis.
• Schedule diagnostic screening for hemochromatosis if you have a family history of it.

SYMPTOMS

• Changes in skin coloration (possibly a bronze or slate-gray appearance) due to increased melanin and iron deposits in the skin.
• Symptoms of chronic liver disease, including abdominal enlargement and pain.
• Joint pain.
• Drowsiness, weakness, and lethargy.
• In men, a decrease in the size of the testes, loss of sexual desire, and impotence.
• Symptoms of congestive heart failure, such as shortness of breath, irregular heartbeat, and swelling of the feet.
• Excessive thirst and urination and other symptoms of diabetes (see Diabetes Mellitus).

Hemophilia

WHAT IS IT?

Hemophilia is a common inherited blood coagulation disorder, in which one of the factors needed to clot the blood is lacking. It affects nearly one out of every 10,000 males. (Females may inherit the gene and be carriers for the disease, but are otherwise unaffected.) Outcome varies; the lower the amount of coagulation factors, the more severe the disease. Mild hemophilia may go undiagnosed until adulthood when prolonged bleeding occurs following surgery or an injury; moderate cases may be associated with bouts of uncontrolled bleeding; severe cases are marked by frequent episodes of bleeding into the joints and soft tissues.

The development of hematomas—accumulations of blood inside an organ, muscle, soft tissue, or body cavity—can cause potentially serious secondary symptoms. For example, bleeding into the brain may cause severe headaches, personality changes, paralysis, coma, or even death. About half of all hemophiliacs experience bleeding into the joints, resulting in arthritis-like symptoms. Also, because hemophiliacs often require numerous transfusions of blood products, they are at increased risk for blood-borne infections such as hepatitis or AIDS, although such risks have diminished due to improvements in the methods of blood-product preparation and the screening of donated blood. With current medical treatment and vigilant self-care, even patients with severe hemophilia may live relatively normal lives.

SYMPTOMS

- Frequent and extensive bruises.
- Prolonged bleeding that may not occur until several days after an injury or a procedure such as tooth extraction.
- Spontaneous bleeding for no apparent reason.
- Painful uncontrolled bleeding into joints or muscles, causing swelling, tenderness, and possibly deformity. Joint pain may precede external evidence of bleeding.
- Blood in the urine or stool.
- Headache, paralysis, or coma from bleeding into the brain.

WHAT CAUSES IT?

- Hemophilia A, accounting for 80 percent of cases, results from genetic deficiency of Factor VIII, also known as antihemophilic factor. Hemophilia B results from a deficiency in Factor IX. Both factors are necessary for normal blood coagulation. Because the genes for the factors are carried on the X chromosomes, hemophilia only affects males; women may be carriers and pass the disorder to their offspring.

PREVENTION

- There is no way to prevent hemophilia, although those with a family history of it may benefit from genetic counseling when considering having a child.

DIAGNOSIS

- Patient history (including family history) and physical examination are necessary.
- Blood tests are taken to measure clotting time and blood levels of Factors VIII and IX.

HOW TO TREAT IT

- Avoiding activities that carry a high risk of injury as well as medications (such as aspirin) that promote bleeding is recommended.
- A bleeding episode can be stopped by intravenous infusion of the missing coagulation factor. Factor VIII can often be administered by the patient himself; early treatment is best.
- Regular preventive doses of clotting factors may be taken in severe cases, but such treatment is very expensive and may induce antibody formation. Patients on a home care regimen require clinical evaluation every six months to a year.
- Episodes of uncontrollable bleeding require hospitalization and prolonged infusions of the missing clotting factor.
- Physical therapy may be advised to rehabilitate damaged joints. Activities such as swimming are encouraged; contact sports should be avoided.
- In 10 to 15 percent of patients, development of an inhibitor to Factor VIII renders treatment ineffective.

WHEN TO CALL A DOCTOR

- See a doctor if you have a bout of uncontrolled bleeding. ▲

Hemorrhoids

WHAT IS IT?

Hemorrhoids (also called piles) are distended varicose veins in the anus. All veins are lined with valves
that permit blood to flow in only one direction
(back to the heart). Excess pressure on these valves
can cause them to weaken and fail, allowing blood
to flow in the wrong direction or to stagnate. The
vein may engorge with blood, which, in the anus,
results in a hemorrhoid.

Although hemorrhoids are often painless, the
swollen wall of the vein is fragile and thus is prone
to rupture and bleeding. Stagnant blood promotes
formation of clots in the vein, which are typically
painful and, in severe cases, may require surgery.
Hemorrhoids usually affect people between the ages
of 20 and 50 and are especially common in those
who are constipated, pregnant, or obese, owing to
increased pressure within the veins of the lower
abdomen.

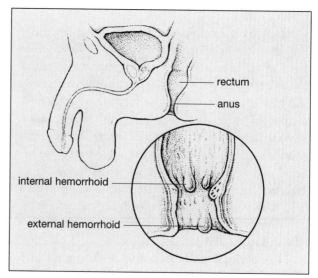

External hemorrhoids affect veins in or near the anal opening; internal
hemorrhoids are located farther up, in the rectum.

WHAT CAUSES IT?

• Straining during bowel movements is a primary
cause. (A diet low in fiber can result in constipation,
which in turn encourages the tendency to strain
during bowel movements.)
• Pregnancy, childbirth, and obesity increase the risk
of hemorrhoids.
• Prolonged standing or sitting may be causes.
• Loss of muscle tone due to old age, an episiotomy,
or rectal surgery can promote hemorrhoids.

PREVENTION

• A high-fiber diet including fresh fruit, vegetables,
and whole-grain breads and cereals is recommended.
• Drink plenty of water.
• Don't strain during bowel movements or stay on
the toilet longer than necessary.

SYMPTOMS

• Bright red blood on the toilet paper, the stool,
  or in the toilet bowl after a bowel movement.
• Pain, especially during bowel movements.
• Anal itching.
• Mucus discharge from the anus.

DIAGNOSIS

• Patient history and examination of the anus and
rectum are necessary. A doctor may detect internal
hemorrhoids with a special scope.
• Barium enema x-rays may be ordered.

HOW TO TREAT IT

• Wash the anal area gently but thoroughly after each
bowel movement, using a soft tissue and warm
water. To dry, dab (don't scrub) the area with a soft
cloth.
• For external hemorrhoids, apply an ice compress.
• Frequent warm baths or sitz baths can relieve mild
symptoms of pain and itching.
• Anesthetic ointment and topical corticosteroids
(such as hydrocortisone) may ease pain and swelling.
• An injection of a solution that turns the hemorrhoid to scar tissue may be used (sclerotherapy).
• Some hemorrhoids may be tied off using a rubber
band (rubber band ligation).
• In severe cases surgical removal (hemorrhoidec-
tomy) may be necessary.

WHEN TO CALL A DOCTOR

• If you experience rectal bleeding or if hemorrhoids
do not improve with home treatment, see a doctor. ▲

Hepatitis, Acute Viral

WHAT IS IT?

Acute viral hepatitis is the most common of the serious infectious diseases of the liver. It is caused by several types of viruses that produce inflammation of the liver. Infection with hepatitis A virus usually results in complete recovery and immunity to future type A infection. The symptoms of hepatitis B, a more serious infection, are usually more severe and persistent (although all types of viral hepatitis may be symptomless). Hepatitis C (formerly known as non-A, non-B hepatitis) is the most common cause of chronic hepatitis. Hepatitis E is similar to type A but is only found near the Indian Ocean, and hepatitis D only infects people already infected with type B.

Although there is no specific treatment for these disorders, most patients recover over time. Some people become carriers of hepatitis B, C, or D—that is, they remain infectious long after all symptoms have cleared. In some cases, both hepatitis B and hepatitis C may lead to chronic hepatitis, cirrhosis, and liver cancer.

WHAT CAUSES IT?

• Viruses cause acute hepatitis.
• Hepatitis A and E are spread by contact with the fecal matter of an infected person, via contaminated fingers, food, or water.
• Raw shellfish from polluted waters may cause hepatitis A.
• Hepatitis B, C, and D may be spread by exposure to contaminated blood (both fresh and dried) on infected needles, during a blood transfusion, or during sexual intercourse.

SYMPTOMS

• General discomfort.
• Fever.
• Fatigue.
• Loss of appetite.
• Nausea and vomiting.
• Aching muscles or joints.
• Abdominal discomfort or pain.
• Jaundice (yellowish tinge to the eyes and skin).
• Dark urine and pale stools.

• Hepatitis B or C may be transmitted to an infant at childbirth by an infected mother.

PREVENTION

• Hepatitis types A and B vaccines are advised prior to traveling to areas where hepatitis infection rates are high. Type B vaccine is also recommended for all children and adults in high-risk categories, such as health-care workers, people with multiple sexual partners, and renal dialysis patients.
• Wash your hands with warm water and soap after a bowel movement or before handling food, especially if you have hepatitis A or E or if you are caring for someone with the infection. (Because hepatitis is contagious for weeks before symptoms develop, people may carry and spread the disease without realizing it.)
• When traveling abroad or in areas with poor sanitation, drink only bottled water or other bottled beverages and eat only cooked foods and fruit you can peel yourself.
• Use condoms during sexual intercourse to help prevent the spread of hepatitis B. Avoid intimate contact with infected persons if possible.
• Sterile or disposable needles should be used in acupuncture, ear piercing, or tattooing. Ask about sterilization procedures in advance.

DIAGNOSIS

• Blood tests for the virus or antibodies to the virus are taken.

HOW TO TREAT IT

• Avoid alcoholic beverages during recovery.
• Rest as needed.
• Increase caloric intake. Several small meals daily rather than a few large ones may help combat nausea and loss of appetite.
• In severe cases, temporary intravenous feeding may be necessary.

WHEN TO CALL A DOCTOR

• Call a doctor if you develop symptoms of acute viral hepatitis.
• Call a doctor if you have been exposed to someone known to have acute viral hepatitis.

Hepatitis, Chronic

WHAT IS IT?

Chronic hepatitis is characterized by ongoing inflammation of the liver and destruction (necrosis) of liver cells that persists for more than six to 12 months. Symptoms may be mild or vague. Chronic hepatitis may progress slowly and can subside spontaneously over months or even years. In some patients, it can be a more dangerous condition because the destruction of liver cells results in the development of scar tissue in the liver (cirrhosis) and may ultimately lead to liver failure. However, for some patients, therapy can cure the disease or retard its progression.

WHAT CAUSES IT?

• An acute infection of hepatitis B or C may develop into chronic hepatitis.
• Years of excessive alcohol consumption may lead to chronic hepatitis.
• Autoimmune disorders (in which the immune system attacks body tissues) and, rarely, metabolic disorders (such as iron accumulation in the liver or Wilson's disease, in which excess amounts of copper are stored in the liver; see Wilson's disease for more information) may be causes.
• In rare instances some medications, such as dantrolene, nitrofurantoin, and the sulfonamides, may lead to chronic hepatitis, as may long-term use of aspirin.
• In some cases the cause is unknown.

PREVENTION

• Consume no more than two alcoholic drinks a day. If you suspect that you may have a drinking problem, seek help at once.
• A hepatitis B vaccination is recommended for those at high risk, such as health-care workers, and before traveling to areas where hepatitis is common.

DIAGNOSIS

• Patient history and physical examination.
• Specific blood tests for hepatitis B and C.
• A liver biopsy (removal of a tissue sample for microscopic examination) is almost always necessary for an accurate diagnosis.

HOW TO TREAT IT

• Do not consume alcoholic beverages.
• Corticosteroids, with or without an immunosuppressant drug such as azathioprine, may be prescribed to treat cases of autoimmune chronic hepatitis.
• Alpha-interferon sometimes in combination with ribavirin may be prescribed to treat chronic hepatitis caused by the hepatitis B or C virus.
• Your doctor may change your prescription(s) to relieve hepatitis caused by medications.
• Lifelong treatment of any underlying metabolic disorder (such as Wilson's disease) is necessary.
• Liver transplantation may be recommended when the liver has been severely damaged.

WHEN TO CALL A DOCTOR

• Call a doctor if you develop symptoms of chronic hepatitis.
• Call a doctor if you have had jaundice or an acute hepatitis infection and symptoms persist despite treatment.

SYMPTOMS
• General discomfort.
• Fatigue.
• Loss of appetite.
• Nausea and vomiting.
• Jaundice (yellowish tinge to the eyes and skin).
• Small, red, spidery veins on the surface of the skin (spider telangiectasias).
• Pain or tenderness in the upper right abdomen.
• Abdominal swelling caused by fluid accumulation (when cirrhosis develops).
• Fever.
• In women (especially when autoimmune chronic hepatitis is involved): cessation of menstruation (amenorrhea), acne, the appearance of male-pattern facial hair (hirsutism), and joint pain.

Herpes Zoster Shingles

WHAT IS IT?

Herpes zoster, also known as shingles, is a disorder caused by varicella zoster, the same virus that causes chicken pox. After an attack of chicken pox, usually a childhood disease, the virus does not die but rather lies dormant in the nerve cells that extend from the spinal cord or the brain. Years later, the virus may be reactivated and migrate along the path of a nerve to the surface of the skin, where it causes a rash of painful blisters. While it is generally not a dangerous condition, shingles can be extremely painful and often causes lingering nerve pain (postherpetic neuralgia) for months or even years after the rash is gone. This disorder only affects those who have previously had chicken pox and usually strikes after the age of 50. Usually only one attack occurs, lasting for two or three weeks. Outlook is good unless the virus spreads to the brain or spinal cord.

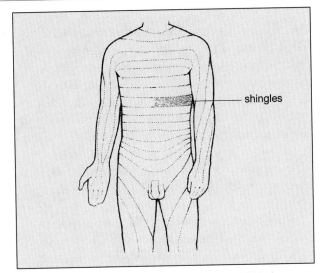

shingles

The lines demarcate the regions of skin supplied by individual nerves branching from the spinal cord. When shingles strikes, the rash is usually confined to one of these narrow bands.

WHAT CAUSES IT?

• How or why shingles occurs is uncertain. It is believed that the virus reactivates when the immune system—owing to age, illness, stress, or the use of immunosuppressant drugs—becomes too weak to keep the virus in a state of dormancy. Indeed, immunosuppressed patients (those with disorders such as Hodgkin's disease or treated with immuno-suppressive drugs) are at increased risk for shingles.

PREVENTION

• There is no known way to prevent herpes zoster.

SYMPTOMS

• In early stages, a sensation of tingling followed by pain (often accompanied by fever and headache), preceding the development of the rash by several days.
• Severe pain and itching in a bandlike rash of small, red, fluid-filled blisters on one side of the torso, arms, legs, or face lasting from about one to four weeks. About 10 days after their appearance, blisters dry up into scabs.
• Pain that persists for months or years after skin lesions have healed (postherpetic neuralgia).

DIAGNOSIS

• Appearance of typical skin lesions and a prior history of chicken pox or shingles indicate herpes zoster.
• A culture of the skin lesions may be taken to confirm the diagnosis.

HOW TO TREAT IT

• Apply cool, wet compresses or ice packs.
• Use over-the-counter pain relievers.
• Calamine lotion and oatmeal or cornstarch baths can help relieve itching.
• During the early stages, acyclovir, an antiviral drug, may stem progression of the rash and speed healing.
• Medications that impede nerve impulses, such as carbamazepine, gabapentin, and amitriptyline, may be used for more serious cases of postherpetic neuralgia.
• In the most severe or persistent cases, injections of blocking agents directly into nerves may be used to prevent pain signals from reaching the brain.

WHEN TO CALL A DOCTOR

• Call a doctor if you develop symptoms of shingles.
• See a doctor or ophthalmologist immediately if herpes zoster is accompanied by eye pain.

Hydrocele

WHAT IS IT?

A hydrocele is a fluid-filled swelling around one or both testicles. Each testicle is surrounded by a two-layered sheath or sac (not to be confused with the scrotum, the pouch of skin in which the testicles hang). The small amount of lubricating fluid that is normally present between the layers of the sheath allows the testicles to move freely. If too much fluid is produced, or too little is absorbed, an excess amount may accumulate between the two sheath layers, forming a hydrocele. (A hydrocele is thus not an enlargement of the testicle itself.)

This disorder is more common among men of middle age or older. However, some young boys may have a hydrocele associated with an inguinal hernia, a localized protrusion of a portion of the abdominal lining, located in the channel where the testicles descended from the abdomen. In these cases the channel did not close properly after descent of the testicles, and excess fluid may leak into the hydrocele sac from the abdominal lining. In rare cases hydroceles are associated with testicular cancer. Hydroceles seldom cause pain, and, in adult men, require treatment only when the swelling causes discomfort.

SYMPTOMS
• A soft, painless swelling in the scrotum.

WHAT CAUSES IT?

• In most cases the cause of a hydrocele is unknown, but overproduction or decreased absorption of the normal cushioning fluid appears to be involved.
• Injury to the testicles may lead to a hydrocele.
• An inguinal hernia may produce a hydrocele in young boys.

PREVENTION

• There is no known way to prevent hydrocele.
• Regular self-examination of the testes aids in early diagnosis and treatment of any abnormalities (see Testicular Cancer for more information on performing a self-examination).

DIAGNOSIS

• The doctor will gently palpate the testicles to determine the size and consistency of any lumps.
• The doctor may shine a bright light on the scrotum to determine the nature of the swelling. Because hydroceles are composed of watery fluid, they are relatively transparent and allow the light to shine through. (A tumor or other mass would appear opaque.)
• An ultrasound examination may confirm the diagnosis.

HOW TO TREAT IT

• In young boys, surgery (through a small incision in the abdomen) to close the inguinal hernia eliminates the cause of the hydrocele.
• Excess fluid may be removed with a needle and syringe (needle aspiration) under local anesthesia; however, with this method the hydrocele tends to recur. Needle aspiration also carries the risk of infection.
• In adult men, surgery (through a small incision in the scrotum) may be used to tighten or remove the testicle sheaths and permanently eliminate a hydrocele.

WHEN TO CALL A DOCTOR

• Call a doctor if you notice an unusual growth or swelling in the testicles. While a hydrocele is not a health risk, an examination by a doctor is warranted to rule out more serious disorders.

Hydrocephalus

WHAT IS IT?

Hydrocephalus is an uncommon disorder involving the overaccumulation of cerebrospinal fluid (CSF) in the fluid-filled spaces, or ventricles, within the brain. CSF is secreted into the ventricles, circulates around the brain tissue, and is then absorbed by tiny finger-like projections from the membranes surrounding the brain. If the flow of CSF is blocked, or if a defect interferes with fluid reabsorption, pressure increases upon the brain. Newborns and the elderly are most susceptible to this disorder. In infants, increased CSF pressure forces the soft bones of the head apart, producing an abnormally large head. The onset of hydrocephalus may be sudden or gradual; in either case it can cause permanent brain damage in all age groups, so prompt treatment is essential.

WHAT CAUSES IT?

• In infants, causes include congenital malformations, injury during birth, bacterial meningitis, and viral infections.
• In both children and adults, causes include brain hemorrhage and brain tumor.
• In adults, causes include head injury and meningitis (an inflammation of the membranes surrounding the brain due to infection).
• In adults, the cause is sometimes unknown.

PREVENTION

• There is no known way to prevent hydrocephalus.

SYMPTOMS

• Abnormal enlargement of the head (in infants).
• Projectile vomiting (in infants).
• Convulsions or seizures (in infants).
• Severe headache.
• Loss of appetite.
• Mental confusion and deterioration, including irritability, loss of memory, anxiety, paranoia, apathy, impaired judgment, or speech disturbances.
• Unsteadiness when walking.
• Urinary incontinence.

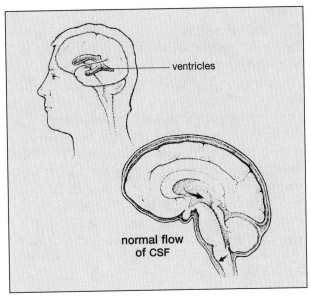

Cerebrospinal fluid (CSF) is produced in the ventricles deep within the brain and then flows into the spaces around the brain and spinal cord. Hydrocephalus is marked by blockage of the normal flow of CSF and consequential enlargement of the ventricles.

DIAGNOSIS

• The circumference of a newborn's head is measured at birth. Enlargement suggests hydrocephalus.
• X-rays, CT (computed tomography) scans, and MRI (magnetic resonance imaging) of the skull.
• Lumbar puncture (spinal tap).

HOW TO TREAT IT

• Surgical insertion of a drainage tube, or shunt, is necessary to circumvent blockage or to drain excess CSF in both children and adults. The shunt allows excess CSF to flow into a vein in the neck, and thus into the bloodstream, or the abdominal cavity, where it is reabsorbed. The shunt is usually permanent. If placed in an infant, the shunt must be periodically replaced as the child grows.

WHEN TO CALL A DOCTOR

• Symptoms of hydrocephalus warrant immediate medical attention to prevent or minimize potential brain damage.
• **EMERGENCY** Call a doctor immediately if a child with a shunt for hydrocephalus exhibits vomiting, irritability, or convulsions. These may be signs of shunt malfunction. ▲

Hypercholesterolemia High Cholesterol

WHAT IS IT?

Hypercholesterolemia is a disorder characterized by high levels of blood cholesterol. Cholesterol is manufactured primarily in the liver and then carried to the cells throughout the body by low-density lipoprotein (LDL). (Because cholesterol and other fats do not dissolve in water, they cannot travel through the body unaided. Lipoproteins are particles formed in the liver to transport cholesterol and other fats through the bloodstream.) Cholesterol is returned to the liver from other body cells by another lipoprotein, high-density lipoprotein (HDL). From there, cholesterol is secreted into the bile, either unchanged or after conversion to bile acids.

Cholesterol is essential for the formation of cell membranes and the manufacture of some hormones, but it is not required from the diet because the liver produces all the cholesterol the body needs. If blood cholesterol levels are elevated, large amounts of LDL (so-called "bad") cholesterol deposit in the arterial walls. These deposits represent the first stage of atherosclerosis, or narrowing of the arteries. Because hypercholesterolemia causes no symptoms, preventive measures and regular measurement of cholesterol levels are important for people in high-risk categories. Hypercholesterolemia is especially dangerous when HDL ("good") cholesterol levels are low. Left untreated, hypercholesterolemia can eventually lead to a heart attack due to coronary artery disease or a stroke due to narrowed arteries supplying the brain.

WHAT CAUSES IT?

• Hereditary factors are the most common cause.
• A diet high in saturated fat and cholesterol increases blood cholesterol levels.

SYMPTOMS

• Unfortunately, the only symptoms (angina, heart attack, stroke) result from the complications of high cholesterol. When cholesterol levels are very high, cholesterol may be deposited as yellow nodules (xanthomas) in tendons or just beneath the skin under the eyes.

• Other disorders, such as diabetes mellitus, Cushing's syndrome, and hypothyroidism, may promote hypercholesterolemia.

PREVENTION

• Eat a diet low in saturated fats and cholesterol. A diet rich in water-soluble fiber tends to lower blood cholesterol.
• Exercise regularly, and try to lose weight if you are more than 20 percent overweight.
• Drink alcoholic beverages in moderation—no more than two a day. Moderate alcohol consumption raises levels of beneficial HDL cholesterol; however, consumption of more alcohol than this amount can have harmful effects.

DIAGNOSIS

• Patient history and physical examination.
• Measurement of blood levels of cholesterol, triglycerides, and HDL cholesterol.

HOW TO TREAT IT

• Lifestyle changes alone are frequently all that is necessary (see Prevention).
• Medications specifically designed to reduce blood cholesterol levels, such as cholestyramine, colestipol, statins (lovastatin, pravastatin, simvastatin, fluvastatin, atorvastatin, and cerivastatin), or niacin, may be prescribed when dietary modifications prove inadequate.
• In rare cases in which cholesterol levels are extremely high (familial hypercholesterolemia), repeated removal of blood plasma may be recommended to lower blood cholesterol levels.

WHEN TO CALL A DOCTOR

• Make an appointment with your doctor to check your cholesterol levels if you are at high risk for coronary artery disease or if any member of your immediate family has hypercholesterolemia.

Hyperparathyroidism

WHAT IS IT?

Hyperparathyroidism is marked by overactivity of one or more of the parathyroid glands, the four pea-size glands embedded in the corners of the thyroid gland at the base of the neck. These glands produce parathyroid hormone (PTH), a chemical that, along with vitamin D and calcitonin (a hormone manufactured in the thyroid gland), regulates blood calcium levels. Excess PTH due to hyperparathyroidism results in unusually high levels of blood calcium (hypercalcemia), most of which is released from the calcium stores in the bones. Eventually, calcium loss may lead to weakened bones (see Osteomalacia for more information).

Excess calcium in the blood may also lead to calcinosis—the deposition of calcium salts in various body tissues, including the kidneys, skin, tendons, and cartilage—resulting in kidney disorders, arthritis, or other problems. The kidneys excrete large amounts of calcium in the urine, which can, over time, cause kidney stones or renal damage. Two other problems associated with hyperparathyroidism are peptic ulcers and pancreatitis. In many cases, hyperparathyroidism causes few if any symptoms and is only discovered during a routine blood test. However, a sudden attack of severe hypercalcemia can be a life-threatening emergency. This relatively rare disorder is most common among women over age 40.

SYMPTOMS

- Generalized discomfort.
- Muscle aches or weakness; arthritic joint pain.
- Heartbeat irregularities.
- Constipation, nausea, vomiting, loss of appetite, weight loss.
- Fatigue, lethargy, confusion, depression, psychosis, or other mental changes, possibly resulting in coma (due to hypercalcemia).
- Increased thirst and urine output (due to kidney involvement).
- Frequent or unexplained bone fractures.
- Chronic low back pain or upper abdominal pain (due to peptic ulcer or pancreatitis).
- Kidney stones.

WHAT CAUSES IT?

- Most often, a benign tumor (adenoma) on one or more of the parathyroid glands is the cause. (Hyperparathyroidism may run in families with a history of multiple endocrine tumors, such as those of the pituitary or pancreas.)
- The disorder may be due to generalized enlargement (hyperplasia) of all four parathyroid glands.
- Other disorders, including chronic renal failure and vitamin D deficiency (rickets), can cause secondary hyperparathyroidism by lowering blood calcium levels. The parathyroids then secrete excessive amounts of PTH to return blood calcium levels to normal.
- Long-term use of certain drugs such as laxatives and the anticonvulsant phenytoin may play a role.

PREVENTION

- There is no way to prevent hyperparathyroidism.

DIAGNOSIS

- Patient history and physical examination are needed.
- Calcium levels in the urine are measured.
- High blood levels of calcium and low levels of phosphorous indicate primary hyperparathyroidism.
- Measuring blood levels of PTH confirms diagnosis.
- Bone densitometry may be taken to assess bone loss.

HOW TO TREAT IT

- In cases producing no obvious symptoms, careful, regular monitoring may be all that is required.
- High fluid intake is recommended in patients with high levels of calcium in their blood or urine.
- In symptomatic cases, surgical removal of abnormal parathyroid tissue usually cures the disorder. If more than one gland is enlarged or if the parathyroid abnormal growth cannot be located, all but half of one of the four parathyroid glands may be removed. (The remaining parathyroid tissue may produce insufficient amounts of PTH, requiring treatment for hypoparathyroidism.) Surgery is indicated if blood calcium levels are too high or if there is evidence of bone or kidney damage.

WHEN TO CALL A DOCTOR

- See a doctor for regular checkups or if you experience symptoms of hyperparathyroidism.

Hyperprolactinemia

WHAT IS IT?

Hyperprolactinemia is a disorder marked by the overproduction of prolactin (one of eight hormones produced by the pituitary gland) in both men and nonpregnant women. Affecting about 1 percent of the general population—but nearly 25 percent of women with amenorrhea (absent menses)—it is the most common form of overproduction of hormones by the pituitary (hyperpituitarism).

The pituitary, a peanut-size organ located at the base of the brain, is the most important gland in the body's endocrine, or hormonal, system. Prolactin induces milk production in women following birth, so levels are high in pregnant women. Although the hormone is also present in small quantities in men and nonpregnant women, elevated levels in these individuals can signal a pituitary tumor and cause other serious problems, such as infertility. Hyperprolactinemia should be evaluated by your doctor.

WHAT CAUSES IT?

• A benign pituitary tumor (adenoma or prolactinoma) is the most common cause of abnormal prolactin overproduction.
• Prolactin levels are typically kept in check by the neurotransmitter dopamine, a substance produced in the brain by the hypothalamus. Decreased dopamine levels, due to a disease of the hypothalamus or a dopamine-blocking drug (such as MAO inhibitors and some antipsychotic drugs), may lead to increased levels of prolactin.
• Many other drugs can raise prolactin levels.

SYMPTOMS

• In women: cessation of menstrual periods (amenorrhea), decreased menstrual flow (oligomenorrhea), abnormal production of breast milk when not breastfeeding (galactorrhea), excess facial hair (hirsutism).
• In men: impotence, infertility, decreased libido, and rarely, enlarged breasts (gynecomastia) and galactorrhea.
• Headaches and impaired vision may occur as tumor growth exerts pressure within the skull.

• High-dose estrogen (such as oral contraceptives, but not estrogen replacement therapy) can raise blood prolactin levels.
• People with an underactive thyroid (see Hypothyroidism) may have elevated levels of prolactin.
• Chronic kidney failure or cirrhosis (see Cirrhosis) may be associated with hyperprolactinemia.

PREVENTION

• There is no way to prevent prolactin-producing pituitary tumors.

DIAGNOSIS

• Patient history and physical examination (including an evaluation of thyroid, kidney, and liver function).
• Blood tests to measure elevated levels of prolactin.
• MRI (magnetic resonance imaging) to detect a pituitary tumor.

HOW TO TREAT IT

• Treatment for hyperprolactinemia depends on the cause and the severity of the disorder. In some patients, prolactin levels spontaneously revert to normal. Some pituitary tumors may be small enough that treatment is not required, although regular follow-up evaluations are necessary.
• When the disorder is caused by a tumor, the first line of treatment is medication, either bromocriptine or cabergoline. Pergolide may be used as a second-line agent. Therapy may even shrink the tumor. Levels of prolactin usually fall within days of beginning therapy.
• If medication is not tolerated or is unsuccessful in reducing the size of a tumor and lowering prolactin levels adequately, surgical removal may be required.
• Treatment for causes other than tumors varies. Your doctor will determine the appropriate therapy.

WHEN TO CALL A DOCTOR

• See a doctor if you develop symptoms of hyperprolactinemia. Leakage of milk from your breast should be evaluated by your doctor. ▲

Hypertension High Blood Pressure

WHAT IS IT?

Hypertension is characterized by a persistent increase in the force that the blood exerts upon the walls of the arteries. It is normal for this force to increase with stress or physical exertion, but with hypertension the patient's blood pressure is high even at rest.

Blood pressure is measured with two numbers: systolic (the top number in a reading) and diastolic (the bottom number). It is measured in millimeters of mercury (abbreviated mm Hg) using a device called a sphygmomanometer. Systolic pressure refers to the force of blood against the walls of the arteries when the heart contracts to pump blood to the rest of the body. Diastolic pressure refers to the pressure within the arteries as the heart relaxes and refills with blood (which explains why the diastolic number is always lower than the systolic measurement). Hypertension is defined as systolic pressure greater than 140 mm Hg or diastolic pressure greater than 90 mm Hg; optimal blood pressure is less than 120/80 mm Hg.

Some 60 million Americans have hypertension, but only about half of them know it, primarily because it so rarely causes any noticeable symptoms and is usually detected only incidentally during a routine physical examination. But left untreated, hypertension promotes atherosclerosis (narrowing of the arteries) and increases the risk of heart attack, stroke, kidney damage, and destruction of tiny blood vessels in the eye, which can result in vision loss. For these reasons hypertension is often called "the silent killer." Fortunately, if detected early and treated properly, the prognosis is good.

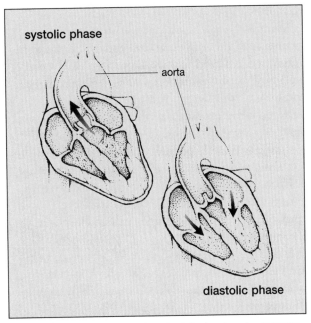

During the systolic phase of the heartbeat, the heart contracts powerfully to pump blood out to the rest of the body; during the diastolic phase, it relaxes as its lower chambers fill with blood to be expelled during the next contraction.

WHAT CAUSES IT?

• In more than 90 percent of cases, no single identifiable cause can be pinpointed, but risk factors include a family history of hypertension, gender (women are at one-half to two-thirds the risk of men), race (incidence is up to twice as great among blacks as among whites), emotional stress, sedentary lifestyle, and aging. Obesity, excessive alcohol consumption, cigarette smoking, and a high-sodium diet also increase the risk of hypertension.

• When an underlying cause can be identified, the condition is known as secondary hypertension. Such causes include kidney disorders, adrenal tumors, and pregnancy.

PREVENTION

• Keep weight within a healthy, normal range.

• Avoid cigarettes and restrict alcohol intake to no more than two drinks a day.

• Aim to get at least 20 minutes of vigorous aerobic exercise (like jogging, biking, dancing, or swimming) a day, three or four days a week.

• Limit intake of sodium to less than 2,500 mg a day.

SYMPTOMS

• Symptoms are rare with uncomplicated hypertension. However, the following may occur when blood pressure is dangerously high:

• Headaches.

• Dizziness or ringing in the ears.

• Palpitations.

• Nosebleeds.

• Numbness or tingling in the hands or feet.

• Drowsiness or confusion.

Hypertension High Blood Pressure *continued*

DIAGNOSIS

• Diagnosis requires accurate measurements of elevated blood pressure on at least three different occasions over a period of a week or more. Some people exhibit "white coat hypertension," wherein blood pressure is consistently high in a clinical setting but is normal when measured at home. Other people sporadically alternate between normal and high readings (known as labile hypertension). Some patients may be asked to wear a portable monitor that automatically records their blood pressure periodically over the course of a day or so, or to measure their blood pressure periodically at home with an electronic monitor.

• Blood and urine tests to look for kidney damage and electrocardiogram (ECG) to check for heart damage (both possible complications of hypertension) will be performed.

HOW TO TREAT IT

• The first line of treatment for essential hypertension involves adopting healthy lifestyle measures (see Prevention). Mild hypertension may respond positively to these measures and thus require no further medical therapy. For example, some studies indicate that as many as 30 percent of those with high blood pressure (specifically, the type known as sodium-sensitive hypertension) can control it by lowering their salt intake.

• If lifestyle changes prove inadequate, your doctor will prescribe one or more of the many available drugs. Diuretics (or "water pills") increase elimination of salt and water and thus reduce overall body-fluid volume. (Some diuretics deplete the body's levels of potassium, thus requiring potassium supplementation.) Beta-blockers interfere with nerve receptors in the heart, causing it to beat less forcefully. Calcium channel blockers reduce the ability of arterial walls to constrict. ACE inhibitors prevent the formation of a hormone that constricts blood vessels. Alpha-blockers and central alpha agonists interfere with nerve impulses that cause arteries to constrict. Vasodilators relax and so dilate the arterial walls.

• For secondary hypertension, the underlying disease must be identified and treated.

WHEN TO CALL A DOCTOR

• All adults should have their blood pressure checked at least once a year. This practice is especially applicable if you are male, over age 40, overweight (particularly if you have been overweight since youth), sedentary, or if you have a family history of hypertension or heart disease.

• Notify your doctor if you experience any unpleasant side effects from antihypertensive medications. Adjustments in your prescription may eliminate the problem; never elect to stop taking your medication without consulting your doctor.

• Get prompt medical attention if you experience symptoms such as ringing in the ears, dizziness, or recurrent headaches or nosebleeds—these may be signs of dangerously high blood pressure. ▲

Hyperthyroidism

WHAT IS IT?

Hyperthyroidism is a disorder caused by excessive secretion of thyroid hormone by the thyroid, a gland in the neck that regulates body growth and metabolism. Normally, the pituitary gland, located at the base of the brain, produces a hormone (thyroid-stimulating hormone or TSH) that regulates the thyroid gland's output of thyroid hormone. Most often, hyperthyroidism is due to autonomous (unregulated by TSH) overproduction of thyroid hormone by an enlarged gland (Graves' disease). This is an autoimmune disorder. Less commonly, hyperthyroidism is caused by the growth of a single thyroid nodule that produces abnormally high amounts of thyroid hormone. Excess thyroid hormone speeds up all metabolic activity in the body (including the rate at which calories are burned) and may result in a myriad of symptoms; some can be mistaken as the result of stress or anxiety. While hyperthyroidism is eminently treatable, severe cases can be fatal if not adequately controlled. The disorder most commonly affects those between 30 and 40 years of age and is five times more frequent in women than men.

WHAT CAUSES IT?

• Graves' disease is an autoimmune disorder, wherein an abnormal antibody is produced that stimulates a constant production of thyroid hormone.

• Hyperthyroidism and other thyroid disorders run in families, although the exact genetic mechanisms are unknown.

• An excessive amount of iodine in the diet and possibly, emotional stress may trigger the disorder in those predisposed to it.

PREVENTION

• There is no known way to prevent hyperthyroidism.

DIAGNOSIS

• Patient history and physical exam often point to the correct diagnosis. Indicators of hyperthyroidism include elevated heart rate, nervousness, tremor, sweating, appearance of goiter, and bulging eyes.

• Blood tests show high levels of thyroid hormones and low levels of TSH.

• A thyroid scan is taken following the administration of radioactive iodine to determine the cause of hyperthyroidism.

HOW TO TREAT IT

• Orally administered radioactive iodine is now the preferred method of treatment. As the thyroid absorbs the iodine, radiation destroys parts of the gland, so that it produces less thyroid hormone.

• Propylthiouracil or methimazole, two drugs that inhibit production of thyroid hormone, may be prescribed. Although symptoms often subside within several weeks, drug therapy must usually be continued for at least a year.

• Surgery to remove a large portion of the thyroid may be recommended for some patients with extreme thyroid enlargement.

• Hyperthyroid patients will require frequent medical supervision throughout their lives. One risk of radioactive iodine treatment or surgery is that the thyroid will end up producing too little thyroid hormone (hypothyroidism), which then requires lifelong supplemental therapy with thyroid hormone.

WHEN TO CALL A DOCTOR

• Contact your doctor if you experience the symptoms of hyperthyroidism.

SYMPTOMS

• Weight loss despite an increase in appetite and food consumption.
• Anxiety, restlessness, and insomnia.
• Rapid heartbeat or palpitations.
• Tremors in the fingers or tongue.
• Increased sweating and intolerance to heat; insensitivity to cold.
• Bulging, watery eyes that feel gritty; an increased sensitivity to light.
• Swelling in the neck (goiter).
• Fatigue and muscle weakness.
• Increased frequency of bowel movements or diarrhea.
• Unusually light or absent menstrual periods.

Hyphema

WHAT IS IT?

Hyphema is a visible accumulation of blood in front of the iris (the colored portion of the eye), usually resulting from an injury. While the outermost layers or whites of the eyeball contain capillaries (small blood vessels), the internal chambers of the eye contain no blood vessels. Instead, the eye has its own special circulatory system, consisting of a transparent liquid known as aqueous humor. If a capillary over the iris bursts, blood may seep into the aqueous humor and cause visual problems.

Fortunately, aqueous humor flows constantly across the iris and is reabsorbed by a network of small veins that empty into the bloodstream. The blood from a hyphema is usually carried away from the eye by the flow of the aqueous humor within a matter of days, and vision returns to normal.

However, a blood clot may block the small veins responsible for reabsorbing the aqueous humor, causing pressure to build up in the eyeball. This may result in damage to the optic nerve from glaucoma, a sight-threatening increase in pressure within the eye (see Glaucoma for more information). The risk of glaucoma is greater with larger hyphemas or in cases when, after the blood has disappeared, there is subsequent bleeding and recurrence of hyphema.

WHAT CAUSES IT?

• An injury to the eye, with a blunt instrument or by a puncture, is the most common cause of hyphema.
• Severe inflammation of the iris may lead to hyphema.
• A blood vessel abnormality may cause blood to leak into the front portion of the eye.

SYMPTOMS
• A visible pool of blood in front of the iris (the colored portion) of the eye sometimes can be seen. Usually, the bleeding is small enough that it is only apparent with a slit lamp (a special magnifier to examine the eye).
• Vision problems.
• Eye pain.

PREVENTION
• Take care to avoid accidents involving the eyes.
• Be sure to wear protective eyewear when playing racquet sports.

DIAGNOSIS
• Patient history and eye examination are needed.
• A thorough eye examination is performed by an ophthalmologist if injury has occurred or if inflammation or blood vessel abnormality is a suspected cause.

HOW TO TREAT IT
• Bed rest and hospitalization may be required to allow damaged blood vessels in the eye to heal and to check for further bleeding and glaucoma. Administration of eyedrops that prevent movement of damaged blood vessels in the eye make the eye extremely sensitive to light. Therefore, a patch may be placed over the eye during recuperation. Sometimes, a clot-stabilizing drug, aminocaproic acid, is used to reduce further bleeding.
• To prevent glaucoma, your ophthalmologist may prescribe eyedrops, such as timolol and acetazolamide, which reduce pressure inside the eyeball, or hyperosmotic agents (which draw fluid away from the inside of the eye), such as mannitol, glycerol, or sorbitol.
• Surgery may be required to evacuate blood from the eye in severe cases. The ophthalmologist will create a small temporary opening, or drain, in the eye, so that the bloody aqueous fluid may be drawn out. This drain may be surgically reopened if hyphema recurs.

WHEN TO CALL A DOCTOR
• Call an ophthalmologist immediately if you injure your eye and hyphema is suspected, or if hyphema recurs after treatment. ▲

Hypoglycemia

WHAT IS IT?

Hypoglycemia is an abnormally low blood sugar level, arising from an imbalance in the rates of glucose release from the liver and its use by other body tissues. Glucose (a simple sugar) is absolutely essential as an energy source for the cells of the central nervous system. Insulin regulates blood glucose levels by slowing the release of glucose by the liver and stimulating its entry into other cells. Low blood glucose levels trigger the release of adrenaline, which produces the symptoms of a hypoglycemic episode, characterized by a sudden attack of anxiety, shakiness, dizziness, hunger, and excessive perspiration. Such episodes are generally not dangerous, because the symptoms incite people to ingest a sugar-containing food or drink, and the adrenaline (and other hormones) released tend to help restore blood sugar levels to normal.

However, prolonged, severe hypoglycemia may be very dangerous, as it gradually and insidiously starves the brain of glucose, which may lead to disorientation and confusion, eventually progressing to seizures, partial paralysis, or loss of consciousness. If left untreated, hypoglycemia may ultimately result in permanent brain damage and, in rare cases, even death. There are two types of hypoglycemic episodes: those that occur two to five hours after eating, known as postprandial hypoglycemia, and those that occur after an extended period without food (usually overnight), known as fasting hypoglycemia.

Postprandial hypoglycemia may be unpleasant, but is usually not serious; it can be corrected easily by eating or drinking and by the action of hormones. Fasting hypoglycemia—which most commonly occurs among people with diabetes when too much insulin is administered—is potentially very dangerous, because of the risk of brain damage. In addition, people with long-standing diabetes often do not have typical symptoms of hypoglycemia. In many cases, however, hypoglycemia can be prevented by carefully following specific diet and lifestyle guidelines (see Diabetes Mellitus for more information).

WHAT CAUSES IT?

• In most cases of postprandial hypoglycemia, the cause is unknown. It may occur, however, as one of the early manifestations of diabetes mellitus, or following stomach surgery.

• The most common cause of fasting hypoglycemia is the administration of too much insulin to a person with diabetes. Risk is increased when these patients exercise or miss meals.

• Other causes of fasting hypoglycemia include excessive alcohol ingestion, insulin-producing tumors of the pancreas (insulinoma), tumors in other organs, adrenal or pituitary insufficiency, rampant leukemia, congestive heart failure, chronic kidney failure, severe liver failure, and some childhood metabolic disorders, such as fructose intolerance and galactosemia.

• Occasionally, hypoglycemia may be triggered by excessive amounts of certain medications, including oral hypoglycemic agents and aspirin (especially among children), and beta-blockers.

PREVENTION

• People with diabetes should carefully abide by their regimen of diet, medication, exercise, and blood glucose monitoring, and should always carry some fast-acting carbohydrate (glucose tablets, hard candies, gumdrops, or fruit juice) to consume at the first sign

---

SYMPTOMS

• Adrenaline-triggered symptoms: anxiety, hunger, a tingling sensation in the hands, palpitations, profuse perspiration, shakiness, or weakness. These symptoms may not occur in people taking beta-blocker drugs and in those with long-standing diabetes.

• Symptoms of nighttime hypoglycemia: nightmares, restlessness, and profuse perspiration.

• Slower-onset symptoms, due to inadequate supply of glucose to the brain: agitation, amnesia, confusion, dizziness, disorientation, feeling cold, headache, impaired vision, lack of coordination, numbness, or personality changes.

• Emergency symptoms: seizures, temporary paralysis of one side of the body, or loss of consciousness.

Hypoglycemia   *continued*

of symptoms. Also, people with diabetes who use insulin should never drive or travel in a car, plane, or train without having some sort of carbohydrate food (such as peanut butter crackers) available for a snack.

• Those who experience postprandial hypoglycemic episodes should eat five or six small meals a day that are low in simple carbohydrates and high in protein, fat, and fiber.

DIAGNOSIS

• In those who do not have diabetes, diagnosis requires demonstration of low blood glucose levels accompanied by the usual symptoms. Depending on the type of hypoglycemia, blood glucose is measured either during a glucose tolerance test or after an overnight fast. Further tests and a detailed patient history are then necessary to determine the underlying cause of hypoglycemia.

• Those with diabetes can verify and document episodes of hypoglycemia with home blood glucose monitoring.

HOW TO TREAT IT

• If you sense a hypoglycemic episode coming on, stop all activity. If you are driving a car, for example, pull over.

• Consume one portion of any fast-acting carbohydrate: four ounces of fruit juice or sugared drink; some candy, such as six or seven jelly beans, or three large marshmallows; or one-half of a tube of Glucose (80 gram container). If you do not feel better quickly, consume one more portion. However, do not eat chocolate because the fat in it slows absorption of sugar into the bloodstream.

• Instruct your family and friends to give you a small drink of fruit juice or to smear syrup inside your mouth if you become disoriented or uncooperative (symptoms of worsening hypoglycemia).

• Instruct your family and friends how to administer an injection of glucagon, a hormone that helps raise your blood sugar level, in the event you lose consciousness from hypoglycemia. After the injection they should call an ambulance and, in the meantime, not attempt to give food or fluids, and most certainly not administer insulin.

• Your doctor may adjust or change your medication if you are receiving too much insulin or if you are taking one of the other drugs that sometimes triggers hypoglycemia in those who are susceptible.

• Surgery is required to treat a pancreatic tumor (insulinoma) that causes hypoglycemia. This sometimes involves removing most of the pancreas. In cases where surgery is not an option, chemotherapy may be used to destroy cancerous cells.

WHEN TO CALL A DOCTOR

• **EMERGENCY** Call an ambulance immediately if someone loses consciousness.

• Consult a doctor if you develop symptoms of hypoglycemia.

Hypoparathyroidism

WHAT IS IT?

Hypoparathyroidism is a disorder that occurs when the parathyroid glands (the four pea-size glands embedded in the corners of the thyroid gland at the base of the neck) fail to produce sufficient quantities of parathyroid hormone (PTH), which helps regulate the blood level of calcium by its actions on the bones and the kidneys. Lack of PTH results in reduced levels of calcium in the blood, which can produce a variety of neurological and muscle abnormalities, from paresthesia (numbness or a burning or prickling sensation) to tetany (hyperexcitability of the nerves, characterized by painful spasms, twitching, and cramps in the face, hands, arms, throat, and sometimes the feet). Such symptoms usually subside with treatment, although the disorder tends to develop gradually, so that by the time it is treated, it may have already caused certain irreversible complications such as cataracts or basal ganglion calcifications. When hypoparathyroidism occurs during childhood and is not treated properly, it may result in poor tooth development and, sometimes, mental retardation. Otherwise, when diagnosis is established early in the course of the disorder, prognosis is good.

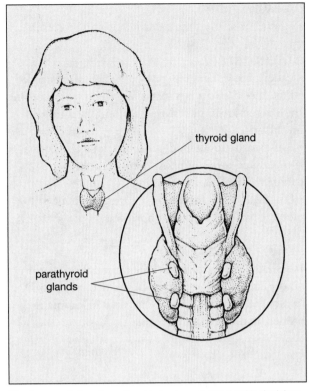

The four, small, round parathyroid glands are located within the lobes of the thyroid gland, which sits atop the trachea (windpipe).

WHAT CAUSES IT?

• The most common causes of hypoparathyroidism in adults are the accidental removal of parathyroid tissue during thyroid or other neck surgery and the removal or destruction of substantial portions of the parathyroid glands during the treatment of hyperparathyroidism.

• In children, hypoparathyroidism most often results from destruction of the thyroid gland as a result of an autoimmune disorder. This may be associated with type 1 diabetes mellitus and thyroid disorders.

• Hypoparathyroidism may occur when the parathyroid tissue is destroyed by amyloidosis (the buildup of a waxy substance in tissues and organs), hemochromatosis (excess iron storage), or malignant (cancerous) tumors.

• In rare cases, an infant may be born without parathyroid glands or with a congenital malfunction of the glands (DiGeorge's syndrome).

• Rarely, a child may not be responsive to PTH and may have symptomatic low calcium levels despite an elevated level of PTH (pseudohypoparathyroidism). Frequently, other characteristics such as short stature, obesity, round face, and shortened fourth and fifth fingers may be present.

SYMPTOMS

• Tingling and numbness or burning and prickling sensations in the face, hands, fingertips, or elsewhere.
• Painful, uncontrollable muscle spasms or cramps in the face, hands, and feet (tetany).
• Breathing or swallowing difficulty.
• Dry, lusterless skin and hair; split, cracked nails.
• Abnormal tooth development in children.
• Cataracts.
• Psychosis (in very severe cases).
• Seizures (in rare cases).
• Mental retardation when the disorder is left untreated in children.

Hypoparathyroidism *continued*

PREVENTION
• There is no way to prevent hypoparathyroidism.

DIAGNOSIS
• Patient history and physical examination are needed.
• Low blood calcium is suspected when tetany of the hand is produced by inflating a blood pressure cuff on the arm.
• Abnormally low blood concentrations of calcium and elevated levels of phosphorus indicate hypoparathyroidism.
• Diagnosis is confirmed by the measurement of low blood levels of parathyroid hormone.

HOW TO TREAT IT
• Therapy usually involves lifelong supplementation with calcium and very large amounts of vitamin D (which, along with PTH, is essential in maintaining proper blood levels of calcium).

• Severe muscle spasms (tetany) or convulsions may require hospitalization. Intravenous infusions of calcium may be given to provide temporary but immediate relief. Sedatives and anticonvulsants may also be administered.
• A spasm of the upper lip may be relieved by tapping on the cheek.
• Regular periodic monitoring of blood calcium levels is essential.

WHEN TO CALL A DOCTOR
• Consult a doctor if you experience painful muscle spasms or cramps, or recurrent tingling, numbness, or burning sensations, especially if occurring in conjunction with other symptoms of hypoparathyroidism.
• **EMERGENCY** Get immediate medical attention if breathing difficulty or seizures occur.

Hypopituitarism

WHAT IS IT?

Hypopituitarism is a rare disorder involving under-production of hormones by the pituitary gland. The pituitary, deep in the brain, is the most important gland in the body's endocrine, or hormonal, system. One of the six hormones produced by the anterior portion of the pituitary is human growth hormone (HGH). In children, HGH deficiency may lead to impaired growth, or dwarfism. Early diagnosis and administration of HGH can correct this hormonal deficiency and result in near-normal height. Deficiencies in other pituitary hormones produce a wide variety of symptoms; in panhypopituitarism, deficiencies occur in all pituitary hormones. Because pituitary hormones stimulate hormone production in other glands, hypopituitarism may have a snowball effect, resulting in deficiencies of adrenal, thyroid, and sex hormones (see Diabetes Insipidus, Addison's Disease, and Hypothyroidism for more information).

WHAT CAUSES IT?

• A tumor in or near the pituitary gland is the most common cause of hypopituitarism.

SYMPTOMS

• Growth retardation (children and adolescents).
• Partial or total sexual maturation impairment.
• Weakness; dizziness or lightheadedness.
• Nausea and vomiting; hoarseness.
• Slow heartbeat; intolerance to cold.
• Slowed or impaired thinking.
• Extreme thirst combined with excessive urination (due to diabetes insipidus), dehydration, constipation.
• Fine wrinkles next to the eyes and mouth, dry skin, depigmentation of the skin, loss of axillary and pubic hair.
• In women: cessation of menstruation (amenorrhea), breast atrophy, vaginal dryness, absence of milk production in new mothers (Sheehan's syndrome).
• In men: loss of libido and potency, reduced muscular strength, shrinking and softening of the testes, decreased secondary hair growth.

• Pituitary surgery or radiation is a potential cause.
• Hypopituitarism may develop in the postpartum period (Sheehan's syndrome) because of necrosis (tissue death) in the pituitary as it outgrows its blood supply during pregnancy.
• Inflammatory processes such as those that occur with tuberculosis are a possible cause.
• Infiltration of the pituitary by a starchy protein (amyloidosis) or iron (hemochromatosis) may result in hypopituitarism.

PREVENTION

• There is no way to prevent hypopituitarism.

DIAGNOSIS

• Patient history and physical examination.
• Blood tests to measure levels of pituitary, gonadal, thyroid, and adrenal hormones.
• X-rays, MRI (magnetic resonance imaging), or CT (computed tomography) scans to detect a tumor.

HOW TO TREAT IT

• Lifelong hormonal replacement therapy is necessary. The specific hormones needed will depend on the nature of the deficiency. To treat adult panhypopituitarism, it is necessary to replace thyroid, adrenal, and gonadal hormones.
• HGH replacement therapy is necessary for children and adolescents to obtain near-normal growth. HGH is also recommended for adults to maintain normal metabolism.
• In some cases, doses of corticosteroids (such as hydrocortisone or prednisone) must be increased during periods of stress, illness, infection, or surgery.
• It may be necessary to reduce insulin dosage in people with diabetes who develop hypopituitarism.
• If a tumor causes hypopituitarism, surgery or radiation therapy may be warranted.

WHEN TO CALL A DOCTOR

• Call a doctor if you or your child develop any of the symptoms of hypopituitarism.
• **EMERGENCY** Nausea, vomiting, extreme weakness, dehydration, and fever suggest adrenal insufficiency that may require emergency medical care. ▲

Hypothermia

WHAT IS IT?

Hypothermia is a drop in internal body temperature to a below-normal level. When the body's core temperature drops too low, the heart rate and metabolism slow dramatically, oxygen consumption decreases, loss of consciousness may ensue, and eventually, cardiac arrest may occur. Body temperature below 90°F indicates moderate to severe hypothermia; temperatures between 90°F and 97°F indicate mild hypothermia. The lower the temperature, the more severe the symptoms. (Incidentally, most household thermometers do not register temperatures below 94°F and thus are not reliable indicators of severe hypothermia.) Hypothermia may develop even at moderate external temperatures of 30°F to 50°F, especially in windy or wet weather. (Water conducts heat away from the body about 25 times faster than air.) The elderly are particularly vulnerable, because the ability to regulate body temperature diminishes with age. Hypothermia is a common killer of outdoor recreationists and constitutes a medical emergency.

WHAT CAUSES IT?

• Exposure to cold weather, especially in wind and rain. Hypothermia may also occur in moderate cold or indoors, especially among infants or the elderly.
• Immersion in cold water rapidly leads to hypothermia, but even water as warm as 70°F may lead to hypothermia if exposure is prolonged.
• Risk factors include alcohol use; diabetes mellitus; disorders of the pituitary, thyroid, or adrenal glands;

fatigue; and use of beta-blocking drugs (often prescribed to treat high blood pressure).

PREVENTION

• Wear several layers of warm, nonrestrictive clothing in cold or wet weather. Keep your head warm. Don't stay out too long in the cold if you can help it. Be aware that fatigue, poor nutrition, and illness may increase your risk.
• Alcohol, drug use, and lack of oxygen at high altitudes may impair judgment and lead to increased cold exposure. Alcohol also increases heat loss.
• Check often on elderly relatives or friends during cold weather.

DIAGNOSIS

• Suspect hypothermia when severe, uncontrollable shivering is present, or when cold exposure leads to confusion, stuttering, or drowsiness.
• A doctor may use a special low-reading thermometer to measure body temperature.

HOW TO TREAT IT

• Call an ambulance or proceed to the nearest emergency room immediately.
• Someone suffering from hypothermia outdoors should go, or be brought, inside as soon as possible. Wet clothing should be removed and replaced with dry clothing, blankets, or a warm sleeping bag. Make sure the top of the head is covered.
• Skin-to-skin contact or careful use of an electric blanket are effective for rewarming. Concentrate on rewarming the torso, since rewarming the limbs may in fact draw blood away from the vital organs.
• Warm, nonalcoholic drinks may be given.
• Be very cautious moving an unconscious victim because heart arrhythmias may result from jarring or dropping the victim.
• Warm intravenous fluids may be given in the emergency room. In severe cases, directly warming the patient's blood may be employed.

WHEN TO CALL A DOCTOR

• **EMERGENCY** Call an ambulance or rescue squad if hypothermia develops. Administer the measures described above until emergency help arrives. ▲

> ### SYMPTOMS
> • Shivering.
> • Numbness.
> • Pallor, or a bluish or grayish tinge to the skin (cyanosis).
> • Slurred speech or stuttering.
> • Confusion.
> • Stumbling.
> • Emergency symptoms: drowsiness, dramatically decreased pulse and breathing rate, dilated pupils, loss of consciousness.

Hypothyroidism

WHAT IS IT?

Hypothyroidism occurs when the thyroid, a gland in the neck that controls body growth and metabolism, produces insufficient amounts of thyroid hormone, thereby slowing all metabolic processes in the body. Symptoms depend on the degree of thyroid deficiency and may develop slowly over many years. (When full-blown symptoms do occur, the condition is known as myxedema.) Although hypothyroidism can occur at any age and in both sexes, it is most common in women over age 50. The disorder can be completely controlled with proper treatment. In rare cases, however, severe untreated hypothyroidism may result in myxedema coma, a life-threatening condition that may be precipitated by illness, sedatives, cold weather, surgery, or injury. Untreated hypothyroidism occurring during infancy results in mental retardation and dwarfism (cretinism).

WHAT CAUSES IT?

• Hypothyroidism is frequently due to an autoimmune disorder (such as Hashimoto's disease), wherein the body's natural defenses against infection mistakenly attack healthy tissue (in this case, the thyroid).
• Hypothyroidism may also occur when the pituitary gland, located at the base of the brain, fails to produce sufficient quantities of thyroid-stimulating hormone (TSH), a regulator of the thyroid gland. (Paradoxically, when hypothyroidism is caused by a defect in

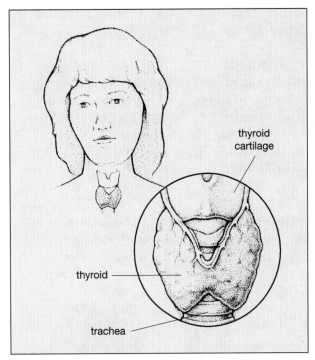

The thyroid (from the Greek word for "shield," referring to the gland's shape) sits atop the trachea (windpipe) at the base of the neck.

the thyroid gland itself, the pituitary releases increased quantities of TSH in an attempt to compensate for low levels of thyroid hormone.)
• The disorder may occur following surgical removal of the thyroid gland to treat hyperthyroidism or thyroid cancer.
• Medical treatments for hyperthyroidism may cause hypothyroidism. Radioactive iodine treatment results in permanent hypothyroidism in more than 50 percent of patients; hypothyroidism due to antithyroid drugs persists only for as long as the drugs are taken (see Hyperthyroidism for more information).
• Certain drugs such as lithium can interfere with thyroid function.
• In rare cases an insufficient dietary intake of iodine may cause hypothyroidism.
• Infants may be born with thyroid defects.
• Risk of hypothyroidism is greater in women over the age of 50.

PREVENTION

• There is no known way to prevent hypothyroidism, although diagnostic screening allows for early detec-

SYMPTOMS

• Fatigue, lethargy, and slowed movement.
• Intolerance to cold.
• Unusual weight gain.
• Constipation.
• Dry, thickened, flaky skin.
• Muscle cramps and weakness.
• Deepened voice.
• Lack of interest in sex.
• Possibly, goiter (swelling in the neck).
• Unusually heavy, prolonged menstrual periods.
• Puffiness around the eyes.
• Dry, brittle hair or hair loss.
• Impaired mental faculties.

Hypothyroidism *continued*

tion and treatment in those at risk for congenital hypothyroidism.

DIAGNOSIS
• Patient history and physical examination are needed. Slowed heart and pulse rates, low blood pressure, and low body temperature suggest hypothyroidism.
• Blood tests are taken to determine levels of thyroid hormone and TSH. (Measuring TSH is the most sensitive test for hypothyroidism.)

HOW TO TREAT IT
• Lifelong hormone replacement therapy with thyroid hormone (thyroxine) is usually necessary. The lowest effective dose is determined and then maintained. (In the elderly and those with coronary artery disease, hormone replacement is started with a small dose and gradually increased. It is controversial whether to initiate such therapy at all in those with slightly elevated TSH but no symptoms.)
• If a large goiter causes breathing or swallowing difficulty, surgical removal may be required.
• Hospitalization is necessary for treatment of myxedema coma. Intravenous thyroid hormone replacement, as well as steroid therapy, will usually be administered. In addition, oxygen, artificial respiration, fluid replacement, and other intensive care measures may be warranted.

WHEN TO CALL A DOCTOR
• If you experience the symptoms of hypothyroidism, consult a doctor as soon as possible. ⚕

IgA Deficiency

WHAT IS IT?

IgA deficiency is a defect in the immune system characterized by an inadequate amount of the antibody class known as immunoglobulin A (IgA). Antibodies are large proteins produced by the body to fight infections caused by invaders, such as bacteria, viruses, fungi, parasites, and other foreign agents. The immune system responds to the protein component (antigens) of these invaders by producing large quantities of specific antibodies, including IgA. These antibodies bind to the antigens on the surface of an invader (bacteria, for example) and prevent them from multiplying, thus halting the spread of disease in the body.

IgA is found in the saliva, mucous membranes, and intestinal secretions, where it may serve as the first line of defense against various sinus, respiratory, and gastrointestinal infections. Consequently, a deficiency of IgA heightens one's vulnerability to such infections. People with IgA deficiency are also more susceptible to certain other disorders, including autoimmune diseases such as rheumatoid arthritis, systemic lupus erythematosus, and chronic hepatitis; respiratory allergies and asthma; irritable bowel syndrome; and some types of cancer, such as squamous cell carcinoma of the lungs and thymoma (cancer of the thymus gland). However, many people with IgA deficiency are relatively healthy and do not suffer from these infections and disorders as much as might be expected.

It is important to note that 40 to 50 percent of people with IgA deficiency develop antibodies to IgA itself, which can cause serious reactions to blood transfusions or other blood products. There is currently no cure for IgA deficiency, so treatment is aimed at easing symptoms and controlling associated diseases. IgA deficiency is the most common immunodeficiency disorder among Caucasians, affecting roughly one in every 600.

SYMPTOMS

- Frequent or chronic infections of the sinuses, lungs, ears, upper respiratory tract, or gastro-intestinal tract.

WHAT CAUSES IT?

- IgA deficiency is most often a hereditary disorder.

PREVENTION

- There is no known way to prevent IgA deficiency.

DIAGNOSIS

- The diagnosis is made by detecting low levels of IgA in the blood and the saliva.

HOW TO TREAT IT

- Antibiotics are prescribed to treat bacterial infections. These should be taken for the full term prescribed.
- Nonprescription pain relievers may be taken to treat minor pain and fever. Acetaminophen (not aspirin) should be given to children.
- Measures must be taken to control underlying disorders that may be associated with IgA deficiency. These include malignant tumors, asthma, and autoimmune disorders (such as rheumatoid arthritis and systemic lupus erythematosus).

WHEN TO CALL A DOCTOR

- Make an appointment with a doctor if you or your child develop frequent or persistent infections.

Impacted Teeth

WHAT IS IT?

An impacted tooth is one that cannot emerge normally from the gums and/or becomes displaced. Most often, the third molars (wisdom teeth) that emerge in the late teens or early twenties become impacted because the jaw is too small to properly accommodate any more teeth. A tooth may also be positioned at an angle before it emerges and thus travel sideways instead of straight. Finally, another tooth may stand as an obstacle and cause a new tooth to emerge crookedly or prevent it from surfacing altogether.

Although wisdom teeth are most frequently affected, any tooth may be impacted. An improperly placed or partially emerged tooth may easily trap food debris and encourage infection and inflammation of the gums. When impaction produces such complications, extraction of the tooth is generally advised. Cysts and tumors may occur around impacted teeth. Any impacted teeth that are likely to become infected or cause damage should be removed.

WHAT CAUSES IT?

• Overcrowding of the teeth within the jaw may cause impacted teeth.
• Faulty alignment of teeth may result in misplacement and impaction.

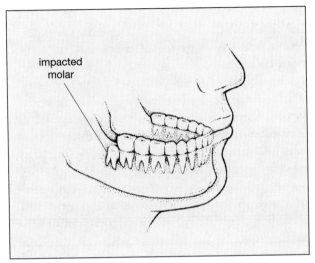

Impacted third molars (wisdom teeth) are very common. Perhaps one explanation is that modern man has a smaller jaw than his hominidal ancestors but similar-size teeth.

DIAGNOSIS

• Dental examination.
• Dental x-rays.

HOW TO TREAT IT

• Until you can see a dentist, over-the-counter pain relievers can be taken for minor tooth pain and discomfort. Rinsing with mouthwash or a solution of warm salt water may be soothing as well.
• Antibiotics are prescribed when bacterial infection occurs at the site of the impacted tooth.
• Surgical extraction is the definitive treatment for an impacted tooth that causes problems. Depending upon the position of the tooth, extraction may be performed in the dentist's office under local anesthesia; more complicated extractions are performed by an oral surgeon and may require general anesthesia.

WHEN TO CALL A DOCTOR

• Make an appointment with a dentist if you develop tooth or gum pain or if a tooth fails to emerge.

SYMPTOMS

• Tooth or gum pain.
• Recurring infections at the site of the impacted tooth.
• Foul taste in the mouth and bad breath, due to trapped food debris or gum infection.
• Headaches.

PREVENTION

• Proper dental care during childhood and adolescence, including orthodontic braces if necessary, may prevent impaction.
• See a dentist at least once a year for an examination and professional cleaning.

Infectious Arthritis

WHAT IS IT?

Infectious arthritis is joint inflammation due to infection by one of a number of microorganisms. The infectious organism may enter the joint directly from a wound, or the infection may spread from a nearby site (such as a boil), but most often it travels to the joint via the bloodstream from an infection elsewhere in the body. The knee and other weight-bearing joints are the ones most commonly affected.

Infectious arthritis is not a permanent condition and does not lead to other forms of joint inflammation, such as osteoarthritis or rheumatoid arthritis. However, if left untreated, it may cause lasting stiffness and limitation of movement in the affected joint or joints.

WHAT CAUSES IT?

• A bacterial infection in another part of the body may invade a joint (usually only one) and result in infectious arthritis, typically accompanied by severe joint pain and swelling, fever, and a general feeling of illness. Staphylococcus, the strain of bacteria that causes skin infections (boils), is the most common underlying cause, but various other strains may produce infectious arthritis too, including those that cause strep throat, gonorrhea, and tuberculosis. Most cases of bacterial arthritis tend to be acute but relatively short-lived, except for those associated with tuberculosis, which tend to be more mild and progress gradually over a period of months.

• Gonococcal bacterial arthritis affects people who do not have a previously damaged joint or bloodstream infection. The gonococcal organism is the most common cause of infectious arthritis among sexually active young women and men. It is rare after age 45. Unlike the other types of bacterial arthritis, it may affect several joints at once, especially those in the hands and wrists.

• Nongonococcal bacterial arthritis affects patients with specific risk factors—including abnormal joint anatomy (such as in rheumatoid arthritis), previous joint trauma or surgery, advanced age, diabetes, corticosteroid or other immunosuppressive use, and endocarditis (infection of heart valves).

• Viral infection, including the viruses that cause hepatitis B, rubella, mumps, infectious mononucleosis, and herpes, may cause infectious arthritis. In some cases, the rubella vaccine may be a cause as well. Viral arthritis often affects multiple joints but generally leaves no permanent damage.

• Fungal infection may cause infectious arthritis; it typically progresses more slowly and is milder than bacterial arthritis.

• Lyme disease, transmitted by a tick bite, may cause recurrent bouts of infectious arthritis (Lyme arthritis) despite initial treatment.

• Syphilis may cause infectious arthritis, although this is now quite rare.

PREVENTION

• Obtain prompt treatment for infections elsewhere in the body.

DIAGNOSIS

• Patient history and physical examination.

• Fluid culture from the swollen joint. Fluid may be withdrawn with a needle and syringe (arthrocentesis). Surgery (arthrotomy) may be required to obtain fluid from some joints (such as the hip) and to treat prosthetic joint infections.

• Blood culture.

• X-rays, CT (computed tomography) scans, or MRI (magnetic resonance imaging).

HOW TO TREAT IT

• Antibiotics are prescribed to treat bacterial infections and Lyme arthritis. These drugs should be taken for the full term prescribed—which may be as long as six weeks or more in severe cases—even if symptoms subside before that time. Failure to do so can permit the strongest, most virulent strains of the

---

SYMPTOMS

• A painful, red, warm, swollen, and stiff joint. (In some cases, multiple joints are affected.)
• Fever (possibly as high as 104°F) and chills.
• Fatigue.
• Skin rash (with Lyme arthritis, as well as gonorrheal, syphilitic, and some varieties of viral arthritis).

Infectious Arthritis *continued*

underlying organism to survive and multiply, which may result in an even more severe rebound infection that is harder to treat. For acute bacterial infections, antibiotics are often initially delivered in very high doses by intravenous injection.

• Aspirin or other nonsteroidal anti-inflammatory drugs (NSAIDs) may be administered to reduce pain and inflammation in viral infections.

• More potent painkillers, such as narcotics, may be prescribed in severe cases.

• Amphotericin B, an antifungal drug, may be used for fungal infections.

• For antibiotics to work, the infected joint must be drained—as often as necessary to control swelling (sometimes as often as several times a day).

• Surgery (arthrotomy) may be required for fluid drainage of some joints, such as the hip or shoulder.

• Infection in a prosthetic joint usually requires

removal of the prosthesis. A new joint can be implanted after intensive treatment cures the infection.

• Immobilization of the joint is necessary during the healing process. This may require bed rest in addition to a cast or splint.

• Physical therapy may be necessary after the infection has subsided, to regain mobility and strength in the affected joint.

WHEN TO CALL A DOCTOR

• Call a doctor immediately if you develop symptoms of infectious arthritis. Prompt treatment may help prevent permanent damage to the joint.

• Consult your doctor immediately if you have rheumatoid arthritis or gout and you develop arthritic symptoms that do not respond to the medication prescribed for flare-ups. █

Influenza

WHAT IS IT?

Influenza, commonly known as the flu, is a highly contagious viral infection of the respiratory tract. Often occurring as an epidemic, the flu results from three kinds of Orthomyxoviruses: influenzae types A, B, and C. Type A viruses tend to be the most virulent, and constantly mutate into new strains, making permanent immunization against them difficult. Type A influenza is most often responsible for large epidemics. The type B virus, generally a less severe variety, mutates occasionally, causing smaller, more localized outbreaks. Type C, which causes only mild illness resembling a common cold, is a very stable virus. During an initial bout with a type C infection, the body produces antibodies that confer immunity against future infections. Symptoms of all types of influenza usually appear following an incubation period of one to four days after initial exposure, and run their course over a period of seven to 10 days. Occasionally, the virus may lead to further, potentially serious complications such as bacterial bronchitis, pneumonia, or sinusitis; the elderly, the very young, and those who suffer from major chronic illnesses are particularly vulnerable to such risks.

WHAT CAUSES IT?

• Influenza is usually contracted by inhaling contaminated droplets expelled into the air during coughing or sneezing by an infected person. Most often, outbreaks occur in winter, when people tend to remain inside and are in close proximity to one another.

PREVENTION

• A yearly flu vaccination is recommended for people at high risk of developing complications, including those with chronic heart or kidney disease; chronic lung disease (including asthma, emphysema, chronic bronchitis, tuberculosis, or cystic fibrosis); diabetes mellitus or other chronic metabolic disorders; severe anemia; and depressed immunity due to diseases (such as AIDS) or medical treatments (such as chemotherapy for cancer). People over age 65 or who live in a nursing facility are also at heightened risk. The vaccine should be administered before the start of flu season, between October 1 and the middle of November.

• Avoid close contact with those infected with influenza.

• Amantadine or rimantadine may be prescribed by a physician during local influenza epidemics, to be taken daily if high-risk patients have not been immunized for that year.

DIAGNOSIS

• Diagnosis is usually self-evident from symptoms; a visit to a doctor is rarely necessary.

HOW TO TREAT IT

• Get plenty of bed rest, preferably in a warm, well-ventilated room.

• Take over-the-counter pain relievers to ease aches and reduce fever. (Give acetaminophen, not aspirin, to children.)

• Drink plenty of fluids to keep mucus secretions thin and easy to expel.

• Drink warm liquids or gargle with salt water to alleviate a sore throat.

• A cool-mist humidifier may help to thin mucus secretions.

• For the elderly or those with a serious chronic illness, the antiviral drugs amantadine or rimantadine may help reduce the severity of symptoms from type A infections, if administered within 24 hours of onset.

WHEN TO CALL A DOCTOR

• See a doctor if flu symptoms do not improve after a week to 10 days.

• Those with any of the conditions that carry a high risk of complications (see Prevention) should consult a doctor immediately if flu exacerbates an underlying illness. ▲

SYMPTOMS

• Sudden onset of chills and fever (usually between 101°F and 104°F).

• Muscle aches; headache.

• Dry cough; sore throat and hoarseness.

• Loss of appetite.

• Nasal congestion or runny nasal discharge.

• Chest pain.

Inguinal Hernia

WHAT IS IT?

A hernia (sometimes referred to as a rupture) is a protrusion of soft tissue, such as a portion of the intestine, through a weak spot in a muscle, usually in the abdominal wall. The most common type—the inguinal hernia—occurs where the abdomen meets the thigh in the groin region. Men are more susceptible to this type of hernia because of a residual weakness along the path (inguinal canal) where the testicles descended into the scrotum prior to birth. But any weakness in the abdominal wall—whether due to injury, strain, aging, or a congenital defect—can promote the formation of one of the two types of inguinal hernia.

In a direct inguinal hernia (the more common of the two), the abdominal organs push through a weak spot in the abdominal wall to create a visible bulge in the groin area. In an indirect inguinal hernia, which occurs almost exclusively in men, the tissue protrudes farther down through the inguinal canal, entering the scrotum. In either case, if the hernia can be pushed back into the abdominal cavity, it is said to be "reducible," which, while not an immediate health threat, eventually requires surgical repair.

If it cannot be pushed back, the hernia is "nonreducible" (or incarcerated), a condition that may lead to dangerous complications including the obstruction of the flow of the intestinal contents or obstruction of intestinal blood supply (strangulation), leading to tissue death. Intestinal obstruction produces nausea, vomiting, loss of appetite, and abdominal pain and usually requires prompt surgery. A strangulated her-

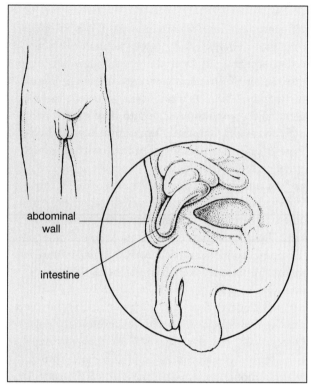

In a direct inguinal hernia, a portion of the intestine pushes through a weak spot in the abdominal wall and may result in a visible bulge in the groin.

nia is extremely painful and requires immediate emergency surgery.

WHAT CAUSES IT?

• Congenital or age-related weakness in the abdominal wall.
• In males, improper closure of the abdominal cavity during gestation.
• Increase in abdominal cavity pressure owing to heavy lifting, straining, obesity, or pregnancy.

PREVENTION

• When lifting heavy objects, bend your knees, keeping the object close to your chest. Lift using your leg muscles and keep your back straight. Don't strain or hold your breath while lifting.

DIAGNOSIS

• Patient history and physical examination are usually all that are required. Observation of a protrusion in

---

SYMPTOMS

• A lump in the groin area that may be evident only when standing or straining and that disappears when reclining.
• Pain at the site of the lump, especially when lifting a heavy object.
• Swelling of the scrotum.
• Excruciating abdominal pain (if strangulation occurs).
• Nausea, vomiting, loss of appetite, and pain (if intestinal obstruction occurs).

Inguinal Hernia   *continued*

the groin when the patient strains or coughs during examination indicates diagnosis of an inguinal hernia.

HOW TO TREAT IT

• In simple cases, the preferred treatment is herniorrhaphy, in which soft tissue is pushed back into the abdominal cavity, the weak spot is sewn closed, and a piece of nylon mesh is sutured into place to reinforce the abdominal wall. New muscle eventually grows over the mesh. This is now one of the safest and most common of all major operations. Formerly, it required hospitalization, several days of bed rest, and weeks of restricted activity. Thanks to improved techniques, the procedure is now usually done on an outpatient basis under local anesthesia, and the patient can usually return to a normal schedule within a week.

• Although it requires a general anesthetic, laparoscopic surgery (using a lighted tube inserted through a small hole in the abdominal wall) may cause less postoperative pain.

• Strangulated hernias require surgical removal of the affected portion of intestine and several days in the hospital.

• An externally worn truss, once a common remedy, is generally no longer recommended, as it does nothing to address the risk of intestinal strangulation or other associated problems. However, a truss may be useful for those who are too frail to withstand an operation.

WHEN TO CALL A DOCTOR

• See a doctor if you develop the symptoms of inguinal hernia.

• **EMERGENCY** Severe lower abdominal pain warrants immediate medical care; it may be a sign of intestinal obstruction or strangulation. ⚠

Insomnia

WHAT IS IT?

Insomnia—difficulty in falling or staying asleep, or waking up too early—is the most common sleep disorder. It may affect people of any age, but prevalence increases with advancing years. Sleep requirements vary greatly: Some people need nine hours of sleep a night; others do fine with five. Many who complain of insomnia sleep more than they think they do. Although persistent insomnia may be frustrating and even debilitating, self-treatment is often successful.

WHAT CAUSES IT?

• Psychological distress—due to emotional upset, a different or noisy sleeping environment, or worrying about the next day—is the most common cause of insomnia. Anxiety, depression, and mania cause more persistent sleep disturbances.
• Caffeine and other stimulants are common causes. Even a single cup of coffee or tea during the day can lead to insomnia in susceptible people.
• Diuretic medications taken later in the day can cause frequent awakenings to urinate.
• Alcoholic beverages disrupt the sleep cycle and cause frequent awakenings. Chronic alcoholism may cause sleeping problems that persist for years, even after drinking is discontinued.
• Paradoxically, sleeping pills cause insomnia. They tend to lose their effectiveness after a few weeks, and withdrawal may cause rebound insomnia.
• Physical disorders—heart and lung diseases, hyperthyroidism, gastroesophageal reflux, arthritis, and many more—cause insomnia. Prostate disorders, kidney disease, and diabetes may cause frequent awakenings throughout the night to urinate.
• Other causes include a sedentary lifestyle, exercising vigorously late in the day, recent surgery, and pregnancy (especially the last month).

SYMPTOMS
• Difficulty falling asleep.
• Waking often during the night or waking significantly earlier than desired.
• Daytime fatigue, drowsiness, inability to concentrate, or irritability.

PREVENTION

• Avoid or minimize caffeinated beverages.
• Within three hours of going to bed, do not drink alcoholic beverages, smoke, or eat a large meal (although a small bedtime snack may be advised).
• Avoid amphetamines or other stimulants (unless directed otherwise by your doctor).
• Exercise moderately during the day; this should help you feel tired at night.
• If possible, go to bed and get up at set times each day, and resist the temptation to take long naps.
• Prior to bedtime, restrict reading and television watching. Try to avoid worrying (it may help to set aside a regular time during the day to think about problems and possible solutions.) Take a warm bath or drink a glass of warm milk to relax.
• Use your bed only for sleeping and intimacy; don't watch television, talk on the phone, or do paperwork in bed. If you awaken in the middle of the night and cannot fall back to sleep, get out of bed to read. Return to bed when tired.

DIAGNOSIS

• In cases with no obvious cause, the doctor may advise an overnight stay at a sleep-study laboratory to monitor brain-wave patterns, breathing, muscle activity, and other body functions.

HOW TO TREAT IT

• Follow preventive tips.
• If you are unable to fall asleep or if you wake up and cannot get back to sleep, get out of bed and stay up until you feel tired and drowsy.
• Psychological counseling may help relieve the anxiety or depression that prevents sleep.
• Your doctor may ask you to keep a log of sleeping patterns to identify causes of sleeplessness.
• When a short-term stressor such as an upcoming event or a recent grief is present, your doctor may prescribe a sedative tranquilizer (such as zolpidem, lorazepam, or alprazolam) to be taken on a short-term basis under his or her supervision.

WHEN TO CALL A DOCTOR

• Make an appointment with a doctor if insomnia persists or interferes with normal activities. ▲

Intervertebral Disk, Herniated

WHAT IS IT?

A herniated disk, also known as a slipped disk, is a protrusion of the central portion of one of the flat, circular pads found in the joints between the bones of the spine (vertebrae). A slipped disk can cause symptoms by pressing either on a nerve leaving the spinal cord or on the spinal cord itself.

Each disk has a soft and gelatinous inner portion surrounded by a tough outer ring that allows it to act as a shock absorber between the bones of the spine. Weakness or trauma may allow the inner portion to push through the outer ring (in some cases compressing one of the spinal nerves and causing pain and numbness in the neck or along an arm or leg). A herniated disk may then rupture. In a rupture, the soft gel squeezes through the outer shell and may press on the nerves. The intervertebral disks in the neck and especially the lumbar spine are the most likely to rupture.

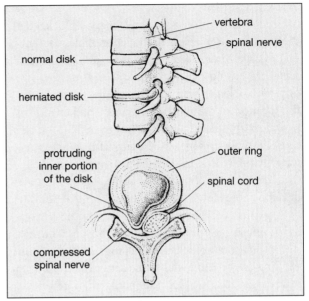

If one of the disks between a pair of vertebrae becomes herniated, it may press on a spinal nerve or the spinal cord, causing symptoms.

WHAT CAUSES IT?

• Neck or back injury is the most common cause.
• Weak muscles, obesity, or a sedentary lifestyle may put uneven stress on the spine and cause a slipped disk.
• Herniated disks are more prevalent among men under age 45, after which the growth of extra fibrous tissue around the disks affords greater stability.
• Risk increases again among the elderly, owing to disk degeneration.

PREVENTION

• Bend and lift objects from the knees, not the waist. Do not strain to lift things that are too heavy.
• Follow a program of moderate, regular exercise to strengthen back and abdominal muscles.
• Lose weight if you are overweight.

DIAGNOSIS

• Patient history and physical examination.
• CT (computed tomography) scans or MRI (magnetic resonance imaging).

HOW TO TREAT IT

• Restricting activity by lying flat for a few days may help relieve symptoms. Avoid activities such as lifting or pushing that aggravate symptoms.
• Ice or heat packs should be used for pain. Muscle relaxants and anti-inflammatories may be prescribed.
• In some cases, various types of surgery may be done to remove the disk. Rarely, in severe cases, the adjoining vertebrae may be fused.
• During recovery, a supportive collar and an extra-firm mattress may be advised. A back brace may be used to provide support during activity.

WHEN TO CALL A DOCTOR

• See a doctor if you have herniated disk symptoms.
• **EMERGENCY** Call an ambulance immediately if someone suffers a serious back or neck injury. Keep the patient still until help arrives.

SYMPTOMS

• Back or neck pain that worsens with movement, coughing, sneezing, or straining.
• Pain that radiates from the spine down the arm or leg.
• Pain, tingling, or numbness in the buttocks, a leg (sciatica), or an arm, usually on one side.
• Back pain not relieved by over-the-counter pain relievers.

Intestinal Obstruction

WHAT IS IT?

Intestinal obstruction is a partial or total blockage of the small or large intestine, which impedes the normal passage of digested matter through the intestinal tract, preventing the excretion of feces and, in cases of total blockage, even gas. Symptoms depend on the location of the obstruction and whether it is partial or complete. Blockage in the small intestine causes intense episodes of abdominal pain and vomiting that may lead to dehydration and possibly shock. Symptoms (intractable constipation and pain) develop more slowly in large-bowel obstruction.

A partial blockage that allows only liquid to pass can result in diarrhea instead. The most obvious feature of intestinal obstruction is progressive abdominal swelling as gas, fluid, and fecal matter build up. If the obstruction restricts blood supply to the intestine, there is an increased risk of tissue death or intestinal perforation, both life-threatening conditions. Complete blockage of the small intestine, if left untreated, can cause death within hours to days.

WHAT CAUSES IT?

• Adhesions (internal scar tissue) from prior abdominal surgery (the most common cause of bowel obstruction).
• A strangulated hernia (a portion of small intestine protruding through a weak spot in the abdominal wall, so that its blood supply is cut off).
• Colon cancer.
• Diverticulitis (inflammation of small pouchlike ulcerations along the wall of the colon).

SYMPTOMS
• Intermittent bouts of painful cramping.
• Vomiting.
• Increasingly painful abdominal swelling.
• Progressive constipation, leading to an inability to pass feces or, sometimes, even gas.
• Uncontrollable hiccupping or burping.
• Diarrhea (occurs with partial obstruction).
• Low-grade fever (less than 100°F).
• Weakness or dizziness.
• Bad breath.

• Volvulus (a twist or knot in the bowel).
• Intussusception (collapse of one segment of intestine into another, much like a telescope).
• Impacted food or feces.
• Gallstones.
• Rarely, a swallowed foreign object that becomes lodged in the digestive tract.
• In paralytic (or adynamic) ileus, as opposed to mechanical blockage, the intestine is not blocked, but ceases to contract and move its contents along. It almost always follows abdominal surgery and lasts a few days before, unlike other causes, resolving on its own.

PREVENTION
• Follow a high-fiber diet.

DIAGNOSIS
• Patient history and physical examination.
• X-rays to locate the site of obstruction.
• Colonoscopy (use of a flexible, lighted viewing tube to inspect the large intestine).
• Barium enema. (Barium provides a clear image of the colon on an x-ray.)

HOW TO TREAT IT
• Intestinal obstruction is a medical emergency requiring immediate professional treatment. Do not attempt to treat it yourself using enemas or laxatives.
• Initially, doctors decompress the distended abdomen by removing fluid and gas through a flexible tube passed through the nose or mouth.
• In most cases, surgery is necessary to clear a mechanical intestinal obstruction. Six to eight hours of preoperative preparation are often necessary to restore fluid and electrolyte (essential mineral) balances, in order to prevent dehydration and shock.
• Bowel resection may be necessary. After removal of the affected portion of the intestine, the severed ends may be rejoined, although ileostomy or colostomy (surgeries in which an abdominal opening is made so that intestinal waste products may empty into an external bag) may be necessary.

WHEN TO CALL A DOCTOR
• **EMERGENCY** If you have symptoms of intestinal obstruction, get immediate medical attention. ▲

Irritable Bladder

WHAT IS IT?

Irritable bladder is a general term for any persistent condition that provokes the muscles in the bladder to contract involuntarily, resulting in a sudden, urgent, uncontrollable need to urinate (urge incontinence). Numerous stimuli can intermittently irritate the bladder and override conscious attempts to inhibit the voiding reflex, sometimes resulting in large-volume accidents that may occur either during the day or while sleeping. The mechanisms that trigger irritable bladder are sometimes difficult to determine; identifying an underlying cause often leads to effective treatment. Irritable bladder is fairly common, especially among women.

WHAT CAUSES IT?

- Urinary tract infections.
- Bladder stones.
- Pregnancy.
- Damage to the nerves that control bladder function, causing excessive contraction of the bladder.
- Obstruction of the outflow of urine, for example, because of a tumor, urethral stricture, or an enlarged prostate.
- A reaction to the use of a urinary catheter.
- In many cases the cause is unknown.

PREVENTION

- Because it is difficult to identify its underlying cause, irritable bladder is difficult to prevent.

DIAGNOSIS

- Patient history and physical examination.
- A "voiding diary," or record of the time, amount, and circumstances of urination.
- Catheterization of the bladder to measure the amount of urine remaining after urination.
- Observation of the effects of filling the bladder through a catheter.
- Microscopic examination and culture of urine, to determine if a urinary tract infection underlies the problem.
- Cytoscopy (use of a lighted scope to view the bladder).
- Voiding cystogram (an x-ray taken while the patient urinates).

HOW TO TREAT IT

- When irritable bladder is due to bacterial infection, antibiotics are given.
- In some cases bladder control can be regained or improved with a technique known as bladder training. The technique begins by scheduling a bathroom visit every two hours, whether the patient needs to urinate or not. The interval is gradually increased by a half hour at a time, toward a goal of four-hour intervals. In many cases the body adapts to this schedule, eliminating incontinence.
- Antispasmodics, antihypertensives, and other drugs may be prescribed to relax bladder muscles and so prevent uncontrolled contractions of the bladder.
- Although adult diapers and pads are widely advocated by advertisers, they may actually promote complications, so they are not recommended for anything but very short-term use unless otherwise advised by a doctor.

WHEN TO CALL A DOCTOR

- Consult a doctor for any repeated episodes of urinary incontinence.

SYMPTOMS

- Sudden, urgent need to urinate.
- Accidental voiding of urine, sometimes in large volumes.
- Frequent urination, both during the day and at night.

Irritable Bowel Syndrome

WHAT IS IT?

Irritable bowel syndrome (IBS) is the most common gastrointestinal disorder in the United States. It is characterized by intermittent periods of constipation or diarrhea and often pain or bloating. After partly digested food leaves the stomach, it is moved through the small and then the large intestine by regular contractions (peristaltic motility) of the muscles in the intestinal wall. In IBS, these muscles may go into spasm and move residues either too quickly (causing diarrhea) or too slowly (causing constipation). IBS should not be confused with the more serious inflammatory bowel diseases (see Colitis, Ulcerative and Crohn's Disease). There is no cure for IBS; however, it is often possible to relieve symptoms with a combination of diet and stress management. Medications are also sometimes helpful. IBS is more common in women than men, and symptoms may worsen in relation to menses.

WHAT CAUSES IT?

• The cause of IBS is unknown, though it is felt to be a disorder of gastrointestinal motility (a disorder of the function of the gastrointestinal tract rather than a structural problem).
• Emotional stress may be a contributing factor.
• Certain foods may trigger flare-ups. Common irritants include high-fat foods such as bacon, poultry skin, vegetable oils, and margarine; dairy products; and gas-producing foods such as beans and broccoli.

PREVENTION

• There is no known way to prevent irritable bowel syndrome; however, symptomatic episodes can often be minimized through dietary modifications and stress management techniques (see Treatment).

DIAGNOSIS

• Patient history and physical examination are needed. Diagnosis is made by ruling out other disorders, such as cancer and inflammatory bowel diseases.
• A barium enema may be necessary. Barium creates a clear image of the colon on an x-ray.
• A small, lighted viewing tube may be used to inspect part (sigmoidoscopy) or all (colonoscopy) of the large intestine.

HOW TO TREAT IT

• A low-fat diet is recommended (high-fat foods may aggravate symptoms).
• Experiment with fiber intake in the diet. Some people find that symptoms are relieved by a diet rich in high-fiber foods (raw fruits and vegetables, bran, whole-grain breads, and dried legumes). Others find that a high-fiber diet increases symptoms.
• Smaller, more frequent meals may be easier to digest.
• Psychological counseling, meditation, or biofeedback may aid in the management of stress. Regular, moderate exercise may also reduce stress and relieve symptoms.
• Your doctor may prescribe laxatives, antidiarrheal medications, antispasmodics, bulk-forming agents (psyllium), or tranquilizers.
• Smoking may act as a trigger and should be avoided.

WHEN TO CALL A DOCTOR

• Make an appointment with a doctor if symptoms of IBS interfere with normal activities. ◪

SYMPTOMS
• Constipation or diarrhea, or alternating bouts of both.
• Abdominal discomfort, pain, bloating, or cramps.
• Excess gas.
• A feeling that the bowels do not empty completely.
• Nausea.

Jaw Dislocation or Fracture

WHAT IS IT?

Dislocation of the jaw occurs when the lower jaw-bone (mandible) becomes displaced from one or both of the joints connecting it to the base of the skull (temporomandibular joints). Because these joints tend to be unstable, they are the ones most commonly dislocated, and recurrences are likely following an initial incident. A jaw fracture is a break in the mandible, usually due to a forceful blow. A severe jaw fracture warrants immediate emergency medical care.

WHAT CAUSES IT?

• Automobile crashes, industrial accidents, and falls are the most common causes of jaw injury. Sports injuries and physical assault are also common causes.
• Some people have especially weak temporo-mandibular joints, so that opening the mouth very widely—for example during yawning or eating a large sandwich—may cause the jaw to dislocate.

PREVENTION

• Wear seat belts in the car.
• Use a helmet if you ride a motorcycle or bicycle.
• Wear protective head gear when playing sports.

DIAGNOSIS

• Patient history and physical examination.
• X-rays of the jawbone (mandible) and temporo-mandibular joints.
• CT (computed tomography) scans of the facial and skull bones.

HOW TO TREAT IT

• A simple dislocated jaw often may be snapped back

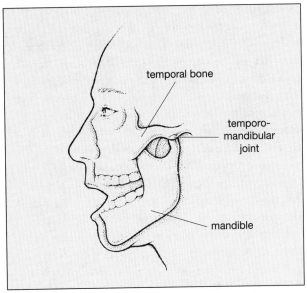

The mandible (jawbone) can become dislocated from the temporo-mandibular joint fairly easily; extreme force may fracture the mandible.

into place. However, recurrent dislocations warrant examination and evaluation by a doctor.
• Get to an emergency room for more serious jaw injuries (fractures or very painful dislocations).
• The doctor or oral surgeon may insert a tube through the mouth and into the throat to ease breathing.
• The doctor will reset the jaw manually (for a minor dislocation) or surgically (for a severe dislocation or fracture). After it is reset, a fractured jaw is immobilized by wiring the upper and lower teeth together while the bones heal. Recurrent dislocations require similar treatment.
• A liquid diet is necessary during recovery (a fracture may take up to six weeks to mend). Do not eat solid foods without your doctor's permission.
• Analgesics and muscle relaxants may be prescribed.
• During recovery from a dislocation, avoid opening your mouth too widely. For example, put your fist under your jaw when yawning, and try not to talk too much.

WHEN TO CALL A DOCTOR

• **EMERGENCY** See a doctor, oral surgeon, or call an ambulance if you sustain a serious jaw injury. ⚠

SYMPTOMS

• Inability to close the mouth normally.
• Painful, swollen, or numb jaw.
• Misalignment of teeth.
• Speaking difficulty.
• Drooling.
• Emergency symptoms: breathing difficulty, heavy bleeding.

Kidney Cancer

WHAT IS IT?

Kidney cancer is the growth of malignant cells in a kidney. The two kidneys, located deep in the body at about the middle of the back, regulate the fluid and electrolyte balance in the body and filter wastes out of the blood into the urine. Urine collects in the portion of the kidney known as the renal pelvis; from there it passes through a narrow conduit (the ureter) to the bladder. There are three distinct types of kidney cancer: Renal cell carcinoma (RCC) and transitional cell cancer (TCC) affect adults almost exclusively, while Wilms' tumor usually affects children under age five. RCC (previously called hypernephroma), which arises in tiny tubules deep within the kidney, accounts for 85 percent of all kidney cancers. TCC arises in the renal pelvis and may also be found in the ureter and bladder. The affected kidney may be removed. Only one kidney is necessary to support life so the remaining kidney compensates for the missing one. With early diagnosis and treatment, the outlook for kidney cancer is optimistic, especially for Wilms' tumor.

WHAT CAUSES IT?

- The cause of kidney cancer is unknown.
- Hereditary factors are thought to play a role in some kidney cancers.
- Smokers have a greater risk of kidney cancer.
- Patients on dialysis for many years have a greater risk of RCC.

SYMPTOMS

- Blood in the urine. Urine may appear dark, smoky, or cloudy. However, early in the development of the cancer, the blood may only be detected by urinalysis.
- Abdominal, back, or flank pain.
- Abdominal mass in an infant or child may indicate Wilms' tumor.
- General feeling of poor health.
- Fever (with RCC).
- Loss of appetite and weight loss.
- A variety of systemic symptoms due to hormones produced by RCC.

- Overuse of pain relievers is associated with greater risk of TCC.
- Toxic industrial chemicals may promote TCC.

PREVENTION

- Don't smoke.
- Avoid high doses or long-term use of analgesics unless recommended by a doctor.

DIAGNOSIS

- Patient history and physical examination are needed. The doctor will press upon the flanks and abdomen to detect any abnormal solid masses.
- Urine is examined for blood or the presence of cancer cells.
- An x-ray of the kidney may be taken after injection with a contrasting dye (intravenous pyelogram).
- Ultrasound, CT (computed tomography) scans, or MRI (magnetic resonance imaging) may be done to determine the nature of a kidney abnormality and to see if cancer has spread.
- Cystoscopy (the use of a thin, lighted tube inserted through the urethra into the bladder) may be used to exclude bladder cancer or to inject contrasting dye into the ureters.
- Chest x-rays and bone scans may be used to determine if cancer has spread.

HOW TO TREAT IT

- For RCC, surgical removal of the affected kidney (nephrectomy) is almost always recommended, unless the cancer has spread to distant sites. For TCC, the renal pelvis or the ureter and part of the bladder may need to be removed.
- Radiation and chemotherapy may be used to destroy cancer cells prior to, in conjunction with, or (if cancer has spread to distant sites) instead of surgery.
- Experiments with various forms of immunotherapy (interferon, interleukin-2, activated lymphocytes) have shown some promise for RCC that has spread.
- Wilms' tumor responds well to a combination of nephrectomy, radiation, and chemotherapy.

WHEN TO CALL A DOCTOR

- Call a doctor if you notice blood in the urine or develop other signs suggestive of kidney cancer. ⚠

Kidney Cysts

WHAT IS IT?

Cysts (spherical, thin-walled fluid-filled sacs) may develop within the tissues of the kidneys singly or in groups. Single kidney cysts are not a health risk and are common after age 50. While cancer or infection may develop within one cyst, such complications are very rare. However, polycystic kidney disease, a common inherited disorder, may lead to the formation of hundreds of cysts, abnormally enlarged kidneys, and eventual kidney failure. (The disease may also cause cysts to develop in many other organs, especially the liver.) Some children are born with the full-fledged disorder and others develop it early in life. More often, however, symptoms of polycystic kidney disease begin by ages 30 to 40. Major complications include kidney failure, high blood pressure, and bleeding around the brain from a ruptured aneurysm. There is yet no cure for polycystic kidney disease; goals of treatment are to preserve kidney function as long as possible, to prevent or treat complications, and to alleviate symptoms. Renal failure rarely occurs before age 40, and normal kidney function is maintained in about half of patients who reach age 70.

WHAT CAUSES IT?

• The cause of single kidney cysts is unknown.
• In most adults, polycystic kidney disease is inherited and, in fact, is the most common hereditary disease in the United States. Occasionally, it occurs without a family history of the disease.

SYMPTOMS

• Pain or tenderness in the back or abdomen.
• Blood in the urine.
• Frequent need to urinate at night (nocturia).
• In infants, abdominal or flank masses.
• Burning on urination and abdominal pain due to associated urinary tract infections (see Bladder Infection for more information).
• Frequent urination, fatigue, swollen ankles, shortness of breath, and itching skin due to end-stage renal disease (see Renal Failure, Chronic for more information).

PREVENTION

• There is no known way to prevent either kidney cysts or polycystic kidney disease.
• If you have a family history of polycystic kidney disease, be sure to get regular checkups to aid in early diagnosis.

DIAGNOSIS

• Patient and family history and physical examination. The doctor will press on the flanks and abdomen to detect any solid, abnormal masses.
• Blood and urine tests.
• Ultrasound or CT (computed tomography) scans of the kidneys.
• A test, known as gene linkage analysis, can detect the genetic abnormality responsible for polycystic kidney disease, but it is rarely necessary.
• Diagnosis of polycystic kidney disease in infants is confirmed by the presence of large bulges in the back below the ribs on either side of the body.

HOW TO TREAT IT

• Asymptomatic cases do not require treatment.
• Antibiotics may be prescribed to treat associated urinary tract infections. Antibiotics should be taken for the full term prescribed.
• Antihypertensive drugs are prescribed to treat associated high blood pressure.
• Rarely, needle aspiration, in which the doctor inserts a needle into the kidney to drain an enlarged or painful cyst, may be done.
• Dialysis is necessary should kidney failure occur. This procedure filters the blood artificially, removing waste products and excess fluid when the kidney can no longer perform these functions (see Renal Failure, Chronic for more information).
• A kidney transplant is an alternative to dialysis in cases of kidney failure.

WHEN TO CALL A DOCTOR

• Call a doctor if you develop symptoms of kidney cysts or polycystic kidney disease.
• Make an appointment with a doctor if you have a family history of polycystic kidney disease. Genetic counseling may be advised for those considering having children. ▲

Kidney Infection Pyelonephritis

WHAT IS IT?

Pyelonephritis is an infection of the kidneys, most often caused by bacteria. The kidneys filter waste products from the blood and produce urine, which passes to the bladder via the ureters (see illustration). The bladder stores urine, which leaves the body via the urethra. Normally, urine is sterile; it contains no bacteria or other microorganisms. But bacteria may enter the urethra and travel back up the urine stream to the kidneys, causing an infection. (In most cases, these are bacteria that normally inhabit the anal area with no ill effect.) Bacteria may also travel to the kidneys from infections elsewhere in the body via the bloodstream. Typically, acute pyelonephritis resolves without treatment, but it also responds well to antibiotics. However, recurrent or persistent kidney infection, known as chronic pyelonephritis—while rare and usually associated with stones or other abnormalities of the urinary system—may lead to scarring of the kidneys and, in severe cases, kidney failure. Kidney infections are more common in women, because the urethra is considerably shorter and so provides less of a barrier to bacteria.

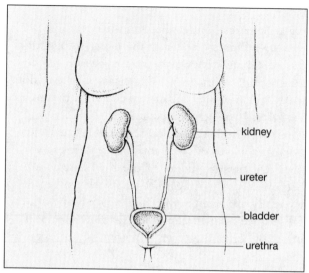

Most urinary tract infections remain confined to the urethra or bladder, but sometimes an infection ascends the ureters to involve the kidneys.

WHAT CAUSES IT?

• Most often, pyelonephritis is caused by a bacterial infection; a fungal infection may also be a cause.
• Risk is associated with kidney stones, bladder tumors, enlargement of the prostate, obstructive lesions of the urinary tract, venereal disease, diabetes mellitus, or the use of a urinary catheter.
• In women, the risk of kidney infection increases with pregnancy and sexual activity.

PREVENTION

• Women should practice careful hygiene. After using the toilet, wipe from front to back to avoid spreading fecal bacteria to the urethra.
• Drink plenty of fluids to stay hydrated.

DIAGNOSIS

• Patient history and physical examination.
• Urine sample for culture and microscopic analysis.

HOW TO TREAT IT

• Take over-the-counter pain relievers to reduce fever and discomfort, and get sufficient bed rest.
• Drink eight or more glasses of water a day.
• Antibiotics are often prescribed to fight the infection and should be taken for the full term indicated.
• Surgical correction may be needed if a urinary tract obstruction causes recurrent pyelonephritis.

WHEN TO CALL A DOCTOR

• Call a doctor immediately if you develop symptoms of a kidney infection. ▲

SYMPTOMS

• Fever and chills.
• Sudden, intense, persistent pain in the abdomen, middle back, or flank. Pain may be worse on one side and may intensify with movement.
• Joint and muscle pain; fatigue.
• Nausea and vomiting.
• Burning on urination; frequent and urgent urination; cloudy or discolored urine, possibly with a strange odor.
• Chronic pyelonephritis generally causes no symptoms until enough damage occurs to induce kidney failure.

Labyrinthitis

WHAT IS IT?

Labyrinthitis is an inflammation of the semicircular canals—the three small, curved tubes in the inner ear that help maintain balance. Each canal is filled with a fluid called endolymph and contains tiny calcium stones known as otoliths. The walls of these canals are lined with crops of specialized cells capped with hairlike fibers. Movement of the head causes the fluid and the otoliths to move and press upon the fibers. When bent, these fibers send signals to the brain so it can calculate the head's position. Inflammation of the semicircular canals interferes with this process, sending conflicting signals to the brain, which causes severe dizziness and nausea. Although the symptoms may be frightening, labyrinthitis is not serious, and full spontaneous recovery is common.

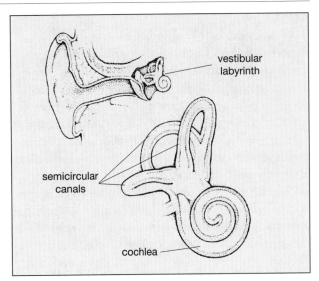

The vestibular labyrinth, deep in the inner ear, is comprised of several structures necessary for balance, including the semicircular canals.

WHAT CAUSES IT?

- Bacterial or viral infections.
- Allergies.
- Certain medications, such as aminoglycosides.
- Head injury.
- Alcohol abuse may produce symptoms similar to labyrinthitis.
- Labyrinthitis may occur as a complication of cholesteatoma (see Cholesteatoma).

PREVENTION

- Obtain prompt treatment for ear infections, bacterial infections elsewhere in the body, and allergies (especially allergies of the upper respiratory tract).
- Drink alcoholic beverages in moderation.

DIAGNOSIS

- Patient history and physical examination are needed.
- A culture of any ear discharge will be taken.

SYMPTOMS

- Acute onset of vertigo (severe dizziness or a spinning sensation, and loss of balance).
- Nausea and vomiting.
- Ringing in the ears (tinnitus).
- Hearing loss (when labyrinthitis involves the hearing portion of the inner ear).

HOW TO TREAT IT

- No specific cure exists for labyrinthitis. Treatment is aimed at easing symptoms as recovery occurs spontaneously, usually after a period of several weeks.
- Labyrinthitis caused by a bacterial infection may require large doses of antibiotics.
- Fluid replacement is needed to prevent dehydration if severe vomiting has occurred. This may be done orally or, in severe cases, intravenously.
- Medications such as meclizine (an antihistamine with an antinausea effect), prochlorperazine (an antinausea drug), scopolamine (a motion-sickness drug), and diazepam (a tranquilizer) may be prescribed.
- Rarely, surgery may be required to drain pus from the middle ear or to remove a cholesteatoma (see Ear Infection, Middle and Cholesteatoma for more information).
- A balance rehabilitation program may help patients compensate for the loss of the ear's balance inputs.
- During recovery, try to avoid positions that trigger or exacerbate dizziness. Rest in bed in a dark, quiet room with your head immobilized between pillows.
- Until vertigo subsides, do not drive or perform other activities in which loss of balance may be dangerous.

WHEN TO CALL A DOCTOR

- See your doctor if you experience persistent dizziness or other symptoms of labyrinthitis. ▲

Lactose Intolerance

WHAT IS IT?

Lactose intolerance is an impaired ability to digest lactose, a type of sugar found in milk and other dairy products. During digestion, lactose is broken down into two simple sugars by lactase, an enzyme found in the small intestine. However, if an insufficient amount of this enzyme is produced, lactose cannot be properly digested, resulting in abdominal discomfort within 30 minutes to two hours after consuming milk or milk-based foods.

The degree of lactose intolerance varies from person to person. In most cases, the ability to digest lactose was present at birth but was lost, either suddenly or gradually, between the ages of three and 20. The condition is very common; indeed, it is estimated that over 70 percent of the world's adult population cannot digest lactose, with the exception of people of northern European descent, of whom less than 20 percent are lactose-intolerant. Most African American, Asian, and Native American adults produce little or no lactase. Lactose intolerance is not a health risk, and symptoms may be controlled by following simple dietary measures.

WHAT CAUSES IT?

• Hereditary factors play a role in lactose intolerance.
• Some chronic gastrointestinal disorders, such as irritable bowel syndrome, Crohn's disease, and ulcerative colitis, may cause lactose intolerance.
• In infants, an intestinal infection such as gastroenteritis may cause temporary lactose intolerance.

PREVENTION

• There is no known way to prevent the development of lactose intolerance (although treatment can prevent symptoms).

SYMPTOMS

• Abdominal pain, cramps, and bloating.
• Excessive gas.
• Diarrhea.
• Audible bowel noises.
• Weight loss or slow growth in infants and young children.

DIAGNOSIS

• Lactose intolerance is suspected when stomach upset occurs shortly after consuming milk or other dairy products.
• Ability to absorb lactose can be determined by administering lactose orally and measuring the resulting rise in blood glucose (lactose tolerance test), or by measuring the amount of hydrogen subsequently exhaled in the breath (hydrogen breath test).

HOW TO TREAT IT

• Eliminate or reduce the amount of dairy products in your diet, including milk, cream, cheese, butter, and ice cream.
• Experiment: You may be able to tolerate moderate amounts of milk if consumed with a meal. Lactose-reduced milk is available.
• Add lactase drops to milk or swallow lactase tablets or caplets just prior to meals. The lactase in these over-the-counter supplements will break down most lactose in dairy products.
• Try yogurt with live cultures. Yogurt contains less lactose than milk, and the bacteria predigest much of what remains. Look for live or active cultures listed on the label.
• Substitute soy milk (a liquid made from soybeans) for cow's milk. Soy milk may be fed to babies, poured on cereal, and used in baking.
• Make sure to get enough calcium in your diet. Broccoli, calcium-fortified orange juice, amaranth (a grain), and legumes are good choices. Your doctor may advise calcium supplements as well.
• Be aware that lactose is commonly found in many foods, including baked goods such as breads, cookies, and cakes; pancake mixes; some powdered drinks such as cocoa and flavored coffees; processed meats such as frankfurters; and some canned and powdered soups.
• Hard, aged cheeses, like cheddar and Parmesan, are very low in lactose.
• Many medications contain lactose as an additive—check with your pharmacist.

WHEN TO CALL A DOCTOR

• See your doctor if self-treatment for lactose intolerance does not relieve abdominal discomfort. ▲

Laryngeal Cancer

WHAT IS IT?

Laryngeal cancer is the growth of malignant cells in the larynx (also known as the voice box), an organ composed of the vocal cords and a structure known as the epiglottis, a flap of tissue that prevents food from entering the airway while you swallow. The larynx is located between the pharynx, or throat, and the trachea (the windpipe). Laryngeal cancer can almost always be cured if detected early enough. Thus, it is essential to be alert to persistent hoarseness—the disease's cardinal and often only symptom.

Treatment is most successful when the tumor is restricted to the vocal cords. The outlook is less optimistic for cancers that have spread from the larynx to nearby lymph nodes or through the bloodstream to other parts of the body. Some 11,000 cases of laryngeal cancer are diagnosed each year, mostly in those over age 50, and nearly 4,000 people die from it annually. Men are affected far more often than women—accounting for about 9,300 annual cases.

WHAT CAUSES IT?

• Like other cancers of the oral and respiratory system, the risk of laryngeal cancer is higher among those who smoke or otherwise use tobacco.
• Heavy use of alcohol is also associated with laryngeal cancer. The combination of drinking and smoking significantly increases risk.

PREVENTION

• Avoid tobacco use as well as excessive alcohol consumption.

SYMPTOMS

• Hoarseness or other changes in voice quality that persist more than a week or recur.
• Symptoms of cancer arising in parts of the throat other than the vocal cords: swallowing difficulty and pain; a lump or swelling in the neck.
• In late stages: pain, a cough, and breathing difficulty.
• Unintentional weight loss.

DIAGNOSIS

• Patient history (including alcohol and tobacco habits) and physical examination are needed.
• You may be sent to an otolaryngologist (ear, nose, and throat specialist), who will do an indirect laryngoscopy (examination of the throat using a bright light and a pair of mirrors). A direct laryngoscopy (use of a flexible lighted scope to inspect the larynx) may be done if the visual exam is suspicious (usually performed under sedation or general anesthesia).
• A biopsy (microscopic examination of a tissue sample) may be taken to confirm the diagnosis when cancer is suspected.
• CT (computed tomography) scans or MRI (magnetic resonance imaging) may be done to determine the extent of a tumor.

HOW TO TREAT IT

• Early tumors confined to the vocal cords can be treated successfully with radiation, which can destroy the tumor while leaving the voice intact.
• Laser surgery can also treat some early tumors without affecting the ability to speak.
• More advanced cancers often require a laryngectomy—removal of the larynx. Most often, this will cure the cancer but will result in the loss of normal speaking ability. In such cases a speech therapist can teach the patient alternate means of speaking, such as using the esophagus (the tube through which food passes) as a substitute for the vocal cords, sometimes with the assistance of a surgically placed valve. Speech may also be synthesized with vibrating electromechanical aids placed against the throat.
• Surgery is often followed by radiation.
• Chemotherapy may be tried in advanced cases to prevent or arrest the spread of cancer and to ease symptoms.
• Administration of isotretinoin may reduce the likelihood of recurrence.
• Cure of laryngeal cancer is unlikely if the patient continues to smoke.

WHEN TO CALL A DOCTOR

• Call a doctor if hoarseness persists for more than a week or recurs frequently.

Laryngitis

WHAT IS IT?

Laryngitis is inflammation of the larynx or voice box, the structure in the throat containing the vocal cords. It occurs in two forms: acute, which lasts only a few days; and chronic, which persists over a period of weeks or months. The most common symptom of either form is hoarseness that may, within several days, progress to partial or total loss of the voice. Fever, sore throat, and swallowing difficulty may occur as well. Children face the added risk of encountering breathing difficulty, because the opening of a child's larynx is narrow to begin with, and inflammation restricts the air passages even further (see Croup for more information). Laryngitis may result from prolonged straining of the voice. It may also occur as an isolated local infection of the larynx or as part of another, more serious underlying disorder, such as pneumonia or tuberculosis. In most cases, however, it is a minor ailment and clears up on its own within a few days or weeks.

WHAT CAUSES IT?

• Acute laryngitis is most often due to a viral infection, including the common cold and influenza. Bacterial infections (such as tonsillitis, bronchitis, and pneumonia) less commonly cause laryngitis.
• Acute laryngitis may result from excessive strain on the vocal cords, as occurs with activities such as yelling, cheering, singing, or public speaking.
• Postnasal drip, allergies, or inhalation of smoke, fumes, or caustic chemicals can irritate the larynx and cause inflammation.
• Chronic laryngitis may be caused by excessive alcohol consumption, smoking, or constant exposure to dust or chemical irritants like paint remover.
• Long-term upper respiratory tract disorders such as sinusitis, bronchitis, nasal polyps, and allergies can cause chronic laryngitis.

SYMPTOMS
• Hoarseness; sore throat; weak or absent voice.
• Sensation of a lump in the throat or constant desire to clear the throat.
• Dry cough; possibly fever.

• Repeated episodes of acute laryngitis may eventually lead to chronic laryngitis.
• Laryngitis due to gastroesophageal reflux, or heartburn, a common cause of chronic laryngitis in adults, may occur without the sensation of heartburn.

PREVENTION

• Prompt treatment for upper respiratory infections is important.
• Smokers should abstain from smoking.
• Straining the voice should be avoided.

DIAGNOSIS

• Physical examination and patient history.
• Laryngoscopy (viewing the larynx with a mirror or a flexible, lighted scope).
• Throat culture (if bacterial infection is suspected).

HOW TO TREAT IT

• Avoid speaking during recovery; write notes instead. Be aware that whispering puts greater strain on the vocal cords than normal speaking. Avoid clearing your throat; cough gently instead.
• Inhale steam from a bowl of hot water.
• Drink plenty of liquids, especially warm, soothing nonalcoholic drinks, to stay hydrated.
• Try a cool-mist humidifier; increased moisture in the air may ease a sore throat. Avoid air-conditioning.
• Nonprescription pain relievers and throat lozenges can ease discomfort.
• Smokers should avoid cigarettes—at the very least until symptoms have subsided.
• If laryngitis is caused by a bacterial infection, antibiotics will be prescribed.
• Speech therapists may be able to assist voice overusers with chronic laryngitis.
• The underlying cause of chronic laryngitis must be diagnosed and treated.

WHEN TO CALL A DOCTOR

• If you have the symptoms of laryngitis for more than two weeks despite self-care measures, see a doctor.
• Chronic hoarseness warrants a doctor's attention; it may be an early symptom of laryngeal cancer.
• Call a doctor if symptoms appear in a child who is three months old or younger.

Legionnaire's Disease

WHAT IS IT?

Legionnaire's disease is a form of bacterial pneumonia that may occur in sporadic isolated cases or, more commonly, as a localized epidemic affecting groups of people. Symptoms develop within two days to a week after infection. Progressively severe pneumonia frequently occurs soon thereafter and lasts an additional week. This is followed by either a gradual recovery or by progressively worsening congestion in the lungs that causes serious breathing difficulty. (In a milder form of the disease known as Pontiac syndrome, symptoms subside in a few days, although fatigue may persist for several weeks.)

The prognosis for Legionnaire's disease largely depends on the age and the general health of the patient. Younger people usually recover fully, while the elderly or those in poor health are at risk for potentially fatal respiratory failure. Legionnaire's disease most often affects those who are middle-aged or older and is most prevalent in late summer or early fall.

WHAT CAUSES IT?

• Legionnaire's disease is caused by the *Legionella pneumophila* bacterium, which breeds readily in warm, moist places. Most outbreaks of the disease occur when these bacteria contaminate the air-conditioning or hot-water systems of large public buildings and are transmitted via airborne vapor droplets. Outbreaks have also been described in hospitals. The infection does not spread from person to person.

SYMPTOMS
• Headache.
• High fever and shaking chills.
• Muscle aches and stiffness.
• Dry cough in early stages; cough with bloody sputum later.
• Shortness of breath.
• Chest pain.
• Diarrhea.
• Nausea and vomiting.
• Mental confusion; disorientation.
• Delirium.

• Smoking and excessive alcohol consumption increase the risk of infection among those exposed to the bacterium.
• Many chronic illnesses, such as kidney failure, emphysema, or diabetes mellitus, increase the risk.

PREVENTION

• Cooling and heating systems should be cleaned and inspected regularly and all filters changed as needed.

DIAGNOSIS

• Patient history and physical examination are needed for proper diagnosis.
• A culture of respiratory mucus may be taken.
• Blood cultures and/or a urine specimen may also be taken.
• A chest x-ray will be done.
• A lung biopsy may be performed (rarely).

HOW TO TREAT IT

• Hospitalization is usually required.
• A macrolide antibiotic (such as erythromycin or azithromycin) or a fluoroquinolone antibiotic is often given intravenously. This usually alleviates symptoms quickly.
• Intravenous replenishment of fluids and electrolytes (essential mineral salts) may be required.
• Aspirin or aspirin-like drugs are used to reduce fever and ease discomfort.
• Supplementary oxygen may be administered, or in severe cases, a mechanical respirator may be required.

WHEN TO CALL A DOCTOR

• If you develop the symptoms of Legionnaire's disease, call your doctor immediately.
• If, during or after treatment, you experience severe chest pain, bluish nails, lips, or skin, or bloody sputum, see a doctor. 🄰

Leukemias

WHAT IS IT?

Leukemia is a disease of the blood-producing structures—the bone marrow and the lymphatic system (the spleen, liver, and lymph nodes)—in which a large number of abnormal white blood cells are produced. These malignant cells are released into the blood, where they circulate throughout the body and may infiltrate other body tissues.

Blood contains three broad types of cells: Red cells carry oxygen; platelets are crucial for clotting; white cells fight infections and are part of the body's immune system. White cells are further subdivided into two major types. Myelocytes destroy bacteria and other foreign invaders by engulfing them; lymphocytes produce antibodies that bind to infectious agents to prevent them from multiplying. Immature white cells, known as blasts, are produced by the bone marrow and lymphatic system but are not released into the bloodstream until they mature. Normally, the body produces only enough white cells to replace the ones that have died. However, in leukemia, too many blasts and mature white cells are produced. Excessive numbers of white cells in the bone marrow interfere with the production of other types of blood cells. The resulting lack of red cells starves body tissues of oxygen; deficiency of platelets greatly increases the risk of hemorrhage; lack of certain white cells can compromise the immune system. Leukemic cells may spread from the blood to other structures in the body, including the liver, the skin, and the central nervous system.

The different types of leukemia are classified as acute and chronic, according to how quickly the disease tends to progress, and by the type of white cell affected. The acute leukemias are rapidly progressing diseases, usually requiring immediate treatment. The chronic leukemias have two phases, gradual and acute. During the gradual phase, which may last for years, symptoms often do not occur, and treatment may be unnecessary; however, the symptoms and rapid progress of the acute phase of chronic leukemia resemble those of the acute leukemias.

Acute and chronic leukemias are further distinguished by the type of white cell affected: acute and chronic myelogenous leukemia (AML and CML) affect myelocytes; acute and chronic lymphocytic leukemia (ALL and CLL) and hairy cell leukemia affect lymphocytes; acute monocytic leukemia affects monocytes. Hairy cell leukemia is a rare chronic leukemia marked by the production of abnormal lymphocytes with irregular hairlike protrusions.

Overall, leukemias account for about 5 percent of cancers in the United States. Half of the cases of leukemia are the acute leukemias; ALL is the most common cancer in children, while over 80 percent of cases of AML occur in adults. Of the chronic leukemias, CLL is the most common overall, comprising over one-third of cases in the United States, and CML accounts for one-fifth of cases. Despite leukemia's reputation as a childhood disease, it mainly affects people over 60, especially men. Treatment can bring about remission, although relapse is

SYMPTOMS

- No symptoms associated with the early stages of the chronic leukemias.
- General feeling of poor health (ALL, AML, CLL, CML, hairy cell leukemia).
- Fever and night sweats due to associated bacterial, viral, or fungal infections. Infections may be frequent because of the weakened immune system and the absence of enough myelocytes for proper defense (ALL, AML, CLL, CML, hairy cell leukemia).
- Severe fatigue, pallor, and breathing difficulty, due to anemia (ALL, AML, CLL, CML).
- Headaches and seizures due to associated meningitis (ALL, AML).
- Increased bruising and bleeding (ALL, AML, CML).
- Bone pain, especially in the legs (ALL, CML, hairy cell leukemia).
- Abdominal pain, nausea, and abdominal distention (ALL, CML, hairy cell leukemia).
- Loss of appetite and weight loss (AML, CLL, CML).
- Swollen glands due to enlarged lymph nodes and spleen (AML, CLL).
- Palpitations (CLL).
- Joint pain due to gout (CML).

Leukemias   *continued*

common. In children, the treatment of acute lymphocytic leukemia is a modern success story: 50 to 70 percent achieve long-term remission and are considered cured.

WHAT CAUSES IT?
• The cause of leukemia is unknown.
• Hereditary factors play a role. A genetic abnormality known as the Philadelphia chromosome leads to CML; 10 percent of people with ALL have also been shown to have the Philadelphia chromosome.
• Some industrial chemicals, such as benzene, a petroleum derivative, may be associated with leukemia.
• Prolonged exposure to x-rays or radiation (as used in cancer treatment) may lead to leukemia.
• Some medications used in chemotherapy, such as the alkylating agents mechlorethamine, chlorambucil, cyclophosphamide, and busulfan, may carry a higher risk of leukemia.
• The human T-cell leukemia virus is involved in a rare type of leukemia known as adult T-cell leukemia.

PREVENTION
• Limit exposure to toxic chemicals, as well as to x-rays and other forms of radiation, to reduce the risk of ALL, AML, and CML.

DIAGNOSIS
• Examination of the number of red cells, platelets, and different types of white cells in the blood.
• Bone marrow aspiration or biopsy. A sample of bone marrow is usually taken from the hip bone.
• Cytological (cell) studies are performed to determine the presence of the Philadelphia chromosome.

HOW TO TREAT IT
• Chemotherapy is used to treat the acute leukemias and the acute phases of the chronic leukemias. High doses are used to induce remission, and in the case of ALL, lower maintenance doses may be continued for months or years to prevent relapses. Bone marrow from the patient may be extracted during a remission and preserved in a frozen state. Removal protects the bone marrow from damage during treatment of a relapse with high doses of chemotherapeutic drugs, after which the preserved marrow cells are given back to the patient.
• Radiation therapy may be used to destroy leukemia cells in the cerebrospinal fluid, central nervous system, spleen, and lymph nodes (ALL, CLL, CML).
• Corticosteroids, usually prednisone, may be prescribed prior to or in addition to chemotherapy (ALL, CLL, the acute phase of CML).
• Bone marrow transplantation may be used to treat and possibly cure ALL, AML, and CML if a compatible donor can be found. Bone marrow is more difficult to match than blood; the best results occur with a sibling donor. If that is not possible, a search to find a compatible donor may be done through the National Bone Marrow Registry. Before transplant, the patient is given intensive chemotherapy or total body radiation to destroy leukemia cells. Bone marrow may also be extracted from the patient, treated to remove leukemia cells, and then returned after intensive chemotherapy or radiation.
• Interferon has been highly successful in the treatment of hairy cell leukemia, with more than 90 percent of patients expected to survive more than five years. Interferon may also be used to treat CML.
• Surgery to remove an enlarged spleen, one of the sites of white cell production, may be necessary in hairy cell leukemia and CLL.
• For all forms of leukemia, transfusions of blood, red cells, or platelets may be used during treatment to maintain adequate levels of blood components.
• Analgesics may be prescribed for all forms.
• Antibiotics or antifungal medications may be needed to treat associated infections in all forms of leukemia. Common infections are dangerous for the leukemia patient, because both the cancer and its treatment suppress the body's immune system.

WHEN TO CALL A DOCTOR
• Call a doctor if you notice an increased tendency to bruise or bleed, or develop severe fatigue, breathing difficulty, bone pain, appetite or weight loss, abdominal pain, swollen glands, palpitations, or fever.
• Call a doctor if your child develops bone pain, an increased tendency to bruise or bleed, fever, or severe fatigue. ▲

Lice

WHAT IS IT?

Lice are small, yellowish gray, wingless insects that live on the body and feed on human blood. There are three species: head lice, pubic lice (crabs), and body lice. Head lice live on and suck blood from the scalp, leaving red spots that may itch severely. Constant scratching may lead to a secondary skin infection. The females lay small, pale, football-shaped eggs (nits) on the hair shafts close to the scalp. These eggs hatch within seven days and then usually live for several weeks. Head lice are spread through direct contact with an infested person.

Body lice live in and lay their eggs on clothing and go to the body only when they need to feed. They may transmit typhus or relapsing fever (both infectious diseases characterized by a rash and fever), although this is quite rare. Body lice usually affect people who do not change their clothes often enough. Pubic lice live in pubic hair and are usually transmitted during sexual contact. Less commonly, they may infest eyelashes, beards, armpit hair, and hair around the anus.

In general, those at greatest risk for lice infestation are school children and people living in nursing homes or in other crowded or unsanitary conditions. Although lice are terribly annoying and spread quite easily, they are fairly easy to treat and rarely pose a serious health risk. Unfortunately, some head lice have become resistant to currently available over-the-counter treatment.

WHAT CAUSES IT?

• Living in an overcrowded or unhygienic environment increases the risk of lice infestation.
• Schoolchildren are often affected because of their close daily contact with schoolmates and the use of communal closets.

SYMPTOMS
• Intense itching, usually in hair-covered areas.
• Redness and flaking of the skin.
• Tiny red bite marks.
• Visible lice on clothing.
• Visible nits (eggs) on hair shafts.

• Head lice can be transmitted through use of an infested hairbrush, comb, hat, or set of headphones.
• Pubic lice are most often transmitted through sexual contact with an infected partner but may also be transmitted through contact with infested bedding.

PREVENTION

• Check your children periodically for head lice and nits, especially during peak season (August through November).
• Do not wear the same clothes for more than a day or two. Launder clothes often.
• Bathe or shower regularly.
• Do not share combs, hairbrushes, hats, or other headwear with others.

DIAGNOSIS

• Diagnosis is usually based on self-examination. Lice and their eggs, although small, are visible on hair shafts, skin, and clothes.

HOW TO TREAT IT

• Several over-the-counter lotions and shampoos are available to treat lice. These products should be applied to all infected areas of the body (follow label instructions) and washed off. Then, using a fine-tooth comb, remove any dead lice or nits from the hair shafts. One or two more applications of the lotion may be necessary.
• Several shampoos are available for the treatment of head lice. Repeated use of these over several weeks is usually required.
• Combs and hairbrushes should be washed in very hot soapy water to kill any attached eggs.
• Infested clothing should be washed in very hot water and dried on a high heat cycle for at least 20 minutes.
• Items like towels, bedding, rugs, upholstery, mattresses, and children's stuffed toys should be thoroughly cleaned (or burned if necessary) to avoid reinfestation.

WHEN TO CALL A DOCTOR

• Call a doctor if symptoms persist despite self-treatment measures.

Liver Tumors

WHAT IS IT?

A liver tumor is an abnormal growth of cells—at times benign but far more often malignant—in the liver. Benign growths may cause symptoms and require treatment in rare cases, but generally they are not a health risk. Malignant tumors are classified as either primary or secondary. Primary tumors, which are relatively uncommon in North America, originate in the liver, either from the liver cells themselves (hepatoma or hepatocellular carcinoma) or from cells of the bile ducts (cholangiocarcinoma).

Much more common are secondary, or metastatic, tumors that have spread to the liver from cancers elsewhere in the body. Next to the lymph nodes, the liver is the most common site for the spread of cancer. The outlook for both primary and secondary liver cancers is poor; they are usually fatal within six months to one year of diagnosis. Treatment is aimed at relieving symptoms. Benign tumors are more common among women, especially those taking oral contraceptives; malignant ones are more common among men.

WHAT CAUSES IT?

• The cause of primary liver tumors is unknown.
• The risk of primary liver cancer is increased in patients with cirrhosis, whether due to hepatitis B or C infection, hemochromatosis, or alcoholism.
• Exposure to toxic chemicals, such as polyvinyl chloride vapors or arsenic, may lead to liver cancer.
• Aflatoxins (molds that grow on incorrectly stored peanuts and grains) may contribute to liver cancer.
• Metastatic tumors may spread to the liver from other sites, most commonly from cancers of the colon, stomach, pancreas, lung, and breast.
• The use of oral contraceptives is associated with some benign liver tumors, although this is rare.

PREVENTION

• Have no more than two alcoholic drinks a day. If you suspect that you may have a drinking problem, seek help immediately. You will need to avoid alcohol completely if you have cirrhosis; a doctor or support group may help you with this.
• Try to limit exposure to toxic chemicals, like insecticides, herbicides, cleaning solvents, paint thinner, and engine exhaust.
• Get regular checkups (including measurement of blood alpha fetoprotein levels every four months and a liver ultrasound annually) if you have a history of hepatitis B or C, hemochromatosis, or cirrhosis.

DIAGNOSIS

• Patient history and physical examination are needed. The doctor will press upon the liver to detect any swelling or solid masses.
• Blood tests will be taken.
• Ultrasound, CT (computed tomography) scans, or MRI (magnetic resonance imaging) may be done.
• A liver biopsy may be performed. Using local anesthesia, a needle is inserted under the ribs and into the liver to extract a small tissue sample for analysis.
• Exploratory surgery may be necessary.

HOW TO TREAT IT

• Surgery is possible for benign, symptomatic tumors.
• Chemotherapy may be used to destroy cancerous cells, but results are disappointing.
• Surgical removal of a single small malignant tumor may be performed. However, surgery is not advised for large malignant tumors or widespread cancer.
• Radiation therapy is used in some cases.
• Liver transplantation is a rare option.

WHEN TO CALL A DOCTOR

• Symptoms of a liver tumor warrant a doctor's attention. ◢

SYMPTOMS

• Usually no symptoms in early stages.
• Pain or discomfort in the upper-right portion of the abdomen.
• Abdominal swelling.
• General feeling of poor health.
• Loss of appetite and weight.
• Nausea and vomiting.
• Fever; profuse sweating.
• Jaundice.
• Severe fatigue, pale complexion, and breathing difficulty due to associated anemia.

Lung Abscess

WHAT IS IT?

A lung abscess is a cavity within the lungs partially filled with pus. Now uncommon, lung abscesses usually result from a severe infection such as pneumonia or tuberculosis or from the aspiration of infectious material through the mouth. An abscess may also develop if a bronchial passage becomes blocked by vomit, food, or some other foreign matter that has trapped lung secretions, allowing them to accumulate and become infected. Generally, coughing expels material that may potentially block the lungs, preventing the formation of abscesses. However, loss of consciousness, for example, owing to a head injury, anesthesia for surgery, or the abuse of drugs or alcohol, may allow infectious material to be aspirated into the lungs and remain there. A tumor may also block bronchial passages and lead to an abscess. An embolus (blot clot) in the blood vessels of the lungs can lead to death of lung tissue. The dead tissue acts as fertile soil for germs, which may enable an abscess to form. Symptoms may develop over a period of days or weeks. The incidence of lung abscesses has decreased substantially since the advent of antibiotics. Lung abscesses are not contagious and generally respond well to a prolonged course of antibiotics.

WHAT CAUSES IT?

• Lung abscess may occur as a complication of a bacterial infection, such as pneumonia or tuberculosis (although this has become less common).
• Fungal infection of the lungs may lead to abscess.
• Inhalation of foreign matter into the lungs may

---

lead to an abscess, especially in the presence of a tooth abscess or an infection of the gums (see Periodontitis for more information).
• A lung tumor may block bronchial passages (see Lung Cancer for more information).
• Immunocompromised patients, such as those with AIDS or those undergoing treatment for cancer, are prone to lung abscesses.

PREVENTION

• Upper respiratory infections should be treated.

DIAGNOSIS

• Patient history and physical examination.
• Blood and sputum cultures.
• CT (computed tomography) scans.
• At times, bronchoscopy (passage of a thin, hollow, flexible tube through the mouth into the windpipe to allow the main bronchial passages to be viewed).
• Chest x-rays. If a lung abscess is found, x-rays will be taken periodically throughout treatment to monitor progress.

HOW TO TREAT IT

• Antibiotics are prescribed to treat a lung abscess involving a bacterial infection (including tuberculosis or bacterial pneumonia). These should be taken for the full term prescribed (often six weeks or more), even if fever and cough subside in less time.
• Antifungal drugs may be prescribed to treat an underlying fungal infection.
• Your doctor may show you how to drain mucus from your lungs by assuming various positions that lower your head below your torso (a technique known as postural drainage).
• Bronchoscopy may be used to aid drainage in some cases, depending upon the location and size of the abscess. Pus may be drawn out through the scope.
• Surgery may be performed to drain the abscess or, more often, to remove the infected lobe of the lung if the abscess does not respond to antibiotics.

WHEN TO CALL A DOCTOR

• Call a doctor for shortness of breath, wheezing, high fever with chills, or fainting spells, or if a respiratory infection worsens despite treatment. ▲

> ## SYMPTOMS
> • Fever and chills.
> • Profuse sweating.
> • General feeling of poor health.
> • Loss of appetite and weight loss.
> • Chest pain.
> • Deep cough that may produce foul-tasting or bloody sputum.
> • Clubbing of the fingers.
> • Fatigue.

Lung Cancer

WHAT IS IT?

Lung cancer, the growth of malignant cells in the lungs, is the leading cause of death from cancer in the United States for both men and women. In 1998 an estimated 178,000 new cases of lung cancer were diagnosed, and 160,000 deaths were attributed to the disease. The types of primary lung cancer (cancer that originates in the lungs) may be grouped into two broad categories: small-cell carcinoma and several forms of lung cancer collectively termed non-small-cell carcinoma (which make up 80 percent of cases). Although the outlook is poor in all types of lung cancer, small-cell carcinoma spreads especially quickly and is more difficult to treat; the majority of patients die within a year of diagnosis.

Primary lung cancer can spread to essentially any organ, where it may produce more disabling symptoms. Most cases occur between ages 45 and 75, after years of exposure to cigarette smoke or other pollutants. In many instances, the disease is preventable: Over 90 percent of cases are caused by smoking. Nonsmokers have only a small risk, and those who quit smoking—even after smoking for years—greatly reduce their risk. The lungs are also a frequent site of secondary cancer, which has spread from elsewhere in the body. Such tumors are almost always incurable.

WHAT CAUSES IT?

• Cigarette smoking is by far the most common cause of primary lung cancer.
• Air pollution, including so-called passive or second-hand smoke, traffic fumes, and smokestack emissions, may contribute to lung cancer.
• Exposure to toxic substances, such as radon and other radioactive gases, asbestos, and arsenic, may cause lung cancer.
• Chronic bronchitis is associated with an increased risk of lung cancer (see Chronic Obstructive Pulmonary Disease for more information).

PREVENTION

• Abstain from smoking; try to limit your exposure to second-hand smoke and air pollution.
• Homes may be tested for radon using a kit available in most hardware stores.

DIAGNOSIS

• Patient history and physical examination.
• Sputum sample.
• Chest x-rays, CT (computed tomography) scans, and MRI (magnetic resonance imaging).
• Bronchoscopy (passage of a thin, hollow, flexible tube through the mouth into the windpipe to allow the main bronchial passages to be viewed).
• A biopsy of cancerous tissue is essential for diagnosis and to guide treatment decisions.

HOW TO TREAT IT

• Surgical removal is the preferred treatment for localized non-small-cell carcinomas (those that have not yet spread). Part or all of the affected lung may be removed, depending on tumor size and location, as well as the patient's physical condition.
• Radiation therapy may be used to treat non-small-cell carcinoma in addition to surgery, or for patients ineligible for surgery.
• Chemotherapy is used to treat localized small-cell carcinomas. Several chemotherapeutic agents are used in an attempt to destroy the tumor. Recent studies have shown a clear benefit of adding radiation therapy to chemotherapy in treating this form.

WHEN TO CALL A DOCTOR

• Call a doctor if you develop symptoms of lung cancer, especially cough, weight loss, or fatigue.
• Get regular lung examinations if you are age 45 or over and smoke heavily. ▲

SYMPTOMS

• Cough, sometimes with bloody sputum.
• Wheezing and shortness of breath.
• Chest pain.
• Pain in the shoulder and arm.
• Fatigue.
• Weight loss.
• Clubbed fingers.
• Hoarseness.
• Swollen neck and face; swallowing difficulty.
• Enlarged lymph nodes in the neck.

Lyme Disease

WHAT IS IT?

Lyme disease is an infection caused by a bacterial spirochete (a corkscrew-shaped organism) spread by a bite from an infected tick. It is named after the community of Old Lyme, CT, where the disease was first identified. Lyme disease may affect several organ systems, and symptoms vary, some arising months or even years after a bite. Left untreated, the infection may affect the brain, heart, or joints, resulting in a type of chronic arthritis (see Infectious Arthritis for more information). The common deer tick carries the infection and is prevalent in New England, along both U.S. coasts, and in the upper Midwest. They are small compared to dog ticks: Adults are the size of a pinhead; nymphs smaller still. Between 20 and 60 percent of ticks carry the bacteria, but infection is rare if the tick is removed within 48 hours of attachment. Lyme disease is preventable; it responds well to treatment, especially if caught early. In some cases, it subsides spontaneously.

WHAT CAUSES IT?

• A bacterial infection causes Lyme disease. Ticks acquire the disease from infected mice and deer and may then transfer the bacteria to humans.

PREVENTION

• Cover exposed skin when in grassy or wooded areas where ticks may be present. Tuck long pants into socks, wear shoes instead of sandals, and wear long-sleeved shirts. Light-colored clothing makes ticks easier to see.
• Use an insect repellent containing DEET (diethyltoluamide) during outdoor summer activities.
• Check skin, clothing, and pets for ticks after an outing. Pets should wear tick-repellent collars.
• Use fine-tipped, curved tweezers to remove a tick attached to your skin. Grasp the tick as close to your skin as possible and pull steadily to remove it. Avoid squeezing the bloated abdomen, as this may inject bacteria into your skin or bloodstream. Do not touch the tick, because bacteria from a crushed tick may penetrate even unbroken skin. Preserve the tick by dropping it in rubbing alcohol. Wash your hands and apply antiseptic to the bite.
• Do not use petroleum jelly, kerosene, or a lighted match or cigarette to remove the tick.
• A new vaccine (Osp A) has been approved for use in adults; it appears to decrease the transmission rate of Lyme by 80 percent following an infected bite.

DIAGNOSIS

• Patient history and physical examination.
• Blood tests. Cument antibody tests used to detect Lyme disease may be inconclusive, especially with early infection. As such, Lyme disease remains a clinical diagnosis to be made only by a physician.
• A preserved tick may be examined to determine if it is the type that carries the infectious bacteria.

HOW TO TREAT IT

• Antibiotics are prescribed for as long as three weeks to treat early stages; others, given intravenously, may be needed to treat chronic arthritis or neurologic forms of the disease.
• OTC pain relievers reduce fever and inflammation.

WHEN TO CALL A DOCTOR

• Call a doctor if you develop symptoms. 🔺

SYMPTOMS

• Within two to 30 days after a bite: a small, red, flat or slightly raised lesion at the site, surrounded by a round, bull's-eyelike, red rash with a pale center. The rash may increase in size for some weeks before fading; similar lesions may appear at other sites. The affected area does not itch but may feel warm to the touch. The rash does not always occur and may be missed.
• Within 30 days: flulike symptoms of fever and chills, extreme fatigue, headaches, muscle and joint aches.
• Within several weeks or months: heart palpitations, shortness of breath, temporary facial paralysis, joint pain and swelling.
• Within two years: chronic joint pain and swelling, especially in knees (Lyme arthritis).
• Not all symptoms occur with every case or in any set order.

Lymphoma, Hodgkin's Hodgkin's Disease

WHAT IS IT?

Hodgkin's lymphoma is an uncommon form of cancer involving lymphatic tissue in the lymph nodes and spleen. Lymph nodes produce lymphocytes, a type of white blood cell that is crucial in regulating and carrying out most of the activities of the immune system. In Hodgkin's disease, cells in the lymphatic tissues grow in a rapid and uncontrolled manner—the defining characteristic of cancer. If not treated in time, the cancer may spread to other organs, such as the lungs, liver, and bone marrow. In addition, the proliferation of abnormal lymphocytes reduces the number of healthy lymphocytes. The resulting impairment of the immune system leaves the body susceptible to serious infection. However, with prompt detection and treatment, prognosis is good (more than 75 percent of adults diagnosed with Hodgkin's are curable). The mortality rate is dropping more rapidly for this disease than for any other type of cancer in the United States, largely because of advances in therapy. Hodgkin's disease, more common among men, most often affects those between ages 15 and 35, and those older than 55.

WHAT CAUSES IT?

• The cause of Hodgkin's disease is unknown, although hereditary factors may play a role. The incidence appears to be higher among those with immune system disorders or those receiving immunosuppressant drugs (used after organ transplants, for example).

PREVENTION

• There is no way to prevent Hodgkin's lymphoma.

SYMPTOMS

• Painless, gradual swelling of lymph nodes, especially in the neck, underarms, or groin. (In a few cases lymph nodes enlarge rapidly and painfully or may fluctuate in size.)
• Fever, chills, or night sweats.
• Persistent fatigue.
• Weight loss and loss of appetite.
• Itching that worsens as the disease progresses.

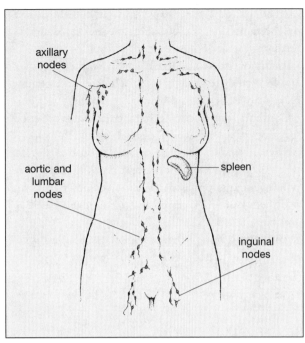

The lymphatic system (which includes the spleen) is comprised of a vast network of glands or nodes essential to the immune system.

DIAGNOSIS

• Patient history and physical examination.
• Lymph node biopsy, in which a portion of an enlarged lymph node is removed and examined under the microscope. Presence of a specific type of cell (Reed-Sternberg cell) characteristic of Hodgkin's disease provides a definitive diagnosis.
• Other tests, including blood tests; liver, spleen, and bone marrow biopsies; chest x-rays; abdominal CT (computed tomography) scans; and bone or lung scans may be done to determine the extent of lymph node and other organ involvement.

HOW TO TREAT IT

• Successful treatment is based heavily upon a process known as staging, which depends upon the presence or absence of general symptoms, use of a battery of tests to determine how far the cancer has spread, and the microscopic appearance of the lymphatic tissue.
• Radiation therapy alone is used for Stage I as well as for Stage II cancers. Stage I is the earliest and least serious stage, involving only one lymph node region or one organ outside the lymph nodes. Stage II involves two or more lymph node regions or one

Lymphoma, Hodgkin's Hodgkin's Disease *continued*

extralymphatic organ and its nearby nodes, grouped on the same side of the diaphragm muscle, which separates the abdominal and chest cavities.

• Radiation is used in combination with chemotherapy for Stage III Hodgkin's, in which cancer affects lymph nodes above and below the diaphragm.

• Combinations of chemotherapeutic drugs are used for patients with Stage IV disease (in which cancer has spread widely to other organs), as well as those who relapse after radiation alone. Such therapy, while generally producing the worst side effects of all treatment options, often leads to prolonged or even complete remission.

• Autologous bone marrow transplantation, in which healthy bone marrow is removed prior to treatment and replaced afterward, may be recommended to preserve bone marrow cells while the rest of the body is subjected to intensive chemotherapy or radiation.

WHEN TO CALL A DOCTOR

• While most incidences of enlarged glands are not a sign of cancer, see a doctor if the swelling persists longer than two weeks, especially if accompanied by fever or night sweats.

• **EMERGENCY** See a doctor immediately for the sudden onset of a high fever, loss of bladder or bowel control, or numbness in the arms or legs—all potential signs of Hodgkin's disease complications.

Lymphoma, Non-Hodgkin's

WHAT IS IT?

Lymphoma is a relatively rare form of cancer involving lymphatic tissue in the lymph nodes and spleen. Lymph nodes produce lymphocytes, a type of white blood cell that is crucial in regulating and carrying out most of the activities of the immune system. In lymphoma, cells in the lymphatic system begin to grow in a rapid and uncontrolled manner—the defining characteristic of cancer.

Non-Hodgkin's lymphoma (nHL), the most common form of lymphoma, is a collective grouping of the types of lymphoma that differ from Hodgkin's lymphoma (see Lymphoma, Hodgkin's for more information). The more than 10 kinds of nHL are categorized according to cell type and how fast they grow: low-grade (slow growing), intermediate-grade, and high-grade (rapidly growing). (Paradoxically, low-grade nHL is considered incurable with conventional therapy while high-grade nHL is potentially curable.) The proliferation of abnormal lymphocytes reduces the number of healthy lymphocytes. The resulting impairment of the immune system leaves the body susceptible to serious infection. Prognosis depends upon the grade and the extent of the disease but is generally not as favorable as that for Hodgkin's disease. This is because nHL is more likely to spread to other organs and has usually done so by the time it is diagnosed.

WHAT CAUSES IT?

• The cause of nHL is unknown, although there is evidence that a viral component may be involved.
• Incidence appears to be higher in those with immune system disorders or those receiving immunosuppressant drugs (used after organ transplants, for example).

PREVENTION

• Non-Hodgkin's lymphoma is not preventable.

DIAGNOSIS

• Patient history and physical examination.
• Lymph node or bone marrow biopsies, in which tissue is removed for microscopic examination.
• Other tests, including blood tests, liver and spleen scans, chest x-rays, or abdominal CT (computed tomography) scans to determine the extent of lymph node and other organ involvement.

HOW TO TREAT IT

• Treatment choices are based upon a process known as staging, which depends upon the presence or absence of general symptoms, use of a battery of tests to determine how far the cancer has spread, and the microscopic appearance of the lymphatic tissue.
• Radiation therapy alone is used for lymphomas (especially low-grade varieties) confined to a single lymph node region or well-defined organ site.
• Since nHL has usually spread by the time it is diagnosed, chemotherapy with a combination of several anticancer agents (like cyclophosphamide, doxorubicin, and vincristine) and corticosteroids may be used, with or without radiation.
• In more severe cases autologous bone marrow donation (in which healthy bone marrow is removed prior to treatment and replaced afterward) may be recommended to preserve marrow while the rest of the body is subjected to intensive chemotherapy or radiation.

WHEN TO CALL A DOCTOR

• While most incidences of enlarged glands are not a sign of cancer, see a doctor if the swelling persists longer than two weeks, especially if accompanied by fever or night sweats.
• **EMERGENCY** See a doctor immediately for the sudden onset of a high fever, intractable constipation, urinary incontinence, or numbness in the arms or legs—potential signs of lymphoma complications. ▲

SYMPTOMS
• Painless, gradual swelling of the lymph nodes, especially in the neck, underarms, or groin.
• Enlarged tonsils and adenoids.
• Fever, chills, or night sweats.
• Breathing difficulty and coughing in children.
• Persistent fatigue.
• Weight loss and loss of appetite.
• Itching, which worsens as disease progresses.
• Rarely, nausea, vomiting, or abdominal pain.

Macular Degeneration, Age-Related

WHAT IS IT?

The macula is the central and most sensitive portion of the retina, the layer of tissue in the back of the eye that contains the light-receptive nerve cells essential for sight. For some people in their 50s, the macula begins to break down to some extent, resulting in the condition known as age-related macular degeneration (AMD). In AMD, central vision and the ability to distinguish fine detail become increasingly impaired, but peripheral vision remains unaffected. If macular function is lost completely, activities such as reading become impossible.

There are two forms of AMD: "dry" (also known as nonexudative or atrophic) and "wet" (exudative or neovascular). About 90 percent of those with AMD have the dry form, which—although irreversible and essentially untreatable—tends to progress slowly and may stabilize, so that most patients experience no serious vision loss. In wet AMD, however, fine blood vessels at the back of the eye proliferate and begin to leak or exude fluid, possibly scarring the macula and resulting in permanent central vision loss within days or weeks. Wet AMD may develop suddenly in patients with dry AMD. Both forms are painless and most often affect one eye at a time. AMD is the leading cause of severe and irreversible vision loss in older Americans.

WHAT CAUSES IT?

• The cause is unknown, although aging is clearly a risk factor. Some evidence of AMD can be detected in approximately one-quarter of all people over the age of 65 and in one-third of those over age 80.

• Other risk factors include hyperopia (farsightedness), cigarette smoking, light-colored eyes, and a family history of AMD. High blood pressure, lifetime sunlight exposure, dietary factors, and genetic susceptibility may increase wet AMD risk.

PREVENTION

• There is no known way to prevent macular degeneration. Presumably, avoidance of smoking, treatment of hypertension, and minimal sun exposure (wear sunglasses and a hat with a wide brim) might help.

DIAGNOSIS

• Eye examination by an ophthalmologist is needed.

• Wet AMD is confirmed with fluorescein angiography (injection of a special dye into the bloodstream to allow clear photographic images of the blood vessels in the eye to be taken).

HOW TO TREAT IT

• There are no ways to arrest or reverse the course of dry AMD. A research study is testing the use of vitamin and mineral supplements as a treatment. Retinal cell transplants do not yet work, but are being tested.

• People with dry AMD should be monitored for the onset of wet AMD. In the meantime, low-vision optical aids may be useful, including: high-power reading glasses; a small telescope mounted on one lens of your eyeglasses; a pocket telescope for reading street signs; and a closed-circuit television hookup that can magnify a written page as much as 60 times and display the image on a television screen.

• If detected early enough, wet AMD can often be treated with laser surgery to destroy the new leaking blood vessels. Such surgery should be performed only by an ophthalmologist with special training and experience in the procedure.

• New treatments being tested include new lasers, surgery to remove or move abnormal vessels, and new drugs that may control new vessel growth.

• Careful follow-up is essential for all AMD patients.

WHEN TO CALL A DOCTOR

• See an ophthalmologist if you have blurred or distorted vision.

• A simple home test (the Amsler grid) can help monitor visual changes. Any worsening of vision warrants an immediate visit to an ophthalmologist. ▲

SYMPTOMS

• Increasingly blurred central vision.
• Haziness, grayness, or blank spots in the central field of vision.
• Visual distortion: Straight lines appear bent; objects may appear smaller than in actuality.
• Dulled color perception.
• Difficulty reading or doing close work.

Malabsorption

WHAT IS IT?

Malabsorption is a term for any condition in which one or more essential nutrients or minerals are not properly digested or absorbed by the intestines. Lipids (fats) are the most commonly malabsorbed nutrients, but proteins, carbohydrates, electrolytes (such as sodium and potassium), vitamins, and minerals (such as iron and calcium) may be poorly absorbed as well. A multitude of different disorders can result in malabsorption; outlook depends upon the success in treating the underlying cause. Symptoms may range from bouts of gas, diarrhea, and stomach cramps that occur only when certain foods are consumed and maldigested (see Lactose Intolerance for more information) to emaciation and other signs of severe malnutrition.

WHAT CAUSES IT?

• Any defect in the functioning of the digestive system (for example, an inadequate production of bile salts by the liver, or digestive enzymes by the pancreas, or cells lining the intestine, or damage to the intestinal absorptive cells) can prevent the proper breakdown of foods and the absorption of adequate amounts of nutrients.

• Inflammation or other abnormalities (see Crohn's Disease and Amyloidosis for more information) in the mucous membrane that lines the intestine may

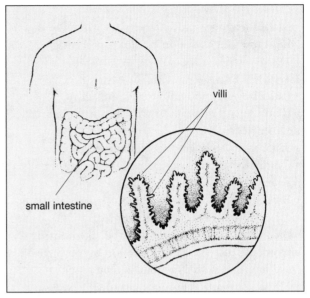

The small intestine is lined with tiny projections, called villi, that afford optimal surface area for the absorption of fluids and nutrients.

prevent nutrients from being absorbed through the intestinal wall.

• Surgery to remove diseased segments of the intestine may result in an inadequate amount of absorptive surface. This is called short bowel syndrome.

• Infections (including acute infectious enteritis) and tapeworm or other parasites may inhibit proper digestion. Some infections may result in an overgrowth of intestinal bacteria, which may also lead to malabsorption. Those with AIDS are particularly prone to malabsorption, since the disease damages immune defenses against secondary infections that may cause digestive problems.

• Any obstruction of the lymphatic system, as may occur with lymphomas and tuberculosis, may also interfere with nutrient absorption.

• Certain cardiovascular problems may result in malabsorption (see Congestive Heart Failure and Pericarditis for more information).

• Malabsorption may be induced by certain medications, such as cholestyramine (a cholesterol-lowering drug), neomycin (an antibiotic), colchicine (an antigout drug), and certain laxatives.

• Other diseases, including diabetes mellitus, hyper- and hypothyroidism, and carcinoid syndrome, may cause malabsorption for reasons that are unclear.

SYMPTOMS

• Diarrhea.
• Stools that float and are bulky, greasy, and unusually malodorous.
• Excessive gas.
• Abdominal discomfort or cramps, especially after eating.
• Fatigue.
• Weight loss or emaciation.
• Night blindness (vitamin A malabsorption).
• Easy bruising (vitamin K malabsorption).
• Bone pain and painful muscle contractions (calcium malabsorption).
• Paleness (pallor) and other symptoms of anemia.

Malabsorption   *continued*

PREVENTION

• Malabsorption is preventable only when the underlying cause (such as an infection) is preventable.

DIAGNOSIS

• Patient history and physical examination.
• Blood tests for anemia and other nutritional deficiencies.
• Stool samples looking for undigested fat.
• Culture of the microorganisms inhabiting the intestine.
• Breath tests to detect lactose intolerance or bacterial overgrowth in the small intestine.
• Biopsy of intestinal tissue (may be taken during endoscopy; that is, visual inspection of the upper small intestine with a flexible, lighted scope).
• Upper GI (gastrointestinal) and small bowel series (use of barium to create a clear image of the intestine on x-ray).

HOW TO TREAT IT

• In some cases the only treatment necessary is to avoid certain foods that trigger or exacerbate symptoms. For example, those with lactose intolerance should avoid milk products; those with nontropical sprue (celiac disease) may be cured by avoiding all foods containing gluten (a protein found in wheat, rye, oats, and barley).
• The underlying disorder causing malabsorption must be diagnosed and treated. For instance, antibiotics are given to cure an infection.
• Nutritional supplements may be prescribed. Common supplements include calcium, magnesium, iron, and vitamins A, D, E, and K.
• Pancreatic enzymes may be prescribed to correct insufficient production of them.
• Corticosteroids may improve absorption in some cases of inflammatory diseases.
• In many cases a high carbohydrate, low-fat diet is recommended; it is easiest to digest and absorb.

WHEN TO CALL A DOCTOR

• Call a doctor if diarrhea or other digestive problems persist for longer than three days. ▲

Malaria

WHAT IS IT?

Malaria is an acute infectious disease, usually transmitted by the bite of a mosquito. Single-celled parasites (plasmodia) carried by the mosquito enter the bloodstream and travel to the liver. There they mature and proliferate for several days or weeks and cause no symptoms. Eventually, however, the plasmodia reenter the bloodstream and infect the red blood cells. After multiplying for two to three days the parasites cause massive destruction of the red cells. This initiates the classic cycle of malaria symptoms that last 12 to 24 hours. It begins as a period of uncontrollable shivering and chills, followed by a fever as high as 105°F. Finally, a period of profuse sweating occurs, which helps the body temperature return to normal. The patient is left exhausted but otherwise temporarily free of symptoms.

However, plasmodia released from dying red cells and those continuing to multiply in the liver infect other red cells and cause repeated attacks, usually every two to three days. If untreated, attacks can continue for years and may be fatal, although the body gradually builds up defenses against the disease. While malaria is rarely life-threatening, one form of the disease, caused by the parasite *Plasmodium falciparum,* releases all of the parasites into the bloodstream at once and produces a single severe attack that is sometimes fatal. Falciparum malaria may be complicated by kidney failure or disseminated intravascular coagulation (DIC).

WHAT CAUSES IT?

• Malaria is caused by single-celled parasites (plasmodia), usually transmitted to their human hosts via the bite of an infected female anopheles mosquito. This disease is most common in tropical areas.
• Malaria may be spread during a blood transfusion or by sharing needles for intravenous drug use.
• Pregnant women with malaria can transmit the infection to their unborn children.

PREVENTION

• Before departing for a tropical or subtropical area, see your doctor or, preferably, go to a travel clinic where you can obtain information on the types of malaria (including drug-resistant malaria) presently found in the area of your destination. Recommendations may include taking the antimalarial drug chloroquine before leaving and for at least four weeks after returning. In a growing number of areas, such as Southeast Asia, Colombia, and Africa, plasmodia are resistant to chloroquine. For trips to such places, other drugs, such as mefloquine or doxycycline are necessary.
• When in mosquito-infested areas, put mosquito netting over beds, use insect repellents, and install window screens. Wear long-sleeve-shirts and long pants if you go out during mosquito-prone hours. Stay indoors between dusk and dawn, the hours when mosquitoes feed.

DIAGNOSIS

• Patient history and physical examination are needed.
• Blood smears are examined for parasites.

HOW TO TREAT IT

• Hospitalization is often required. The drug chloroquine is administered to kill parasites in the blood. To kill chloroquine-resistant plasmodia, other drugs, such as quinine or quinidine, are used.
• For malaria other than that due to *P. falciparum* (which causes only one attack), an additional drug, primaquine, must be taken for two weeks. This kills parasites in the liver, thereby preventing recurrent attacks.

WHEN TO CALL A DOCTOR

• Contact your doctor before traveling to areas where malaria is prevalent.
• See a doctor if malaria symptoms develop or recur. ▲

SYMPTOMS
• Headache.
• Sudden chills and uncontrollable shivering.
• High fever.
• Nausea and vomiting.
• Rapid, shallow breathing.
• Profuse perspiration accompanied by a drop in body temperature.
• Muscle aches and pain.

Measles Rubeola

WHAT IS IT?

Measles (also known as rubeola) is a highly contagious viral infection that primarily affects the respiratory tract. Symptoms appear in a predictable sequence: After an incubation period of eight to 12 days (at which time the disease is most communicable), fever, runny nose, and a dry cough develop. By the third day, fever subsides somewhat and tiny gray-white bumps (Koplik's spots) appear inside the mouth. On subsequent days, fever rises again and the spotted skin rash characteristic of measles appears, in addition to cough, conjunctivitis, nasal drainage. Typically, within a week of onset, all symptoms (including the rash) begin to fade and the disease is no longer contagious.

Measles is one of the most serious preventable childhood illnesses. Risk of severe disease is increased in children who are malnourished, immunocompromised, or have HIV infection. Large-scale immunization efforts in the United States and Canada have, over the past 25 years, reduced the incidence of measles by 99 percent—although it is still a major cause of childhood mortality in underdeveloped countries. Although the outlook is very optimistic, on rare occasions spread of the virus or a secondary bacterial infection can lead to serious complications, including middle ear infections (otitis media), pneumonia, and encephalitis (inflammation of the brain).

SYMPTOMS
- Cough; sore throat.
- Watery nasal discharge; red, watering eyes.
- Fever.
- Aversion to light.
- Loss of appetite.
- Muscle aches.
- General feeling of poor health.
- Small grayish-white bumps (Koplik's spots), surrounded by a red halo, on the lining of the mouth (appearing three or four days after the onset of initial symptoms).
- Red, slightly itchy bumps that gradually spread all over the body, usually within five days of the onset of symptoms.

WHAT CAUSES IT?
- Measles is caused by the paramyxovirus, which is most commonly spread by airborne respiratory droplets from an infected person.

PREVENTION
- Children should be inoculated with the MMR (measles, mumps, rubella) vaccine between the ages of 12 and 15 months. A booster shot is generally recommended between ages four and six years. Those not reimmunized at school entry should receive their second dose by 12 years of age.
- Gamma globulin (a substance derived from human blood containing antibodies to most types of infection) may be given to those who have been exposed to measles but have not been properly immunized or are immunocompromised, such as those with symptomatic HIV infections.

DIAGNOSIS
- Physical examination and patient history are needed.
- Blood, mucus, or urine samples, or a blood test for antibodies against the measles virus may be taken to identify the measles virus.

HOW TO TREAT IT
- There is no specific treatment for measles except to make the patient as comfortable as possible. In most cases, the disease remits on its own after about 10 days. In the meantime, bed rest, over-the-counter pain relievers, and humidified air are advised.
- Vitamin A may be given to some children.
- In some cases, doctors may administer an injection of gamma globulin antibodies, which battle the virus and thus may ease the severity of the infection.
- Antibiotics may be required if a secondary bacterial infection (such as bacterial pneumonia) occurs.

WHEN TO CALL A DOCTOR
- Call a doctor if symptoms do not begin to ease after one week, or if earache, cough, or severe lethargy develop—all signs of impending complications.
- **EMERGENCY** Get medical help immediately if, in extremely rare cases, generalized bleeding from skin lesions (hemorrhagic measles) or seizures occur. ⚠

Megacolon, Toxic

WHAT IS IT?

Toxic megacolon is a serious condition characterized by swelling and dilation of the large intestine due to inflammation of the intestinal wall and accumulation of excessive amounts of gas. It primarily occurs in association with a severe attack of inflammatory bowel disease—either ulcerative colitis or Crohn's disease (see Colitis, Ulcerative and Crohn's Disease for more information). Bacterial infections of the colon and certain drugs can also cause toxic megacolon. The disorder produces extreme illness and is life-threatening; treatment requires hospitalization, and surgery may be required to remove the affected portion of the intestine.

For adults, the prognosis for toxic megacolon varies; there is a danger of widespread blood poisoning (see Septic Shock), extensive hemorrhaging from the colon, perforation of the colon (see Peritonitis), and blockage of the arteries that supply blood to the lungs (see Pulmonary Embolism).

WHAT CAUSES IT?

• Ulcerative colitis or Crohn's disease in the colon are the most common causes of toxic megacolon. In such patients episodes may be triggered by a worsening of the disease, other superimposed diseases resulting in prolonged bed rest, or discontinuing or decreasing prescribed dosages of anti–inflammatories such as sulfasalazine or the 5-aminosalicylic acid (5-ASA) drugs.

• Some medications—including narcotics (such as morphine and codeine), anticholinergic agents (such as scopolamine and atropine), and some antidepressants—may lead to toxic megacolon.

PREVENTION

• Do not discontinue medications for ulcerative colitis or Crohn's disease unless otherwise advised by your doctor.

DIAGNOSIS

• Patient history, especially of prior diagnosis of inflammatory bowel disease.
• Blood tests for anemia and for high white-blood-cell count.
• Abdominal x-rays.
• Stool cultures to detect an underlying infection.
• Colonoscopy (insertion of a thin, lighted viewing tube through the anus) may be performed to inspect the colon and rectum. A biopsy of the colon lining may be taken during colonoscopy.

HOW TO TREAT IT

• Prompt hospitalization is required. Doctors will attempt to relieve the distended bowel and prevent intestinal perforation (which results in peritonitis) by passing a small tube through the nose or mouth into the intestine to remove gas and fluids.
• Intravenous solutions and nutrients are given.
• Blood transfusions are given if necessary.
• Antibiotics may be prescribed to prevent or treat associated bacterial infection or blood poisoning due to septic shock.
• Surgery may be required if other treatment fails to relieve the distention and symptoms of toxicity. The affected portion of the large intestine is removed, and the remaining sections are sewn together (bowel resection). In some cases it is necessary to create a temporary or permanent colostomy, in which the end of the remaining upper portion of the colon is brought through an opening created in the abdominal wall. Wastes pass through this opening into a bag, instead of being eliminated rectally.

WHEN TO CALL A DOCTOR

• **EMERGENCY** See a doctor right away for severe abdominal pain and distention with fever.

SYMPTOMS

• Acute illness most often preceded by increased intensity of ulcerative colitis or Crohn's disease symptoms, which include abdominal pain, diarrhea possibly leading to dehydration, and blood in the stool.
• Abdominal distension and tenderness.
• High fever.
• Rapid heart rate.
• Paleness (pallor).
• Mental changes.
• Shock.

Melanoma

WHAT IS IT?

Melanoma is the least common form of skin cancer but by far the most deadly. Unfortunately, the incidence of melanoma has been increasing for many decades. In women, for example, only the incidence of lung cancer is rising more quickly and melanoma is the most common cancer diagnosed in women between ages 29 and 34.

Melanoma develops from melanocytes, cells located primarily in the skin that produce the dark pigment melanin, which serves to protect the skin from ultraviolet radiation. People with darker skin produce more melanin and generally are at less risk for all skin cancers, including melanoma, than those with pale skin. There is a relationship between sunburn (especially repeated sunburns before age 20) and skin cancers. However, other factors, including family history and skin type, also figure into the equation of who gets skin cancer.

Melanomas may develop anywhere on the body. The most common sites are areas intermittently exposed to the sun, such as the trunk and legs. One type of melanoma, however, is associated with chronic sun exposure and occurs most often on the face and arms. (Melanoma in the eye is fortunately uncommon; see Eye Cancers.) Left untreated, melanoma may quickly metastasize, or spread, to

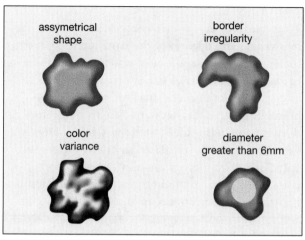

Melanomas can be characterized by the acronym ABCD: *asymmetrical* shape; *border* irregularity; *color* variation; *diameter* larger than a pencil eraser.

other parts of the body. Metastasized melanoma is potentially and frequently fatal, making detection and treatment critical.

WHAT CAUSES IT?

• The cause of melanoma is unknown; however, it is likely a combination of genetic factors and environmental sun exposure.
• Exposure to ultraviolet (UV) radiation from the sun or from artificial sources (such as sunlamps) may promote melanoma. Skin damage and melanoma risk increase with cumulative UV exposure.
• Hereditary factors play a role in some forms of melanoma; a family history of melanoma increases the risk.
• Those with pale skin, blue or green eyes, and red or blond hair are most at risk for skin cancer. However, anyone of any age or skin color may develop melanoma.
• The presence of atypical moles (as differentiated by the acronym ABCD; see Symptoms) increases risk.
• Having many moles on the skin is a risk factor.
• A congenital mole (a mole present at birth) has an increased chance of developing a melanoma within it. With very large moles, this may occur before age five; with small moles, this may occur at any time, even in old age.
• The risk of melanoma increases steadily with age.
• People's relatively recent tendency to spend more

SYMPTOMS

• Any change in a mole's appearance. Such changes are characterized by the acronym ABCD: *asymmetrical* shape; *border* irregularity; *color* variation; *diameter* larger than a pencil eraser.
• An irregularly shaped flat spot or raised bump anywhere on the skin. The spot or bump may be brown, black, blue, tan, red, white, or multicolored; it usually has no symptoms. Only occasionally will it be tender, itchy, or ooze or bleed.
• A black or brown spot on the color portion (iris) or the white (sclera) of the eye; change of color of the iris; gradual loss of vision; pain and redness in the affected eye.

Melanoma   *continued*

time in the sun with less clothing coverage is believed to be a factor in the increasing incidence of skin cancer.

PREVENTION

• Perform regular skin self-examinations: once every few months for those with a low risk of skin cancer; more often for those in high-risk categories. To perform: Stand in front of a mirror and slowly inspect the entire surface of the skin, checking for changes in existing moles and for the appearance of any new skin lesions or spots. Do not neglect hard-to-see areas; a second mirror may help. Regular self-examination aids in early diagnosis and treatment.
• Whenever possible, avoid exposure to direct sunlight between 10 a.m. and 2 p.m.
• Block the sun's rays by wearing protective clothing, such as hats and long-sleeved shirts.
• Apply a waterproof sunscreen lotion with a sun protection factor (SPF) of 15 or higher before going outside. Reapply often, especially after swimming or perspiring heavily.
• Avoid sunlamps and tanning booths.
• Using yourself as an example, make sure children follow steps for proper sun protection. Sun exposure and sunburn during childhood and adolescence increase the likelihood of skin damage later in life.
• People who have had one episode of melanoma are at greater risk of developing a second melanoma. For this reason, preventive measures are especially important after initial diagnosis.

DIAGNOSIS

• A skin biopsy is done by removing part or all of a suspicious skin growth; the tissue is sent to a laboratory for analysis.

• If melanoma in the eye is suspected, a complete eye examination is conducted by an ophthalmologist, possibly with the patient under general anesthesia.

HOW TO TREAT IT

• Surgery to remove a melanoma (and usually at least half an inch of normal surrounding skin) is required. In some cases, neighboring lymph nodes may be removed to prevent the cancer from spreading.
• Chemotherapy and radiation therapy may be used in advanced cases of melanoma to forestall cancer growth and thus ease symptoms (although these treatments rarely result in a cure).
• Laser surgery, cryosurgery (in which liquid nitrogen is used to freeze the targeted tissue), or radiation therapy may be used to destroy cancerous cells within the eye.

WHEN TO CALL A DOCTOR

• Make an appointment with a dermatologist if you notice a change in the appearance of a mole or a new unidentified growth. Most skin growths are harmless, but if there is any question, a simple skin biopsy may be done to determine the presence or absence of cancer.
• Schedule regular follow-up appointments with a dermatologist after an episode of melanoma, because of the increased likelihood of subsequent episodes.
• Have regular skin cancer screenings with a dermatologist if you have a family history of melanoma or are in a high-risk category for melanoma or other skin cancers. Relatives of high-risk people should also be screened regularly.
• See an ophthalmologist if you develop symptoms of melanoma in the eye.

Ménière's Disease

WHAT IS IT?

Ménière's disease is characterized by a buildup of excess fluid in the inner ear. The excess fluid leads to increased pressure that distorts (and occasionally ruptures) the labyrinth, or inner ear, membranes, causing episodes of severe vertigo (the sensation of spinning), ringing in the ears, and fluctuating hearing loss. The disorder is characterized by spells of symptoms in one ear, but in about a third of cases symptoms may occur in the other ear as well.

Symptoms arise in periodic acute attacks, which may last from several minutes to several days. Attacks may occur as often as every few weeks or as infrequently as every few years. In most cases, the disorder is mild and will disappear spontaneously; in other cases, attacks may become increasingly frequent and severe. Over time, hearing loss and ringing in the ears may persist between attacks. In rare cases, deafness in one or both ears may occur. Ménière's disease usually strikes between ages 30 and 60 and affects men slightly more than women.

WHAT CAUSES IT?

• Ménière's disease may result from the overproduction or decreased absorption of endolymph, a fluid produced naturally in the ear. Why this occurs, however, remains unclear.
• In some women with the disease, premenstrual retention of fluid may precipitate an attack.

SYMPTOMS

• A sudden attack of vertigo. These spells frequently trigger nausea and vomiting as well.
• Hearing impairment or loss.
• Ringing or buzzing in the ears (tinnitus).
• Pressure, fullness, or a feeling of blockage in the affected ear.
• In "classic" Ménière's disease, fullness, hearing loss, tinnitus, and vertigo cluster together. Clearly, however, there are many atypical forms of the disease in which only some of these symptoms occur on a periodic basis.
• Sweating.
• Giddiness.

PREVENTION

• There are no known ways to prevent Ménière's disease.

DIAGNOSIS

• Patient history and physical examination.
• Audiometry (measurement of hearing ability).
• X-rays to rule out other disorders that may cause similar symptoms.
• A caloric stimulation test, in which water of different temperatures is instilled into the ear canals, causing the eyes to reflexively flicker in a predictable way (nystagmus). This indicates whether or not there is nerve damage in the ear.

HOW TO TREAT IT

• Most cases of Ménière's disease can be managed with medications and dietary changes.
• Lie still during an acute attack. Avoid reading and bright lights, as these may exacerbate dizziness and nausea.
• Drugs such as atropine may be prescribed to control nausea and vomiting and to reduce vertigo.
• Antihistamines such as diphenhydramine may help to ease symptoms during a severe attack, or they may be taken preventively to ward off attacks.
• Mild sedatives may be prescribed for those who suffer anxiety during a severe attack.
• Diuretics and a low-sodium diet may be recommended to reduce the overall amount of fluid in the body, and thus reduce the accumulation of endolymph fluid in the ear.
• If the disorder persists and causes very severe or frequent attacks, several surgical options are available, including severing the nerve involved or removing the affected portion of the labyrinth. Such methods are effective but may result in irreversible hearing loss.

WHEN TO CALL A DOCTOR

• Call your doctor or an otolaryngologist (ear, nose, and throat specialist) if you have persistent dizziness, ringing in the ears, or fluctuating hearing loss. ▲

Meningitis

WHAT IS IT?

Meningitis is inflammation of the meninges, the three thin layers of tissue that cover the brain. It is almost always due to an infection—usually one that has spread to the meninges from elsewhere in the body. (In rare cases meningitis may also be caused by tumors or exposure to chemical irritants.)

Three major types of infections cause meningitis—bacterial, viral, and fungal—and the nature and severity of symptoms vary depending on the specific microorganism involved. For example, viral meningitis (the most common type) typically causes mild symptoms such as headache and malaise and usually gets better on its own in a week or two. On the other hand, bacterial meningitis (usually affecting infants and young children) is a serious medical emergency that may cause brain damage or even be fatal if left untreated.

Other types of meningitis (such as those caused by a fungus or tuberculosis) tend to progress slowly but may also lead to brain damage and death if not treated. Immediate treatment should thus be sought even for mild symptoms of meningitis. Prompt diagnosis and treatment allow most people to recover fully, with no permanent neurological damage.

WHAT CAUSES IT?

• Bacterial, viral, or fungal infection causes meningitis. Meningococcal meningitis (a bacterial variety that is the most dangerous) may occur in epidemic outbreaks.

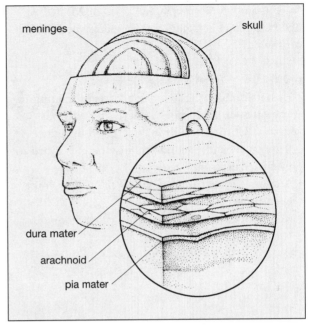

Between the brain and skull are three protective membranes: the meninges. Swelling due to inflammation of the meninges (meningitis) may exert potentially harmful pressure on the brain.

• A higher risk of meningitis is associated with head injury, brain surgery, cancer in or around the brain, acute otitis media (middle ear infection), pneumonia, syphilis, tuberculosis, exposure to chemical irritants, and alcoholism.
• Anyone whose immune system is weakened—for example, by AIDS or cancer chemotherapy—is at greater risk of meningitis.

PREVENTION

• Obtain prompt treatment for bacterial infections elsewhere in the body, especially ear and upper respiratory infections.
• Vaccines can protect against outbreaks of meningococcal meningitis in groups such as military recruits.
• Antibiotics may be administered to prevent infection in those who are in close contact with others infected with meningococcal meningitis.

DIAGNOSIS

• Lumbar puncture (spinal tap) to examine under the microscope spinal fluid for cells and organisms and to culture for bacterial or fungal growth.
• Blood cultures.

SYMPTOMS
• Fever (may be very high in cases of bacterial meningitis).
• Headache, possibly severe.
• Stiff neck.
• Nausea and vomiting.
• Aversion to light.
• Poor feeding in infants.
• With bacterial meningitis: mental confusion, drowsiness, seizures, and loss of consciousness.
• With meningococcal meningitis: red, blotchy skin rash.

Meningitis   *continued*

• CT (computed tomography) scans or MRI (magnetic resonance imaging) may be performed during treatment.

HOW TO TREAT IT

• Hospitalization is required for bacterial meningitis. Antibiotics are given in large doses, often intravenously. Corticosteroids may be given to reduce inflammation and tranquilizers may be prescribed to prevent seizures.

• A respirator may be necessary if the patient loses consciousness.

• Antibiotics are ineffective against viral meningitis, which is usually mild anyway and is overcome by the body's own defenses within a week or two. Treatment is thus aimed at relieving symptoms: Bed rest, plenty of fluids, and over-the-counter pain relievers are recommended.

• Antifungal medication is prescribed to treat a fungal infection.

• Antitubercular medications are given for tubercular meningitis.

WHEN TO CALL A DOCTOR

• **EMERGENCY** Call a doctor immediately if you or your child develops symptoms of meningitis. ▲

Mesenteric Ischemia

WHAT IS IT?

Mesenteric ischemia is an uncommon condition characterized by obstruction of one of the arteries to the intestines. Blockage occurs when a blood clot forms at a site already narrowed by atherosclerosis (mesenteric thrombosis), when plaques gradually build up in the arterial walls, or when an embolus (a blood clot from a distant site) lodges in an artery. Less often, mesenteric ischemia results from blockage of a vein leading away from the intestine. Total obstruction of a mesenteric artery due to severe atherosclerosis may be preceded by a period of "abdominal angina"—abdominal pain that begins 20 to 30 minutes after eating and lasts for several hours. Obstruction resulting from an embolus occurs without warning.

Complete blockage of a mesenteric artery causes death of the affected portion of the intestine. Treatment involves removing any permanently damaged portion of the intestine and, if possible, removal of the embolus or bypassing the portion of the artery obstructed by the clot; prognosis is generally grim.

WHAT CAUSES IT?

• Mesenteric thrombosis occurs in people with far-advanced atherosclerosis (see Coronary Artery Disease for more information).
• An embolus in the mesenteric arteries is most common in patients with atrial fibrillation (see Cardiac Arrhythmias), artificial heart valves, and valvular heart disease (see Valvular Heart Disease).
• Oral contraceptives may increase the danger of occlusion of mesenteric veins.

PREVENTION

• As much as possible, observe heart-healthy behaviors, such as maintaining a healthy diet, engaging in regular aerobic exercise, and avoiding cigarettes.

DIAGNOSIS

• Patient history and physical examination.
• Abdominal x-ray.
• For "abdominal angina," a barium-swallow test (use of barium to help create a clear image of the intestines on an x-ray) or a CT (computed tomography) scan may be followed by angiography (x-ray of the blood vessels after injection of a contrast agent).
• If complete blockage of a mesenteric artery is suspected, immediate angiography is done to locate the blockage, followed by emergency surgery if diagnosis is confirmed. When the diagnosis is strongly suspected, surgery may be initiated without angiography.

HOW TO TREAT IT

• When blockage of the mesenteric blood supply is only partial, surgical options include arterial bypass graft (rerouting blood flow around the damaged portion of the artery) and percutaneous transluminal angioplasty (inflation of a tiny balloon, routed via a catheter, at the narrowed point inside the artery to compress the plaque and widen the passageway).
• Complete occlusion requires immediate surgery. The damaged portion of the intestine is removed and the remaining ends sewn together (bowel resection).
• A second operation is often needed 24 to 36 hours later to remove dead bowel tissue that was not apparent at the time of the first procedure.
• Heparin, an anticoagulant, may be administered after surgery to reduce the risk of subsequent clots.

WHEN TO CALL A DOCTOR

• **EMERGENCY** Call an ambulance immediately if you experience severe, unremitting abdominal pain or cramping, especially if accompanied by other symptoms of mesenteric ischemia. ▲

SYMPTOMS

• Abdominal angina: intermittent dull or cramping pain beginning 20 to 30 minutes after a meal and lasting several hours.
• Severe, cramping abdominal pain, usually beginning around the navel. Pain later becomes steady throughout the abdomen.
• Weight loss.
• Abdominal swelling.
• Nausea and vomiting.
• Fever.
• Diarrhea or constipation.
• Rectal bleeding or bloody stools.
• Rapid heartbeat.

Mitral Valve Prolapse

WHAT IS IT?

In mitral valve prolapse (MVP)—also known as floppy valve syndrome—the valve between the heart's left atrium (upper chamber) and left ventricle (lower chamber) does not close normally and balloons outward, or prolapses, into the atrium. Disquieting as a heart valve abnormality may sound, MVP is typically harmless and causes no symptoms. However, in less than 4 percent of cases, blood may flow backward through the valve from the ventricle to the atrium (mitral regurgitation). Rarely, when severe, this can interfere with blood supply to the body, which may produce mild to serious symptoms and require treatment. Often discovered in early adulthood, MVP affects nearly 5 percent of the population.

WHAT CAUSES IT?

• The cause of MVP is most likely genetic.
• Women are twice as likely to develop MVP as men, especially women who are thin or who have scoliosis (curvature of the spine) or other types of skeletal abnormalities of the chest.

PREVENTION

• There is no known way to prevent MVP.

DIAGNOSIS

• MVP is typically discovered during a routine checkup, as the condition produces characteristic sounds that can be heard through a stethoscope.
• Echocardiography (the use of ultrasound to map the structure and motion of the heart) confirms the diagnosis.

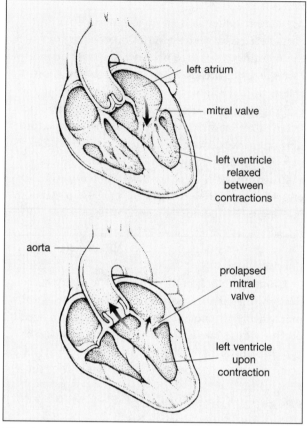

When the heart contracts, a prolapsed mitral valve may allow blood to reflux back into the left atrium, rather than enter the aorta exclusively.

SYMPTOMS

• In the majority of cases, MVP causes no symptoms. In more serious cases, however, the following may occur:
• Heart palpitations (in 10 to 15 percent of cases).
• Shortness of breath, especially when lying flat.
• Recurrent lightheadedness, especially when arising from a chair or bed; possible fainting.
• General fatigue or weakness.

HOW TO TREAT IT

• Treatment is rarely needed, but people with MVP should have regular checkups. Periodic echocardiograms may help evaluate a patient's status.
• Those with MVP are at increased risk for endocarditis (infection of a heart valve), and so may be given antibiotics prior to some dental or surgical procedures to help prevent infection.
• Beta-blocking drugs (often used for high blood pressure) may be prescribed for patients with frequent or bothersome palpitations. However, these drugs may exacerbate fatigue.
• For the most severe and debilitating cases of MVP, surgery to reconstruct or replace the prolapsed valve may be recommended.

WHEN TO CALL A DOCTOR

• See a doctor for frequent dizziness or palpitations.

Mononucleosis, Infectious

WHAT IS IT?

Infectious mononucleosis is an acute infection stemming from the Epstein-Barr virus or, more rarely, the cytomegalovirus, both members of the herpes family. It most often affects children, adolescents, and young adults and is particularly common among college students in the early fall and again in the spring. Once the virus enters the body, it multiplies in lymphocytes, a type of white blood cell. The characteristic sore throat, fever, and debilitating fatigue usually emerge after an incubation period of about 10 days in children and from 30 to 50 days in adults. Acute symptoms usually disappear after about six to 10 days, although some residual weakness and fatigue may linger for two to three months. Mononucleosis is usually not serious; major complications—which may include infection of the brain or heart or rupture of the spleen—are very rare.

WHAT CAUSES IT?

• Mononucleosis is frequently transmitted via saliva, hence the nickname "the kissing disease." It may also be spread via mouth-to-hand-to-mouth contact or by sharing towels or utensils.
• The infection may be transmitted during a blood transfusion.

PREVENTION

• Avoid mouth-to-mouth or hand-to-mouth contact as well as sharing towels or utensils with persons known to be infected with mononucleosis.

SYMPTOMS

• Headaches.
• Weakness and fatigue.
• Sore throat and enlarged tonsils.
• Swollen lymph glands in the neck, armpits, and groin.
• Fever (with fluctuating temperatures that peak during the evening at about 101°F to 102°F).
• Loss of appetite.
• Stiff or sore muscles.
• Temporary jaundice, due to mild, reversible liver damage.

DIAGNOSIS

• Diagnosis is suspected in those who exhibit the classic triad of symptoms—sore throat, swollen lymph glands, and fever—upon physical examination. An enlarged spleen may also be identified.
• A high white cell count and the presence of "atypical" lymphocytes in the blood are characteristic findings.
• A positive heterophile antibody test (a blood test that reveals the presence of specific antibodies against the virus) confirms the diagnosis.
• Liver function tests may be done.

HOW TO TREAT IT

• There is no specific treatment for infectious mononucleosis; however, the vast majority of people recover on their own within four to six weeks. Bed rest is essential when symptoms are most acute. A normal schedule of activity can be gradually resumed as symptoms subside.
• Take over-the-counter analgesics to reduce fever and to relieve headaches, body aches, and sore throat. (Children should be given acetaminophen instead of aspirin.)
• Drink water and fruit juice to help relieve fever and prevent dehydration.
• Gargle with one-half teaspoon of salt in a glass of warm water several times a day to relieve sore throat.
• In rare cases corticosteroids may be prescribed to reduce tonsil inflammation, should it become severe enough to obstruct breathing.
• Approximately 20 percent of those with infectious mononucleosis will also be simultaneously infected with strep throat, which requires antibiotic therapy for at least 10 days.
• In rare cases mononucleosis causes a rupture of the spleen, requiring immediate emergency surgery.

WHEN TO CALL A DOCTOR

• If you experience any of the symptoms of infectious mononucleosis, call a doctor.
• **EMERGENCY** If you have been diagnosed with infectious mononucleosis and you feel sudden sharp pains in the upper left side of your abdomen, get professional medical care immediately. This may be an indication of a ruptured spleen. ⚠

Multiple Myeloma

WHAT IS IT?

Multiple myeloma is a form of cancer resulting from the overproduction of a single clone of plasma cells, a type of white blood cell produced in the bone marrow. Plasma cells proliferate in the marrow, infiltrate adjacent bone tissue, and may spread throughout the skeleton, resulting in bone pain and fractures of fragile, brittle bones. (Some patients develop a single plasma cell tumor, known as a plasmacytoma, in a bone or elsewhere.) Proliferation of plasma cells interferes with the formation of red cells (causing anemia), platelets (increasing the risk of hemorrhage), and white cells (increasing susceptibility to infection). Symptoms may arise from kidney failure, hypercalcemia (high levels of blood calcium, due to bone breakdown), and compression of the spinal cord due to collapse of the vertebrae. Myeloma also involves the production of large amounts of a type of immunoglobulin (antibody) termed myeloma protein. Multiple myeloma most often affects those over age 60 and is usually fatal within two years of diagnosis. Although there is no cure, treatment can prolong life and improve the quality of life of the patient.

WHAT CAUSES IT?

- The cause of multiple myeloma is unknown, although genetic factors may play a role.
- Risk increases with age and exposure to radiation.

PREVENTION

- Try to minimize exposure to radiation.

DIAGNOSIS

- Patient history and physical examination.
- Blood tests for myeloma protein, calcium levels, and numbers of red cells, platelets, and white cells.
- Urine examination for myeloma protein.
- Bone marrow biopsy, usually taken from the hip.
- X-rays of the chest, spine, or other sites of pain.

HOW TO TREAT IT

- Stay as active as possible to maintain bone strength (inactivity hastens bone loss). Because bones may be brittle, your doctor or physical therapist should supervise any program of activity.
- A combination of chemotherapeutic agents, often including corticosteroids (usually prednisone), is used to destroy cancerous cells.
- Radiation therapy is effective for plasmacytomas.
- Radiation is also used to relieve bone pain and spinal cord compression.
- Surgery may be necessary to repair bone fractures.
- Plasmapheresis, a procedure that filters excess waste products out of the blood artificially, may be performed in the event of an increase in the blood viscosity due to excess protein, produced by myeloma cells (hyperviscosity syndrome).
- Analgesics are administered to reduce pain.
- Antibiotics may be prescribed to treat associated bacterial infections.

WHEN TO CALL A DOCTOR

- Call a doctor for bone pain or for the emergency symptoms of hypercalcemia or kidney failure. ▲

SYMPTOMS

- Bone pain, especially along the spine, that worsens with movement.
- Unexplained bone fractures. The collapse of affected vertebrae may cause loss of height and compression of the spinal cord, which may result in the inability to urinate and pain or paralysis of the legs.
- Fatigue, paleness (pallor), and shortness of breath, due to associated anemia.
- Frequent bacterial infections, due to a weakened immune system.
- Increased bruising and bleeding (for example, from the nose or gums).
- Headache and visual disturbances.
- Symptoms of hypercalcemia (high blood levels of calcium), which include generalized discomfort; muscle aches or weakness; arthritic joint pain; heartbeat irregularities; constipation, nausea, vomiting, and loss of appetite; and fatigue, lethargy, confusion, depression, psychosis, or other mental changes. These symptoms may possibly result in coma.
- Symptoms of kidney failure (see Renal Failure, Acute).

Multiple Sclerosis

WHAT IS IT?

Multiple sclerosis (MS) is a disorder characterized by destruction of the protective outer casings of the nerves within the central nervous system (the brain, optic nerves, and spinal cord). The nerve casings, known as myelin sheaths, are composed mostly of fats; they insulate the nerves and preserve the speed of electrical transmissions. In MS, patchy areas of the sheaths are destroyed (demyelinated) and replaced by scar tissue (called plaques)—a process known as sclerosis—at multiple sites throughout the central nervous system (hence the name of the disorder). Sclerosis impairs electrical conduction, thus reducing or eliminating transmission of nerve impulses within the affected areas. When severe, the disease may destroy the inner cables of the nerves (axons), causing irreversible damage.

Symptoms wax and wane unpredictably and vary widely from patient to patient. For example, sclerosis of the optic nerves may cause vision disturbances, and sclerosis of the nerves that control the muscles may lead to spasticity, weakness, muscle spasms, or paralysis. Different symptoms may occur in combination and may vary greatly over time.

SYMPTOMS

- Muscle weakness and stiffness in the arms and legs.
- Muscle spasms.
- Eye pain and visual disturbances, including blurry vision, loss of vision in one eye, or a sudden inability to distinguish colors (optic neuritis).
- Double vision.
- Tingling or prickling sensations.
- Disturbances in gait; loss of coordination.
- Vertigo with nausea and vomiting.
- Slurred speech.
- Loss of bladder control and constipation.
- Severe fatigue.
- Emotional depression and mood swings.
- Mental confusion or loss of memory.
- Paralysis of one side of the face.
- Partial or complete paralysis of the body.

The initiating cause is unknown; however, current research indicates that MS is an autoimmune disorder, in which the immune system attacks some of the body's own cells, mistaking them for foreign invaders. MS is rare in children and in people over 60; the first episode usually occurs between the ages of 20 and 50.

MS occurs in two major forms. In relapsing/remitting MS, which afflicts about 70 percent of MS patients, a series of flare-ups or attacks are separated by periods of normal or near-normal health. Such remissions may be short or may last for months or years. In a few cases, remission is permanent, but many patients gradually accumulate permanent neurological deficits.

The other type of MS, chronic/progressive, gradually worsens without remission. Rarely is progression so rapid or severe that survival is limited to only months or a few years. Women are affected more often than men. Average survival after diagnosis is more than 35 years, but destruction of the myelin sheaths eventually results in a combination of nerve, muscle, and, occasionally, brain damage. However, many people retain much of their function for years and are able to pursue a wide range of normal activities with the help of supportive therapy. Current treatment is aimed at reducing the frequency and severity of attacks, relieving the problems caused by neurological deficits, and providing psychological support.

WHAT CAUSES IT?

- The cause of multiple sclerosis is unknown.
- Hereditary factors may play a role.
- Environmental factors may be associated with multiple sclerosis; the majority of cases occurs in temperate climates.
- Some theories suggest that multiple sclerosis may be triggered by a virus or other infectious agent.
- There is abundant evidence of an autoimmune component to the disease.

DIAGNOSIS

- Patient history and careful neurological and eye examination.
- Lumbar puncture (spinal tap).

Multiple Sclerosis *continued*

- MRI (magnetic resonance imaging) to detect plaques of scar tissue even in the absence of associated symptoms.
- Tests to detect abnormalities of vision and other sensory modalities.
- No single diagnostic test is definitive for MS, and several attacks may occur before diagnosis is certain.

PREVENTION
- There is no known way to prevent the onset of MS.

HOW TO TREAT IT
- Oral corticosteroids, such as prednisone, or intravenous corticosteroids, such as methylprednisolone, may be prescribed to shorten the duration and reduce the severity of attacks.
- Your doctor may prescribe interferon beta-1b or interferon beta-1a injections, a form of biological therapy, to treat MS. These medications are synthetically engineered to be identical to a naturally occurring protein and reduce the frequency and severity of attacks by altering many of the body's immune responses. Alternatively, your doctor may prescribe glatiramer acetate injections to modulate the immune dysfunction in MS. The choices among these therapies are complex and usually require the assessment of an MS specialist.
- Your doctor may prescribe antispasmodics or tran-quilizers, including diazepam or baclofen, to relax spastic muscles and provide pain relief, or antidepressants to treat associated depression.
- A variety of medications may be administered to treat incontinence, frequency, hesitancy, and other bladder-control problems.
- Try not to become overheated. Avoid excessive sunbathing, heavy exertion, and hot baths, and obtain prompt treatment for fevers; a raised body temperature may trigger or worsen symptoms. Taking a cool shower, swimming, or sitting in an air-conditioned room may relieve the severity of symptoms during an attack.
- Pursue a program of moderate exercise to help keep muscles as flexible and strong as possible.
- Physical and occupational therapy may help patients adjust to muscular and sensory changes.
- Psychological counseling may help patients and their families cope with depression and the lifestyle changes imposed by MS.
- Be wary of unproven remedies, such as bee venom.
- Obtain more information by contacting your local chapter of the National Multiple Sclerosis Society.

WHEN TO CALL A DOCTOR
- Call a doctor if you develop any of the symptoms of MS, especially if you have suffered several episodes or attacks. ▲

Mumps

WHAT IS IT?

Mumps is an acute illness characterized by swelling of the parotid glands, just below and in front of the ear, and at times, the salivary glands under the jaw. It occurs most often in children ages two through 12, although unvaccinated adults are susceptible too. The patient is contagious for about one week before and two weeks after the onset of symptoms, which occurs about two to three weeks after exposure to the mumps virus. Preliminary symptoms (headache, sore muscles, appetite loss, and low-grade fever) usually persist for 24 hours, followed by an earache that is aggravated by chewing, soreness and swelling of the parotid glands on either or both sides, and moderate fever. About 20 percent of men and adolescent boys experience pain and swelling in one or both testes (orchitis), which in rare cases may cause sterility.

Although uncomfortable, mumps is usually harmless, and symptoms normally subside within 10 days. Occasional complications include arthritis, kidney involvement, meningitis (inflammation of membranes around the brain) and pancreatitis (inflammation of the pancreas); these usually resolve with no permanent adverse effects. The incidence of mumps in the United States has drastically diminished over recent decades owing to increased childhood immunization efforts. In almost all cases, those who do get the mumps have lifelong immunity to reinfection.

WHAT CAUSES IT?

• The disorder is transmitted by direct contact with infectious saliva or by inhalation of airborne moisture droplets containing the paramyxovirus.

PREVENTION

• The MMR (measles, mumps, rubella) vaccine should be given to children between the ages of 12 and 15 months and a second dose at four to six years. Those not reimmunized by entry to school should receive the second dose by age 12.
• Immunization within 24 hours of mumps exposure.

DIAGNOSIS

• Patient history and physical examination are needed. Diagnosis is generally based on the presence of the characteristic symptoms (particularly glandular swelling).
• Because children may have swelling of the parotid gland from other causes, diagnosis should be confirmed by a saliva or urine culture or with a blood test for antibodies against the mumps virus.

HOW TO TREAT IT

• Use acetaminophen or ibuprofen to reduce fever and relieve discomfort. Aspirin should not be given to children; it may increase the risk of Reye's syndrome, a rare, but life-threatening inflammation of the brain and liver in children (see Reye's Syndrome).
• Bed rest is advised for the duration of the fever.
• Ice packs or heating pads may ease the pain of swollen glands.
• Adequate fluid intake is essential to prevent dehydration due to fever. Extreme swallowing difficulty may warrant intravenous fluid replacement.
• For males with orchitis, doctors may prescribe stronger pain medications.

WHEN TO CALL A DOCTOR

• See a doctor if symptoms occur in conjunction with severe headache, unusual drowsiness, persistent vomiting or abdominal pain, or convulsions.

SYMPTOMS

• Soreness and swelling of the parotid or salivary glands on one or both sides. Discomfort may range from vague tenderness to obvious pain when opening the mouth or swallowing.
• Fever, usually lasting two or three days.
• Sore muscles; joint pain.
• Loss of appetite.
• Earache that is aggravated by chewing.
• In men and adolescent boys, swelling in one or both testes (may subside within four days).
• Headache with aversion to light, lethargy, and a stiff neck (which may indicate meningitis).
• Upper abdominal pain, nausea, and vomiting (which may indicate pancreatitis).
• Lower abdominal discomfort in women (may indicate swelling of the ovaries, which is rare).
• Children with mumps may have no symptoms.

Muscular Dystrophy

WHAT IS IT?

Muscular dystrophy (MD) is a general term used to describe a number of inherited disorders characterized by progressive weakness and wasting of the muscles. The most common and severe type is Duchenne's MD, in which a genetic defect leads to severe depletion of the muscle protein called dystrophin. Becker's MD is similar to Duchenne's MD, but milder, resulting from a defect in the same gene. Others include facioscapulohumeral MD, myotonic MD, and various types of limb-girdle MDs.

The types of MD are classified according to the location of muscles involved, the age when symptoms appear, the rate that symptoms progress, and the manner in which the defective gene is passed on. (For example, the genes for Duchenne's and Becker's MD are X-linked recessives; that is, they generally affect males only but are carried and passed on by women.) Symptoms and prognosis vary, depending on the type of MD. The disease may affect some or all muscles, may develop during childhood or adulthood, may progress very gradually or rapidly, and may or may not become severely disabling. Boys with Duchenne's MD are usually dependent on a wheelchair by the age of 12 and rarely live past age 20; on the other hand, people with facioscapulohumeral MD often have a normal life span and, because the leg muscles are only mildly affected, usually remain able to walk. Some forms of MD affect the heart and thus result in cardiomyopathy.

WHAT CAUSES IT?

• All forms of MD result from some type of genetic defect. In most cases, the defect is inherited and affects various relatives throughout a family. In some cases, a new genetic mutation is responsible.

PREVENTION

• If you have a family history of MD, you may choose to see a genetic counselor before planning to have a child. Genetic tests can determine whether you carry an MD gene or an unborn child has MD.

DIAGNOSIS

• Patient history and physical examination are needed.
• A muscle biopsy (removal of a small tissue sample for microscopic examination) may be performed to check that the weakness is due to muscle disease.
• Electrical activity in the muscles may be measured and analyzed (electromyography).
• DNA tests can prove the exact diagnosis.

HOW TO TREAT IT

• There is no specific treatment to cure or halt the progression of MD.
• In Duchenne's MD, corticosteroids such as prednisone can slow the early course of weakness only.
• Physical therapy, exercise, orthopedic devices (such as braces or wheelchairs), or corrective orthopedic surgery may help to preserve muscle function, reduce joint contractures, and improve quality of life.

WHEN TO CALL A DOCTOR

• If you or your child appears to be exhibiting the symptoms of muscular dystrophy, call a doctor.
• Consult a doctor if there is a history of muscular dystrophy in your or your spouse's family and you are considering having a child.

SYMPTOMS

• Progressive muscle weakness, wasting, and loss of function. (The muscle groups affected depend on the type of MD.)
• In Duchenne's MD, delayed development of basic muscle skills and coordination in children. Signs include poor balance with frequent falls, walking difficulty with waddling gait, and limited range of movement. Muscular and skeletal deformities, including curvature of the spine with protruding abdomen, are likely. Respiratory failure may occur.
• Joint contractures and calf enlargement (in Duchenne's and Becker's MD).
• Cataracts, frontal baldness, drooping eyelids, gonadal atrophy, and mild mental impairment (with myotonic dystrophy).
• Intellectual impairment (most common in Duchenne's MD).

Myasthenia Gravis

WHAT IS IT?

Myasthenia gravis is a chronic autoimmune disorder characterized by weakness and rapid fatigue of the muscles. Antibodies, which normally fight infection, attack and inactivate muscle cell receptors that, in response to nerve impulses, permit the muscles to contract. Muscles with a reduced number of functioning receptors become weak or easily fatigable. In almost all cases, muscles behind the eye or in the face are involved first, causing double vision, drooping eyelids, and changes in speech and facial appearance. In about 85 percent of patients, muscles in the arms and legs are affected later. Muscles tend to tire after brief periods of use but recover with rest. The degree of weakness tends to fluctuate throughout the day, but is often worse in the afternoon or evening.

Cycles of partial remissions alternating with debilitating relapses are common throughout the course of the disease. While there is no cure, highly effective treatments allow most patients to return to full, productive lives. The disorder may, however, become life-threatening and require emergency care in the case of myasthenic crisis, when severe muscle weakness interferes with breathing or swallowing. Myasthenia gravis most often affects women between ages 20 and 30 and, less often, men between 50 and 70.

WHAT CAUSES IT?

• Myasthenia gravis occurs when, for reasons that remain unclear, antibodies produced by the body's immune system begin to inactivate receptors for acetylcholine that allow muscle fibers to respond to nerve impulses. The thymus (a gland in the chest and a component of the immune system) appears to play a role. Overgrowth of the thymus (hyperplasia) appears in 65 percent of cases, while tumors in the gland (thymomas) appear in 10 percent.

PREVENTION

• There is no way to prevent myasthenia gravis.

DIAGNOSIS

• Patient history and physical exam. Injection of a drug that temporarily improves muscle function in myasthenia gravis patients may be given. Immediate gains in muscle strength suggest a positive diagnosis.
• Blood tests for acetylcholine-receptor antibodies.
• Measurement of the electrical activity of the muscles, including repetitive nerve stimulation and single fiber electromyography.
• CT scan or MRI of the upper chest to look for thymus enlargement or a tumor.

HOW TO TREAT IT

• Acetylcholine released from nerves is rapidly inactivated by the enzyme cholinesterase. Agents that block this enzyme (anticholinesterase drugs) allow high levels of acetylcholine to persist at muscle receptor sites, thus enhancing the responsiveness to nerve impulses. These drugs alleviate symptoms but become less effective as the disease progresses.
• Removal of the thymus (thymectomy) combined with immunotherapy results in improvement in most patients and complete remission in 35 to 50 percent.
• Long-term use of corticosteroids, azathioprine, cyclosporine, or other immunosuppressive drugs may reduce autoimmune activity and improve strength.
• Plasmapheresis (a procedure involving partial removal of blood plasma while blood cells are returned to circulation) may be used to remove the antibodies that inactivate muscle receptors.
• Hospitalization and intensive care are needed in myasthenic crisis (swallowing and breathing problems).

WHEN TO CALL A DOCTOR

• Call a doctor if you develop the symptoms of myasthenia gravis.
• **EMERGENCY** Swallowing or breathing difficulty requires immediate medical attention. 🅰

SYMPTOMS

• Drooping eyelids; double vision.
• Facial weakness characterized by a "snarling" expression when attempting to smile.
• Difficulty chewing.
• Slurred and nasal-sounding speech.
• Regurgitation of liquids through the nose.
• Muscle weakness in the arms and legs, making it difficult to walk, stand up, or grasp objects.
• Severe breathing and swallowing difficulty.

Myelofibrosis

WHAT IS IT?

Myelofibrosis is a disorder characterized by a progressive replacement of normal bone marrow cells with useless fibrous tissue. This impairs the marrow's ability to manufacture healthy blood cells (marrow hematopoiesis), including red cells, white cells, and platelets. In some types of myelofibrosis, failure of marrow hematopoiesis is associated with the initiation of blood production in the spleen, liver, and lymph nodes, which causes these organs to enlarge. Myelofibrosis may develop gradually, usually in people over the age of 50 with no apparent cause; this is known as primary myelofibrosis.

Symptoms normally do not appear until several years after the onset of the disease. The most common initial symptoms—fatigue, weakness, and appetite loss—are due to the anemia that results from insufficient red cell production. But eventually, other complications such as infection and bleeding occur. Average survival time is estimated at four to five years after diagnosis of myelofibrosis, but one-quarter of patients live up to 15 years. Treatment is aimed at relieving symptoms.

Secondary myelofibrosis is the term used when the disorder results from some other disease that damages the bone marrow. It may also occur if bone marrow is exposed to certain industrial toxins or to radiation.

SYMPTOMS

- Weakness and fatigue; heart palpitations; shortness of breath; paleness (pallor); loss of weight and appetite (due to anemia).
- Easy bleeding and bruising; clusters of pinpoint-size hemorrhages (petechiae) on the skin (due to platelet insufficiency).
- Fever and night sweats (due to overactive blood formation in the spleen and liver, or infection).
- Bone pain (in some cases).
- Attacks of gouty arthritis or kidney stones.
- Abdominal pain, fullness, or breathing difficulty (due to enlargement of the spleen and liver).

WHAT CAUSES IT?

- The cause of primary myelofibrosis is unknown.
- Secondary myelofibrosis arises as a result of some other disease that affects the bone marrow (such as metastatic cancer, Hodgkin's disease, polycythemia vera, lymphoma, HIV infection, chronic myelogenous leukemia, multiple myeloma, and acute leukemia), or from exposure to certain toxins (such as benzene) or to radiation, including x-rays.

PREVENTION

- There is no known way to prevent myelofibrosis, except in cases caused by exposure to radiation or industrial chemicals.

DIAGNOSIS

- Patient history and physical examination are necessary. An enlarged spleen and, in later stages, an enlarged liver are characteristics of the disease.
- Blood tests show abnormal numbers and appearance of blood cells.
- A bone marrow biopsy is necessary for a definite diagnosis, as myelofibrosis is often difficult to distinguish from certain other blood disorders.

HOW TO TREAT IT

- There is currently no effective treatment to cure or slow the progression of primary myelofibrosis.
- Blood transfusions may be administered, as needed, to treat anemia.
- Occasionally, treatment with recombinant human erythropoietin will combat anemia.
- Supplemental folic acid should be given to meet an increased need for this vitamin.
- The antigout drug allopurinol is prescribed when uric acid levels are elevated, to avoid kidney stones.
- Surgical removal of the spleen (splenectomy) may be indicated in cases where spleen enlargement causes severe problems for the patient, such as pain or difficulty eating.
- Treatment of the underlying disease is essential for correction of secondary myelofibrosis.

WHEN TO CALL A DOCTOR

- If you experience the symptoms of myelofibrosis, call a doctor. 🅰

Myocardial Infarction Heart Attack

WHAT IS IT?

A myocardial infarction, commonly known as a heart attack, is a medical emergency that occurs when a portion of the heart is deprived of oxygen because of blockage of one of the coronary arteries, which supply the heart muscle (myocardium) with blood. Lack of oxygen causes characteristic chest pain and death of myocardial tissue.

Heart attacks are more likely to occur when arteries have already been substantially narrowed by years of coronary artery disease (see Coronary Artery Disease for more information). Plaque—composed of cholesterol-rich fatty deposits, collagen and other proteins, and excess smooth muscle cells—builds up in the arterial walls, a process known as atherosclerosis. Arterial walls thicken and narrow, inhibiting the flow of blood into the heart. When arterial walls have been roughened by plaque deposits, it becomes much easier for blood clots to form along the surface of the plaque. If the clots grow, or if they detach from their place of origin and are carried along to a narrower section of artery, they may block a coronary artery completely, causing a heart attack. Arteries may also narrow suddenly as a result of an arterial spasm.

One-third of all heart attacks occur with no prior warning signs. In the remainder, attacks of chest pain

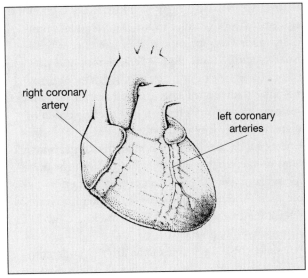

right coronary artery

left coronary arteries

If a blood clot forms in a coronary artery narrowed by atherosclerotic plaque, the blockage may starve heart tissue of oxygen-rich blood, causing the chest pain and tissue death associated with a heart attack.

(angina) brought about by stress or exertion occur periodically for months or years prior to a heart attack. In some cases a mild heart attack produces no symptoms—a so-called silent heart attack.

Prompt emergency medical attention is crucial: If treatment is received within a few hours of the onset of a heart attack, chances for survival are good. Improved treatment methods—including the administration of thrombolytic (clot dissolving) drugs and angioplasty (inflation of a tiny balloon at the site of the blockage to widen the artery and permit the flow of blood through the artery)—have led to a steady decrease in mortality from heart attacks. However, the best treatment remains prevention. The process of atherosclerosis may be halted or even reversed with fairly simple measures, and the risk of myocardial infarction can thus be reduced.

WHAT CAUSES IT?

• Blood clots that block a coronary artery are the most common cause of heart attacks. Clots develop on plaque in a coronary artery. Pieces of a clot may also be carried along the coronary artery and cause an obstruction.

• Severely narrowed arteries due to atherosclerosis underlie the development of a heart attack.

SYMPTOMS

• Chest pain or pressure, tightness, squeezing, burning, aching, or heaviness in the chest, lasting longer than 10 minutes. The pain or discomfort is usually located in the center of the chest just under the breastbone and may radiate down the arm (especially the left), up into the neck, or along the jaw line.

• Shortness of breath.

• Profuse sweating.

• Dizziness.

• Muscle weakness.

• Nausea and vomiting.

• A choking sensation.

• Anxiety, or a feeling of impending doom.

• No symptoms occur with a silent heart attack.

Myocardial Infarction Heart Attack *continued*

• Cigarette smoking, high blood pressure, high blood cholesterol levels, a diet rich in saturated fat (especially animal fat), obesity, lack of exercise, and diabetes mellitus all promote atherosclerosis and thus increase the risk of heart attacks.

• A family history of early or premature heart attacks (before the age of 55 in men and 65 in women) increases the risk of heart attack.

• Men have a significantly higher risk of heart attack than premenopausal women. But the risk for post-menopausal women approaches that of men as estrogen production decreases with menopause.

• Risk increases with age: Heart attacks are most common after age 65.

• A spasm of the muscles of the arterial walls may cause a heart attack by narrowing an artery. Spasms may be triggered by smoking, extreme emotional stress, or exposure to very cold air or water.

• Abuse of cocaine or amphetamines may cause a sudden heart attack even in those with no signs of heart disease.

• Heavy exertion, such as shoveling snow or carrying heavy objects up stairs, and severe emotional stress may trigger a heart attack.

• Having had one heart attack increases the risk of future heart attacks.

PREVENTION

• Don't smoke. Your doctor may recommend methods for quitting, including nicotine replacement.

• Eat a diet low in fat, cholesterol, and salt.

• See your doctor regularly for blood pressure and cholesterol monitoring.

• Pursue a program of moderate, regular aerobic exercise. People over age 50 who have led a sedentary lifestyle should check with a doctor before beginning an exercise program.

• Lose weight if you are overweight.

• Your doctor may advise you to take a low dose of aspirin regularly. Aspirin reduces the tendency for the blood to clot, thereby decreasing the risk of heart attack. However, such a regimen should only be initiated under a doctor's expressed recommendation.

• Women at or approaching menopause should discuss the possible cardioprotective benefits of estrogen replacement therapy with their doctors.

DIAGNOSIS

• Patient history and physical examination are needed. Diagnosis will often be made immediately by a doctor or emergency response technician.

• An electrocardiogram (ECG) will be performed. This test measures changes in the electrical activity of the heart that result from abnormalities in the flow of blood.

• Blood tests measure the release of enzymes from damaged heart muscle into the bloodstream.

• A coronary angiography (using a tiny catheter inserted into an artery in a leg or arm and threaded up the artery to the heart) is performed to locate the arterial blockage prior to angioplasty or bypass surgery. A contrast material is then injected from the end of the catheter into the coronary arteries, and a high-speed series of x-rays is taken.

HOW TO TREAT IT

• It is advised to chew on an aspirin at the onset of the symptoms of a heart attack. It may help break up the clot.

• Emergency treatment and immediate hospitalization is necessary.

• A stopped heartbeat must be restarted immediately by cardiopulmonary resuscitation (CPR) or by a device known as an electrical defibrillator.

• Thrombolytic, or clot-dissolving, drugs such as tissue plasminogen activator (tPA), streptokinase, or urokinase may be injected immediately to dissolve arterial blockage. This technique is most effective within three hours of the onset of a heart attack.

• Painkillers such as morphine or meperidine are administered to relieve pain.

• Nitroglycerin may be given to reduce the heart's oxygen demands and to lower blood pressure.

• Antihypertensive drugs such as beta-blockers, ACE inhibitors, or calcium channel blockers may also be administered to lower blood pressure and to reduce the heart's oxygen demand. The effect of these drugs may be enhanced by diuretics.

• Oxygen may be administered through nasal tubes.

• Anticoagulants such as heparin, aspirin, or warfarin may be administered to reduce the risk of blood clots.

• Digitalis glycosides may be prescribed in some cases to strengthen heart muscle contraction. (In the

Myocardial Infarction Heart Attack *continued*

United States, digoxin is the most commonly pre-scribed type of digitalis.)
• Dopamine or dobutamine may be administered to increase blood flow to the heart and strengthen the heartbeat.
• Blocked arteries may be opened or widened by percutaneous transluminal coronary angioplasty (PTCA). A small balloon is inserted into an artery, guided with a catheter to the narrowed point in the coronary artery, and then inflated. This compresses the plaque, widens the passageway, and improves blood flow.
• Coronary bypass surgery may be performed to restore adequate blood flow to the heart muscle. A mammary artery or a vein from the leg is grafted onto the narrowed coronary artery to circumvent the blocked portion.
• Electronic implants such as a pacemaker or a defibrillator may be attached to the heart to maintain strong, regular contractions of the heart muscle.

• A heart transplant may be advised in severe cases when heart tissue has been badly damaged. The sur-vival rate for heart transplant is 80 percent after one year and over 60 percent after four years.
• During recovery, follow prevention tips to reduce the risk of another heart attack.
• Contact your local chapter of the American Heart Association for information about support groups.

WHEN TO CALL A DOCTOR
• **EMERGENCY** Call an ambulance if you experience crushing chest pain, with or without nausea, vomit-ing, profuse sweating, breathlessness, weakness, or intense feelings of dread.
• **EMERGENCY** Call an ambulance if chest pain from previously diagnosed angina does not subside after 10 to 15 minutes.
• **EMERGENCY** Call an ambulance the first time you experience intense chest pain. ▲

Myocarditis

WHAT IS IT?

Myocarditis is an inflammation of the heart muscle (myocardium), usually due to a viral infection. In many cases myocarditis produces no noticeable symptoms, although severe cases may cause serious disturbances of the heartbeat (cardiac arrhythmia), weakness of the heart muscle (cardiomyopathy), heart failure, or sudden cardiac arrest. While in most instances the inflammation subsides on its own without treatment and without causing permanent damage, more severe cases or those that become chronic may require hospitalization and medical treatment. Myocarditis can affect people of all ages. Because it is often asymptomatic, it is sometimes diagnosed only after a young adult with heart damage due to chronic myocarditis dies unexpectedly during strenuous exercise. Patients with viral myocarditis often exhibit pericarditis (inflammation of the lining around the heart; see Pericarditis) as well.

WHAT CAUSES IT?

• Viral infections, including Coxsackie virus, measles, rubella, influenza, and polio-, adeno-, and echoviruses, are the most common cause of myocarditis in the United States.
• Bacterial infection is a rare cause.
• Radiation therapy for cancer (especially lung or breast carcinoma and Hodgkin's disease).
• Excessive alcohol consumption.
• Certain chemicals and drugs (such as immuno-suppressants).
• Parasitic infections such as trichinosis and toxoplasmosis (both rare in the United States).
• Chagas' disease, due to the parasite *Trypanosoma cruzi* (a common cause of heart disease in Central and South America).

SYMPTOMS
• In many cases there are no symptoms.
• Fatigue.
• Shortness of breath.
• Heart palpitations or rapid heartbeat.
• Fever.
• Chest pain.

• Toxins released in the course of diphtheria infections.
• Rheumatic fever.
• Lyme disease.

PREVENTION

• Vaccinations for diphtheria, tetanus, measles, rubella, and polio should be kept current.
• Get prompt treatment for infections, especially those of the upper respiratory system.

DIAGNOSIS

• Patient history and physical examination.
• Blood tests.
• Electrocardiogram (ECG), which measures the electrical activity of the heart.
• Endomyocardial biopsy (removal of a small sample of heart muscle with a needle for microscopic analysis) provides a definitive diagnosis.

HOW TO TREAT IT

• Most cases subside in a few weeks without medical treatment. Studies have indicated that exercise may be risky for those with myocarditis, so all strenuous activity should be avoided. Bed-rest is generally recommended in severe cases during convalescence to minimize the workload on the heart. A low-salt diet and abstinence from alcohol may also be advised.
• Antibiotics are prescribed for bacterial infection.
• In some cases corticosteroid drugs may be prescribed to reduce inflammation of the myocardium and to speed recovery.
• Appropriate medications may be needed to treat congestive heart failure or arrhythmias.
• In very severe cases heart transplantation may be recommended for congestive heart failure.

WHEN TO CALL A DOCTOR

• Call a doctor if you develop the symptoms of myocarditis, especially if you have a recent history of infection.

Nasal Polyps

WHAT IS IT?

Nasal polyps are usually benign growths or swellings in the lining of the nasal cavity. (However, a single nasal polyp that bleeds may represent a rare nasal cancer.) Nasal polyps are caused by an overproduction of fluid in the cells of the mucous membrane, usually due to persistent irritation from an underlying chronic allergy or recurrent nasal or sinus infections. Polyps typically form when sinus passages are narrow and swollen tissues meet.

Polyps may occur singly, but they more often appear in clusters in both sides of the nose. They are generally not a serious health threat but may grow large enough or numerous enough to obstruct the airways and cause breathing difficulty. Also, they may block drainage of the sinuses and foster recurrent sinus infections. Nasal polyps usually respond well to treatment, although they tend to recur. Incidence is higher among adults than children.

WHAT CAUSES IT?

• Nasal polyps usually result from persistent irritation caused by a chronic allergy (allergic rhinitis), which triggers swelling and fluid retention in the mucous membrane of the nasal cavity.
• Recurrent or persistent nasal and sinus infections increase the risk of developing nasal polyps.

PREVENTION

• Prompt and aggressive treatment of nasal allergy or chronic sinusitis may slow nasal polyp development.

DIAGNOSIS

• Patient history and physical examination are necessary. The doctor may use a nasal speculum, a device that distends the nostrils to view the nasal cavity.

SYMPTOMS

• Feeling of blockage in the nose or sinuses.
• Loss of the sense of smell.
• Dull pain or pressure in the face.
• Recurrent headaches.
• Nasal discharge.
• Breathing difficulty.

• X-rays may be taken of the nasal passages and sinuses.

HOW TO TREAT IT

• The first line of treatment is the same as for allergies: antihistamines, nasal decongestants, inhaled corticosteroid spray, or allergy shots. These measures are most successful when polyps are small. A dose of oral corticosteroids usually reduces the size of polyps. However, relief is likely to be temporary.
• Antibiotics may be prescribed if an infection is diagnosed.
• The most reliable and long-lasting treatment of polyps is surgical removal (polypectomy). A single polyp may be removed in the doctor's office with local anesthesia. Multiple polyps are best treated with endoscopy, a procedure using a slender optical viewing tube that can be inserted into the nose.
• In addition to polyp removal, narrow passages in the sinuses are corrected during the polypectomy in order to permit a more precise and complete excision of the polyp, thereby reducing the likelihood that polyps will recur at the same site.
• After a polypectomy, nasal steroids should be used, even if they were previously ineffective. With the polyps removed, the medication will reach the mucous membrane.
• Over-the-counter pain relievers may be used. A special note: People who are prone to nasal polyps should use acetaminophen rather than aspirin. For reasons that remain unclear, people with nasal polyps also tend to be allergic to aspirin.

WHEN TO CALL A DOCTOR

• If you experience symptoms of nasal polyps, make an appointment to see a doctor. You will most likely be referred to an otolaryngologist (ear, nose, and throat specialist) for further examination and treatment.
• If you experience persistent or excessive bleeding, high fever, or unrelenting pain after surgical removal of nasal polyps, contact a doctor immediately.

Nephrotic Syndrome

WHAT IS IT?

Nephrotic syndrome is a condition marked by the loss of large amounts of protein through the urine. A number of diseases can result in the syndrome; however, in many cases it is caused by kidney damage of unknown origin, especially in children, in whom it is most common. The syndrome arises from damage to the glomeruli, the tiny structures in the kidneys that filter blood. Small chemical substances, including waste products, pass through the glomerular membrane; most proteins are normally too large to cross an intact membrane. But if the glomeruli are damaged, proteins may escape into the urine.

Loss of large amounts of protein through the urine lowers albumin levels in the blood, thus preventing fluid in the body tissues from returning to the bloodstream and partially producing the swelling (edema) characteristic of this syndrome. Swelling is exacerbated by an abnormal retention of salt by the kidneys. Major complications include protein malnutrition, massive swelling, occlusion of major veins by blood clots, and renal failure. Children with nephrotic syndrome are more vulnerable to systemic infections. The outcome depends on the underlying cause of the syndrome.

WHAT CAUSES IT?

• Disorders that can cause the syndrome include diabetes mellitus, systemic lupus erythematosus, amyloidosis, syphilis, hepatitis B, HIV, and cancer.
• Some toxins and medications, such as heroin, gold, mercury, lead, mesantoin, and perchlorate, can damage the kidneys.

SYMPTOMS

• Swelling of the feet and ankles and, if severe, the abdomen and the tissues around the eyes due to fluid retention.
• Weight increase owing to fluid retention.
• Shortness of breath due to fluid retention in the lungs.
• Decreased amount of urine; foamy, sometimes discolored urine.
• Diarrhea; loss of appetite; fatigue.

• Allergic reactions to bee stings and poison ivy may result in nephrotic syndrome.
• The cause of many cases is unknown.

PREVENTION

• Treatment of potential underlying causes (such as lupus) may prevent the onset of nephrotic syndrome.

DIAGNOSIS

• Blood tests show a reduction in albumin and an increase in triglycerides and cholesterol.
• Urine protein loss is measured. Urine is also examined for red and white blood cells.
• A kidney biopsy may be performed. Under local anesthesia a needle is inserted into the kidney through the back to extract a small tissue sample.

HOW TO TREAT IT

• A low-salt diet may help reduce fluid retention.
• Diuretics are used to reduce excess fluid retention and increase urine output.
• Long-term anticoagulant treatment may be needed in those with the tendency to form blood clots.
• Antihypertensive drugs, such as ACE inhibitors (which may help decrease urine protein and prevent the loss of renal function), may be prescribed to reduce associated high blood pressure.
• Antibiotics may be needed for bacterial infections.
• Corticosteroids may reduce protein loss in the urine if no known cause is found. Usually, a kidney biopsy is performed prior to the use of this medication which has many side effects.
• Intravenous albumin may be given to increase plasma protein levels when extremely low blood albumin levels cause severe swelling. However, the albumin is rapidly excreted in the urine.
• Chemotherapeutic drugs used to treat cancer or medications used in transplant patients may be effective in preventing relapses.

WHEN TO CALL A DOCTOR

• Call a doctor for symptoms of nephrotic syndrome.
• **EMERGENCY** Call your doctor immediately if symptoms of kidney failure develop, including fatigue, nausea and vomiting, appetite loss, itching, headaches, impaired vision, or blood in the urine.

Neuralgia

WHAT IS IT?

Neuralgia refers to a range of disorders marked by spasms of pain along the path of a nerve. Neuralgia tends to afflict people over age 50. Some forms are named for the nerves they affect. For example, trigeminal neuralgia, also known as tic douloureux, affects the trigeminal (fifth cranial) nerve that supplies sensation to the face, causing brief but intense spasms of pain on one side of the lips, gums, cheek, chin, or, rarely, around the eyes. Other forms of neuralgia are associated with specific diseases. Postherpetic neuralgia can arise after a case of shingles; it causes a dull, burning pain that may persist for months or even years. Facial neuralgia may also be a feature of multiple sclerosis or migraines. Trigeminal neuralgia is fairly common, particularly in older women; postherpetic neuralgia is also common, while the other forms of neuralgia are rare. Although painful, neuralgia is not life-threatening.

WHAT CAUSES IT?

• In most cases the cause is unknown.
• Some cases may be due to compression of the nerve by blood vessels or a tumor.
• Herpes zoster infection (shingles) precedes postherpetic neuralgia.
• Multiple sclerosis is a cause of neuralgia in those younger than 50.

PREVENTION

• There are no known ways to prevent neuralgia.

SYMPTOMS

• Brief, staccato bursts of excruciating pain, typically lasting from a few seconds to a minute or two.
• Recurrent pain in the same location, often in bouts lasting weeks at a time. Between bouts, there may be weeks or months with no pain.
• Pain triggered by touching specific areas of the skin or by talking, chewing, shaving, brushing the teeth, or swallowing. Bursts of dull dental or sinus pain may be an early sign of trigeminal neuralgia.

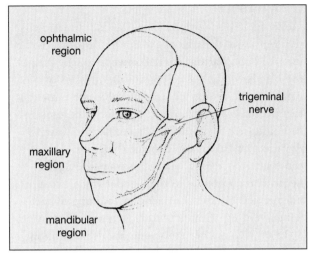

The trigeminal nerve has three distinct branches. Neuralgia in any one of them produces pain within the regions indicated.

DIAGNOSIS

• Neuralgia is identified by symptom presence.
• X-rays or MRI (magnetic resonance imaging) may be done to rule out other conditions.

HOW TO TREAT IT

• Over-the-counter pain relievers may help.
• A topical cream containing capsaicin (such as Zostrix or Axsain), along with physical therapy, may ease postherpetic neuralgia.
• The most effective medications for neuralgia are nortriptyline, amitriptyline, and carbamazepine.
• More invasive procedures may be warranted if drug treatment fails. The most common approach delivers high-frequency sound waves or electrical currents to the nerve to reduce its sensitivity. This often helps but causes lingering numbness and, if the region around the eye is involved, may result in corneal damage. Also, neuralgia may recur.
• Another approach involves exploratory surgery to look for and loosen any blood vessels that may be compressing the nerve. This approach provides long-term relief in most cases but can require up to a week of hospitalization and, like all major surgeries, carries significant risks.

WHEN TO CALL A DOCTOR

• Call a doctor if you experience persistent pain that does not respond to over-the-counter treatment.

Neurogenic Bladder

WHAT IS IT?

Neurogenic bladder is impaired bladder function resulting from damage to the nerves that govern the urinary tract. Various nerves converge in the area of the bladder and serve to control the muscles of the urinary tract, which include the sphincter muscles that normally form a tight ring around the urethra to hold urine back until it is voluntarily released. A variety of factors can damage these nerves and cause urinary incontinence. In some cases spontaneous nerve impulses to the bladder trigger spastic, unexpected bladder contractions, resulting in accidental voiding of sometimes large amounts of urine.

In other types of neurogenic bladder conditions, the bladder may become flaccid and distended and cease to contract fully, resulting in only partial emptying and continual dribbling of small amounts of urine. Rashes may erupt in areas of skin irritated by urine. Stagnant urine in the bladder also increases the risks of bladder stone formation and urinary tract infections. Such infections, when severe, can lead to life-threatening kidney failure. In some patients there is partial loss of anal sphincter control as well. Neurogenic bladder can occur at any age, but it is especially common among the elderly.

WHAT CAUSES IT?

• Spinal cord injuries resulting in paralysis.
• Other disorders that may produce neurogenic bladder as they progress; these include syphilis, diabetes mellitus, brain or spinal cord tumors, stroke, ruptured or herniated intervertebral disk, and degenerative neurological diseases such as multiple sclerosis and amyotrophic lateral sclerosis (or Lou Gehrig's disease).
• A congenital spinal cord abnormality (that is, one that is present at birth), such as spina bifida.
• Long-term effects of alcoholism.

PREVENTION

• There are no known ways to prevent this condition.

DIAGNOSIS

• A thorough patient history is essential. It is useful to keep a 24-hour record of urination patterns, including the approximate volume of urine voided, how urgently you felt the need to urinate, and any factors that may aggravate incontinence. It is also important to report any medications you are taking.
• Physical examination will likely include a rectal, genital, and abdominal check to look for enlargement of the bladder or other abnormalities.
• A complete neurological exam is essential.
• X-rays or an ultrasound scan may be taken during urination (voiding cystography).
• Tests to measure urine output are conducted. To determine whether urine is retained after voiding, the doctor may insert a catheter into the bladder. To determine whether leakage occurs, a full-bladder stress test may be necessary: The bladder is filled to capacity via a catheter, and the patient is then asked to bend over, cough, or walk.
• Urine and blood samples may be taken in order to look for abnormalities, including infections and underlying disorders that might be causing or aggravating the condition.
• Spinal x-rays may be ordered.

HOW TO TREAT IT

• Patients suffering from bladder paralysis can be taught to insert a catheter several times a day to drain the bladder completely and so prevent urine retention that may lead to bladder stones and infections.
• A urinary catheter (drainage tube) can be used continuously by patients who have sudden, unexpected bladder contractions. Women usually fare better with such therapy; men are more prone to developing urinary tract infections and complications, including abscess formation.

SYMPTOMS

• Urinary incontinence, characterized by either the involuntary release of large volumes of urine or continuous dribbling of small amounts. Bed-wetting may occur.
• Frequent urination.
• Persistent urge to urinate despite recent voiding; constant feeling that the bladder is not completely empty.
• Pain or burning on urination.

Neurogenic Bladder   *continued*

• Various medications may help to improve bladder muscle control and to prevent involuntary muscle contractions. Muscle relaxants, antispasmodics, and anticholinergic drugs (which block the neurotransmitter acetylcholine), such as propantheline, oxybutynin, and imipramine, are helpful in some cases.

• A device that stimulates bladder contraction with electrical impulses may be used, although such therapy is considered experimental.

• Surgery may be performed to widen the sphincter to decrease resistance in the bladder outlet and thus maximize bladder emptying. In other cases the sphincter or lower pelvic muscles may be surgically tightened to improve bladder control. An artificial sphincter may also be permanently implanted.

• In very severe cases surgery may be done to reroute the flow of urine so that it empties into the intestine or into an externally worn receptacle.

WHEN TO CALL A DOCTOR

• Call a doctor if you experience recurrent urinary incontinence. Don't allow embarrassment to prevent you from seeking professional help. ▲

Obesity

WHAT IS IT?

Obesity is conventionally defined as an excess of stored fat resulting in a body weight that is 20 percent or greater than what is accepted as ideal for a person's height and body type. It is not in itself a disease, but obesity does represent a serious health risk. Mortality rates and the incidence of high blood pressure, coronary heart disease, and diabetes mellitus are substantially higher in obese adults, especially in those whose excessive fat is stored in the abdomen rather than in the hips. Excess weight increases the risk of gallbladder disease and places greater stress on the back, hips, and knees, which may aggravate arthritis. Certain types of cancer may also be more common in overweight people. Obesity is often accompanied by poor self-image, psychological distress, and diminished quality of life. Health-care professionals have come to realize that losing weight and keeping it off is extraordinarily difficult. Nonetheless, a sensible balanced diet and a regular regimen of moderate exercise confer valuable health benefits and so are advised for everyone, regardless of weight.

WHAT CAUSES IT?

• Obesity results from an imbalance between caloric intake and energy expenditure, possibly from habitually excessive food intake or from extremely limited physical activity. Some people may gain weight because they have lower basal metabolic rates: They burn fewer calories to maintain body functions, such as breathing, heart contractions, and digestion.
• Hereditary, environmental, and psychological factors all play a role in obesity.

PREVENTION

• Establish healthy eating habits; maintain a nutritious, low-fat, high-carbohydrate diet.
• Exercise regularly and stay as active as possible.

SYMPTOMS

• Symptoms such as chest pain or shortness of breath from heart disease, knee or hip pain, or abdominal pain from gallstones all result from the complications of obesity.

DIAGNOSIS

• Obesity is formally defined by a body mass index (BMI) greater than 30. The BMI is found by dividing your weight in pounds by your height in inches squared, and then multiplying by 705.
• In one approach, actual weight is compared to an ideal weight for a patient's height and body type.
• Blood tests are obtained for complications of diabetes, such as high blood glucose and triglycerides.
• Waist and hip circumferences are taken; a waist-to-hips ratio greater than 1.0 in men or 0.8 in women indicates the more-dangerous abdominal obesity.

HOW TO TREAT IT

• Your doctor or nutritionist may advise a diet of no less than 1,200 calories a day, made up of nutritious, low-fat, low-calorie foods (fruits, vegetables, whole grains, lean meat or fish, and low-fat dairy products).
• Crash diets, fasting, and appetite suppressants (which may produce short-term weight loss, but rarely sustained weight loss) should be avoided.
• Engaging in regular, vigorous aerobic exercise, such as running, biking, or swimming—or even walking or gardening—for at least 30 minutes a day four days a week is helpful.
• Modest weight loss may be achieved with the prescription weight-loss drug sibutramine (Meridia). The drug should be combined with the dietary and lifestyle measures described above.
• For the grossly obese, doctors may advise a very low-calorie liquid diet program (800–900 calories a day) to be followed under close medical supervision.
• In rare cases when obesity is life-threatening, doctors may resort to extraordinary measures, including surgery to staple the stomach and reduce its size, or cutting or suctioning away fat (liposuction). The long-term success of liposuction is questionable, and severe complications are possible.
• Therapy or counseling may help to confront underlying psychological and emotional reasons for overeating. Support groups are often helpful.

WHEN TO CALL A DOCTOR

• If you are obese and unable to change your eating and exercise habits to lose weight, see a doctor or nutritionist. 🔳

Optic Neuritis

WHAT IS IT?

Optic neuritis, an inflammation or demyelination (progressive loss of the protective sheaths around a nerve) of the optic nerve in one or both eyes, may interfere with the transmission of nerve impulses from the optic nerve to the brain, causing sudden blurring or other visual impairment. Usually, central vision and color perception are affected the most. Although rare, some cases progress from blurring to total temporary blindness in the affected eye(s) within a matter of days.

Underlying conditions that can damage the optic nerve include multiple sclerosis and various infections, such as syphilis. In the majority of cases, symptoms disappear spontaneously and normal or nearly normal vision is restored within a few months. But attacks may recur and eventually lead to permanent vision loss, depending on the cause.

WHAT CAUSES IT?

• An episode of optic neuritis may be one of the earliest indications of multiple sclerosis (MS), a disease in which the protective sheaths (myelin) surrounding the nerves are gradually destroyed. An estimated 35 percent of men and 75 percent of women who develop optic neuritis will develop MS within the ensuing 15 years, and 40 percent of MS patients experience at least one episode of optic neuritis.
• The condition may also result from inflammation due to infection of the tissues near the optic nerve.

PREVENTION

• There are no known ways to prevent optic neuritis.

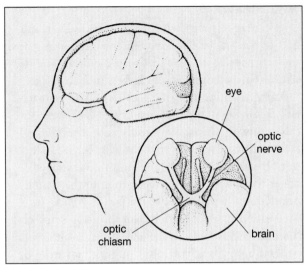

At the optic chiasm, some of the fibers of either of the two optic nerves cross over to the optic tract on the opposite side. Optic neuritis is characterized by inflammation of any part of this nerve structure.

DIAGNOSIS

• A thorough eye examination is required. Inspection with an ophthalmoscope (a lighted instrument that permits viewing of the internal structures of the eye) often reveals only normal conditions during the early stages, but later examinations may uncover characteristic signs of optic neuritis.
• Visual field and color perception tests may be performed; the reaction of the pupil to light is carefully assessed.
• Tests may be required to rule out serious underlying diseases associated with optic nerve damage. If multiple sclerosis or temporal arteritis is suspected, the doctor will recommend further testing.

HOW TO TREAT IT

• In most cases, partial or full recovery of vision will occur within several months without treatment.
• Corticosteroids may be prescribed to speed natural recovery. Side effects, including increased recurrences, keep this treatment limited to select patients.

WHEN TO CALL A DOCTOR

• If you experience any vision loss or impairment, contact an ophthalmologist immediately. ▲

SYMPTOMS

• Impaired central vision or color perception in one or both eyes.
• Partial or total vision loss within a period of several hours to several days. If both eyes are involved, the second eye may be affected several days or weeks later.
• Pain when moving or touching the affected eye or eyes, especially in the first several days after the onset of symptoms.

Oral Cancers

WHAT IS IT?

Oral cancer is the growth of malignant cells in any part of the oral cavity, which includes the lips, gums, tongue, cheeks, floor or roof of the mouth, and tonsils. The most common site is the lip, followed by the tongue, and then other locations. The primary risk factor for all types of oral cancer is the use of tobacco in any form. Symptoms vary depending on the location of the cancer but usually include ulcerations that are initially painless. In more advanced stages the cancer spreads, most often to the lymph nodes in the neck or under the jaw.

Treatment depends on the location and stage of the malignancy and the age and overall health of the patient, but it usually involves surgery, radiation, or both. Prognosis is good if the cancer is detected and treated in its early stages, before it has spread. In most cases lip cancer is very treatable because it is easier to detect, while prognosis for tongue cancer is not as good, particularly if the lesion is near the rear of the mouth and hard to see. Oral cancers account for about 5 percent of all cancers. Risk increases with age; the majority of cases occur in people over age 45, with men at twice the risk as women.

WHAT CAUSES IT?

The cause of oral cancer is unknown. However, a number of risk factors have been identified; these factors include:
• The use of tobacco in any form (smoking, chewing, or dipping).
• Long-term heavy alcohol use.
• Nutritional deficiencies (including lack of iron, vitamin A, and certain B vitamins).
• Years of exposure to sunlight (a risk factor for lip cancer).
• Infections with herpes simplex or human papillomavirus.

PREVENTION

• All tobacco products should be avoided.
• Excessive alcohol use is discouraged.
• Regular dental checkups and periodic self-examination of the mouth may help detect cancer in its early stages.

DIAGNOSIS

• Patient history and examination of the mouth and neck are necessary.
• A small sample of affected tissue is removed for microscopic examination of the cells (biopsy) to determine if cancer is present.
• X-rays of the head or chest may be taken to detect if the cancer has spread.

HOW TO TREAT IT

• Surgery to remove the tumor, the surrounding tissue, and possibly the lymph nodes in the neck is generally recommended.
• Radiation therapy is often advised when there is suspicion that cancer may have spread. It may be administered externally (for example, with x-rays) or internally (by implanting pellets into the tumor).
• Speech therapy and other kinds of occupational therapy may be part of rehabilitation.
• A wide variety of plastic surgery techniques are available to correct surgical scars and radiation damage to normal tissues.

WHEN TO CALL A DOCTOR

• Contact your doctor or dentist if you develop any mouth lesion that fails to heal within two weeks to a month. 🔺

SYMPTOMS

• A skin lesion or ulcerations in some area of the mouth that persist or worsen over time. In early stages such lesions are often painless.
• In more advanced cases, difficulty speaking, eating, and swallowing.
• Bad breath.
• Abnormal sense of taste.
• An enlarging growth on the lip that crusts over and bleeds when the crust is removed.
• A sore throat or burning sensation in the mouth during advanced stages, especially when eating or drinking.
• White patches (leukoplakia) or velvety red patches (erythroplakia); these must be watched carefully, as they may be precancerous.

Oral Herpes Cold Sores

WHAT IS IT?

Oral herpes is a viral infection characterized by outbreaks of mouth lesions commonly known as cold sores or fever blisters. The initial infection typically occurs in childhood. Although a large majority of the population has been infected by herpes, most do not show signs or symptoms. The people who do get sick with the initial infection develop painful sores inside the mouth, affecting the back of the throat, roof of the mouth, tongue, and sometimes the cheeks and inside of the lips. Usually people feel quite sick, with fever, enlarged lymph nodes, sore throat, and bad breath. Though the symptoms completely subside within 10 to 21 days, the virus remains in the body and lies dormant (inactive) until reactivated by certain factors such as stress, menses, or sun exposure. Subsequent flare-ups or reactivation of the virus, known as recurrent herpes simplex, affects the outside, as opposed to the inside, of the mouth, usually at the edge of one area of the lip. These recurrences are much milder and generally last for eight to 10 days.

WHAT CAUSES IT?

• Herpes simplex virus type 1 (HSV-1) is the most common cause of cold sores.
• Herpes simplex virus type 2 (HSV-2), the virus that commonly causes genital herpes, may also cause cold sores.
• The reason some people get recurrent cold sores while others do not is unclear. However, in people who do develop recurrences, factors that seem to induce them include anxiety, stress, wind, sunlight, menstruation, and fever.

SYMPTOMS

Recurrent HSV infection:
• A tingling sensation or discomfort one to two days prior to the appearance of the cold sore.
• Small, raw, open sores appearing on the outside edges of the lips.
• Scabbing of the sores within 48 hours. The sores usually heal completely within eight to 10 days.

• People with weakened immune systems, such as those undergoing cancer treatment or who have HIV or AIDS, are at greater risk for more severe and more frequent recurrences.

PREVENTION

• Avoid intimate contact with someone who has active sores, to prevent the transmission of the virus.
• Try to determine which factors precipitate a flare-up and plan to avoid them or to lessen their severity. For example, if sunlight is a factor, apply sunblock to your lips before going outdoors, or wear a wide-brimmed hat.

DIAGNOSIS

• Patient history and physical examination are needed.
• Microscopic examination of scrapings from a lesion, or of a culture of fluid from blisters or sores, is sometimes required when the diagnosis cannot be made by history and physical examination alone.

HOW TO TREAT IT

• Because open sores increase the risk of bacterial infection, a topical antibacterial ointment applied several times daily is prudent. If bacterial infection does develop, your doctor may prescribe an antibiotic.
• The antiviral drugs acyclovir, famciclovir, or valacyclovir may be prescribed for persons with primary infection inside the mouth and also for persons with severe or prolonged recurrences. Antiviral medications help tremendously in relieving symptoms
• Application of topical penciclovir cream, an antiviral drug, may speed the healing process in some people.

WHEN TO CALL A DOCTOR

• Call your doctor if you have a primary infection (affecting the inside of the mouth and throat).

Orchitis

WHAT IS IT?

Orchitis is the inflammation of one or both of the testicles because of infection. Indeed, orchitis is the most common complication of mumps in adult males, occurring in up to one-fourth of men who contract mumps after puberty. Orchitis is characterized by swelling and severe pain in the testes, which usually begins to subside after three to seven days. Most of the time the affected testicles return to normal size and function, but complications may include testicular atrophy and, rarely, infertility. Two-thirds of cases affect only one testicle; involvement of both carries a higher risk of infertility. Orchitis is most common among males 15 to 25 years old.

WHAT CAUSES IT?

• Orchitis is most often caused by a viral infection, especially the virus responsible for mumps.
• Bacterial infections of the epididymis (the long, tightly coiled sperm conduit that rests on the back of each testicle) or the prostate may spread to the testes.
• Testicular inflammation may be a manifestation of sexually transmitted diseases such as syphilis and chlamydia.

PREVENTION

• Be sure you have been immunized with the MMR (measles, mumps, rubella) vaccine.
• Practice safe sex behaviors, such as monogamy and condom use.

DIAGNOSIS

• Patient history and a physical examination are necessary.
• Urinalysis and urine culture are performed to screen for an underlying bacterial infection.

SYMPTOMS

• Severe pain in the scrotum or in the affected testicle.
• Swelling and a feeling of heaviness, usually on one side of the scrotum.
• Fever.

HOW TO TREAT IT

• Antibiotics are prescribed for bacterial infections. Sexual partners may also need to be treated.
• If orchitis is caused by a virus, treatment is aimed exclusively at relieving symptoms (as antibiotics are effective against bacterial but not viral infections). Analgesic drugs, bed rest with support of the scrotum on a rolled towel, and application of ice packs may help to ease the pain of orchitis.

WHEN TO CALL A DOCTOR

• Call your doctor if you develop any persistent pain or swelling in the scrotum. It is likely that you will be referred to a urologist. A careful urological evaluation is necessary to rule out other disorders such as epididymitis and testicular torsion, which produce similar symptoms to orchitis.

Osteoarthritis

WHAT IS IT?

Osteoarthritis—also known as degenerative joint disease—is the gradual age-related deterioration of cartilage within the joints, causing pain and sometimes deformity. (Joint inflammation is uncommon.) It is the most common form of arthritis: nearly all people have developed some degree of osteoarthritis in one or more joints by the age of 60. It can occur in any joint, but most commonly osteoarthritis affects the fingers, neck, spine, hips, knees, and feet.

As the elastic cartilage that serves as a cushion between bones breaks down, bone ends may rub together, causing them to develop uneven outgrowths called osteophytes, or spurs, that may grind against each other as the joint moves. Damage usually develops gradually over a period of years. In some people, symptoms remain mild or even fade; in others, symptoms grow progressively worse until they are severely disabling. Affected joints may begin to lose their shape and alignment. Weakness and wasting of the muscles surrounding the joints may occur if pain and stiffness prevent normal motion.

Osteoarthritis has no impact on longevity (unlike some other forms of arthritis), but it can diminish overall quality of life. There is no cure, but a number of treatments can ease pain and minimize disability.

WHAT CAUSES IT?

• Osteoarthritis occurs as a part of aging, owing to years of cumulative wear and tear on the joints.

SYMPTOMS

• Joint pain that is aggravated by movement and relieved by rest.
• Stiffness, especially in the morning or after exercise; loss of flexibility in the affected joints.
• Knobby overgrowths on the joints closest to the fingertips (Heberden's nodes) or on the fingers' middle joints (Bouchard's nodes).
• Audible crackling noises upon movement of the joints.
• Changes in gait.
• Rarely, redness, warmth, and swelling of a joint.

Obesity increases the risk of developing osteoarthritis in weight-bearing joints, such as the hips, knees, and those of the back.
• Trauma or overuse of a joint can hasten the development of osteoarthritis. This is common among athletes and those whose occupations require constant repetitive motions, such as pianists, typists, machinists, and dancers.

PREVENTION

• Maintain a healthy weight.
• Avoid repetitive activities that may lead to joint overuse as much as possible.

DIAGNOSIS

• Patient history and physical examination are needed.
• X-rays may be taken.
• In rare cases when diagnosis is in question, fluid may be drawn from the affected joint through a needle for laboratory analysis.

HOW TO TREAT IT

• Cold packs, warm compresses, heat lamps, and warm baths or showers may bring relief.
• Splints, braces, neck collars, crutches, or canes may provide support and limit stress on the affected joint.
• A regular exercise program under the guidance of a doctor or physical therapist is recommended. The right program can help to maintain flexibility, strengthen muscles (and thus lessen stress on joints), and improve overall fitness. Therapists can also evaluate the performance of daily activities (such as dressing, brushing teeth, preparing a meal) and recommend ways to improve function.
• The primary indication for drug treatment is pain relief. Acetaminophen and nonsteroidal anti-inflammatory drugs (NSAIDs such as ibuprofen, naproxen, and salsalate) may be very helpful. New medicines, dubbed COX-2 inhibitors, are becoming available that have pain-relieving and anti-inflammatory effects with a low risk of bleeding or stomach ulcers (common side effects of NSAIDs). Celecoxib (Celebrex) is the first of this new class to gain Food and Drug Administration (FDA) approval.
• A new type of treatment for knee osteoarthritis is now available. The therapy, called viscosupplementa-

Osteoarthritis   *continued*

tion, is designed to reduce joint pain by supplementing or enhancing the natural lubricating and shock absorbing properties of synovial (joint) fluid. Two drugs derived from hyaluronan (a substance found naturally in joint fluid) have been approved by the FDA. These drugs (Hyalgen and Synvisc) are recommended for the treatment of knee osteoarthritis after traditional therapies have failed.

• A variety of surgical procedures may be warranted in severe cases, including arthroscopy (insertion into the affected joint of a thin, flexible viewing scope that can be used to smooth or repair cartilage) and arthroplasty (total joint replacement). Most joint replacements are of the hip or knee. Discussion of the activities the patient would like to continue after the replacement aids the surgeon in selecting the appropriate type of prosthesis and makes the patient more aware of the risks and limitations of surgery.

• Researchers are studying new agents that may halt or repair the damage done by osteoarthritis. Glucosamine and chondroitin sulfate have received much media attention. These naturally occurring substances play important roles in forming and maintaining joint cartilage and may initiate repair. Although these agents seem to cause few or minimal side effects, studies are needed to determine their long-term benefits and safety.

• Corticosteroid injections into the joint space may be advised for relief of severe pain, particularly if only one or a few joints are involved.

WHEN TO CALL A DOCTOR

• If the symptoms of osteoarthritis begin to interfere with the enjoyment of normal activities, make an appointment with a doctor. ▲

Osteomalacia and Rickets

WHAT IS IT?

Osteomalacia is a disorder marked by inadequate or defective mineralization of the skeleton, resulting in soft or fragile bones. It typically occurs either when there are insufficient amounts of vitamin D in the diet or, more commonly, when the body is unable to properly absorb and metabolize vitamin D, which is essential for the absorption of the calcium needed to maintain strong, healthy bones. It can also occur with calcium and phosphorus deficiency. When the disease occurs in children, it is known as rickets and tends to produce obvious skeletal deformities such as bowed legs. The disease has more subtle manifestations in adults and may be difficult to diagnose or to differentiate from osteoporosis. In some cases repeated pressure on soft bones can lead to fractures or mild deformities. In adults, when osteomalacia is due to a vitamin D deficiency, treatment usually cures the problem within six months. In children, the disease may be arrested with treatment, although skeletal deformities may be permanent. Although common in underdeveloped countries, rickets is now rare in Western nations.

WHAT CAUSES IT?

• A chief cause of osteomalacia is intestinal malabsorption of vitamin D, which may result from a number of causes (see Malabsorption).
• Low levels of vitamin D lead to secretion of excessive amounts of parathyroid hormone, which in turn mobilizes calcium from the bones and increases the loss of phosphorus in the urine.
• Dietary deficiency of vitamin D is rarely a cause; however, inadequate exposure to sunlight reduces the amount of vitamin D produced naturally by the skin.
• Chronic renal failure and complications of hemodialysis are potential causes.
• Chronic acidosis (an abnormal state of reduced alkalinity in the blood or body tissues, usually due to renal failure) may lead to osteomalacia.
• Osteomalacia may occur as a side effect of some anticonvulsant drugs used to treat epilepsy. They interfere with normal activation of vitamin D.
• Several rare hereditary disorders can cause low phosphorus levels in the blood (hypophosphatemia), resulting in osteomalacia.
• Hypophosphatemia may result from chronic use of nonabsorbable antacids.

PREVENTION

• Dietary intake of vitamin D-fortified foods (such as milk products) and adequate exposure to sunlight help prevent vitamin D deficiency.

DIAGNOSIS

• Patient history and physical examination.
• X-rays to evaluate bone mass and fractures.
• Blood tests to measure vitamin D, calcium, phosphorus, and parathyroid hormone levels.
• Bone biopsy in some cases.

HOW TO TREAT IT

• Oral supplements of vitamin D are given, sometimes in conjunction with calcium.
• For osteomalacia due to intestinal malabsorption, large doses of oral vitamin D or vitamin D injections may be needed. Such patients may also benefit from calcium supplements.
• Osteomalacia due to chronic renal failure requires correction of the acidosis.
• Disorders leading to low blood phosphorus are treated with large doses of oral phosphate supplements plus vitamin D metabolites.
• Skeletal deformities may be corrected surgically.

WHEN TO CALL A DOCTOR

• Consult a doctor if you or your child experiences bone pain, unexplained fractures, or apparent limb deformities. ▲

SYMPTOMS
• Bone pain in the arms, legs, spine, and especially the hips.
• Muscle weakness, waddling gait.
• Unexplained bone fractures or deformities.
• Painful spasms or cramps in the face, hands, and feet due to low levels of calcium in the blood (rare).
• In rickets: bowed limbs (especially the legs), pot belly, waddling gait, disturbed growth.

Osteomyelitis

WHAT IS IT?

Osteomyelitis is infection of the bone. The infection can originate in another part of the body (in the throat or skin, for example) and spread to the bones via the bloodstream, or it can develop after a bone fracture has broken the skin, infecting the bone directly. It may also spread from an adjacent area of infection, or settle in an area with inadequate circulation. The infected bone becomes inflamed, resulting in severe bone pain, fever, and the formation of pus. Single episodes of the disorder, known as acute osteomyelitis, are most common in the arm and leg bones of rapidly growing children.

Chronic osteomyelitis, a rare and stubborn form of the condition, causes persistent bone pain for years. This form of the disease may also lead to complications, including skin abscess, bone deformity, cessation of bone growth in children, and amyloidosis (the deposition of a waxy substance into tissues and vital organs). Chronic osteomyelitis is more prevalent among adults and most often affects the vertebrae or pelvis. With prompt attention, acute osteomyelitis can usually be treated successfully with antibiotics. Chronic osteomyelitis, however, is more difficult to treat and normally requires surgery to remove the affected bone.

WHAT CAUSES IT?

• Acute osteomyelitis occurs when infectious organisms—usually bacteria—invade bone tissue. (Rarely, a fungal infection is the cause.) A bone is more susceptible to infection after a blunt physical trauma or fracture.

• Possible causes of chronic osteomyelitis include an acute case that is ignored or fails to respond to treatment; a compound bone fracture; and tuberculosis that spreads to the bone from elsewhere in the body.

SYMPTOMS

• Pain, often excruciating, in the affected bone.
• Heat, swelling, tenderness, redness, and restricted movement in the affected area.
• High fever.
• Fatigue and malaise.

PREVENTION

• Get prompt and thorough medical treatment for any bacterial infection before it can spread to the bones or other organs.

DIAGNOSIS

• Patient history and physical examination are needed.
• Blood cultures may identify the organism responsible for infection.
• Bone scans can provide early detection of osteomyelitis.
• Bone x-rays may also detect osteomyelitis, but usually only two to three weeks after infection.
• Biopsy (a small sample of tissue or pus removed for microscopic examination) can be taken to identify the infectious organism if blood cultures fail.

HOW TO TREAT IT

• Acute osteomyelitis can usually be cured with an extended course of antibiotics, given orally or intravenously over a period of weeks or months.
• Bed rest and immobilization of the affected area may be advised.
• If antibiotics fail to cure the infection, surgery to drain pus and remove infected or dead tissue may be warranted.
• The only effective treatment for chronic osteomyelitis is surgical removal of the affected bone tissue and any foreign bodies such as prosthetic devices. Bone grafting may be necessary in such cases.

WHEN TO CALL A DOCTOR

• If you experience the symptoms of osteomyelitis, see a doctor right away.
• If you develop any sign of complication during treatment for osteomyelitis (including formation of or increased drainage from an abscess, fever, unbearable pain), see a doctor immediately.
• If you previously had osteomyelitis and experience any of the symptoms of recurrence, see a doctor as soon as possible. ⬛

Osteoporosis

WHAT IS IT?

Osteoporosis is characterized by a loss of bone mass due to an imbalance of bone formation and bone resorption, a depletion of calcium and phosphorus essential to bone formation, or both. Affected bones become porous and brittle and susceptible to fractures. The wrists and hips, and vertebrae in the spine are the most common fracture sites. The disorder is very common among people over age 70; it affects women four times more often than men, owing to hormonal changes that occur with menopause.

WHAT CAUSES IT?

• Some degree of loss of bone mass is a normal consequence of aging, but a number of factors hasten osteoporosis: reduced estrogen levels after menopause; dietary calcium deficiency; physical inactivity; smoking; excessive alcohol use; and being underweight.

• Hereditary factors may be involved. For example, Caucasian women have a higher incidence of osteoporosis than others.

• Osteoporosis may occur as a consequence of an underlying condition, such as hyperthyroidism, premature menopause (before age 45), chronic lung diseases, and Cushing's disease (excessive production of corticosteroids by the adrenal glands). It may also arise from long-term use of corticosteroid drugs or heparin (an anticoagulant).

PREVENTION

• Estrogen replacement is highly effective in preventing osteoporosis in postmenopausal women. Estrogen must be started soon after menopause because bone loss accelerates rapidly at that time.

• A diet rich in calcium and vitamin D protects against osteoporosis. Older men and postmenopausal women should get 1,500 milligrams of calcium daily through diet and calcium supplements.

• Regular weight-bearing exercise is important.

SYMPTOMS
• Lower back pain.
• Gradual loss of height and stooping posture.
• Wrist, hip, or vertebral fractures.

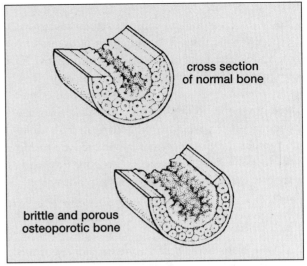

Rich stores of calcium make normal bones remarkably strong. Osteoporosis weakens bone by robbing it of its mineral content.

DIAGNOSIS

• Patient history and physical examination.
• Bone density scan.
• Blood or urine tests or a bone biopsy to detect or rule out other causes of bone loss.
• X-rays or other imaging tests, such as CT (computed tomography) scans. Routine x-rays, however, do not detect osteoporosis until 25 percent or more bone mass has been lost.

HOW TO TREAT IT

• Over-the-counter analgesics are effective for pain.
• Prompt estrogen replacement therapy can slow the progress of osteoporosis in postmenopausal women.
• Bisphosphonate therapy (with drugs such as alendronate and etidronate) slows bone resorption and builds bone. Calcium supplements may be advised.
• High doses of calcitonin (a hormone that regulates the body's calcium usage) can slow bone loss and possibly add bone mass.
• The drug raloxifene (Evista) may be an option for some people.
• Exercise and physical therapy may preserve function.

WHEN TO CALL A DOCTOR

• See a doctor with any symptoms of osteoporosis.
• If you have osteoporosis and pain develops after any strain or injury, call a doctor immediately.

Otosclerosis

WHAT IS IT?

Otosclerosis is a disorder caused by abnormal growth of spongy bone tissue at the junction of the inner ear and middle ear, resulting in gradual hearing loss. The overgrowth of bone impedes and, in the majority of cases, eventually immobilizes the stapes, one of the three tiny bones in the middle ear that mechanically conduct sound waves into the inner ear. This condition results in what is known as conductive hearing loss. In some cases, however, excess bone growth may eventually spread to the inner ear, impairing function of the inner ear (sensorineural hearing loss), which is far more difficult to treat than conductive hearing loss.

Otosclerosis may occur in one ear alone, but most often it affects both, either simultaneously or in succession. In general, hearing loss progresses gradually over a period of 10 to 15 years, usually leading to total deafness. Partial or total hearing can be restored, however, with a surgical procedure called a stapedotomy. Otosclerosis is fairly common, affecting one out of every 200 people, usually between the ages of 15 and 30, and is especially prevalent among Caucasians. Incidence is twice as high in women as in men.

WHAT CAUSES IT?

• Otosclerosis appears to be an inherited disorder; many of those who develop it report a family history of hearing loss.
• Pregnancy may trigger the onset of symptoms or accelerate the rate of hearing loss in those with active otosclerosis.

SYMPTOMS
• Gradual and progressive hearing loss.
• Ringing or noises in the ears (tinnitus).
• Dizziness.
• A tendency to speak softly.
• Improved ability to perceive spoken words in environments with background noise. (The opposite is true with many other types of hearing loss, including that which commonly occurs with age.)

PREVENTION
• There is no known way to prevent otosclerosis.
• Fluoride therapy may limit the progression of otosclerosis in the inner ear.

DIAGNOSIS
• Diagnosis is suspected in patients who have a blood relative with known otosclerosis or early hearing loss.
• Hearing tests will be performed to determine the type and degree of hearing loss. If the doctor suspects otosclerosis, especially if a patient has a family history of the disorder, more specialized hearing tests will be conducted.

HOW TO TREAT IT
• Stapedotomy (surgical removal of a portion of the stapes bone and replacement with an artificial prosthesis) is the only method to restore functional hearing. The procedure is often highly successful, significantly improving hearing in the majority of cases. Because there is a slight risk that the surgery will result in total deafness in the operated ear, stapedotomy is usually performed on one ear at a time.
• Hearing aids can be very effective for people with otosclerosis when stapedotomy is not possible. Also, a hearing aid may be required to augment hearing after stapedotomy.

WHEN TO CALL A DOCTOR
• Contact an otolaryngologist (ear, nose, and throat specialist) or ask your regular family practitioner to recommend one if you experience any degree of hearing loss.
• If you have had stapedotomy surgery for otosclerosis and you experience any sign of postoperative infection (pain, dizziness, or fever), call a doctor immediately.

Ovarian Cancer

WHAT IS IT?

Ovarian cancer occurs when cancer cells form malignant tumors in one or often both ovaries. With about 20,000 new cases diagnosed each year, ovarian cancer is the seventh most common type of cancer in women. Although the overall incidence is relatively low, the death rate from ovarian cancer is very high. It is the most deadly of all gynecologic cancers and the fourth most common cause of cancer-related death in women. The reason for the low survival rate is that ovarian cancer usually produces no noticeable symptoms in its early stages, and there is currently no simple test to screen for it. Consequently, the disease is usually not diagnosed until symptoms appear and the cancer has spread. Occasionally, the disease is first suspected during a routine pelvic examination. Prognosis varies depending on the type and the stage of the disease, but the overall five-year survival rate is between 30 and 40 percent. It is therefore important to keep up with regular pelvic examinations; diagnosis and treatment of ovarian cancer in the earliest stages yields nearly a 75 percent five-year survival rate. Owing to recent advances in treatment, the survival rate has improved even among women with late-stage disease, and some types of ovarian cancers can now be cured.

WHAT CAUSES IT?

• The cause of ovarian cancer is unknown. It is most common among postmenopausal women. Women who have not had children are at increased risk; those who have used oral contraceptives are at decreased risk.

SYMPTOMS

- In early stages there are usually no symptoms.
- Vague abdominal discomfort, indigestion, or other mild gastrointestinal problems.
- Abdominal swelling or bloating.
- Pelvic fullness or pressure.
- Urinary frequency.
- Unexplained vaginal bleeding or abnormal menstrual cycles.
- Weight loss.

PREVENTION

• There are no known ways to prevent ovarian cancer. Scheduling regular pelvic examinations, however, may help to detect ovarian cancer at an earlier, more treatable stage.

DIAGNOSIS

• Patient history and physical examination are needed.
• Abdominal ultrasound or CT (computed tomography) scans are used to locate tumors. However, the diagnosis of ovarian cancer can only be made by obtaining a tissue sample for microscopic examination (biopsy), most likely during surgery.

HOW TO TREAT IT

• When cancer is strongly suspected, surgery (known as exploratory laparotomy) is performed to confirm the diagnosis and determine the extent of the disease (staging) in order to plan the future course of treatment. Tumors found during this procedure are removed, if possible, and biopsied.
• Most often, both ovaries are surgically removed. In addition, the fallopian tubes, uterus, nearby lymph glands, or any other suspect tissues may be removed as well (radical hysterectomy).
• Surgery is typically followed by chemotherapy or radiation treatment to shrink or destroy any remaining cancer sites.
• Follow-up "second-look" surgery may be scheduled at some point during the course of therapy to evaluate the efficacy of treatment and to remove any new malignancies (although the value of second-look surgery is controversial).

WHEN TO CALL A DOCTOR

• If you experience any of the symptoms of ovarian cancer, see a doctor immediately. 🔺

Ovarian Cysts, Benign

WHAT IS IT?

An ovarian cyst is a fluid-filled sac that forms in the ovary. Ovarian cysts are common and, in the vast majority of cases, they are benign (noncancerous). They vary in size and may occur at different sites in the ovary; the most common type develops when an egg-producing follicle does not rupture and release the egg but instead swells with fluid and forms a follicular cyst. Benign ovarian cysts often cause no symptoms and are discovered incidentally during a routine pelvic examination. In some cases, however, they may alter hormone production in the ovaries or grow large enough to produce noticeable symptoms. Cysts often disappear on their own without treatment, but in some cases they may require surgical removal. In rare cases a cyst that twists or ruptures may cause serious complications warranting emergency surgery.

WHAT CAUSES IT?

• The cause of ovarian cysts is unknown.

PREVENTION

• There are no known ways to prevent ovarian cysts.

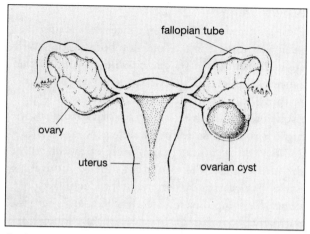

Ovarian cysts are globular sacs filled with fluid or semisolid material. They are typically detected during a routine pelvic examination.

DIAGNOSIS

• Gynecological examination is necessary. If a lump or mass in the ovary is detected, further tests are necessary to rule out the possibility of ovarian cancer.
• Abdominal or pelvic ultrasonography may be performed.
• A minor procedure called laparoscopy (insertion of a scope through a small incision in the abdomen to view the ovaries) may be used to confirm the diagnosis and determine the size and position of the cyst.

HOW TO TREAT IT

• Ovarian cysts often disappear without treatment.
• Surgery to remove the cyst may be needed if cancer is suspected, if the cyst does not go away, or if it causes symptoms. In many cases it can be taken out without damaging the ovary, but sometimes the ovary has to be removed.
• In some cases ovarian cyst may be drained during laparoscopy (see Diagnosis).

WHEN TO CALL A DOCTOR

• If you experience any of the symptoms of ovarian cysts, call a gynecologist.
• **EMERGENCY** If you have been diagnosed with an ovarian cyst and you experience sudden, sharp abdominal pain, fever, or vomiting, see a doctor immediately. ⚠

SYMPTOMS

• In many cases, ovarian cysts produce no symptoms.
• Mild abdominal ache.
• Abdominal swelling or a feeling of fullness or pressure.
• Pain during sexual intercourse.
• Menstrual irregularities including absence of menstrual bleeding (amenorrhea), heavy bleeding (menorrhagia), and painful periods (dysmenorrhea).
• Unusual hair growth on the face and body caused by an increased production of masculinizing hormones (hirsutism).
• Sudden, sharp abdominal pain, fever, and nausea if a cyst becomes twisted or ruptures.
• Rarely, painful, frequent urination—or urinary retention—if a cyst presses against the bladder.

Paget's Disease

WHAT IS IT?

Paget's disease is a slowly progressive bone disorder, most commonly affecting the spine, hip, skull, thigh, shin, and upper arm, although almost any bone may be involved. Bone is continuously broken down and restored. In the initial stages of Paget's disease, too much bone is broken down and, to compensate, new bone is formed at an increased rate. Often, however, the new bone cells are laid down in a disordered pattern, making the bone weak and prone to fractures. In addition, overgrowth of new bone results in deformities in affected areas.

The disease is most common in those over age 40, affecting up to 3 percent of the population in some parts of the world. Most cases are mild and tend to progress slowly. Advanced cases, however, may cause pain, deformity, incapacitation, hearing loss, or heart failure. Malignant bone cancer (sarcoma), the most serious complication, occurs in less than 1 percent of cases.

WHAT CAUSES IT?

• The cause of Paget's disease is unknown, although viral infection strongly appears to play a role. Indeed, the disease has been reported to occur within families but is not transmitted from one generation to another. This finding is consistent with an infectious disorder.

PREVENTION

• There are no specific preventive measures.
• For those with Paget's disease, regular checkups are advised to screen for early bone cancer or to detect hearing loss.

DIAGNOSIS

• X-rays or bone scans are taken.
• Blood or urine tests may point to the diagnosis.
• A bone biopsy may be required.

HOW TO TREAT IT

• Most patients never develop symptoms and so do not require treatment.
• Over-the-counter (OTC) analgesics (aspirin, ibuprofen, acetaminophen) may be used to reduce pain and inflammation.
• Prescription anti-inflammatory drugs may be needed when OTC products prove to be inadequate.
• Drugs (such as calcitonin, alendronate, and pamidronate) that correct the abnormally rapid bone metabolism may be prescribed in serious cases. These medications may completely halt the progress of the disease in some patients, but the damage that has already occurred is usually irreversible.
• Orthopedic surgery may be indicated. For example, if bone deformities lead to difficulty in walking, hip replacement or reshaping the leg bones may be performed to improve gait.

WHEN TO CALL A DOCTOR

• See your doctor if symptoms of Paget's disease develop. 🔺

SYMPTOMS

• Most cases go unnoticed and are discovered incidentally when x-rays or blood tests are taken for another reason. In more severe cases symptoms may occur and are highly variable.
• Bone pain (usually persistent and sometimes severe).
• Neck or back pain (especially the lower back), which may radiate to the buttocks or legs.
• Pain or stiffness in the joints (especially the hips, knees, or shoulders), resembling osteoarthritis.
• Warmth in the skin overlying affected bones.
• Unexplained bone fractures.
• Bone swelling or deformities, including bowed legs, skull enlargement around the eyes and forehead, barrel-shaped chest, or bent spine causing reduced height.
• Hearing loss, ringing in the ears.
• Headache, dizziness.

Pancreatic Cancer

WHAT IS IT?

Pancreatic cancer, currently the fifth leading cause of death from cancer in the United States, is the growth of malignant cells in the pancreas, a pear-shaped organ located just below and behind the stomach. The pancreas secretes digestive enzymes into the small intestine via the common bile duct, and islet cells of the pancreas secrete hormones (insulin and glucagon) into the blood. Pancreatic cancer impairs the digestive process and may block the bile duct as it grows. Most cases occur after age 50; men are affected slightly more often than women. A cure is sometimes possible with early diagnosis and surgical removal. However, pancreatic cancer is extremely difficult to diagnose and has usually spread by the time symptoms appear, so cures are uncommon. Islet cell tumors (insulinomas) are much less common. They release excessive amounts of insulin, causing low blood glucose (hypoglycemia). Only about 10 percent of insulinomas are malignant, and the symptoms of hypoglycemia can be eliminated by surgical removal of the tumor.

WHAT CAUSES IT?

- The cause of pancreatic cancer is unknown.
- Pancreatic cancer is two to three times more common in heavy smokers than nonsmokers.

SYMPTOMS

- Poor appetite; weight loss.
- Pain in the upper-central or right abdomen. The pain may spread to the back and may be relieved by sitting up and leaning forward.
- Jaundice.
- Itching skin.
- Nausea and vomiting.
- Diarrhea or constipation, dark-colored urine, or pale stools.
- A feeling of fullness.
- Fatigue, depression, and mood swings.
- Shakiness, irritability, profuse perspiration, chills, dizziness, or muscle spasms in patients with an islet cell tumor, due to associated hypoglycemia (see Hypoglycemia).

- Exposure to solvents, petroleum, and coal tar compounds may lead to the disease.
- Hereditary pancreatitis may be associated with a greater risk of pancreatic cancer.

PREVENTION

- Minimize exposure to toxic chemicals at home and in the workplace, and avoid cigarettes.

DIAGNOSIS

- Chest and abdominal x-rays are performed initially.
- Ultrasound scans or CT (computed tomography) scans detect about 80 percent of cases. Further tests are performed if diagnosis is questionable.
- ERCP (endoscopic retrograde cholangiopancreatogram) is done using a thin, lighted, viewing tube (endoscope) passed down the throat and into the small intestine. Contrast material is injected into the bile duct, and x-rays are taken. The endoscope may also be used to take a biopsy.
- Diagnosis is confirmed by biopsy of pancreatic tissue, which is extracted with a needle, or in some cases, using exploratory abdominal surgery.

HOW TO TREAT IT

- Surgical removal of the tumor is possible with a relatively small tumor that has not yet spread, which may prolong survival time. Surgery may involve removal of the entire pancreas as well as a portion of the small intestine.
- Surgery to bypass a bile duct blocked by the tumor may be performed to relieve symptoms.
- Chemotherapy in combination with radiation therapy may destroy cancerous cells and ease symptoms.
- Analgesics or narcotics are administered to reduce pain. Antihistamines or amphetamines may be used to enhance analgesic effects. In cases of severe pain, the relevant nerves may be cut or destroyed by an alcohol injection at the time of surgery.
- Tablets containing pancreatic enzymes may be prescribed if food is poorly absorbed because of a blockage of pancreatic secretions.

WHEN TO CALL A DOCTOR

- Call a doctor if you develop symptoms of pancreatic cancer.

Pancreatitis

WHAT IS IT?

Pancreatitis is inflammation of the pancreas, an organ that produces digestive enzymes and hormones (insulin and glucagon). Acute attacks of pancreatitis usually subside within several days to a week but carry the risk of life-threatening complications, including shock and infection in a collection of fluid near the pancreas (pseudocyst). Chronic pancreatitis involving permanent damage to the pancreas may follow recurrent attacks of acute pancreatitis or be due to persistent smoldering inflammation. Possible long-term complications include inadequate absorption of nutrients and diabetes mellitus.

WHAT CAUSES IT?

- Passage of a gallstone that blocks the pancreatic duct is often a cause of acute attacks.
- Alcoholism is commonly associated with both acute and chronic pancreatitis.
- Less common causes of acute attacks: trauma to the pancreas; use of certain drugs (including immuno-suppressants, corticosteroids, and sulfa drugs); high triglycerides; viral infection such as mumps.
- Other causes of chronic pancreatitis: recurrent acute pancreatitis; cystic fibrosis (children); malnutrition.
- In rare cases pancreatitis is hereditary.
- In many cases the cause cannot be determined.

PREVENTION

- Avoid excessive alcohol use.

DIAGNOSIS

- Medical history and physical examination.
- Blood tests.
- X-ray, ultrasound, or CT (computed tomography).

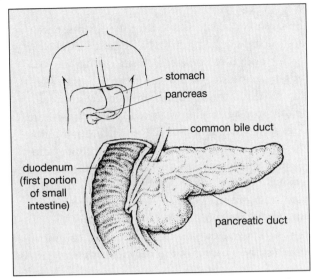

The pancreas, located just below and behind the stomach, manufactures crucial hormones and digestive enzymes.

- ERCP (endoscopic retrograde cholangiopancreatogram) is done using a thin, lighted, viewing tube (endoscope) passed down the throat and into the small intestine. Contrast material is injected into the bile duct and pancreatic duct and x-rays are taken.
- Stool (for fat content), pancreatic-function, and other tests help confirm chronic cases.

HOW TO TREAT IT

- Acute attacks require hospitalization. The stomach is emptied of its contents, and intravenous fluids and painkillers are given. Patients are not allowed to eat for several days to a week. Antibiotics may be given to treat an associated infection.
- Surgery to remove gallstones may be necessary.
- Narcotic painkillers may be needed for severe pain.
- Alcohol and large, fatty meals should be avoided by those with the chronic form of the illness.
- Pancreatic enzyme pills are usually prescribed for patients with chronic pancreatitis, to aid in digestion.
- Insulin may be needed if diabetes develops.
- Chronic pancreatitis occasionally requires partial or total removal of the pancreas (pancreatectomy) or surgery to deaden the nerves that transmit the pain.

WHEN TO CALL A DOCTOR

- Call a doctor if you have symptoms of pancreatitis.

SYMPTOMS

- Acute disease: moderate to severe abdominal pain that may spread to the chest, back, and sides (and is often worse when lying down); nausea and vomiting; abdominal bloating; mild fever; clammy skin.
- Chronic: constant or episodic abdominal pain; weight loss; bulky, floating stools.

Parkinson's Disease

WHAT IS IT?

Parkinson's disease, named after the English physician who first described it in 1817, is caused by the progressive death of nerve cells (neurons) within a layer of gray matter in the brain (substantia nigra). Neurons communicate with one another by releasing highly specialized chemicals called neurotransmitters. The substantia nigra produces the neurotransmitter dopamine, which is essential for fast, smooth, and coordinated movement. In Parkinson's disease, the gradual deterioration of dopamine-producing neurons results in the slowness, shaking, stiffness, and uncoordinated movements characteristic of the disorder. Parkinson's disease, one of the most common degenerative diseases of the nervous system, typically begins between the ages of 55 and 70. Men are affected slightly more often than women. Symptoms usually begin gradually and may not be noticeable at first, or may be mistakenly attributed to aging. Although there is no definitive diagnostic test for Parkinson's disease, worsening of symptoms over time eventually allows a diagnosis to be made with certainty. The cause of Parkinson's disease remains unknown, and there is as yet no cure. However, medications can alleviate many symptoms and greatly improve the quality of life for patients.

SYMPTOMS

- Slowness of movement.
- Rhythmic shaking of the hands (pill-roll tremor), especially at rest or in moments of anxiety.
- Cessation or lessening of the tremor with movement and sleep.
- Muscle stiffness.
- Difficulty in changing position; for example, from sitting to standing or standing to walking, or when getting out of a car or turning in bed.
- A temporary inability to move (in some cases).
- Hesitant gait with small, shuffling steps.
- Loss of balance.
- Stooped posture.
- Decreased facial expression.
- Difficulty swallowing.
- Drooling.
- Oily skin and scalp (seborrhea).
- Small, cramped handwriting.
- Quavering, expressionless voice; mumbling; decreased volume.
- Bowel or bladder dysfunction, including incontinence and constipation.
- Emotional depression and anxiety.
- Gradual confusion, loss of memory, and other mental disorders (only in some severe cases).

WHAT CAUSES IT?

- The cause of Parkinson's disease is unknown. It is believed to be due to genetic and environmental factors combined with the aging process.
- Brain injury, tumors, postinfluenza encephalitis, and possibly carbon monoxide poisoning may cause symptoms and signs resembling Parkinson's disease.
- Certain medications, notably those that interfere with dopamine (such as antipsychotics and antiemetics), may cause symptoms that mimic those of Parkinson's disease (parkinsonism).

PREVENTION

- There are no known measures for preventing Parkinson's disease.

DIAGNOSIS

- Patient history and physical examination by a physician or neurologist experienced in Parkinson's disease.

HOW TO TREAT IT

- Treatment may not be necessary in the early stages if the symptoms are not interfering with functioning.
- Levodopa (L-dopa) is the mainstay of therapy to relieve symptoms of Parkinson's disease. Within the brain, L-dopa is converted to the missing neurotransmitter dopamine. L-dopa is combined with a decarboxylase inhibitor (carbidopa or benserazide) to enhance efficiency and limit side effects of L-dopa by preventing the conversion of L-dopa to dopamine from occurring outside of the brain. (Side effects include nausea and vomiting, and dizziness when sitting or standing up from a reclining position.)

Parkinson's Disease *continued*

Because the effectiveness of L-dopa gradually decreases with time, doctors will often withhold the drug until symptoms interfere greatly with normal activities.

• Deprenyl, also known as selegiline, may be prescribed immediately upon diagnosis. This drug may slow the progression of symptoms, thus postponing the time before L-dopa becomes necessary.

• Anticholinergic drugs such as trihexyphenidyl block certain nerve impulses and may be prescribed to reduce tremor and stiffness.

• Benztropine mesylate and antihistamines such as diphenhydramine may also be used to decrease tremor and stiffness.

• Amantadine, which increases the release of dopamine in the brain, may be prescribed to reduce tremor, stiffness, and difficulty in movement.

• Dopamine agonists (such as bromocriptine, pergolide, pramipexole, and ropinirole), which work directly in the dopamine receptors in the brain, can be added to L-dopa for additional control of symptoms and are being used increasingly as initial therapy for early Parkinson's disease.

• COMT (catechol-O-methyltransferase) inhibitors, such as tolcapone, are added to L-dopa for improved control of symptoms.

• For disabling tremor, consideration should be given to surgical therapy, with either a thalamotomy (in which a small group of cells in the thalamus portion of the brain is destroyed) or the placement of an electrical stimulator in the thalamus cells to short-circuit them.

• For the motor fluctuations that often complicate advanced Parkinson's disease, another surgical option is pallidotomy in which a lesion is made in the globus pallidus to reduce the overactive nerve cells. Electrical stimulation of the globus pallidus and other areas is under investigation and looks promising.

• Implantation of fetal tissue into the basal ganglia has shown promise in a few patients.

• Patients should stay active and exercise regularly to keep muscles as flexible as possible.

• Physical and speech therapy may help patients adapt to the limitations imposed by the disease.

• Psychological counseling may be advised for patients to combat depression and provide emotional support. Family members of Parkinson's patients may also benefit from counseling.

• To allow L-dopa to work better, your doctor may advise dietary changes, such as consuming the majority of the daily protein allotment with the evening meal and maintaining a seven-to-one ratio of carbohydrates to protein.

• Call your local branch of the National Parkinson Foundation, the United Parkinson Foundation, or the American Parkinson's Disease Association for more information, results of current research, and support groups in your area.

WHEN TO CALL A DOCTOR

• Call a doctor if you develop symptoms of Parkinson's disease.

• Call a doctor if new, unexpected symptoms develop during treatment (some medications prescribed may have significant side effects, such as low blood pressure, confusion, and hallucinations).

Pelvic Inflammatory Disease

WHAT IS IT?

Pelvic inflammatory disease (PID), a condition marked by acute, persistent, or recurrent infection of the internal female reproductive organs, is one of the most frequent causes of pelvic pain in women. Infection usually begins in the cervix, extends into the uterus and fallopian tubes, and then involves the pelvic cavity. In most cases proper treatment leads to full recovery within a week, although recurrence is common. If untreated, however, PID may lead to serious complications, including life-threatening abdominal abscess, infection of the abdominal cavity (peritonitis), and blood poisoning. In addition, PID may scar the fallopian tube, significantly increasing the risks of infertility and ectopic pregnancy (which occurs when a fertilized egg becomes trapped in the fallopian tube before it can settle in the uterus).

WHAT CAUSES IT?

• Various infectious agents, especially those that cause chlamydia and gonorrhea, can be transmitted by a sexual partner to cause PID.
• Less often, PID is caused by using an intrauterine contraceptive device (IUD), or may occur in the aftermath of a miscarriage, full-term pregnancy, or a gynecological procedure such as endometrial biopsy or dilatation and curettage (D&C).
• Risk factors include sexual activity at a young age and multiple sexual partners. Use of oral contraceptives appears to reduce risk.
• Occasionally, infection may spread from other organs (for example, as a complication of appendicitis).

SYMPTOMS

• Dull, aching pain and tenderness in the lower abdomen or back.
• Pain during intercourse.
• Low-grade fever, possibly with chills.
• Irregular, absent, or unusually heavy menstrual periods.
• Bad-smelling, excessive vaginal discharge.
• Frequent, painful urination.
• Loss of appetite.
• Nausea and vomiting.

PREVENTION

• Monogamy, abstinence, or the use of condoms helps protect against sexually transmitted infections.
• After minor gynecologic procedures such as D&C, avoid douching, tampons, tub baths, and intercourse for at least seven days. Report any fever, increased vaginal discharge, or pain after such procedures.

DIAGNOSIS

• A gynecologic pelvic exam is needed. PID can be difficult to diagnose, as it is hard to distinguish from other types of infection, such as appendicitis.
• Cultures of swab samples of vaginal discharge may identify underlying infectious agents. However, a patient may be infected with gonorrhea or chlamydia even though the culture does not show growth.
• Inspection of the pelvic organs with a small, slender scope passed through a small abdominal incision (laparoscopy) may be carried out to confirm diagnosis or to drain an abscess.

HOW TO TREAT IT

• If PID appears likely, antibiotics are often prescribed immediately because delaying treatment is risky. Therapy can be adjusted after lab results are known.
• Hospitalization may be advised for more serious cases, if the diagnosis is uncertain, if the patient is pregnant or an adolescent, or if the infection fails to respond to outpatient treatment. Treatment may include intravenous antibiotics and surgical drainage of the abscess. A ruptured abscess is life-threatening and may require a complete hysterectomy with removal of the ovaries.
• Surgery may also be considered for complicated or persistent cases that do not respond to antibiotics.
• A successfully treated woman may become reinfected by an infected partner and so sexual partners—even asymptomatic ones—should be treated for gonorrhea and chlamydia.

WHEN TO CALL A DOCTOR

• If you have PID symptoms, especially high fever with severe pain in the lower abdomen, see your physician or gynecologist immediately. 🔺

Penile Cancer

WHAT IS IT?

Penile cancer is the growth of malignant cells in the skin or underlying tissues of the penis. The cancer cells tend to arise on the glans (head) of the penis or, in uncircumcised men, on the foreskin, although they may arise anywhere on the penis. If left untreated, the cancer typically spreads, first to the deeper layers of penile tissue, then to nearby lymph nodes in the groin or to blood vessels, and finally to distant sites throughout the body. Most penile cancers are slow-growing, although some are highly aggressive, spreading to the lymph nodes over the course of months. Any suspicious growth on the penis therefore requires prompt medical attention. Cancer of the penis is rare in the United States, particularly among circumcised men. As with any malignancy, penile cancer may be life-threatening. However, if detected and treated early (before it spreads to lymph nodes), a cure is likely.

WHAT CAUSES IT?

• The cause is unknown, but the risk is higher in uncircumcised men, particularly in those who do not wash the area around the foreskin thoroughly.
• Risk appears to be greater among cigarette smokers and in those with a history of leukoplakia of the penis (a precancerous condition marked by white, scaly patches of skin), balanitis (an inflammation of the head of the penis), or an epithelial horn (an abnormal skin growth) on the penis.
• Sexually transmitted diseases (especially genital warts) are associated with increased risk.

PREVENTION

• Perform monthly self-examinations to detect penile cancer at an early, more treatable stage.

SYMPTOMS

• A wartlike lump, pimple, sore, or ulcer on the penis, usually near the glans (head).
• Bleeding or unusual discharge from the penis.
• Painful urination (as cancer progresses).
• Enlarged lymph nodes in the groin (indicating spread of cancer).

DIAGNOSIS

• If a growth looks suspicious, a small sample of affected skin (biopsy) is removed for examination.
• If the tissue is found to be cancerous, additional tests are performed to see whether the cancer has spread to other parts of the body (a process known as staging).

HOW TO TREAT IT

• Treatment generally depends on how far the cancer has spread, as well as the age and overall health of the patient.
• Surgery is the most common form of treatment. Cancer confined to the foreskin in uncircumcised men can be cured by circumcision alone.
• Radiation therapy may be effective for slow-growing tumors detected early.
• Surgery is especially warranted for rapidly growing tumors and those that have spread into deeper tissues of the penis. If the cancer does not appear to have spread very far, the surgeon may remove the tumor and a small area of surrounding normal tissue (in case any cancer cells have invaded there), sparing as much of the penis as possible.
• In more advanced cases removal of most or all of the penis and, often, affected lymph nodes in the groin may be required. Subsequent plastic surgery may be performed in such cases to help restore the appearance and function of the penis.
• If cancer has spread to distant sites, radiation or chemotherapy may be used to reduce discomfort.
• Psychological counseling and support groups may be helpful.

WHEN TO CALL A DOCTOR

• Call a doctor if any suspicious sore or growth appears on the penis or if any symptoms of penile cancer arise. ▲

Peptic Ulcer

WHAT IS IT?

Peptic ulcers are craterlike erosions in the lining of the stomach, the duodenum (the part of the small intestine just past the stomach), and rarely, the esophagus. Duodenal ulcers are about three times more common than stomach (gastric) ulcers. Normally, glands in the stomach secrete acid and the enzyme pepsin (hence the name peptic ulcer) that help to break down foods in the digestive process. The stomach and duodenum meanwhile secrete mucus to protect them against harm from pepsin and gastric acid. In peptic ulcer disease the digestive tract's defensive mechanisms break down, often as a result of infection with the bacterium *Helicobacter pylori*. Consequently, even small amounts of stomach acid can cause corrosion.

Each year, about 1 percent of Americans develop peptic ulcers, and overall, up to 10 percent of the population will have an ulcer at some point during their lives. All ages may be affected (including children), although ulcers most often affect those over 30. Ulcers commonly recur: Even after an ulcer has healed, new ones often arise throughout the patient's lifetime, either in the original location or elsewhere. Therefore, current ulcer drugs, which mostly act to reduce levels of stomach acids, must often be taken on a long-term basis. The development of newer,

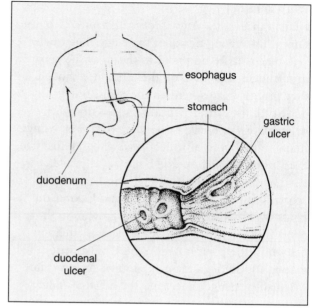

Peptic ulcers may arise anywhere in the lining of the stomach or the duodenum (or, more rarely, the esophagus).

short-term drug regimens directed against *H. pylori* may significantly lower the high rate of ulcer recurrence. Although peptic ulcers are rarely a major health threat, they sometimes lead to serious complications, such as bleeding, obstruction of the digestive tract due to scarring, or the creation of a hole or tear (perforation) in the digestive tract, which can lead to severe, life-threatening infection of the abdominal cavity (peritonitis). In addition, in a small percentage of cases a persistent stomach ulcer may be cancerous. The same is not true for duodenal ulcers. For most ulcers, treatment is highly effective in controlling symptoms and preventing serious complications.

WHAT CAUSES IT?

• At least 80 percent of ulcers are believed to be caused by infection of the digestive tract with *H. pylori* bacteria. It's not known how the infection spreads, although it may be transmitted orally. *H. pylori* infests about 60 percent of Americans by age 60, but most of those infected do not develop ulcers. Rather, the bacteria merely increase the chances of developing an ulcer by weakening the stomach's protective mechanisms and making the lining of the digestive tract susceptible to erosion by

---

SYMPTOMS

• No symptoms in some patients.
• Gnawing pain in the upper stomach area several hours after a meal (duodenal ulcer) or dull, aching pain, often right after a meal (gastric ulcer). Pain may radiate to the back or behind the breastbone, resembling heartburn.
• Indigestion, nausea, vomiting, and weight loss.
• Emergency symptoms: black, tarry, or bloody stools; vomiting of blood or material resembling coffee grounds (signs of potentially serious bleeding). Searing abdominal pain could indicate that an ulcer has eroded completely through the digestive tract (perforation). Such complications require immediate emergency medical attention.

Peptic Ulcer *continued*

stomach acids. Once an ulcer has developed, various secondary factors can aggravate it, including alcohol, caffeine, dietary factors, smoking, and stress.
• In the past, excessive production of stomach acid was thought to be the primary cause of ulcers. It is now recognized that many people with ulcers actually have normal or even slightly less-than-normal amounts of stomach acid. However, because mechanisms that protect the digestive tract lining are weakened (in most cases by *H. pylori*), even small amounts of stomach acid can cause (or delay the healing of) ulcers. The exception is ulcers caused by certain kinds of pancreatic or duodenal tumors, which secrete the hormone gastrin and cause massive amounts of acid secretion (Zollinger-Ellison syndrome).
• Long-term use of aspirin and other nonsteroidal anti-inflammatory drugs (NSAIDs), such as ibuprofen or naproxen, can lead to ulcers primarily in the stomach by irritating its lining.
• Hereditary factors also appear to play a role. The chances of developing an ulcer are greater if a close family member has had one.

PREVENTION
• Avoid long-term use of aspirin or nonsteroidal anti-inflammatory drugs if possible. Anyone who must take these drugs on a long-term basis, such as those with arthritis, may benefit from the prescription drug misoprostol.
• To help prevent ulcer recurrence, carefully follow instructions for any ulcer drugs prescribed. Do not smoke, and avoid foods or drinks that have caused flare-ups in the past.

DIAGNOSIS
• Patient history and physical examination are needed.
• An upper GI series (which involves swallowing a solution containing barium to create a clear image of the digestive tract on x-ray) may show active ulcers or scarring caused by past ulcers.
• Endoscopy (in which a flexible scope is guided down the throat and into the stomach and duodenum) allows ulcers to be viewed directly. A small sample of the ulcer (biopsy) may be taken at the same time to test for cancer.

• Biopsies can also detect the presence of *H. pylori*, but this method is invasive and expensive. Quick office tests for the detection of this bacterium are becoming available.

HOW TO TREAT IT
• For those with mild disease (one or two periods of symptoms a year), prescription drugs that reduce secretion of stomach acid (cimetidine, ranitidine, famotidine, nizatidine, or omeprazole) or that coat the lining of the stomach (sucralfate) usually relieve pain within a week, although ulcers take about eight weeks to heal. Antacids may also help, although they may interfere with the actions of the prescription drugs if both are taken in close succession.
• Antibiotics directed against *H. pylori* bacteria are generally reserved for those with more serious disease who do not respond to other ulcer medications, as the long-term effectiveness and side effects of this approach are still being evaluated. A combination of two antibiotics (usually metronidazole and tetracycline) is usually taken for at least two weeks, along with a bismuth-containing antacid (such as Pepto-Bismol). Antacids or medications that reduce acid secretion may also be given. Combination antibiotic regimens prevent ulcer recurrences in about 90 percent of cases.
• Surgery may be needed for bleeding, obstruction or perforation of the digestive tract, or intractable pain from ulcers.
• Eat a well-balanced diet rich in fiber. Many dietary measures advocated in the past—such as eating bland foods, eating many small meals a day rather than three larger meals, or drinking milk—do not appear to help. Indeed, milk may actually increase stomach acid production, although one or two glasses a day is usually not harmful. Coffee, tea, and caffeinated sodas can increase acid secretion. Avoid excessive alcohol consumption.

WHEN TO CALL A DOCTOR
• Call a doctor for symptoms of peptic ulcer disease.
• **EMERGENCY** For those with ulcers, any signs of bleeding or perforation (including vomiting blood; black, tarry stools; or severe abdominal pain) require immediate emergency medical attention.

Pericarditis

WHAT IS IT?

Pericarditis is inflammation of the pericardium, the membrane that surrounds and protects the heart. It occurs in two forms: acute (sudden and short-lived) and chronic (persistent over long periods). The most common type of acute pericarditis, caused by a viral infection, generally resolves spontaneously with no permanent damage, even without treatment. Acute pericarditis due to bacterial infection, however, may cause fluid to accumulate in the space between the pericardium and the heart (pericardial effusion) and interfere with the heart's ability to function properly. This may result in severe symptoms and may even be fatal unless fluid is promptly removed from the pericardial sac. In chronic pericarditis, ongoing inflammation scars and thickens the pericardium (constrictive pericarditis) so that it constricts the heart and hinders the heart's ability to fill with blood returning from the great veins. Constrictive pericarditis nearly always leads to progressive heart failure; surgical intervention is often beneficial.

WHAT CAUSES IT?

• Acute pericarditis may result from a number of underlying disorders, including: viral, bacterial, or fungal infection; heart attack; rheumatic fever; systemic lupus erythematosus; rheumatoid arthritis; hypothyroidism; metastatic cancer; and kidney failure.
• Acute pericarditis may occur following a chest injury or open heart surgery.
• Chronic pericarditis may develop from recurrent acute cases.

SYMPTOMS
• Acute pericarditis: severe, sudden chest pain that may spread to the neck, back, shoulders, or arms, and is often worse when breathing deeply or changing position and relieved by sitting up or leaning forward; fever.
• Pericardial effusion: breathing difficulty or ill-defined pain or fullness in the chest.
• Chronic pericarditis: swelling in the legs and abdomen due to fluid retention; breathing difficulty; fatigue.

• Chronic cases may result from a chronic infection such as tuberculosis.
• In some cases the cause is unknown.

PREVENTION
• There are no specific measures to prevent this condition.

DIAGNOSIS
• Medical history and physical examination, including listening for abnormal heart sounds with a stethoscope.
• Blood and urine tests.
• Chest x-rays.
• Electrocardiogram (ECG), which measures electrical activity in the heart.
• Echocardiography (ultrasound imaging of the heart).
• Culture of pericardial fluid taken through a needle to identify infectious organisms.

HOW TO TREAT IT
• The underlying cause is treated if possible. For example, antibiotics are given for bacterial infections.
• Analgesics (including aspirin and ibuprofen) are used to reduce pain and inflammation.
• Diuretics may be used to reduce fluid retention.
• Bed rest and restricted activity may be advised.
• Surgical drainage of fluid with a needle (pericardiocentesis) may be required for severe pericardial effusion.
• Partial or total surgical removal of the pericardium (pericardectomy), the treatment of choice for chronic pericarditis, often yields excellent results.

WHEN TO CALL A DOCTOR
• If you experience any symptom of pericarditis, get to a doctor as soon as possible.

Periodontitis

WHAT IS IT?

Periodontitis is inflammation of the periodontia—the tissues that surround and support the teeth, including the gums and the bony tooth sockets in the upper and lower jaw. The disease begins as gingivitis (inflammation of the gums, usually due to inadequate dental hygiene) which progresses without treatment. Gingivitis occurs when dental plaque (a sticky substance made of mucus, food particles, and bacteria) and calculus (the hardened deposit composed of mineralized plaque and saliva) irritate and inflame gum tissue, causing it to gradually erode. Over time, the gums recede and small pockets form between the gums and teeth. As these pockets deepen, they trap increasing amounts of plaque and calculus. Bacteria in the plaques produce enzymes that erode the bones and ligaments that support the teeth, causing the teeth to loosen from their sockets. Pus tends to form as the periodontia fall prey to infection. In some cases an acute infection may cause an abscess to form. Eventually, bone erosion is so extensive that the affected teeth become loose. Indeed, periodontitis—not tooth decay—is the major cause of adult tooth loss in the United States.

WHAT CAUSES IT?

• Periodontitis results when gingivitis is left untreated, and so progresses beyond the gums to affect the deeper tissues of the periodontia.

PREVENTION

• Practice careful oral hygiene (see Gingivitis for more information) and see a dentist at least once a year for a routine cleaning and checkup.

DIAGNOSIS

• A complete dental examination is necessary. The dentist will measure the depth of gum pockets to assess the extent of the disease.
• Dental x-rays are taken to determine how much underlying bone has been lost.

HOW TO TREAT IT

• If the disease is discovered early enough, it may be possible to reverse its progress simply by having a dentist remove plaque and calculus from the root surfaces of the teeth. This is called periodontal scaling and root planing and may require local anesthesia. Afterward, a strict self-care program of brushing and flossing is required. Often, periodontal treatments are required every three months to maintain healthy gums.
• More advanced cases may require flap surgery. In this procedure the tissue is cut and pushed away from the teeth so that the roots and supporting bone may be cleaned and recontoured. The flap of gum is then sutured back into place.
• Occasionally, surgical grafting with bone or a bone substitute may be needed to restore damaged underlying bone.
• Loose teeth may be anchored to other teeth by splinting them together; in some cases affected teeth must be extracted due to the extent of bone loss. Dentures or permanent dental implants may then be used to replace missing teeth.

WHEN TO CALL A DOCTOR

• Make an appointment with a dentist right away if you experience bleeding gums or loose teeth. ⓐ

SYMPTOMS

• Red, shiny, swollen, tender gums that bleed easily.
• Bad breath and an unpleasant taste in the mouth.
• Toothache.
• One or more loose or missing teeth.
• Pus appearing at the gumline.
• Intense toothache and fever (if abscess occurs).

Peripheral Neuropathies

WHAT IS IT?

Peripheral neuropathies are a group of disorders characterized by the degeneration of the nerves involved in the communication between the central nervous system (the brain and spinal cord) and the rest of the body. Peripheral nerves transmit sensory signals back to the central nervous system, and signals from the brain to the muscles. Neuropathies are caused by a wide variety of underlying disorders, and nerve function may be lost in a number of ways: the nerve fibers themselves (axons) may degenerate; the myelin sheaths that cover and protect the nerves may erode; and in some cases there is a loss of blood supply to a nerve.

The mononeuropathies are conditions that affect a single nerve (see Bell's Palsy and Carpal Tunnel Syndrome for more information); polyneuropathies affect multiple nerves that may be distributed throughout the body. Symptoms vary according to which nerves are affected. Most often, symptoms develop gradually over months or years; however, in Guillain-Barré syndrome, an uncommon form of polyneuropathy, severe symptoms appear within days. (Recovery from Guillain-Barré may also be relatively rapid in many cases.)

Peripheral neuropathies are most common in men between the ages of 30 and 50. Symptoms may arise from degeneration of the sensory neurons, the motor neurons, or both. Fortunately, because these disorders often leave the cell bodies of the nerves intact, the nerves can regenerate; thus, chances for recovery

may be good. However, prognosis and specific treatment depend on the underlying disorder.

WHAT CAUSES IT?

• Many disorders, including alcoholism, diabetes mellitus, rheumatoid arthritis, systemic lupus erythematosus, amyloidosis, and uremia, may cause peripheral neuropathy.
• Malnutrition, especially a vitamin deficiency, may lead to peripheral neuropathy.
• A viral infection, rabies and flu vaccines, or surgery may sometimes be associated with Guillain-Barré syndrome.
• A number of medications, especially isoniazid, pyridoxine, and vincristine, can cause peripheral neuropathy.
• Exposure to toxic chemicals, including lead, mercury, arsenic, and the chemicals in pesticides and herbicides, may lead to peripheral neuropathy.
• Nerve damage may be caused by injuries or by repeated jarring, such as that brought on by operating a jackhammer.
• Exposure to cold temperatures can produce nerve damage (see Hypothermia for more information).
• Some cancers, such as multiple myeloma, lung cancer, and leukemia, may cause peripheral neuropathy.
• Some types of peripheral neuropathy are hereditary.
• The cause is unknown in some cases.

PREVENTION

• Consume no more than two alcoholic drinks a day. If you suspect that you may have a drinking problem, seek help from a doctor or support group immediately.
• Eat a healthy, balanced diet.
• Try to reduce or eliminate exposure to toxic chemicals at home and in the workplace.

DIAGNOSIS

• Patient history and physical examination are needed.
• Electromyography may be performed. In this procedure, needle electrodes are inserted into various muscles to measure electrical activity associated with nerve function.
• A variety of tests may be given to evaluate reflexes and nerve performance.

SYMPTOMS

• A tingling sensation followed by numbness and pain, commonly beginning in the hands or feet and spreading toward the center of the body. The facial muscles are also frequently affected. The pain may be severe with diabetes mellitus or alcoholism.
• Muscle weakness.
• Loss of bladder or bowel control.
• Unsteady gait.
• Emergency symptoms: difficulty in breathing, paralysis.

Peripheral Neuropathies *continued*

• Lumbar puncture (spinal tap).
• Blood tests.
• X-rays.
• Biopsies of nerve or muscle tissue.

HOW TO TREAT IT

• Strict control of diabetes through medication, diet, and exercise may allow diabetic neuropathy to subside either partially or completely, depending upon the extent of the nerve damage.
• People with diabetes should practice good foot care and check their feet every day. Peripheral neuropathy reduces sensation in affected areas, so minor foot problems may go unnoticed and develop into major infections.
• Alcohol-induced neuropathy requires complete abstinence from alcohol.
• Multivitamin supplements may be recommended.
• Exposure to toxic chemicals should be reduced or eliminated as much as possible.
• Plasmapheresis (a procedure that involves partial removal of blood plasma while the blood cells are returned to circulation) may be performed to speed recovery from Guillain-Barré syndrome by filtering out irritating or dangerous antibodies from the bloodstream.
• Hospitalization is recommended for treatment of Guillain-Barré syndrome because the condition may worsen unpredictably and be life-threatening before recovery begins. Breathing and swallowing difficulties are treated with supplemental oxygen and intravenous feeding.
• Over-the-counter pain relievers may be taken to reduce pain.
• Physical therapy is advised to help regain muscle function. Canes, walkers, or wheelchairs may be temporarily useful, and rails near stairs and in the bathroom are recommended to prevent falls.

WHEN TO CALL A DOCTOR

• **EMERGENCY** Call an ambulance if you or someone in your presence experiences breathing difficulty, widespread muscle tingling or numbness, or paralysis.
• Call a doctor if you develop symptoms of peripheral neuropathy.
• Call a doctor if, after being diagnosed with peripheral neuropathy, you develop sores or open wounds on the hands and feet. 🖎

Peripheral Vascular Disease

WHAT IS IT?

Peripheral vascular disease results from a narrowing of the arteries in the legs and sometimes the arms, generally due to atherosclerosis, the buildup of plaque in the arterial walls. Plaque—composed of cholesterol-rich fatty deposits, collagen, other proteins, and excess smooth muscle cells—gradually accumulates in the arteries. Thickening of the arterial walls narrows the vascular channels and impedes blood flow. During walking or other activities the narrowed arteries are unable to supply enough blood and oxygen to the muscles, causing pain (intermittent claudication), most commonly in the calves.

Peripheral vascular disease is most common after the age of 50, although one form can affect some male smokers as early as age 20. Diabetes greatly increases the risk of peripheral vascular disease, especially in women. The disease may worsen if left untreated, in some cases even leading to tissue death (gangrene). Peripheral vascular disease shares the same risk factors as the more dangerous coronary artery disease, and the diseases often occur together.

WHAT CAUSES IT?

• Atherosclerosis is the most common cause.
• Smoking is the greatest risk factor.
• Obesity, a sedentary lifestyle, high cholesterol levels, and high blood pressure contribute to atherosclerosis.
• People with diabetes mellitus are at increased risk.

SYMPTOMS

• Muscle pain in the calves or thighs of one or both legs that occurs when walking, especially fast or uphill. Pain subsides with rest. It may also occur in the fingers, arms, buttocks, lower back, or the arch of the foot.
• Impotence (erectile dysfunction).
• Symptoms of severe disease: muscle pain at rest that worsens at night; discolored or blue toes; cold or numb feet; numbness in the affected area when at rest; sores on the feet or legs that do not heal; added sensitivity to cold, or weak or absent pulse in the affected limb; scaly or hairless skin over the affected area.

PREVENTION

• Don't smoke.
• Exercise regularly.
• Eat a diet low in saturated fat, cholesterol, and salt.
• Have your cholesterol and blood pressure checked.
• Lose weight if overweight.

DIAGNOSIS

• Patient history and physical examination.
• Blood pressure measurements in the arms and legs.
• X-rays of the arteries after the injection of a contrast material (angiography).
• Ultrasound or MRI (magnetic resonance imaging).

HOW TO TREAT IT

• Follow prevention tips.
• Each day, take a walk and continue until leg pain develops. Rest for a short time to let the pain subside, then continue walking. Gradually, the distance that can be traveled painlessly will increase.
• Practice good foot care and check your feet every day. Poor circulation due to peripheral vascular disease slows the healing of sores. Spotting problems early may help to prevent minor foot problems from becoming major infections.
• Pentoxifylline (Trental), a blood-viscosity reducing agent, may be prescribed to improve blood flow.
• People with diabetes must maintain scrupulous control over their blood sugar levels.
• Daily doses of aspirin may be prescribed to prevent blood clots that can lead to heart attack or stroke.
• Cholesterol-lowering drugs may be prescribed for those with unhealthy blood cholesterol levels that cannot be controlled by lifestyle changes alone.
• In severe cases angioplasty to dilate the narrowed portion of the artery, or bypass surgery to reroute blood around the narrowed artery may be necessary.
• In extreme cases when gangrene is spreading uncontrollably, amputation of the affected limb may be required.

WHEN TO CALL A DOCTOR

• Make an appointment with a doctor if you repeatedly develop muscle pain when walking or at rest.

Peritonitis

WHAT IS IT?

Peritonitis is a serious disorder caused by an inflammation of the peritoneum, most often due to a bacterial infection. The peritoneum is a two-layered membrane that lines the abdominal cavity and encloses the stomach, intestines, and other abdominal organs. This membrane supports the abdominal organs and protects them from infection; however, occasionally the peritoneum itself may become infected by bacteria or other microorganisms. Infection usually spreads from organs within the abdomen. The inflammation may affect the entire peritoneum or be confined to a walled-off, pus-filled cavity (abscess). A rupture anywhere along the gastrointestinal tract is the most common pathway for entry of an infectious agent into the peritoneum.

Peritonitis is a medical emergency: the muscles within the walls of the intestine become paralyzed and the forward movement of intestinal contents stops (ileus). However, since the advent of antibiotics, most people recover fully from peritonitis with proper treatment.

WHAT CAUSES IT?

• Many different types of bacteria can cause peritonitis, particularly those found within the intestine.
• Tuberculosis and fungal and parasitical infections may cause a less acute form of peritonitis.
• Perforation of the gastrointestinal tract, due to a stab or bullet wound, peptic ulcer, colon cancer, appendicitis, or diverticulitis, may allow bacteria-laden gastrointestinal contents to enter the abdominal cavity and cause peritonitis.
• Abdominal surgery occasionally results in peritonitis.
• Infection of the fallopian tubes, which are adjacent to the peritoneum, may cause peritonitis.
• Cirrhosis of the liver may promote the development of bacterial peritonitis.
• Systemic lupus erythematosus may cause a non-infectious inflammation of the peritoneum.

PREVENTION

• Obtain prompt treatment for any infections or abdominal injuries or diseases.

DIAGNOSIS

• Patient history and physical examination.
• Abdominal x-rays, ultrasound exams, and CT (computed tomography) scans.
• Blood tests will show an elevated white blood cell count.
• Exploratory abdominal surgery (laparotomy) may be necessary.

HOW TO TREAT IT

• Large doses of antibiotics are administered intravenously to treat bacterial peritonitis.
• Surgery is often necessary when peritonitis is due to a disorder that has caused perforation along the intestinal tract; for example, a peptic ulcer or a burst appendix.
• Intravenous fluids and feeding are usually necessary to prevent dehydration and give the intestines a rest.
• Analgesics may be administered to reduce pain.
• A tube passed through the nose into the intestine is attached to a suction device to remove contents from a temporarily paralyzed intestine.

WHEN TO CALL A DOCTOR

• **EMERGENCY** See a doctor or call an ambulance immediately if you experience severe abdominal pain that persists longer than 10 or 20 minutes, accompanied by any other symptoms of peritonitis.

SYMPTOMS

• Acute onset of severe, steady pain throughout the abdomen or localized pain in one area of the abdomen. Pain may persist for several hours and is worsened by movement or pressure on the abdomen.
• Boardlike rigidity of the abdomen, due to contraction of the abdominal wall muscles.
• Swollen or bloated abdomen.
• Chills and fever, with profuse perspiration.
• Nausea and vomiting.
• Weakness.
• Pale, cold skin.
• Shock.

Peritonsillar Abscess Quinsy

WHAT IS IT?

Peritonsillar abscess (also known as quinsy) is a pus-producing infection occurring in the cavity at the back of the throat, near the tonsils. Quinsy is usually a complication of tonsillitis, a bacterial infection of the tonsils. The infection may spread to the soft palate (the back of the roof of the mouth) or may travel down the throat into the chest. If left untreated, the infection may attack the membranes that surround the heart and lungs, known as the pericardium and the pleura, respectively. Infections of these membranes may eventually produce serious, even life-threatening, complications, including fluid accumulation around the heart or lungs, chest pain, and breathing difficulty (see Pericarditis). Also, in rare cases, swelling on the roof of the mouth may become severe enough to interfere with breathing.

Although peritonsillar abscess occurs more often in young adults, it is uncommon even among that age group. This disorder will not respond well to oral antibiotics, and surgical drainage or aspiration with a needle is often needed. An abscess may recur if the tonsils are not removed.

WHAT CAUSES IT?

• Bacterial infection of the tonsils is the underlying cause of peritonsillar abscess.

PREVENTION

• Obtain prompt treatment for sore throats and other upper respiratory infections.

DIAGNOSIS

• Examination of the throat and palate is needed.

HOW TO TREAT IT

• Antibiotics administered to treat peritonsillar abscess should be taken for the full term prescribed.
• In some cases, intravenous antibiotics and fluid may be needed.
• Surgery or needle aspiration may be necessary to drain a large, pus-filled abscess.
• Pain relievers may be taken as necessary to reduce fever and pain.
• Patients should gargle with warm salt water to soothe a sore throat during recovery and consume plenty of additional nonalcoholic liquids.
• Surgery to remove the tonsils (tonsillectomy) may be advised to prevent recurrence of peritonsillar abscess, but the operation is usually delayed until the infected abscess has subsided.

WHEN TO CALL A DOCTOR

• Call a doctor if you develop symptoms of a peritonsillar abscess. 🔺

SYMPTOMS

• A sore throat that suddenly intensifies in severity, often spreading to the soft palate.
• Pain or difficulty in swallowing or opening the mouth. Ear pain may occur during swallowing.
• Drooling.
• Swollen neck.
• Fever.
• Headache.
• Enlarged lymph nodes (swollen glands) in the neck.

Pharyngitis

WHAT IS IT?

Pharyngitis—often simply referred to as a sore throat—is inflammation of the pharynx, the portion of the throat that lies just beyond the back of the roof of the mouth and stretches to the Adam's apple (larynx). It usually occurs when viruses (or sometimes, bacteria) from a cold, flu, or sinus infection involve the throat. Pharyngitis is very common but rarely serious. Most cases clear up on their own after three to 10 days and require no therapy other than pain relievers to ease discomfort. Rarely, though, tissues in the throat may swell considerably and obstruct breathing—a life-threatening condition. In addition, strep throat (caused by streptococcus bacteria) requires antibiotics to prevent complications, including rheumatic fever, a condition that can permanently damage the heart valves. Diphtheria is a rare but serious bacterial variety of pharyngitis.

WHAT CAUSES IT?

• Most cases are caused by viral infection.
• About 5 percent of cases are caused by bacterial infections (including strep) or other microorganisms.
• Some cases are caused by contact with toxic fumes or chemicals, long-term exposure to cigarette smoke or polluted, dry, or dusty air, excessive alcohol consumption, or gastroesophageal reflux (see Gastroesophageal Reflux for more information).
• Persistent infections elsewhere in the head, such as the sinuses or mouth, can cause lingering, or chronic, pharyngitis.

PREVENTION

• Avoid cigarette smoke, excessive alcohol, or other substances that can irritate the throat.

SYMPTOMS
• Sore or red, raw throat.
• Difficulty speaking or swallowing.
• Tender, swollen lymph nodes (glands) in the neck.
• Fever.
• Headache.
• Earache.

• Treat gastroesophageal reflux.
• A humidifier or air purifier may help if dust or dryness causes irritation.

DIAGNOSIS

• A doctor will examine the throat and may take a throat swab culture to test for strep or other bacteria.

HOW TO TREAT IT

• Symptoms such as sore throat and fever can be treated with nonprescription pain relievers. Gargling with a half teaspoon of salt dissolved in a glass of warm water or using antiseptic lozenges or sprays may also provide temporary relief.
• Antibiotics are prescribed for pharyngitis caused by bacteria. These drugs are effective in killing bacteria and certain other microorganisms, but not viruses. If the diagnosis is strep throat, it is very important to continue the antibiotics for at least 10 to 14 days, even if sore throat and other symptoms subside, to assure that all of the bacteria are eliminated. Strep infection can lead to rheumatic fever (which may permanently damage the heart valves).
• Pharyngitis caused by viruses clears up on its own; antibiotics are not effective against viral infections, so treatment is aimed at easing symptoms.
• Smoking should be avoided and alcohol intake curbed. Smoke and alcohol irritate the throat.
• Persistent pharyngitis caused by exposure to toxic fumes, air pollution, or industrial chemicals is treated by reducing or eliminating exposure to the noxious agent.

WHEN TO CALL A DOCTOR

• Call a doctor if a sore throat is unusually severe, is accompanied by high fever, or doesn't seem to be getting better after a few days.
• **EMERGENCY** If sore throat escalates to the point of causing breathing difficulty or inability to swallow liquids, get to an emergency room at once.

Pheochromocytoma

WHAT IS IT?

Pheochromocytoma is a rare type of tumor that usually develops in the inner portion (medulla) of the adrenals, the small glands atop each kidney. The tumor causes excess release of epinephrine (adrenaline) and norepinephrine (noradrenaline), hormones that help to regulate heart rate and blood pressure.

The primary effect of the tumor is to cause intermittent or sustained periods of high blood pressure. Sporadic surges in blood pressure are marked by a rapid or pounding heartbeat, palpitations, headache, sweating, and extreme anxiety. Symptomatic attacks are sometimes brought on by emotional upset, a change in posture, or certain medications and tend to increase in frequency, duration, and severity if the tumor is left untreated. Treatment should be initiated as early as possible to prevent the long-term consequences of high blood pressure, which include heart disease, stroke, and kidney damage. (In patients with sustained high blood pressure, hypertension may persist even after removal of the tumor.)

Pheochromocytomas are most common in young to middle-aged adults. Most cases are benign (noncancerous) and affect only one adrenal gland. Sometimes tumors arise on both adrenals (especially in people with familial pheochromocytoma) or at other sites in the abdomen or chest. About 10 percent of pheochromocytomas are malignant (cancerous) and may spread to distant sites. Tumors that have spread are difficult to treat and prove fatal within five years in more than half of such cases. Benign tumors, on the other hand, are usually curable with surgery.

SYMPTOMS
- Headache, often severe.
- Palpitations, or rapid or pounding heartbeat.
- Excessive sweating.
- Lightheadedness, especially when arising from a sitting position.
- Chest or abdominal pain.
- Constipation.
- Weight loss.
- Nervousness, irritability, or anxiety.
- Mental confusion or psychosis.

WHAT CAUSES IT?
- The cause of pheochromocytomas is unknown.
- Some people with a rare inherited syndrome called multiple endocrine neoplasia develop pheochromocytomas in association with medullary thyroid tumors and overproduction of parathyroid hormone (hyperparathyroidism).

PREVENTION
- There is no way to prevent pheochromocytoma.

DIAGNOSIS
- Blood and urine samples are taken to check for high levels of epinephrine, norepinephrine, and their breakdown products. Blood tests may show a high blood glucose level.
- A computed tomography (CT) scan or magnetic resonance imaging (MRI) of the abdomen usually identifies an adrenal tumor.
- An angiogram (injection of a contrasting material into the blood vessels to make them clearly visible on a series of x-rays) is occasionally performed.
- In rare cases, an octreotide (hormone) or MIBG scan is used to visualize the tumor.

HOW TO TREAT IT
- Surgical removal of the tumor (adrenalectomy) is possible in most cases and usually leads to a cure and full recovery. The earlier the tumor is treated the better. Surrounding tissue may be removed as well if there is concern that the cancer may have spread locally. Drugs are given to control blood pressure for several weeks prior to the operation.
- If a malignant tumor has spread to other sites, radiation or chemotherapy may be tried, although results are generally disappointing.
- In a small percentage of cases, recurrence of tumors after surgery requires additional surgery.
- Drugs to lower blood pressure are used when hypertension persists after removal of a benign pheochromocytoma or in cases of malignant tumors.

WHEN TO CALL A DOCTOR
- See a doctor if you develop symptoms of pheochromocytoma. ▲

Pinworms

WHAT IS IT?

Pinworms are slender, white, threadlike worms, about a third of an inch long, that can infest the intestinal tract. Infestation with these parasites begins when pinworm eggs are swallowed and lodge in the intestine, where they hatch and mature. Two to six weeks later, the adult worm exits the anus to lay new eggs, often during the night when a person is sleeping. Pinworms are more of a nuisance than a serious health problem. The main complaint is intense anal itching, due to the irritation caused by worms migrating across the skin. In general, the body's immune system eliminates pinworms living in the intestine within several months. However, eggs are usually dispersed in bedding material or clothing and may spread via the fingers or even through the air, making reingestion of eggs and a new cycle of infestation common—not just among those who were originally affected but among other members of the household as well. Pinworms are very common, affecting up to 10 to 15 percent of the population, especially children.

WHAT CAUSES IT?

• Swallowing pinworm eggs initiates a cycle of infection. Most often, eggs are spread when a child scratches the anus, allowing the eggs to be transported on the fingers or beneath the fingernails, where they can then contaminate food, dishes, toys, or play areas.

PREVENTION

• It is difficult to prevent an initial outbreak of pinworms. However, the following measures can be used to prevent reinfestation once the first outbreak has occurred:

• Wash the hands thoroughly before eating and after handling potentially infected objects, such as children's toys.
• Keep fingernails short so they are less likely to pick up eggs.
• Shower daily in the morning.

DIAGNOSIS

• Adult worms are sometimes seen around the anal area at night or in bowel movements. A doctor can supply a piece of cellulose tape to be applied to the anal area during the night or in the early morning. The tape is then examined under a microscope for worms or eggs to confirm the diagnosis. Specimens from three consecutive mornings may be necessary to confirm the diagnosis.

HOW TO TREAT IT

• Usually, a single dose of mebendazole or pyrantel pamoate is given, followed by a repeat dose two weeks later. These medicines are very effective in killing worms.
• Creams or ointments that relieve anal itching and that may contain substances that kill the worms can be prescribed.
• There is a high risk of reinfection and recurrence is common. If repeated infections occur, members of the whole household should be treated.

WHEN TO CALL A DOCTOR

• Call a doctor if symptoms of pinworm infestation occur. ⚠

SYMPTOMS
• Anal itching or pain.
• Irritability or fidgetiness.
• Restless sleep.
• Vaginal itching, pain, or discharge. This occurs infrequently when adult worms migrate across the skin to the vagina.

Plantar Fasciitis

WHAT IS IT?

Plantar fasciitis is inflammation, usually due to injury, of the plantar fascia, the ligament between the front of the heel bone and the base of the toes that helps to support the arch. Excess stress absorbed by the foot may irritate or tear the plantar fascia, making this a common disorder among athletes, especially runners. Although plantar fasciitis may take up to a year to heal fully, it is not a serious health risk, and proper rest and stretching techniques may promote faster healing.

WHAT CAUSES IT?

• A tendency for the foot to roll inward (pronation) upon walking.
• Stress on the heel due to repeated hard pounding or quick turns, often from long-distance running, jogging, or basketball.
• Wearing shoes that lack proper heel support or that have thin or stiff soles.
• Age-related loss of resiliency in the ligaments.
• Some forms of arthritis, such as ankylosing spondylitis or Reiter's syndrome.

PREVENTION

• Wear running shoes with proper cushioning.
• Avoid exercising on nonresilient surfaces such as concrete.

DIAGNOSIS

• Patient history and physical examination.

HOW TO TREAT IT

• Rest the foot as much as possible, especially during the first week. Avoid running or jogging; instead, substitute exercises that do not put undue stress on the injured ligament, like bicycling or swimming.
• Take over-the-counter pain relievers to reduce pain and inflammation.
• Apply ice to the tender area daily to reduce inflammation. Try rolling the arch of the foot over an empty tennis-ball can that has been filled with water and frozen; it will cool and stretch the affected area.
• Insert an over-the-counter heel-support cushion into your shoe. Cut a hole in the pad to relieve pressure on the tender area if necessary. Try to avoid walking barefoot because it may put added stress on the plantar ligament.
• Stretch the ligament with the following exercises (each position should be held for 30 seconds, and each exercise repeated six times; the entire series should be performed three times daily if possible):
• Sit on a table with your knees bent. Loop a towel under the ball of the injured foot and pull, flexing the front of your foot upward. Keep your knee bent and try to press your foot against the towel.
• Perform the exercise as above with the leg extended straight out in front of you. Keep the leg straight during the stretch.
• Sit on a chair and cross the ankle of the injured foot over the opposite knee. Slowly push your toes backward with your hand until you feel the stretch in the bottom of the foot.
• Stand facing a wall, about one foot away, with the injured foot about six inches farther back. Put your hands on the wall and gently lean forward, stretching the lower calf of the back leg.
• Stand facing a wall, about two feet away, with the injured foot about six inches farther back. Keep both feet slightly turned out. Put your hands on the wall and gently lean forward, bending the front knee and keeping the back heel on the floor.
• A local injection of a corticosteroid is often helpful. Rarely, surgery may be recommended in chronic cases.

WHEN TO CALL A DOCTOR

• Make an appointment with a doctor if pain does not subside within four to six weeks.
• Call a doctor if pain is severe. 🏃

SYMPTOMS

• Sharp or burning pain directly under the heel. Pain worsens upon running or walking.

Plantar Warts

WHAT IS IT?

Plantar warts are noncancerous skin growths that develop on the soles of the foot. Like all warts, they are caused by a virus (human papillomavirus). Various features set plantar warts apart from so-called common warts (which typically form raised dome-shaped skin lesions on the fingers and other areas) and genital warts.

First, plantar warts arise exclusively on the bottoms of the feet. Pressure from body weight tends to make plantar warts grow inward, just beneath the skin's surface, and a rough, thickened layer of skin (callus) typically grows over the wart. A plantar wart may feel like a pebble in the shoe; however, in some cases it causes intense pain, particularly if it lies on the heel or ball of the foot. Second, plantar warts do not tend to spread to other sites on the body. They usually appear singly, although a variant, the mosaic wart, consists of multiple small, merging lesions.

Finally, unlike genital warts, which have been linked to serious health problems such as genital cancer, plantar warts pose no such risks. Several treatment sessions may be necessary to cure plantar warts, but a doctor can usually eliminate even the most stubborn cases.

WHAT CAUSES IT?

• Plantar warts, like other warts, are caused by the human papillomavirus. The virus incubates in the skin for several months before causing a wart.
• The incidence is highest among adolescents, likely due to going barefoot in public recreational and shower facilities.

DIAGNOSIS

• A doctor can identify a plantar wart by its characteristic appearance. Cutting off the surface layer reveals a soft, cauliflower-like central portion that is speckled with small, clotted blood vessels resembling pinpoint splinters.

PREVENTION

• Wear footwear in public places.

HOW TO TREAT IT

• Treatment is certainly warranted if the wart is painful and interferes with walking. Treatment will also keep a wart from growing or being spread to other people.
• Home treatment can be attempted, although plantar warts (unlike common warts) tend to be rather difficult to treat and often require professional care. One approach involves nightly applications of salicylic-acid plasters, which are available in drugstores.
• Warts that fail to respond to self-treatment and those that develop in people with diabetes require a physician's or podiatrist's care. Usually, the doctor will cut away any thickened skin over the wart before treating it with any of several techniques. (Do not cut off warts or the calluses that cover them on your own; it may lead to infection.)
• Liquid nitrogen may be applied to the wart (cryosurgery), which may cause it to blister and fall off within a couple of days or weeks. Alternatively, the wart may be destroyed using acidic chemicals or surgically removed with a beam of electric current (electrocautery) or laser light. These approaches generally cause some discomfort and, for warts requiring electrocautery or laser surgery, may necessitate local anesthesia. Several treatment sessions may be necessary because the thickness of the plantar surface makes it more resistant to treatment, and because the wart virus may be very resistant to destruction.

WHEN TO CALL A DOCTOR

• See a doctor or podiatrist if you have diabetes and develop a plantar wart, if the wart is painful and interferes with walking, or if the wart does not respond to self-treatment.

SYMPTOMS

• A callouslike, white, tender skin growth on the bottom of the foot, usually surrounded by a callus.
• Pain or discomfort when putting weight on the affected foot.

Platelet Function Disorders

WHAT IS IT?

Various disorders can affect platelets, the components of the blood that help blood to clot and that maintain the integrity of the blood vessel wall. Normally, platelets are formed continuously from megakaryocytes (large bone marrow cells) in the bone marrow. From there, they are released into the blood, where they circulate and help with wound healing. For example, after a simple cut, platelets flowing by the damaged area collect, form a small clot that stanches blood flow, and release various substances that help the wound to heal.

Most platelet disorders are due to an insufficient number of platelets, a condition known as thrombocytopenia. This condition results either from inadequate production of platelets in the bone marrow or from their excessive destruction in the bloodstream. Less often, the number of circulating platelets is normal, but they are defective and function improperly. In either case deficient platelet function can lead to excessive bleeding. The most common result is for blood to leak slowly from minute tears in the smallest blood vessels (capillaries), causing bright or dark red pinpoint-size hemorrhages, called petechiae, to appear on the skin. Petechiae often occur on the lower legs (where gravity exerts increased pressure on blood vessel walls), on the inside of the cheeks (owing to pressure from chewing), or along areas constricted by tight clothing (such as brassiere straps). Petechiae in skin and mucous membranes are harmless, but they may be a harbinger of more serious internal bleeding, particularly bleeding from the gastrointestinal tract or from blood vessels in the brain (a potentially life-threatening complication known as intracranial hemorrhage).

There are a wide variety of causes of platelet disorders, and they can occur at any age. Some are hereditary disorders that may become obvious as early as infancy; for example, there may be excessive bleeding following circumcision. In older people, platelet disorders may become manifest after a dental extraction or surgical procedure. Outcome varies widely, depending on the cause and severity of the disorder. Some forms are mild and lifelong, with only minor bruising or limited periods of excessive bleeding; others arise suddenly and may be fatal. In general, older patients seem to be at higher risk of serious complications like intracranial hemorrhage.

WHAT CAUSES IT?

• In many cases, platelet disorders are believed to be due to an autoimmune disorder (an attack, for unknown reasons, by the body's immune system against its own healthy cells). In this case, platelets are destroyed prematurely as they circulate in the blood. A common unexplained autoimmune disorder is called idiopathic thrombocytopenic purpura (ITP), and platelets are rapidly destroyed in systemic lupus erythematosus, also an autoimmune disorder.
• Certain types of leukemia or bone marrow invasion by cancer can give rise to decreased platelet number and function.
• A number of infections, including rubella, mononucleosis, bacterial blood infections, malaria, hepatitis, tuberculosis (TB), and human immunodeficiency virus (HIV), can cause platelet disorders.
• A wide variety of drugs is capable of causing platelet disorders in a small percentage of people. Some of these drugs are very commonly used, including aspirin, ibuprofen, and antibiotics such as penicillin. Others include quinidine and quinine (used to treat malaria) and illicit intravenous drugs.

SYMPTOMS

• Minor bleeding just under the surface of the skin or in the mouth—usually appears as multiple tiny, pinpoint-size specks (petechiae) on the lower legs or inner cheeks.
• Bleeding of the gums or blood blisters in the mouth.
• Nosebleeds.
• Easy bruising.
• Prolonged menstrual periods.
• Prolonged bleeding after a minor cut or after dental or surgical procedures.
• Emergency symptoms: sudden onset of severe headache, nausea, vomiting, vision loss, or confusion (signs of a brain hemorrhage); black or tarry stools may indicate bleeding from the gastrointestinal tract.

Platelet Function Disorders   *continued*

• In aplastic anemia, a rare but very serious condition, production of platelets (and other blood cells) in the bone marrow is severely suppressed. It can be induced by radiation or chemotherapy drugs (for cancer), gold compounds (used to treat arthritis), the antibiotic chloramphenicol, or exposure to organic solvent fumes, including benzene and glue. It also sometimes occurs in those with acute hepatitis, but in many cases the cause cannot be determined.

• Chronic alcoholism or deficiencies of certain B vitamins can cause platelet disorders.

• Massive blood transfusions can cause a temporary platelet deficiency, exacerbated at times by an immune reaction to the donor's blood that leads to platelet destruction.

• Various genetic defects can cause inherited platelet disorders.

• Disseminated intravascular coagulation (DIC) involves impaired platelet function and direct decline in platelet number.

• Chemotherapy and radiation treatments for cancer or leukemia may destroy platelets.

PREVENTION

• There are no known ways to prevent platelet function disorders.

DIAGNOSIS

• Patient history should include all drugs being taken and family history of bleeding disorders.

• Blood samples will be taken for a platelet count and to test platelet function and presence of platelet antibodies.

• A bone marrow aspiration and biopsy (removal of tissue through a needle inserted into the hip or thigh) may be necessary to determine whether adequate numbers of platelets are being manufactured.

HOW TO TREAT IT

• All patients should avoid aspirin and other drugs that can affect platelets until the condition clears.

Those whose only symptoms are petechiae may need no additional treatment.

• For people with more serious bleeding disorders, transfusions of platelets are given (if no detectable antiplatelet antibodies are present) until the underlying defect is corrected and the body produces enough healthy platelets on its own. Those with chronic or inherited forms of the disease may require transfusions whenever bleeding problems arise or before surgical or dental procedures are performed.

• If a drug is found to be the cause, discontinuation of the drug usually resolves the problem quickly.

• Corticosteroid drugs may be prescribed to suppress the destruction of platelets by the immune system. The disorder often improves within several weeks and may disappear completely. Other immunosuppressive drugs may be tried as well.

• Those who continue to have platelet defects despite corticosteroids or other forms of therapy may benefit from surgical removal of the spleen (splenectomy). The spleen acts to produce helpful antibodies and to remove worn-out blood cells, including platelets. But in those with platelet disorders, it can become enlarged and overactive and thus stall recovery. Splenectomy—used especially in those with ITP—brings about long-term remissions in many patients without causing other long-term side effects.

WHEN TO CALL A DOCTOR

• See a doctor if you have symptoms of a bleeding disorder.

• If you have already been diagnosed with a platelet disorder, call a doctor if you notice increased bruising or new areas of petechiae or if you begin bleeding from the nose or gums.

• **EMERGENCY** Get to an emergency room immediately if symptoms of internal bleeding from the gastrointestinal tract (black, tarry stools) or brain (severe headache, nausea, vision loss) occur. ◢

Pleurisy and Pleural Effusion

WHAT IS IT?

Pleurisy is inflammation of the pleura—the delicate, two-layered membrane that encases the lungs and lines the inside of the chest cavity. The space between the pleural membranes (pleural space) is normally bathed in a thin lubricating fluid that ensures smooth expansion and contraction of the membranes during breathing. With pleurisy, a section of the pleura becomes inflamed and roughened, causing the two layers of the membrane to rub together painfully. Pleurisy can affect people of any age. Most cases are due to infections and, with treatment, clear up in a few days or weeks. However, some cases are caused by more serious underlying disorders, such as systemic lupus erythematosus or a pulmonary embolism.

If inflammation is severe, fluid may accumulate in the pleural space, a condition known as pleural effusion. The excess fluid often provides lubrication that eases the pain, but it may also compress the underlying lung and make breathing difficult. Although pleural effusion is often associated with pleurisy, pleural effusion can exist in the absence of pleurisy (such as with heart failure). Because pleurisy and pleural effusion are not diseases themselves as much as they are manifestations of an underlying disorder, treatment outcome depends on the seriousness of the underlying cause.

SYMPTOMS

- Pleurisy symptoms: Mild but continuous chest pain made worse by deep breathing, coughing, sneezing, or moving the affected area. The pain may radiate to the shoulder, lower chest, or abdomen, but usually affects only one side of the body. Less commonly, the pain is sharp and fleeting.
- Fever and chills.
- Headache.
- Weakness.
- Rapid, shallow breathing.
- Dry cough.
- Generally no symptoms for pleural effusion. If severe, it may cause shortness of breath.

WHAT CAUSES IT?

- Pleurisy is often caused by lung or chest infections, including tuberculosis, pneumonia, and viral infections. Pleurodynia, a viral infection that most often affects children, may cause outbreaks of pleurisy among family members.
- Pulmonary embolism (a blood clot in an artery of the lung) is a life-threatening cause of pleurisy.
- Other causes include autoimmune disorders (such as systemic lupus erythematosus or rheumatoid arthritis), chest injury, and sickle cell disease.
- Pleural effusion may be caused by a tumor in the pleura (mesothelioma), cancer that has spread from the lung or elsewhere, heart failure, liver disease, kidney disease, or pancreatitis.

PREVENTION

- There is no known way to prevent pleurisy or pleural effusions.

DIAGNOSIS

- Patient history and physical examination are needed.
- X-rays, ultrasound, or CT (computed tomography) scans of the chest may be done to detect pleural effusions.
- Aspiration (withdrawal of fluid from the pleural space with a needle) and biopsy may be done.

HOW TO TREAT IT

- Underlying disorders are treated. For example, antibiotics are given for bacterial pneumonias.
- Over-the-counter or prescription pain relievers may be recommended. Wrapping the chest loosely in elastic bandages may also help to ease pain.
- If pleural effusion makes breathing difficult, fluid may be withdrawn with a needle (thoracentesis).
- For very severe cases of recurrent pleural effusion—such as those that may occur with inoperable cancer—doxycycline (an antibiotic) or an anticancer drug is injected into the pleural space. The drugs cause scarring and fusion of the two pleural layers, thus preventing future recurrences.

WHEN TO CALL A DOCTOR

- Call a doctor if symptoms of pleurisy develop. ▲

Pneumonia

WHAT IS IT?

Pneumonia, a general term encompassing many different diseases, is an inflammation of the lungs. Although usually caused by an infectious microorganism, such inflammation may also be caused by the inhalation of irritating gases or particles. The lungs have a complex system of defense: frequent branching and narrowing of the bronchial passages make it difficult for invaders to penetrate the lungs deeply; millions of tiny hairs, or cilia, in the bronchial lining constantly sweep particles out of the airways; the cough reflex forces irritating substances out of the lungs at high speed; and white blood cells, known as phagocytes, engulf and destroy many infectious agents.

Despite these defenses, pneumonia is still common. Inflammation may be limited to the air sacs (alveoli) of the lung (lobar pneumonia) or may occur in patches throughout the lungs, originating in the airways and spreading to the alveoli (bronchopneumonia). An accumulation of fluid in the alveoli impairs transfer of oxygen to the bloodstream. The body's cells may thus become starved of oxygen, and in severe cases respiratory failure may result. Until the development of antibiotics, pneumonia was the number one cause of death in the United States, and recently, strains of the most common cause of bacterial pneumonia *(Streptococcus pneumoniae)* have emerged that are penicillin resistant. Pneumonia, especially among the elderly or those already weakened by underlying illness, remains among the 10 leading causes of death today.

Nevertheless, despite the serious health risks posed by the disease, the outlook for complete recovery is good, especially with early diagnosis and treatment. For the elderly and members of other high-risk groups, a vaccine is available that provides long-term protection against 23 different strains of *S. pneumoniae* (which account for 90 percent of cases of pneumococcal pneumonia).

SYMPTOMS

- Symptoms vary greatly depending on the type of pneumonia involved. The elderly and very sick people tend to have less pronounced symptoms and less fever, even though pneumonia is more dangerous among these patients.
- Fever (over 100°F, possibly as high as 105°F) and chills.
- Cough, possibly with bloody yellow or green sputum. (A cough may persist for six to eight weeks after the infection, especially a viral infection, subsides.)
- Chest pain upon inhalation.
- Shortness of breath.
- Headache, sore throat, and muscle pain.
- Nasal discharge.
- General feeling of poor health.
- Weakness and fatigue.
- Profuse perspiration.
- Loss of appetite.
- In severe cases: breathing difficulty, blue tinge to the skin, mental confusion.

WHAT CAUSES IT?

- Viral or bacterial infections are the most common causes of pneumonia.
- Other microorganisms may sometimes cause pneumonia; for example, fungal and parasitic pneumonia commonly affects those with AIDS.
- Although bacteria are usually inhaled, they may spread to the lungs from elsewhere in the body via the bloodstream.
- Inhalation of chemical irritants, such as poisonous gases, may lead to pneumonia.
- Vomit inhaled into the lungs, which may occur when a person loses consciousness, may cause what is known as aspiration pneumonia.
- Infancy or very old age, smoking, recent surgery, hospitalization, the use of chemotherapy and other immunosuppressive drugs, and the prolonged use of antibiotics are risk factors for pneumonia.
- Other conditions increase the risk both of contracting pneumonia and of encountering more serious complications associated with the disease. These include asthma, chronic bronchitis, poorly controlled diabetes mellitus, AIDS, alcoholism, Hodgkin's disease, leukemia, multiple myeloma, and chronic kidney disease.

Pneumonia   *continued*

PREVENTION

• Don't smoke.

• People at high risk for pneumonia should be immunized against pneumococcal pneumonia. These people include those over age 65; those with heart, lung, or kidney disease, diabetes mellitus, or weakened immune systems; and alcoholics. The vaccine is required only once; it provides long-term protection and is between 60 to 80 percent effective in those whose immune system is functioning normally.

• An annual flu vaccination (particularly for people over age 65) may be recommended because pneumonia is a common complication of severe influenza.

DIAGNOSIS

• Patient history and physical examination.
• Blood and sputum cultures.
• Chest x-rays.
• A biopsy of lung tissue may be performed in complicated cases.

HOW TO TREAT IT

• Antibiotics or other antimicrobial drugs are prescribed to treat a bacterial infection and should be taken for the full term prescribed. Stopping the medication too soon may produce a relapse.

• Antifungal drugs, such as amphotericin B, are prescribed to treat a fungal infection.

• Antiviral drugs such as ribavirin, acyclovir, and ganciclovir sodium are effective against some types of viral infection.

• Your doctor may recommend analgesics to reduce fever and pain. Check with your doctor before taking over-the-counter pain relievers; they are not recommended for some types of bacterial pneumonia.

• Take an over-the-counter cough suppressant containing dextromethorphan if you have a persistent dry cough. However, if you are coughing up sputum, suppressing the cough completely may encourage mucus accumulation in the lungs, potentially leading to serious complications.

• Your doctor will instruct you how to drain mucus from your lungs by assuming various positions that lower your head below your torso (a technique known as postural drainage).

• Drink at least eight glasses of water a day to loosen lung secretions and make them easier to expel.

• Rest in bed until fever subsides.

• Hospitalization may be recommended, especially during the early stages, since pneumonia may unexpectedly become severe within hours.

• Oxygen may be administered through a mask to aid breathing. In severe cases an artificial respirator may be required.

• Excess fluid in the space surrounding the lungs may be removed by aspiration with a syringe and needle inserted through the chest wall (thoracentesis).

WHEN TO CALL A DOCTOR

• Call a doctor if you develop symptoms of pneumonia, especially a fever above 100°F, shortness of breath even when lying down, or bloody sputum from coughing.

• **EMERGENCY** Call an ambulance if you experience difficulty in breathing or if a blue tinge to the lips, nose, or fingernails appears. ▲

Pneumothorax

WHAT IS IT?

Pneumothorax is an accumulation of air in the area between the outer edge of the lung and the inner lining of the rib cage (pleural space), resulting in partial or total collapse of the affected lung. Different types of pneumothorax (spontaneous, secondary, traumatic, and tension) are distinguished by their cause. Treatment and outcome depend upon severity.

WHAT CAUSES IT?

• Spontaneous pneumothorax occurs when an air-filled blister known as a bleb ruptures on the surface of the lung. Blebs are believed to be congenital or hereditary in origin; smoking may be a contributing factor. Scuba diving or high altitudes may precipitate the rupture of a bleb. This type of pneumothorax is most common among tall, thin, and otherwise healthy men between the ages of 20 and 40, and recurs in about one-third of patients.

• Secondary pneumothorax (usually far more serious than spontaneous pneumothorax) occurs as a complication of some underlying lung disorder, including chronic obstructive pulmonary disease, cystic fibrosis, tuberculosis, and certain types of pneumonia.

• Traumatic pneumothorax results from a direct puncture or laceration of the surface of the lung (which may occur with a stab wound, a rib fracture, or as a complication of a medical procedure) when air enters the pleural space.

• A tension pneumothorax develops when air entering the pleural space during inhalation becomes trapped and cannot escape during exhalation.

PREVENTION

• Don't smoke.

• Seek prompt treatment for any existing lung disorders, such as tuberculosis or asthma.

SYMPTOMS

• Sudden shortness of breath (of varying degrees) and tightness in the chest.

• Chest pain, usually sudden and sharp.

• Bluish skin, bulging neck veins, and weak rapid pulse (in severe cases).

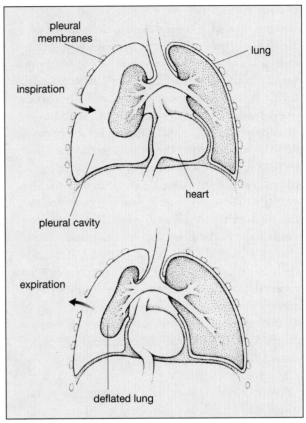

In traumatic pneumothorax, air enters the pleural cavity upon inspiration and exits on expiration, while the lung remains deflated. Tension pneumothorax results when air cannot escape during expiration.

DIAGNOSIS

• Patient history, examination, and chest x-rays.

HOW TO TREAT IT

• A small pneumothorax may heal on its own; a few days of monitoring in a hospital may be advised.

• More serious cases may require removal of air by suction through a needle or catheter. Using this procedure, the lung usually reexpands over several days.

• Recurrent spontaneous pneumothorax may warrant installation of irritants into the pleural space to cause the surface of the lung and the inner surface of the chest wall to fuse together.

• Surgery may be considered to repair a lung lesion causing secondary pneumothorax.

WHEN TO CALL A DOCTOR

• See a doctor immediately if you have symptoms.

Poliomyelitis

WHAT IS IT?

Poliomyelitis, also known as infantile paralysis or polio, is a highly contagious viral infection. In its most severe form, polio may cause rapid and irreversible paralysis and until the late 1950s was one of the most feared infectious diseases, often occurring in epidemics. Postpolio syndrome or postpoliomyelitic progressive muscular atrophy may occur 30 years or more after the initial infection, gradually producing additional muscle weakness, atrophy, and pain. Polio is preventable by immunization and has virtually disappeared in this country; however, the danger from this disease still exists. The dramatic decline in cases of polio has created a false sense of security; fewer children in the United States have been receiving the vaccine, so the number of people vulnerable to the infection is rising. Polio is still common in much of the world, and there is no cure; therefore, until the poliovirus is destroyed, immunization remains essential for protection.

WHAT CAUSES IT?

• Poliomyelitis is caused by a viral infection by one of the three forms of poliovirus.
• The virus may be spread through contact with contaminated food and water, or by infected saliva expelled during coughing or sneezing.

PREVENTION

• A series of vaccines is recommended to begin at two months of age, repeated at four and 18 months of age, and followed by a booster shot when the child enters school (between the ages of four and six).
• In adults, immunization against polio is only recommended before traveling to an area where polio is common.

DIAGNOSIS

• Patient history and physical examination.
• Blood tests.
• Lumbar puncture (spinal tap).

HOW TO TREAT IT

• Bed rest is advised until severe symptoms subside.
• Pain relievers may be administered to reduce fever, pain, and muscle spasms.
• Your doctor may prescribe bethanechol to treat urinary retention and antibiotics to fight an associated bacterial infection of the urinary tract.
• A urinary catheter, a thin tube attached to a storage bag used to collect urine, may be necessary if bladder control has been lost because of paralysis.
• Artificial respiration may be required if breathing is impaired; in some cases a surgical opening (tracheotomy) in the throat may be necessary.
• Physical therapy is needed in cases of temporary or permanent paralysis. Mechanical aids such as braces, crutches, a wheelchair, and special shoes may aid in mobility.
• A combination of occupational and psychological therapy may help patients adapt to the limitations imposed by the disease.

WHEN TO CALL A DOCTOR

• Call a doctor immediately if you or your child develops symptoms of polio, or if you may have been exposed to the virus and have not yet been immunized.
• Make an appointment with your doctor to receive the polio vaccine if you have not been immunized and plan to travel where polio is common.
• **EMERGENCY** Call an ambulance if someone experiences breathing difficulty or develops paralysis in any of the limbs. 🔺

SYMPTOMS

• Fever.
• Headache and sore throat.
• Stiff neck and back.
• Nausea and vomiting.
• Muscle pain, weakness, or spasms.
• Difficulty in swallowing.
• Constipation and urine retention.
• Swollen or bloated abdomen.
• Irritability.
• Emergency symptoms: muscle paralysis; breathing difficulty.

Polycystic Ovaries

WHAT IS IT?

Polycystic ovarian disease is characterized by the formation of follicle cysts (spherical, thin-walled nodules filled with a thin fluid) within both ovaries. Each ovary contains an abundance of structures known as ovarian follicles. Roughly once a month, hormones stimulate a single follicle to grow and rise to the ovarian surface, where it bursts and releases an egg. At the same time, hormones from the follicles cause the uterine wall to thicken to provide support if the egg becomes fertilized. The egg passes out of the ovary, through the fallopian tube, and into the uterus. If fertilization does not occur, the thickened uterine lining is shed and the egg, excess lining, and blood are all released through the vagina during menstruation.

In polycystic ovarian disease the follicle grows but fails to burst. Instead of releasing an egg, the follicle forms a cyst just below the ovary's surface. Normal menstrual periods may be present early in puberty but become widely spaced or cease completely as the ovaries begin to produce cysts instead of releasing eggs. Eventually, both ovaries become filled with tiny cysts. Lack of ovulation results in the cessation of menstrual periods, infertility, and overproduction of the male sex hormone testosterone by the ovaries. Other common features of this disorder are obesity, acne, infertility, a resistance to insulin, and the abnormal growth of male-pattern facial hair (hirsutism).

The reason for cyst development is not fully understood, but it is believed to involve an imbalance in the production of the two pituitary hormones that normally stimulate the ovaries to function: luteinizing hormone (LH) and follicle-stimulating hormone (FSH). Polycystic ovarian disease affects women during their reproductive years. If left untreated, the relative excess of estrogen compared to progesterone may increase the risk of endometrial hyperplasia and uterine cancer later in life. However, the disease often responds well to treatment, which may restore fertility and eliminate symptoms. Specific treatment depends on the individual needs of the patient, especially whether or not she wishes to have children in the future.

WHAT CAUSES IT?

• The cause of this condition is unknown, but it may be genetic.

PREVENTION

• There is no known way to prevent polycystic ovarian disease.

DIAGNOSIS

• Patient history and pelvic examination. The gynecologist may be able to detect enlarged ovaries during a biannual pelvic examination.
• Blood tests can measure levels of LH, FSH, testosterone, and other hormones that affect function of the ovaries.
• Ultrasound scans may be performed.
• Laparoscopic abdominal surgery (use of a lighted scope that is inserted into the abdomen through a small incision) may confirm the diagnosis.

HOW TO TREAT IT

• For those women who wish to become pregnant, clomiphene citrate, a fertility drug, or hormones such as human gonadotropins and human chorionic gonadotropin may be prescribed to induce ovulation. Rarely, laparoscopic surgery to reduce the size of the ovary (wedge resection or ovarian drilling) may be performed to create more favorable conditions for ovulation.
• For those who do not wish to become pregnant, oral contraceptives or progestins such as medroxyprogesterone acetate may be prescribed to suppress ovulation and reduce the risk of endometrial hyperplasia or uterine cancer later in life.

WHEN TO CALL A DOCTOR

• Call your gynecologist if you develop symptoms of polycystic ovarian disease. ▲

SYMPTOMS
• Absent or irregular menstrual periods.
• Infertility.
• Abnormal growth of facial hair (hirsutism).
• Obesity.
• Acne.

Polycythemia Vera

WHAT IS IT?

Polycythemia vera is an uncommon blood disorder characterized by a pathological overproduction of red blood cells, white blood cells, and platelets. Each type of blood cell performs an essential function: red cells carry oxygen, platelets are crucial for clotting, and white cells can engulf infectious agents and thus serve as part of the body's immune system. Red cells, platelets, and most types of white cells are produced by the bone marrow and released into the bloodstream as they mature. Normally, the marrow produces only enough new cells to replace the ones that have died.

However, in polycythemia vera new blood cells are produced in excess. The overabundance of red cells increases the viscosity or thickness of blood, resulting in a greater frequency of blood clots in both the arteries and veins. There is also a higher risk of excess bleeding, due to defective platelets or possibly due to blood vessels that are overengorged with the extra red cells. Late in the disease, the spleen and liver may enlarge markedly. Polycythemia vera is associated with a greater risk of acute leukemia (see Leukemias for more information). Symptoms develop gradually, and the disorder affects people of all ages. Although slightly more common in men than in women, this is not true in patients under age 40.

SYMPTOMS
- Frequent headaches and a feeling of pressure in the head.
- Dizziness and ringing in the ears (tinnitus).
- Fatigue.
- Blurred or double vision.
- Flushed or itching skin.
- Night sweats.
- Frequent nosebleeds and bruises.

If left untreated, polycythemia vera may be fatal; stroke and heart attack are the most common causes of death. However, with treatment and control of the disease, the majority of patients survive more than 25 years after their initial diagnosis.

WHAT CAUSES IT?
- The cause of polycythemia vera is unknown.
- An ethnic component may be involved; for example, people of Jewish descent appear to be at greater risk of polycythemia vera.

PREVENTION
- Polycythemia vera cannot be prevented.

DIAGNOSIS
- There are no widely available diagnostic tests for polycythemia vera. Diagnosis is suggested by patient history and physical examination and by blood tests showing an elevation of red cell, white cell, and platelet counts. Initially, only one of these may be elevated (commonly the red cells). A test called red cell volume measurement may be done.
- Because an elevated red cell count can be caused by diseases of the heart, lungs, liver, or kidneys, evaluation of these organs may be necessary to be sure that the elevated count is due to polycythemia vera.

HOW TO TREAT IT
- Phlebotomy, or blood removal, is performed to eliminate excess red cells and to decrease blood viscosity. At first it may be necessary to withdraw a pint of blood every few days; with time, phlebotomy may only be necessary once or twice a year, to keep hemoglobin at certain levels.
- If possible, exposure to chemotherapy agents (alkylating agents such as busulfan) or radioactivity, or x-rays should be avoided as these agents increase the risk of leukemia. Interferon alpha or hydroxyurea may be given to reduce a high white cell or platelet count or shrink an enlarged spleen.
- Medication to prevent heartburn or to relieve itching (such as antihistamines) may be prescribed. Allopurinol may be given to prevent kidney stones.
- Surgery to remove an enlarged spleen may be necessary if drug therapy fails.

WHEN TO CALL A DOCTOR
- Make an appointment with a doctor if you develop symptoms of polycythemia vera.

Presbycusis

WHAT IS IT?

Presbycusis—the gradual loss of hearing that accompanies aging—is a type of sensorineural or perceptive hearing loss that is brought on by degeneration of specialized receptor cells of the inner ear. (This is in contrast to typically more treatable conductive hearing losses, which occur when earwax, fluid, a tumor, or a tear in the eardrum physically interferes with the transmission of sound through the middle ear.)

Like many types of sensorineural hearing loss, presbycusis is characterized by difficulty understanding speech, especially in the presence of background noise (common in restaurants, for example). Presbycusis is not necessarily an inevitable part of aging; many people in their 80s hear perfectly well. Individual risk factors determine the degree of hearing loss a person will experience with age. A decline in auditory nerve fibers may begin as early as age 40, although presbycusis rarely becomes noticeable before the age of 55. By age 65, one in every three people has some degree of hearing loss.

WHAT CAUSES IT?

• Presbycusis is caused by age-related degeneration of sensory cells of the inner ear.
• Cumulative lifetime exposure to excessive noise can hasten hearing loss.
• Atherosclerosis (the buildup of cholesterol-based plaques in the arteries) may deprive structures in the ear of sufficient blood supply.
• Certain drugs, such as aminoglycoside, may be toxic to tissues in the inner ear.
• A hereditary predisposition appears to be involved.

PREVENTION

• Avoid loud sounds and noisy places as much as possible. Use earplugs whenever you are likely to be exposed to machine-generated noise or weapon fire.

SYMPTOMS

• Progressive hearing loss.
• Inability to discern high-frequency sounds.
• Difficulty understanding speech, especially in noisy or crowded environments.

DIAGNOSIS

• Patient history and hearing tests (audiometry) are necessary. Examination is usually conducted by an audiologist (hearing specialist).
• Other procedures, including blood tests, x-rays, and CT (computed tomography) scans or MRI (magnetic resonance imaging), may be ordered to rule out other possible causes of hearing problems.

HOW TO TREAT IT

• Generally, the only remedy available for presbycusis is a hearing aid. Resist the temptation to go directly to a hearing-aid supplier or to order from companies that advertise on television or in print. They typically cannot provide the flexibility or quality of medical attention you need. Go instead to a certified audiologist, preferably one recommended by your primary-care physician or otolaryngologist (ear, nose, and throat specialist). Advances in technology have made hearing aids more effective and better suited to individual needs than ever before.
• An audiologist may provide counseling and non-medical rehabilitation techniques, such as lip-reading.

WHEN TO CALL A DOCTOR

• Consult your doctor if you experience any degree of hearing difficulty. You will likely be referred to an audiologist or an otolaryngologist for testing and diagnosis.

Presbyopia

WHAT IS IT?

Presbyopia is the inability to focus on close objects, which occurs as the lens of the eye progressively loses its flexibility—a normal consequence of aging. The lens, located just behind the pupil, expands and contracts in response to the tiny ciliary muscle surrounding it, providing clear focus over a range of distances. When the ciliary muscle is relaxed, tension in the area around the lens holds the lens at a thickness adequate for distance vision. When the ciliary contracts, this tension decreases, which allows the lens to expand (thicken) and focus on a close object.

With age, the lens hardens and becomes less flexible and the ciliary muscle may weaken; these changes make it increasingly difficult to focus at close range. Sometime after age 40, most people notice that close objects seem more blurry, and that newspapers and books must be held at arm's length to be read. Prescription reading glasses compensate for this loss of focusing power. Those who already require glasses to correct other vision problems, such as nearsightedness or astigmatism, may need bi- or trifocal lenses when presbyopia develops. Presbyopia is not a serious health risk and does not lead to blindness.

WHAT CAUSES IT?

• Aging causes the lens in the eye to harden and become less flexible. The ciliary muscle may lose some of its ability to contract as well.

PREVENTION

• Presbyopia cannot be prevented.
• Contrary to popular belief, vision cannot be improved by refusing to wear prescription lenses if you need them or by performing so-called vision-strengthening exercises.

SYMPTOMS
• Blurred vision at close range.
• Blurred vision of distant objects after prolonged focusing on nearby objects.
• Eyestrain.
• Headaches.

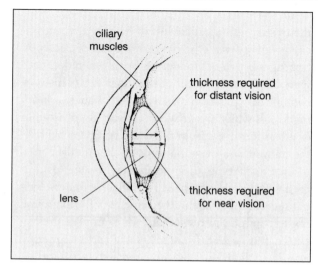

As the lens loses its flexibility with age, it becomes difficult for the ciliary muscles to shape it to the thickness required for near vision.

DIAGNOSIS

• An ophthalmologist will perform a complete eye examination.

HOW TO TREAT IT

• Eyeglasses are prescribed to allow nearby objects to be seen clearly. Some people may need bifocals, trifocals, or multiple pairs of glasses if additional vision problems exist; others may only need reading glasses.
• The prescription for eyeglasses may need to be updated approximately every two years as lens flexibility is progressively lost. After age 65, the eye's lens becomes completely inflexible, so the prescription for corrective lenses usually stabilizes.
• Use goggles or a sports strap to secure glasses during sports or other strenuous physical activities.

WHEN TO CALL A DOCTOR

• Make an appointment with an ophthalmologist or optometrist if it becomes difficult to see nearby objects clearly.

Proctitis

WHAT IS IT?

Proctitis is an inflammation of the rectum. Located at the lower portion of the digestive tract, the rectum connects the large intestine, or colon, to the anus, where fecal matter exits the body. Inflammation may occur owing to a variety of causes; symptoms vary according to the cause and the severity of the inflammation. Proctitis usually responds well to treatment, except in cases caused by genital herpes, as there is currently no cure for herpes. However, in such cases treatment may relieve symptoms, and episodes tend to become milder over time (see Genital Herpes for more information).

WHAT CAUSES IT?

• Inflammatory bowel disease, which may affect much of the lower digestive tract, may cause proctitis (see Colitis, Ulcerative, and Crohn's Disease for more information).

• A bacterial or viral infection, including dysentery, gonorrhea, syphilis, chlamydia, and genital herpes, may cause proctitis (see specific disorders for more information).

• Anal intercourse may lead to proctitis, either by injuring the anus or rectum or by spreading sexually transmitted infections.

• Rare causes of proctitis include tuberculosis, amebiasis, and tissue damage due to radiation.

• The cause of proctitis is sometimes unknown.

DIAGNOSIS

• Your doctor may perform a proctoscopy by passing an illuminated scope though the anus to allow a visual examination of the rectum.

• A biopsy of the colon lining may be taken during proctoscopy.

• A blood test for syphilis is taken if sexually transmitted proctitis is suspected.

• Discharge of mucus or pus is cultured for bacteria and examined under a microscope.

PREVENTION

• Use latex condoms during sexual intercourse to reduce the risk of sexually transmitted disease.

HOW TO TREAT IT

• Antibiotics are prescribed to treat a bacterial infection and should be taken for the full term indicated.

• Corticosteroid suppositories or mesalamine (suppositories or oral tablets) may be prescribed to treat proctitis due to inflammatory bowel disease.

• Treatment for herpes is aimed at relieving symptoms. The antiviral drug acyclovir may be prescribed in topical form to lessen severity and pain, and in oral form to lessen the length and frequency of outbreaks.

• Over-the-counter pain relievers may be taken to reduce pain and inflammation.

• Frequent warm baths may ease rectal discomfort.

WHEN TO CALL A DOCTOR

• Call a doctor if you develop discomfort or pain in the rectum or if bowel movements become difficult, painful, or bloody.

SYMPTOMS

• Painful, frequent bowel movements.
• Straining at stool (tenesmus).
• Rectal pain, itching, and cramps.
• Bloody, pus- or mucus-filled discharge.
• Constipation or diarrhea.
• Fever.
• Blisters or open sores in or around the anus and rectum (due to bacterial or viral infection).
• Pain in the lower back, difficulty in urination, and impotence (due to genital herpes).

Prostate Cancer

WHAT IS IT?

Prostate cancer is the growth of malignant cells in the prostate, a walnut-size gland located just below the bladder in men, which produces about 30 percent of the fluid portion of semen. Prostate cancer is common: Men have a lifetime chance of between one in 10 and one in 13 of developing the disease. It is the most commonly diagnosed male cancer and the second leading cause of male cancer deaths. Indeed, autopsy studies have shown that 60 to 70 percent of all men who reach the age of 80 have at least some microscopic evidence of prostate cancer. Symptoms do not occur until the cancer has spread beyond the prostate, highlighting the importance of regular checkups.

Because prostate cancer tends to grow very slowly and takes years to spread, immediate and aggressive treatment may not be advised in older men. For such patients a diagnosis of prostate cancer may warrant a strategy of "watchful waiting." This involves regular examinations and blood tests, but treatment is undertaken only if evidence indicates tumor growth. The specific treatment plan depends upon a number of factors: the patient's age, the characteristics of the cancerous cells, the size of the tumor, whether cancer appears to have spread to other sites, and the risk of complications. Prostate cancer may be cured by removing the prostate gland before the cancer has spread. However, much controversy prevails about when to advise surgery because it is not possible to predict which cancers will spread and which will not. There is no cure once the cancer has spread beyond the prostate. In some cases though, prostate cancer never spreads, and in general, the outlook is good when the cancer is detected early.

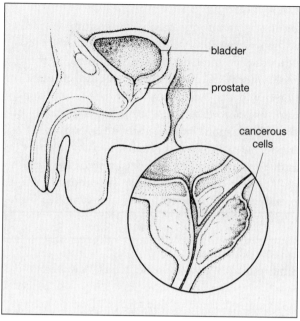

The prostate gland, located just beneath the bladder, commonly enlarges in men over age 50; in some cases, the growth is cancerous.

WHAT CAUSES IT?

• The cause of prostate cancer is unknown, but age, family history, and race are the strongest risk factors.
• Age: The incidence of prostate cancer (rate of newly diagnosed cancer) increases faster with age than any other form of cancer.
• Family history: A family history of prostate cancer and early age at onset (under age 55) within a family increase the risk that a male will develop the disease.
• Race: African Americans have a one-and-a-half times greater incidence of prostate cancer than Caucasian Americans.
• The role of factors such as male hormones, dietary fat, and environmental toxins is not clear.

PREVENTION

• Men over age 50 should have regular digital rectal examinations (examination of the prostate with a gloved finger) and measurements of PSA (see Diagnosis) to aid in early detection and treatment. Men at high risk should begin testing between 40 and 45.

DIAGNOSIS

• Patient history and physical examination, including a digital rectal examination.

SYMPTOMS

• Frequent or urgent need to urinate; delayed or interrupted urinary stream; dribbling.
• Pain upon urination.
• Blood in the urine.
• Painful or bloody ejaculation.
• Erectile dysfunction (impotence).
• Pain in the pelvis or lower back.

Prostate Cancer   *continued*

• Blood tests. The prostate specific antigen (PSA) blood test is the most useful test for early detection. PSA, an enzyme secreted by the cells lining the prostate, functions to liquefy semen after ejaculation. Normally, little PSA enters the blood, but prostate cancer tends to boost levels of PSA in the bloodstream. However, since nonmalignant abnormalities such as benign hyperplasia (prostate enlargement) and prostatitis may also cause increased blood levels of PSA, other tests are necessary to confirm the diagnosis. (See Prostatic Hyperplasia, Benign, or Prostatitis for more information.)

• Multiple biopsies of the prostate are necessary to confirm the diagnosis. Transrectal ultrasonography (ultrasound scan with a rectal probe) allows visual imaging of the prostate and accurate placement of biopsy needles to obtain tissue samples. Small tissue samples are obtained with a needle inserted into the prostate through the rectum, guided by ultrasound.

HOW TO TREAT IT

• Because prostate cancer tends to grow very slowly, a common management strategy is watchful waiting, which involves regular physical examinations and measurements of PSA to monitor the progress of the tumor, with more aggressive treatment advised when warranted. Watchful waiting is often recommended for men in their 70s and 80s who are thought to have localized cancer.

• Total surgical removal of the prostate gland (radical prostatectomy) is the most common treatment; it usually includes removal of nearby lymph nodes. A better understanding of the location of structures important for erectile function and urinary control have greatly reduced the risk of impotence and incontinence. Surgery is generally recommended for men in their 50s and 60s.

• Radiation therapy to destroy cancerous cells may be recommended for somewhat older men or those who are unable to withstand surgery. (Chemotherapy, which is useful in the treatment of some types of cancer, has not been effective in the treatment of prostate cancer.)

• In advanced cases in which the cancer has spread, surgical removal of the testicles (orchiectomy) or hormone therapy (which involves the administration of substances that block the release or function of male hormones) may slow the growth of prostate cancer and thus minimize or arrest the further spread of the cancer.

WHEN TO CALL A DOCTOR

• Call a doctor if you experience difficult, painful, or unusually frequent urination. ▲

Prostatic Hyperplasia, Benign

WHAT IS IT?

Benign prostatic hyperplasia (BPH) is a nodular, irregular enlargement of the prostate, a walnut-size gland located just below the bladder in men, which produces about 30 percent of the fluid portion of semen. Because the prostate surrounds the urethra (the passageway through which urine empties from the bladder), enlargement of the prostate may eventually constrict the urethra and thus interfere with urination. An enlarged prostate may also cause the muscular bladder wall to thicken, as stronger contractions are necessary to push urine through a narrowed urethra. Increased thickness of the wall of the bladder can reduce its ability to store urine and can result in frequent need for urination and sudden strong urges to urinate (urgency). BPH is common, and its incidence increases with age: Evidence of BPH is present in over 50 percent of men by age 60. There is no evidence that BPH leads to prostate cancer; however, symptoms of both disorders are similar, and it is possible to have BPH and prostate cancer at the same time. BPH responds well to treatment.

WHAT CAUSES IT?
• The cause of BPH is unknown.
• Male sex hormones play a role.

PREVENTION
• There is as yet no way to prevent BPH.

DIAGNOSIS
• Patient history and physical examination, which includes a digital rectal examination (DRE). In DRE the doctor inserts a gloved finger into the rectum and presses on the prostate gland to check for enlargement.
• Tests to measure the rate of urine flow.

SYMPTOMS
• Frequent or urgent need to urinate; delayed, weak, or interrupted urine stream; dribbling.
• Pain upon urination.
• Urge to urinate several times a night.
• Blood in the urine.

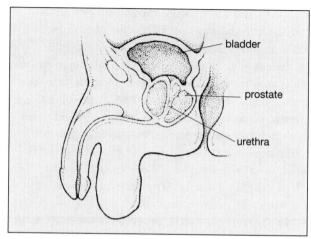

An enlarged prostate (common among men over age 50) may constrict the urethra, impeding the passage of urine from the bladder.

• Urine tests and cultures.
• Measurement of retained urine within the bladder.

HOW TO TREAT IT
• Treatment may be unnecessary for mild symptoms.
• Excess alcohol or fluid intake, especially at night, should be avoided.
• Your doctor may prescribe medication such as finasteride (Proscar) to shrink the prostate or drugs that relax smooth muscle tone in the prostate (alpha-blockers).
• Heat treatment (the application of heat to prostate tissue) can be used to alleviate symptoms of BPH. An advantage of this approach is that it can be administered on an outpatient basis using minimally invasive microwave or radio-frequency energy.
• Removal of excess tissue from an enlarged prostate via transurethral resection of the prostate (TURP) is the most common surgical treatment. A thin, lighted viewing tube is passed through the penis into the urethra. A minuscule cutting tool at the end of the tube is used to excise prostate tissue that is pressing upon the urethra.
• Surgical removal of obstructing prostate tissue via an abdominal incision may be necessary when the prostate is unusually large.

WHEN TO CALL A DOCTOR
• Call a doctor if you develop symptoms of BPH. █

Prostatitis

WHAT IS IT?

Prostatitis is an acute or chronic inflammation of the prostate, a walnut-size gland located just below the bladder in men, which produces about 30 percent of the fluid portion of semen. Inflammation may be caused by an infection. Acute prostatitis is characterized by the sudden onset of symptoms; chronic prostatitis causes persistent, long-term symptoms that are less severe. Chronic prostatitis may affect as many as 35 percent of men over age 50. An inflamed prostate may press upon the urethra and completely block the flow of urine. Additionally, if left untreated, acute prostatitis may lead to a prostate abscess, an infected, pus-filled cavity. Treatment for the acute and chronic forms of prostatitis may differ considerably.

SYMPTOMS

- Fever and chills (with acute prostatitis).
- Urinary difficulty, frequency, or urgency.
- Pain upon urination.
- Blood in the urine.
- Feeling of fullness in the bladder.
- Painful ejaculation, blood in the semen, or impotence (with chronic prostatitis).
- Pain in the pelvis or lower back.

WHAT CAUSES IT?

- The cause of prostatitis is unknown in almost all cases.
- Bacterial infection may cause about 5 percent of cases. Infection usually ascends through the urethra to the prostate. It may be transmitted sexually.
- The use of a urinary catheter increases the risk of prostatitis.
- Acute prostatitis may lead to chronic prostatitis in some cases.
- Risk of acute prostatitis is higher among men between the ages of 20 and 40 who have multiple sex partners and who practice high-risk behaviors such as anal intercourse or failure to use condoms.

PREVENTION

- Get prompt treatment for urinary tract infections.
- Use condoms to prevent the spread of sexually transmitted disease.

DIAGNOSIS

- Patient history and physical examination, which includes a digital rectal examination (DRE). In DRE the doctor inserts a gloved finger into the rectum to press on the prostate gland.
- Microscopic examination and culture of secretions expressed from the prostate during a DRE.
- Culture and microscopic analysis of urine.
- Ultrasound scans, which may be helpful in detecting an abscess.

HOW TO TREAT IT

- Hospitalization is often necessary to treat acute prostatitis. Intravenous antibiotics are given for bacterial infections, and a urinary catheter may be required to permit urination.
- Oral antibiotics are prescribed to treat acute and chronic prostatitis and should be taken for the full term prescribed (from four to 12 weeks).
- Caffeinated and alcoholic beverages should be avoided until symptoms subside, because the diuretic effect of these drinks increases urinary frequency.
- Warm baths may provide some relief from symptoms of chronic prostatitis.
- Over-the-counter analgesics may be taken as necessary to reduce pain and fever.
- If the prostate has become abscessed, surgical drainage is needed.
- Stress reduction techniques may be advised to help patients manage nonbacterial chronic prostatitis.

WHEN TO CALL A DOCTOR

- Call a doctor if you become unable to urinate or if you develop difficult or painful urination.

Psoriasis

WHAT IS IT?

Psoriasis is a common, persistent skin disorder, characterized by patches of raised, red bumps covered with white, flaking scales. It generally develops on the scalp, knees, or elbows, although it may affect any area of the skin. The production of skin cells at affected sites is accelerated, either chronically or intermittently. Normally, new skin cells are constantly produced in the deepest layer of skin. From there, they rise to the top layer—the epidermis—where dead surface cells are shed, a process that typically takes about 28 days. However, in areas affected by psoriasis, new cells only take three to four days to reach the skin's surface, and the accumulation of excess cells causes the characteristic scaly plaques.

Lesions may continue to enlarge slowly, or flare-ups of psoriasis may be separated by periods of remission. First attacks usually begin between the ages of 10 and 30. In rare cases psoriasis may cover the entire surface of the skin—see a dermatologist for immediate treatment. Although most cases of psoriasis can easily be controlled with treatment and do not represent a serious health risk, the disorder cannot be cured and may be itchy or occasionally painful and unpleasant to live with.

WHAT CAUSES IT?

- The cause of psoriasis is unknown.
- Hereditary factors may play a role.
- Flare-ups may be triggered by infection, alcohol, stress, cold temperatures, or skin injury. Certain medications (such as antimalarial drugs and lithium) or initiation and withdrawal of intravenous or oral corticosteroids may produce a severe flare-up of total body (erythrodermic) or pustular psoriasis, which are medical emergencies.

PREVENTION

- There is no known way to prevent psoriasis.
- Avoiding alcoholic beverages and limiting exposure to stress, cold temperatures, and skin injuries (such as cuts and scrapes) may prevent flare-ups of psoriasis.

DIAGNOSIS

- Diagnosis is generally made by viewing the skin.
- A skin biopsy may be needed to confirm diagnosis.

HOW TO TREAT IT

- Moisturizing skin creams can prevent dryness, particularly when applied immediately after bathing to retain the moisture absorbed by the skin.
- Prescription creams or ointments containing cortisone (such as triamcinolone, fluocinolone, and fluocinonide), vitamin D, and/or vitamin A derivatives may be used to clear or control the psoriasis lesions.
- Preparations and shampoos containing coal tar may soothe irritated skin.
- Physician-supervised phototherapy or photochemotherapy (PUVA, using the drug psoralen and UVA radiation) may be needed.
- In severe cases immunosuppressive or antiproliferative drugs such as methotrexate, acitretin, cyclosporine, or other medications may be used to clear or control the psoriasis.
- Check with your doctor regarding any prescriptions you may take for other conditions. Some medications that may worsen symptoms of psoriasis include lithium for bipolar disorder (see Bipolar Disorder) and antimalarial drugs. Ask your doctor about other drugs that may worsen psoriasis.
- Contact the National Psoriasis Foundation for information about support groups in your area.

WHEN TO CALL A DOCTOR

- Make an appointment with a doctor if symptoms do not respond to self-treatment.
- Call a doctor immediately if you suddenly develop widespread psoriasis, with or without fever, joint pain, and fatigue. ▲

SYMPTOMS

- Often itchy or painful patches of red, raised, quarter- to dollar-size plaques with silvery-white, flaking scales, commonly located on the scalp, knees, elbows, navel, or fold of the buttocks.
- Itching skin.
- Loosened, pitted, thickened, and/or discolored nails.
- Joint pain and stiffness (psoriatic arthritis).

Pulmonary Edema

WHAT IS IT?

Pulmonary edema, a medical emergency, is an accumulation of fluid in the lungs. Most often a consequence of congestive heart failure, pulmonary edema typically occurs when the heart is unable to pump blood out through the arteries as quickly as it is returned to the heart through the veins. Failure of the left side of the heart (left ventricle) causes blood to accumulate in the veins of the lungs (pulmonary veins), producing a dangerous rise in blood pressure within these veins. Sustained high pressure in the pulmonary veins eventually forces some fluid from the blood into the surrounding microscopic air sacs (alveoli), which transfer oxygen to the bloodstream. As the alveoli fill with fluid, they can no longer provide adequate amounts of oxygen to the body. Symptoms, especially severe breathing difficulty, develop over the course of a few hours and may be life-threatening. Although the outlook for pulmonary edema is favorable if the disorder is treated in a timely fashion, the overall outcome for the patient depends upon the nature of the underlying disorder. Adults at high risk for heart failure are most commonly affected.

A less common form of the disease, high-altitude pulmonary edema (which may occur while mountain-climbing, for instance), is also life-threatening if not treated quickly. Strenuous activity upon arrival at high altitudes may cause a dangerous rise in the pressure in the pulmonary veins, forcing fluid out of the veins into the alveoli. After people become acclimated to the altitude, strenuous activity does not pose such a risk. High-altitude pulmonary edema most often affects young adults under age 25 who are unacclimatized to the altitude but otherwise in good health. Symptoms appear within 24 to 72 hours and necessitate immediate descent to a lower altitude for treatment. (Air travelers are generally not at risk for this disorder because commercial airplane cabins are pressurized.)

WHAT CAUSES IT?

- Congestive heart failure due to high blood pressure, aortic or mitral valve disease, or cardiomyopathy is a common cause of pulmonary edema (see discussions of these disorders for more information).
- A heart attack may cause pulmonary edema.
- A variety of other conditions, such as lung infections, extensive burns, liver or kidney disease, Hodgkin's disease, pneumothorax, or nutritional deficiencies, may lead to pulmonary edema in some cases.
- Overdoses of heroin, morphine, and other narcotics may lead to pulmonary edema.
- Rapid ascent to high altitudes followed immediately by heavy exertion may cause high-altitude pulmonary edema.

PREVENTION

- To prevent heart disease, don't smoke; eat a low-fat, low-cholesterol diet; exercise regularly; and lose weight if you are overweight.
- Have your blood pressure and cholesterol checked.
- Allow a few days to adjust to a higher altitude before engaging in strenuous physical activity. If you have an existing heart condition, your doctor may alter your medication prior to a high-altitude trip.

DIAGNOSIS

- Patient history and examination of the chest is necessary.
- Blood samples are taken to measure oxygen and carbon dioxide content.
- A chest x-ray may be taken.
- An electrocardiogram (ECG) may be performed to identify a heart rhythm disturbance or evidence of a heart attack.

SYMPTOMS

- Severe breathing difficulty, including wheezing; rapid, shallow breathing; and a feeling of suffocation.
- Cough, dry at first, but later producing pink, frothy sputum.
- Fatigue.
- Profuse perspiration.
- Blue tinge to the nails, lips, or skin.
- Palpitations.
- Anxiety and restlessness.
- Loss of consciousness.

Pulmonary Edema *continued*

• An ultrasound test (echocardiogram) may be performed to evaluate the pumping function and thickness of the heart, and to evaluate the mitral and aortic valves.

• A stress test or angiogram (injection of a contrasting dye into the blood vessels to make them clearly visible on x-rays) may be performed to check for the presence of coronary artery disease or narrowed arteries.

HOW TO TREAT IT

• Call an ambulance or go to the nearest emergency room immediately. While waiting for an ambulance, sit upright. If possible, sit facing backward on an armless chair, with your raised arms resting on the chair back, to ease breathing.

• Pure oxygen is administered through a face mask or nasal tube or by an assisted positive pressure ventilator, which mechanically aids breathing.

• Morphine is given to relieve anxiety and to decrease the force of blood flow through the lungs.

• Diuretics, such as furosemide, bumetanide, or ethacrynic acid, are administered to promote excretion of excess fluids.

• Sodium nitroprusside or digoxin may be prescribed to dilate the arteries and strengthen the contractions of the heart muscle.

• Inhaled bronchodilating drugs, such as aminophylline, may be administered to relax constricted bronchial passages.

• It is imperative to return to a lower altitude immediately to obtain emergency medical care for high-altitude pulmonary edema. If possible, ask a ranger to call a helicopter if someone becomes too disabled to walk.

WHEN TO CALL A DOCTOR

• **EMERGENCY** Call an ambulance immediately if you develop symptoms of pulmonary edema.

• **EMERGENCY** Descend immediately to a lower altitude and call for emergency medical treatment if you develop high-altitude pulmonary edema. ▲

Pulmonary Embolism

WHAT IS IT?

A pulmonary embolism is a blood clot that travels through the veins to block a pulmonary artery, one of the vessels that carry blood to the lungs to be oxygenated. In most cases the blood clot (thrombus) originates in a leg vein, owing to a condition known as deep-vein thrombosis; the next most common sources are the right chambers of the heart. Part or all of a loosened thrombus may be carried into the pulmonary arteries. (Clumps of cancerous cells, fat, or bubbles of air in the bloodstream may also form emboli, although this is rare.) An embolus lodges in the main pulmonary artery or one of the smaller ones, cutting off the blood flow through the affected portion of the lungs.

Symptoms occur suddenly; severity depends on the size and number of emboli. The disorder may quickly turn fatal if a large enough portion of the lungs is affected by either one large embolus or many smaller ones. Approximately one case in 10 results in sudden death. The first hour of a pulmonary embolism is crucial, so emergency treatment should be sought immediately; patients who survive long enough to be hospitalized and diagnosed usually recover. In the United States over a half million cases of pulmonary embolism occur each year. Outlook is most favorable among younger patients. Pulmonary embolism affects significantly more women than men (in an approximately two-to-one ratio).

WHAT CAUSES IT?

• A blood clot dislodged from a leg vein is the most

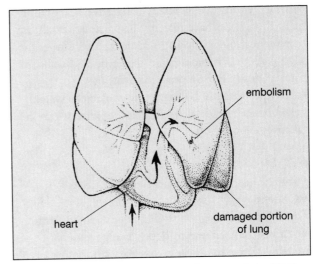

As the heart pumps blood into the lungs to be oxygenated, a blood clot carried in the bloodstream may lodge in a pulmonary artery.

common cause of pulmonary embolism.
• Rarely, an air bubble or a clump of cancerous cells, fat, bacteria, or other material may lodge in a pulmonary artery.
• Risk factors include pregnancy; recent surgery; previous heart attack or stroke; prolonged bed rest (for example, while recovering from an illness); obesity; smoking; bone fractures, especially of the hip or leg bones; cancer, especially of the lungs, breast, or liver; and family history of venous thrombosis, pulmonary embolism, or certain blood clotting disorders.
• People with heart disease, emphysema, or chronic bronchitis are at greater risk of severe consequences from pulmonary embolism (see Coronary Artery Disease or Chronic Obstructive Pulmonary Disease for more information).

PREVENTION

• Prescription elastic support hose may be worn to prevent deep-vein thrombosis in the legs among those at risk. Try not to cross the legs when sitting, as this promotes thrombus development.
• Regular doses of aspirin may be prescribed to prevent the development of blood clots for those at high risk.
• Heparin, an anticoagulant, may be administered in low, continuous doses to decrease the possibility of blood clots in people at risk (for example, those with

---

SYMPTOMS
• Sudden shortness of breath.
• Sudden onset of chest pain, which is usually sharp and made worse by taking a deep breath.
• Cough, possibly with bloody sputum.
• Profuse perspiration.
• Anxiety.
• Palpitations or rapid heartbeat.
• Lightheadedness.
• Emergency symptom: loss of consciousness.

Pulmonary Embolism *continued*

chronic venous insufficiency, congestive heart failure, or in those who have recently had a heart attack) or in people about to undergo surgery. After surgery, such patients are encouraged to get up and walk as soon as possible to improve circulation.
• Another form of heparin, low-molecular weight heparin, may be an alternative to heparin. It can be taken intermittently.

DIAGNOSIS
• Patient history and physical examination.
• Chest x-ray.
• An electrocardiogram (ECG) is performed to rule out a heart attack and to detect evidence of increased pressure in the pulmonary arteries or of other serious cardiovascular conditions.
• Radionuclide scanning, which involves inhaling a small amount of radioactive gas and injection of radioactive particles into the bloodstream, may highlight blocked portions of the blood vessels in the lungs on an x-ray scan.
• Pulmonary arteriography (injection of a contrast dye into the pulmonary arteries prior to taking a series of x-rays) is the only certain way to identify pulmonary embolism and thus establish a definitive diagnosis.

HOW TO TREAT IT
• Anticoagulant drugs, like heparin and warfarin, are administered to prevent further blood clots.
• Thrombolytic (clot dissolving) medications such as tPA (tissue plasminogen activator), streptokinase, or urokinase may be injected into the bloodstream to clear the blockage.
• Analgesics are given to relieve pain.
• Oxygen may be administered via an oxygen mask or, in severe cases, a respirator.
• Emergency treatment is necessary for a suspected pulmonary embolism. Immediate surgical removal may be required when a large embolus is blocking a major pulmonary artery.

WHEN TO CALL A DOCTOR
• **EMERGENCY** Call an ambulance immediately if you or someone in your presence develops sudden, severe chest pain and shortness of breath, along with feelings of great apprehension or dread. In addition to pulmonary embolism, such symptoms may also be indications of a heart attack or other serious cardiovascular crisis.
• **EMERGENCY** Call an ambulance immediately any time someone unexpectedly loses consciousness. ▲

Rabies Hydrophobia

WHAT IS IT?

Rabies is a severe viral infection of the brain that primarily affects animals. Raccoons, skunks, bats, foxes, and other mammals may be rabid; domestic dogs and cats can also become infected. Rabies may be transferred to humans through the saliva of an infected animal, usually by a bite, although the virus can also enter the bloodstream via a lick over broken skin. The rabies virus travels to the brain and attacks the central nervous system. Rabies is fatal in humans unless measures are taken right away to prevent the disease from developing, so if you are bitten by an animal, see a doctor immediately. Do not wait to see if rabies develops—once symptoms appear, the course of the disease is irreversible despite treatment, and death occurs within a few days. Symptoms most often emerge in four to eight weeks, but anywhere from 10 days to six months may lapse between the bite and the appearance of symptoms. Treatment consists of a series of vaccines and is effective only if administered in time.

WHAT CAUSES IT?

• Rabies virus infection causes rabies.

PREVENTION

• Immunize pets against rabies. Human rabies is rare in the United States, thanks to extensive animal-vaccination programs. Rabies in wild animals, such as raccoons, skunks, and bats, remains a problem.
• People at high risk (veterinarians and other animal handlers, hunters, cave explorers, and people planning to live in developing countries where rabies is prevalent) should get an annual rabies vaccine.
• Stray animals in areas where rabies is common are often killed by local authorities to prevent the spread of the disease.
• A quarantine is imposed on imported animals in countries where rabies is not present, including England, Japan, and Australia.

DIAGNOSIS

• Patient history and physical examination.
• Biopsy of nerve tissue.
• Every effort should be made to capture the animal inflicting a bite so that its brain can be tested for the presence of the virus. Healthy-appearing domestic animals are kept under observation for 10 days to watch for any behavioral abnormalities.

HOW TO TREAT IT

• Call a doctor immediately if bitten by an animal.
• Wash the wound gently but thoroughly with soap and water and then apply antiseptic.
• Immunization within two days of a bite usually halts the disease from developing. Two types of immunization are necessary: a passive immunization provides antibodies for immediate protection against the rabies virus; the active vaccine provokes the production of antiviral antibodies for long-term protection against the virus. The passive vaccine is injected around the wound as well as into a muscle. The active vaccine is given in a series of injections. People who have already received the active vaccine need only receive the passive one for treatment.
• Antibiotics and a tetanus booster shot may be given to prevent associated bacterial infections.
• Hospitalization is necessary if symptoms appear; however, the outlook is unfavorable at this point.

WHEN TO CALL A DOCTOR

• **EMERGENCY** See a doctor immediately if you have been bitten by an animal; do not wait for symptoms of rabies to appear. 🔱

SYMPTOMS

• Initial symptoms: fever, muscle aches, headaches, general sense of illness, loss of appetite, difficulty swallowing, tingling and muscle twitches at the site of the bite.
• Violent muscle spasms provoked by swallowing liquids (hence the name hydrophobia).
• Agitation and violent behavior. Periods of rage alternate with periods of calmness, but lucid periods quickly become shorter and less frequent as the disease progresses.
• Drooling due to excessive salivation and difficulty swallowing.
• Mental confusion.
• Seizures, paralysis, and coma.

Refractive Disorders

WHAT IS IT?

Refractive disorders—which include myopia (near-sightedness), hyperopia (farsightedness), and astigmatism—are common, correctable vision problems. Light enters the eye through the cornea, the thin, transparent membrane covering the eye, and then the pupil, the dark area in the center of the iris. The lens, located behind the pupil, focuses the light rays onto the retina, the layer of light-sensitive cells that line the back of the eye. Refractive disorders arise when irregularities in the shape or refractive strength of these structures distort the focus and impair vision. In myopia, objects at a distance appear out of focus; in hyperopia, nearby objects are unclear. In astigmatism, the cornea is unevenly curved, producing blurriness or varying degrees of distortion in portions of the visual field. Astigmatism may be combined with either myopia or hyperopia in the same eye. In addition, the lens becomes progressively less flexible after age 40, impairing close vision (see Presbyopia). Refractive disorders may be corrected with glasses, contact lenses, or laser surgery.

WHAT CAUSES IT?

• Hereditary factors play a role.

PREVENTION

• Contrary to popular belief, vision cannot be improved by refusing to wear glasses if you need them or by performing so-called eye exercises.
• Wear goggles to protect your eyes or a sports strap to secure glasses during sports and strenuous activities.

DIAGNOSIS

• An ophthalmologist will perform an eye examination and determine your eyeglass measurement.

SYMPTOMS
• Blurred vision at a distance (myopia).
• Blurred vision of nearby objects and difficulty reading, possibly causing eyestrain and headaches (hyperopia).
• Uneven degrees of blurriness in portions of the visual field (astigmatism).

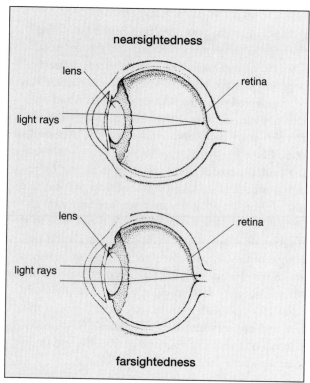

In nearsightedness (myopia), light is focused at a point just short of the retina; in farsightedness (hyperopia), just beyond the retina.

HOW TO TREAT IT

• Glasses or contact lenses are prescribed to correct vision. The prescription is updated as vision changes.
• Two types of laser surgery have been developed to sharpen vision: PRK (photorefractive keratectomy) and LASIK (laser-assisted in-situ keratomileusis). They use a special machine known as an excimer laser to produce pulses of light energy that can alter the shape of the cornea so that light rays from distant objects will focus on the retina with greater precision. Both procedures can be performed to correct myopia, hyperopia, astigmatism, and presbyopia. An older form of surgery, known as radial keratotomy (RK), which helps correct mild to moderate myopia, is now used infrequently.

WHEN TO CALL A DOCTOR

• Make an appointment with an ophthalmologist or optometrist if you or a child has vision problems.

Renal Artery Stenosis

WHAT IS IT?

Renal artery stenosis is a blockage of one of the arteries that supply blood to the kidneys. When the renal artery or one of its branches is blocked, the blood supply to the kidney is partially or completely cut off; the affected kidney tissue may be damaged irreversibly. The unaffected kidney compensates for the decrease in function of the other one. Sudden total occlusion of a renal artery may cause acute onset of vague pain in the flanks, blood in the urine, nausea, and vomiting. These symptoms generally disappear in three to four days. More often, renal artery stenosis has no symptoms. Its most common indication is high blood pressure that responds poorly to regular treatment measures. Although chronic kidney failure may be a possibility if both kidneys are affected (or if someone has only one kidney), in many cases blockage may be reduced or eliminated with treatment, and kidney function may improve.

WHAT CAUSES IT?

• The buildup of plaque in the arteries (atherosclerosis) is the most common cause of renal artery stenosis. It occurs when a piece of plaque breaks off of an artery wall and travels to the kidney.
• An inherited disorder called fibromuscular dysplasia causes abnormal thickening of the arterial walls and may thus block the renal artery. This disorder primarily affects women between ages 20 and 40.

PREVENTION

• Maintaining a healthy weight, diet, and lifestyle to avoid the buildup of plaque in the arteries may help to prevent renal artery stenosis.

SYMPTOMS

• Usually no symptoms. Renal artery stenosis is typically detected only when a physical examination reveals high blood pressure (also symptomless), and further tests are performed to determine the underlying cause.
• Dull flank pain, blood in urine, nausea, and vomiting may occur for a few days if sudden total occlusion of a renal artery occurs.

DIAGNOSIS

• Patient history and physical examination.
• Urine and blood samples.
• Renal artery occlusion is suspected when blood pressure is unusually high, particularly hard to control, or rises suddenly in a person with previously normal blood pressure. Under such circumstances the tests described below may be done.
• An x-ray of the kidney may be taken after injection with a material that creates a clear image of the kidneys (intravenous pyelogram).
• A similar procedure, renal arteriography, allows the exact location of the blockage to be determined.
• Ultrasound, CT (computed tomography) scans, or MRI (magnetic resonance imaging) may be done.

HOW TO TREAT IT

• Fibrinolytic (clot-dissolving) therapy may be administered to break up the artery-blocking clot.
• Percutaneous transluminal angioplasty, in which a tiny balloon on the tip of a catheter is threaded through the artery, may be performed. At the narrowed or blocked point, the balloon is inflated to widen the passageway. If this fails, the surgeon may insert a stent (a hollow rodlike device) at the location of the blockage to help keep the artery open.
• Antihypertensive drugs may be needed to lower associated high blood pressure.
• Surgery may be performed to remove or bypass an extensive or calcified (hardened) blockage. In cases of severe arterial wall damage, tissue from an artery elsewhere in the body is grafted onto the renal artery.
• Long-term administration of anticoagulant drugs may be prescribed to prevent future blood clots.

WHEN TO CALL A DOCTOR

• Call a doctor immediately if you notice a decrease in urine output (an indication of kidney failure) or if you develop lower back pain accompanied by nausea, vomiting, and possibly fever (indications of kidney tissue death due to sudden blockage of a renal artery).

Renal Calculi Kidney Stones

WHAT IS IT?

Renal calculi, also known as kidney stones, form when substances (such as calcium oxalate) in the urine concentrate and coalesce into hard, solid lumps in the kidney. Calcium-containing stones account for about 70 to 80 percent of renal calculi (most of these consist of calcium oxalate or calcium phosphate). Other stones are composed of uric acid or magnesium, ammonium, and phosphate.

During the production of urine, the two kidneys regulate the fluid and electrolyte balance in the body and filter wastes out of the blood. Urine collects in the portion of the kidney known as the renal pelvis; the urine then passes from the kidney to the bladder via a narrow tube called the ureter. Kidney stones may form in the renal pelvis, then pass through the ureter into the bladder before they are eliminated from the body with the urine. Some stones are so small that they cause no symptoms and pass painlessly on their own; large stones may never leave the kidney and can be detected only if an abdominal x-ray is taken for other reasons.

Sometimes, however, a stone enters the ureter and produces intermittent severe pain (known as renal colic) that continues until the stone has reached the bladder; this process may take a few hours or up to several days. The pain of a single attack is usually felt on only one side of the body; however, stones may

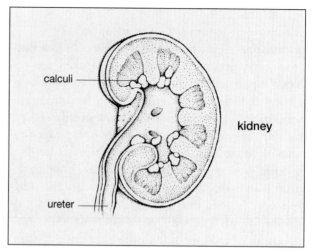

Renal calculi can cause substantial pain if they become lodged in the ureter. Most kidney stones pass spontaneously.

recur or develop in the other kidney, causing pain on that side. Symptoms subside once the stone is passed. Recurrence is common, and treatment is aimed at relieving symptoms, dissolving or removing existing stones, and preventing recurrence. Kidney stones are common, especially among young and middle-aged people, particularly men.

WHAT CAUSES IT?

All stones:
- Mild, persistent dehydration concentrates the urine and may lead to stone formation.
- Hereditary factors may be associated with stone formation.
- In some cases the cause of kidney stones is unknown.

Calcium stones:
- The most common cause of calcium-containing kidney stones is increased calcium in the urine (hypercalciuria). Most patients have unexplained excessive absorption of calcium from the intestine.
- High blood calcium levels (for example, from hyperparathyroidism or vitamin D intoxication) lead to hypercalciuria and kidney stones.
- Irritable bowel disease, Crohn's disease, a diet high in oxalic acid (found in rhubarb, spinach, leafy vegetables, and coffee), or severe dietary calcium restriction increases the excretion of oxalate in the urine and raises the risk of calcium oxalate stones.

SYMPTOMS

- Intermittent pain, sometimes excruciating, beginning in the lower back below the ribs and traveling downward through the lower abdomen to the groin. Men may experience pain in the testes and penis as the stone passes.
- Interruption of the urine stream, inability to urinate except in certain positions, frequent urge to urinate but with only small amounts of urine passed.
- Bloody, cloudy, or darkened urine.
- Nausea and vomiting.
- Burning upon urination; fever (due to an associated bacterial infection—see Kidney Infection for more information).

Renal Calculi Kidney Stones *continued*

Magnesium-ammonium-phosphate stones:
• Urinary tract infections involving certain bacteria that break down urea may create a chemical environment conducive to kidney stone development. Urea is made into ammonium and the urine is made alkaline, which may lead to magnesium-ammonium-phosphate stones.

Uric acid stones:
• Excessively acidic urine is the most common cause of uric acid stones. High uric acid levels in the urine, sometimes associated with symptoms of gout, may also lead to their formation (see Gout).

PREVENTION
• Drink at least eight to 10 cups of water a day, and eat a healthy, well-balanced diet.
• Dietary changes may be advised to prevent recurrence. Specific changes—such as avoiding sodium, animal protein, and foods containing high amounts of oxalic acid (found in rhubarb, spinach, leafy vegetables, and coffee)—will depend on the type of kidney stone involved.
• It is important to note that severe dietary calcium restriction is discouraged.
• Medications such as thiazide diuretics, phosphate-based compounds, allopurinol, sodium or potassium citrate, or large doses of calcium or magnesium may be administered to help prevent recurrence of stones. The type of medication varies according to the exact composition of the stone.
• An effort is made to decrease urine acidity in those with uric acid stones.

DIAGNOSIS
• Patient history and physical examination.
• A blood sample to measure calcium and uric acid levels.
• Urine culture and examination for cells and crystals.
• In cases when stones recur, your doctor may ask you to collect urine over a 24-hour period in order to measure the amount of calcium, sodium, oxalate, citrate, uric acid, sulfate, or urea nitrogen volume.
• Abdominal x-rays, following injection of an iodine-based dye into the kidneys (pyelography).
• Laboratory analysis of the chemical content of any stone that is passed and captured.

HOW TO TREAT IT
• To encourage a small stone to pass, drink at least three liters of water daily to flush the stone into the bladder. Urinate through a piece of gauze or filter to trap the stone when it passes, so it can be analyzed.
• Over-the-counter pain relievers in moderation are recommended.
• Antibiotics may be prescribed to treat an associated bacterial infection.
• In more severe cases hospitalization may be advised, and narcotic painkillers are prescribed to relieve pain.
• Antispasmodic drugs may be prescribed to help the ureter muscles relax and ease passing of the stone.
• Larger stones can be pulverized with a treatment called extracorporeal shock-wave lithotripsy, which aims concentrated bursts of sound waves at the stones. The tiny fragments then pass into the bladder and are excreted.
• Abdominal surgery may be performed to remove the stone.
• Surgery to remove an overactive parathyroid gland may be performed in cases where stones have resulted from hyperparathyroidism.
• Surgery to remove the kidney may be required in advanced cases that do not respond to other forms of treatment. Only one kidney is necessary for normal body function; if a diseased kidney is removed, the remaining one compensates for the loss.

WHEN TO CALL A DOCTOR
• Call a doctor if you develop symptoms of kidney stones.

Renal Failure, Acute

WHAT IS IT?

Acute renal failure—or kidney failure—occurs when both kidneys suddenly stop functioning. The kidneys regulate the chemical and fluid balance in the body and filter waste products out of the blood and into the urine. Acute renal failure may occur via a number of different mechanisms, including kidney disorders, partial or complete blockage of the passage of urine, and a decrease in the blood volume, following severe blood loss for example. Symptoms may develop over several days: the amount of urine passed may be greatly reduced, and fluid that should be excreted accumulates in bodily tissues, producing weight gain and swelling, especially in the ankles.

Acute renal failure is a life-threatening condition, as excessive amounts of water, minerals like potassium, and waste products, all normally eliminated in the urine by the kidneys, accumulate in the body. The disorder usually responds well to treatment; kidney function may be fully regained within several months after normal blood volume is restored or an obstruction to urine flow is released. However, acute renal failure due to a kidney disorder may occasionally progress to chronic renal failure, and the long-term outlook ultimately depends upon the response of the underlying disorder to treatment.

WHAT CAUSES IT?

- Depletion of blood volume from severe injury with associated blood loss or dehydration is a common cause of acute renal failure. Reduced blood flow to the kidneys due to diminished blood volume may damage the kidneys.
- Other kidney disorders, such as acute glomerulonephritis, may cause acute renal failure (see Glomerulonephritis, Acute for more information).
- Tumors, kidney stones, or an enlarged prostate gland may obstruct both ureters or the urethra, impeding urine flow and damaging the kidneys.
- Other disorders may cause the kidneys to fail, including polycystic kidney disease, systemic lupus erythematosus, diabetes mellitus, congestive heart failure, heart attack, liver disease, acute pancreatitis, and multiple myeloma (see specific disorders for more information).
- Poisoning with heavy metals such as cadmium, lead, mercury, or gold may lead to kidney damage.
- Chemotherapeutic agents and certain antibiotics such as streptomycin may lead to kidney failure, especially in those with underlying kidney disease.
- Long-term high doses of nonsteroidal anti-inflammatory drugs (NSAIDs), such as ibuprofen and naproxen, may cause kidney damage.
- The radiographic contrast materials used to highlight blood vessels or organs in some x-ray procedures may induce kidney failure in those at higher risk.
- The release of the protein myoglobin from the muscles because of muscle injury, heat stroke, drug or alcohol overdose, or severe infection may lead to acute kidney failure.
- Those who have had one kidney removed are more vulnerable to severe complications of kidney damage.
- Rarely, women may develop acute renal failure as a complication of childbirth.

PREVENTION

- Treatment of potential underlying causes may prevent acute renal failure.

DIAGNOSIS

- Patient history and physical examination.
- Ultrasound scans.
- Blood and urine tests.
- An x-ray of the kidney may be taken after injec-

SYMPTOMS

- Passing only small amounts of urine.
- Weight gain and swelling of the ankles and face, due to fluid accumulation (edema).
- Loss of appetite.
- Nausea and vomiting.
- Widespread itching.
- Fatigue.
- Late stage symptoms if renal failure is not treated successfully: shortness of breath, due to fluid in the lungs; unexplained bruising or bleeding; drowsiness; mental confusion; muscle spasms or seizures; loss of consciousness.

Renal Failure, Acute   *continued*

tion with a contrasting dye (intravenous pyelogram) to locate an obstruction to urine flow.

• A kidney biopsy may be done. After local anesthesia is administered to the patient, the doctor inserts a needle into the kidney through the back to extract a small sample of tissue for microscopic examination.

HOW TO TREAT IT

• The underlying cause of kidney failure must be treated. Emergency medical treatment may be necessary in the event of severe injury and may include surgery to repair damaged tissues, intravenous fluids to reverse dehydration, and blood transfusion to replace extensive blood loss.

• Surgery may be necessary to remove an obstruction of the urinary tract.

• Diuretics may be prescribed to reduce fluid retention and increase urine output.

• There are a number of postemergency measures that are important to a full recovery. A low-salt, low-protein, high-carbohydrate diet, vitamin supplementation, and restriction of fluid intake may all be recommended.

• Antibiotics may be prescribed to treat associated bacterial infections and should be taken for the full term indicated.

• Antihypertensive drugs may be prescribed to treat associated high blood pressure.

• Glucose, sodium bicarbonate, and other substances may be given intravenously until kidney function is regained, in order to maintain proper levels of these substances in the bloodstream.

• Temporary dialysis, an artificial blood-filtering process, may be necessary until kidney function is regained. There are several types of dialysis. In hemodialysis, blood is pumped from the body into an artificial kidney machine, or dialyzer, where it is filtered before being returned to the body. Hemodialysis is usually performed for about nine hours weekly (typically in three sessions), but may be required daily.

• Peritoneal dialysis is another option. In this procedure a catheter is inserted into the abdomen, and a special fluid, known as dialysate, is circulated through the peritoneum, the membrane lining the abdominal cavity, to draw impurities out of the bloodstream. Peritoneal dialysis must be performed for a total of 30 to 40 hours per week; however, indwelling catheters make it possible for the patient to move about during dialysis. (See Renal Failure, Chronic for more information.)

• Contact your local chapter of the National Kidney Foundation for more information.

WHEN TO CALL A DOCTOR

• **EMERGENCY** Call a doctor immediately if you develop symptoms of acute renal failure, including decreased urine output, nausea, shortness of breath, and swollen ankles. ⚕

Renal Failure, Chronic

WHAT IS IT?

Chronic renal, or kidney, failure occurs when both kidneys gradually cease to function. Within the kidneys are numerous tiny structures (glomeruli) that filter waste products from the blood and retain larger substances, such as proteins. Waste products and excess water then accumulate in the bladder until excreted as urine. In chronic kidney failure, the kidneys suffer progressive damage over a number of months or years. As kidney tissue is destroyed by injury or inflammation, the remaining healthy tissue compensates for the loss of function. The extra work overloads the previously undamaged portions of the kidneys, causing more damage, until eventually the entire kidney may cease to function (a condition known as end-stage renal failure).

The kidneys are resilient organs; over 80 percent of the kidneys may be damaged before symptoms appear (although symptoms may develop earlier if the weakened kidney is subjected to a sudden stress, such as an infection, dehydration, or use of a kidney-damaging drug). As excessive amounts of water, minerals like potassium, and waste products accumulate in the body, chronic renal failure becomes a life-threatening condition. However, if the underlying disease is treated and further damage can be controlled, the onset of end-stage renal failure may be delayed for up to 10 to 20 years. End-stage renal failure may be treated with dialysis or kidney transplantation; either can prolong life and allow participation in many normal activities.

WHAT CAUSES IT?

• Diabetes mellitus and hypertension are the most common causes of chronic renal failure.
• Primary kidney disorders, such as acute and chronic glomerulonephritis, polycystic kidney disease, and kidney infection, may lead to chronic renal failure (see specific disorders for more information).
• High blood pressure can both cause and be caused by progressive damage to the kidneys.
• Tumors, kidney stones, or an enlarged prostate gland may obstruct the urinary tract, impair the flow of urine, and thus damage the kidneys.
• Long-term use of large doses of nonsteroidal anti-inflammatory drugs (NSAIDs), such as ibuprofen or naproxen, may lead to chronic renal failure.
• Poisoning with heavy metals like cadmium, lead, mercury, or gold may lead to kidney failure.
• Certain antibiotics (like streptomycin), antifungal drugs, and immunosuppressants may damage the kidney and lead to kidney failure.
• The contrast substances used in some x-ray procedures may induce kidney failure in those with weakened kidneys.
• Kidneys damaged by any disorder are more prone to chronic infection.
• Hypercalcemia (excess blood levels of calcium, from hyperthyroidism for example) and elevated levels of uric acid may lead to chronic renal failure.
• Those who have had one kidney removed are more vulnerable to severe complications from kidney damage.

PREVENTION

• Treatment of potential underlying causes (especially drug therapy for high blood pressure and scrupulous control of diabetes) may prevent or delay development of chronic renal failure.

SYMPTOMS

• Frequent urination; passing only small amounts of urine.
• General feeling of poor health.
• Symptoms of end-stage renal failure due to the accumulation of waste products in the blood (uremia): swelling of the ankles or the tissues around the eyes, due to fluid retention (edema); shortness of breath, due to fluid accumulation in the lungs; nausea and vomiting; loss of appetite and weight loss; frequent hiccups; bad breath; furred tongue; pain in the chest and bones; overall itching; yellowish or brownish tinge to pale skin; tiny white crystals upon the skin (uremic frost); unexplained bruising or bleeding, including bleeding gums; cessation of menstrual periods in women (amenorrhea); fatigue and drowsiness; mental confusion; muscle spasms or seizures; loss of consciousness.

Renal Failure, Chronic *continued*

DIAGNOSIS

- Patient history and physical examination.
- Blood and urine tests.
- Ultrasound or CT (computed tomography) scans, or MRI (magnetic resonance imaging) of the abdominal area.
- A kidney biopsy may be done. After local anesthesia is administered to the patient, the doctor inserts a needle into the kidney through the back to extract a small sample of tissue for microscopic examination.

HOW TO TREAT IT

- A low-salt, low-protein, high-carbohydrate diet, restricted fluid intake, and vitamin supplements may be recommended.
- Surgery may be necessary to remove an obstruction in the urinary tract.
- Antibiotics may be prescribed to treat associated bacterial infections.
- Antihypertensive drugs are prescribed to control associated high blood pressure.
- Medications may be needed to treat congestive heart failure.
- Anemia can be treated with erythropoietin, which stimulates blood cell formation.
- Sodium bicarbonate or calcium carbonate is administered to treat the excessive accumulation of body acids (renal acidosis).
- Phosphate-binding agents, calcium supplements, and vitamin D are given to prevent secondary hyperparathyroidism, which may produce further kidney damage.
- Dialysis, an artificial blood-filtering process, is necessary once a significant portion of kidney function has been lost. There are several types of dialysis. In hemodialysis, blood is pumped from the body into an artificial kidney machine, or dialyzer, where it is filtered before being returned to the body. Hemodialysis must be performed for about nine to 12 hours weekly (usually in three sessions).
- Peritoneal dialysis is another option. There are two types of peritoneal dialysis: CAPD and APD. CAPD (continuous ambulatory peritoneal dialysis) requires the patient or caregiver to instill two to three liters of a sterile solution through a catheter into the peritoneum three to five times a day, seven days a week. APD (automated peritoneal dialysis) utilizes a small machine the size of a personal computer to automatically instill the sterile fluid through the catheter into the peritoneum while the patient sleeps. This process generally takes about 12 hours a day.
- A kidney transplant offers the best alternative to dialysis in cases of end-stage renal failure. Successful transplantation may cure kidney failure, but potential donors must be matched carefully for compatibility; family members of the patient are most likely to be compatible, but spouses and friends who wish to donate should also be screened. Recipients of a kidney transplant must remain on immunosuppressive drugs to prevent rejection of the transplant.
- Contact your local chapter of the National Kidney Foundation for information about support groups.

WHEN TO CALL A DOCTOR

- **EMERGENCY** Call a doctor if you experience frequent urination, nausea and vomiting, swelling around the ankles, shortness of breath, a yellowish tinge to the skin, or any other symptoms of chronic renal failure.

Renal Vein Thrombosis

WHAT IS IT?

Renal vein thrombosis (RVT), an uncommon disorder, is a blood clot in one or both of the veins that carries blood from the kidneys back to the heart. In infants, the condition may occur suddenly and result in kidney failure and severe acute illness. In adults, the condition may produce no symptoms. In many cases part of the blood clot may separate from the renal vein and lodge in a pulmonary artery, where the clot, known as an embolism, may produce symptoms of chest pain and shortness of breath (see Pulmonary Embolism for more information). In many cases RVT subsides spontaneously over time.

WHAT CAUSES IT?

• In adults, renal vein thrombosis is almost always a result of some underlying illness, most commonly nephrotic syndrome (see Nephrotic Syndrome for more information).
• Diarrhea with severe dehydration is the most common cause in children.
• An injury to the abdomen or lower back may result in RVT.
• Malignant kidney tumors that extend into the renal vein can lead to RVT.
• Pregnancy or the use of oral contraceptives increases the risk.

PREVENTION

• There is no known way to prevent renal vein thrombosis. Some doctors may recommend preventive use of anticoagulant drugs (such as warfarin) in high-risk individuals.

SYMPTOMS
• In adults, there are often no symptoms as the clot develops slowly.
• Pain, usually mild, in the lower back and side. There may be visible blood in the urine.
• In infants: fever and chills; blood in the urine.
• Chest pain, shortness of breath, cough, possibly with bloody sputum, profuse perspiration, anxiety, and palpitations, due to associated pulmonary emboli.

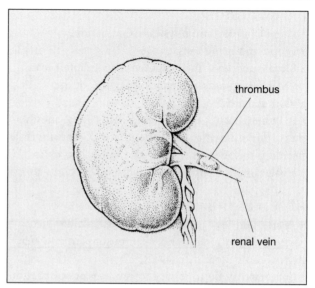

Blood is filtered in the kidneys, then returns to the heart via the renal veins. A thrombus (blood clot) lodged in a renal vein impedes this flow.

DIAGNOSIS

• Patient history and physical examination.
• Urine sample.
• Renal venography (injection of a contrast material into the renal vein prior to x-rays), ultrasound scans, CT (computed tomography) scans, or MRI (magnetic resonance imaging) may be performed to locate a blood clot.

HOW TO TREAT IT

• Streptokinase or urokinase (enzymes) may be administered to dissolve blood clots in severe cases of renal vein thrombosis of both renal veins associated with acute kidney failure.
• Anticoagulant medications may be prescribed on a long-term basis to reduce the risk of a pulmonary embolus.
• In infants with life-threatening cases, surgical removal of the affected kidney may be required.

WHEN TO CALL A DOCTOR

• Call a doctor if you develop nagging, persistent pain in the lower back or side, or if you experience shortness of breath and chest pain. ▲

Restless Legs Syndrome

WHAT IS IT?

Restless legs syndrome has been characterized as "an unusual, almost indescribable sensation" deep within the leg that leaves its sufferers with an irresistible urge to move their legs for relief. The sensation is usually reported as uncomfortable, but occasionally it may be painful. The arms, shoulders, or torso are also sometimes affected. Worse at night, the condition may keep patients from falling asleep or cause them to awaken from sleep.

Symptoms come on with rest and are relieved with walking. Sufferers find that the only way to ease the sensation is to kick their legs or get up and walk around, making it a common underlying cause of insomnia. Restless legs syndrome affects between 2 and 5 percent of the general population. Although the syndrome can occur in all age groups, its incidence seems to increase with age. The condition, though unpleasant and annoying, does not constitute a major health risk, nor is it an early warning sign of a more serious neuromuscular disorder such as Parkinson's disease.

WHAT CAUSES IT?

• The exact cause of restless legs syndrome is unknown, but some studies suggest the symptoms are related to low levels of the neurotransmitter dopamine in the brain.
• Hereditary factors may play a role.
• Emotional stress or regular use of caffeine, antihistamines, or tobacco may trigger or worsen symptoms.

SYMPTOMS

• An uncomfortable sensation deep within one or both legs, often worse at night and relieved by walking.
• Irresistible urge to move the legs (or other affected muscles).
• Involuntary jerking movements of the legs if the person does not voluntarily move them. Such leg movement may occur during sleep as well.
• Insomnia caused by a worsening of symptoms during the night.

• It is associated with iron deficiency anemia, pregnancy, dialysis, and peripheral neuropathy (see Anemia, Iron Deficiency and Peripheral Neuropathies for more information).

PREVENTION

• There is no way to prevent restless legs syndrome.

DIAGNOSIS

• Diagnosis is based upon the symptoms.
• A polysomnagram may be conducted to study sleep behavior if symptoms occur only during sleep.
• Physical examination may be performed to rule out other disorders such as neuropathy, myopathy, or arthropathy.
• Blood tests to measure iron levels may be conducted.

HOW TO TREAT IT

• Although some nondrug therapies are outlined below, the only consistently successful treatments are with medications.
• Walk around for 10 to 15 minutes prior to going to bed, to stretch the leg muscles and promote restful sleep. Contracting, massaging, or keeping the leg muscles warm before going to bed may relieve symptoms.
• Many medications appear to be effective: the dopamine-related medications (such as levodopa, pergolide, pramipexole, and ropinirole), analgesics (such as codeine, propoxyphene, and tramadol), clonazepam, and gabapentin.
• Antipsychotic medications (neuroleptics), antiemetics (nausea preventives), and antidepressants may aggravate the symptoms, as may long-term use of levodopa (see your doctor for an alternative).
• Some cases caused by iron deficiency may respond to iron supplements, but these should not be taken without your doctor's guidance.

WHEN TO CALL A DOCTOR

• Make an appointment with a doctor if restless legs symptoms interfere with sleep. ▲

Retinal Detachment

WHAT IS IT?

Retinal detachment is a vision-threatening condition that results when the retina, the layer of light-sensitive cells lining the back surface of the eye, becomes separated from the back wall of the eye, which contains blood vessels that nourish the retina. The retina is also attached in places to the vitreous humor, a transparent, jellylike substance that fills the eye. In many cases detachment follows a small tear or hole in the retina, which occurs when there is age-related shrinkage or degeneration of the vitreous humor that causes part of it to pull away from the retina. As this detachment of the vitreous humor occurs, the retina may tear at points where the retina and vitreous meet. Once a tear forms, vitreous humor seeps between the retina and the back wall of the eye, causing a progressively larger area of detachment over a period of hours or days. The retina must be reattached as soon as possible to minimize or prevent permanent vision loss in the affected eye.

WHAT CAUSES IT?

- Eye injury may tear the retina.
- The risk of spontaneous retinal detachment increases with age.
- Hereditary factors may play a role.
- A disease called cytomegalovirus retinitis, common among AIDS patients, may cause retinal detachment.
- Those with severe myopia (nearsightedness), tumors or inflammation in or around the eye, diabetes mellitus, or a family history of retinal detachment are at greater risk.
- Cataract surgery may increase risk.

PREVENTION

- Regular eye examinations may aid in early detection.
- Use protective gear, such as goggles or helmets

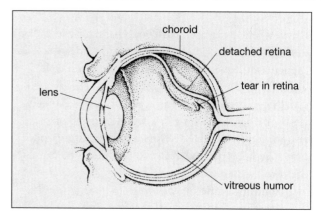

If the retina becomes detached from the choroid (the thin, blood-vessel-rich membrane surrounding the eye), vitreous humor may seep in and behind the retina and cause further detachment.

with face shields, during vigorous activities like motorcycling or racquet sports.

DIAGNOSIS

- Eye examination by an ophthalmologist.
- Ultrasound scans or fluorescein angiography (injection of a special dye into the bloodstream that allows clear photographic images to be taken of the blood vessels in the eye) may be necessary.

HOW TO TREAT IT

- In some cases the retina may be reattached by laser surgery or cryosurgery (use of liquid nitrogen to freeze the targeted tissue) and sometimes by the installation of a gas bubble into the eye. These procedures produce scarring around the edges of the retinal tear, sealing it into place.
- In cases of more severe detachment, more complex surgical procedures may be necessary.
- Medicated eyedrops and ointments may be prescribed to aid healing following surgery.
- A silicone-based oil can be injected into the eye to hold the retina in place; this treatment is reserved for the most complicated cases that have failed to be corrected by standard surgery.

WHEN TO CALL A DOCTOR

- **EMERGENCY** See an ophthalmologist immediately if you develop sudden symptoms of flashing lights, black spots in the field of vision, or visual loss. ▲

SYMPTOMS

- Sudden appearance of floating spots or flashes of light in the visual field.
- Blurred or wavy vision.
- Vision loss. It may seem as if a cobweb or curtain obscures part of the field of vision.

Retinal Vessel Occlusion

WHAT IS IT?

Retinal vessel occlusion is a blockage in one of the arteries or veins of the retina—the layer of light-sensitive cells lining the back surface of the eye. The condition is more common among older individuals. Occlusion of the major, or central, retinal artery produces sudden, painless vision loss and is a sight-threatening emergency. If blood flow is not reestablished within a few hours, death of the light-sensitive cells produces permanent vision loss in the affected eye. Most blockages are caused by a blood clot formed at the site or by a fragment of atherosclerotic plaque (embolus) that broke away from its original site and traveled through the bloodstream to lodge in the artery. Blockage in the central retinal artery or one of its branches will choke off the blood supply to the affected eye or portion of the retina.

By contrast, sudden occlusion of the central retinal vein is not a medical emergency—though it too affects vision and warrants prompt evaluation. In retinal vein occlusion, a vessel that normally drains blood from the retina becomes blocked, causing fluid and blood to build up in the retina. The worse the buildup, the greater the degree of visual disturbance. In some cases, vision may clear spontaneously; in others it may remain permanently clouded. In both retinal artery and retinal vein occlusion, temporary episodes of partial vision loss may precede the event. Because the cause needs to be identified, all cases of sudden vision loss require immediate attention for prompt diagnosis and possible treatment.

WHAT CAUSES IT?

• Arterial occlusions are caused by a blood clot, a piece of atherosclerotic plaque (embolus) that traveled to the site, or cancerous cells.
• Venous occlusions may be linked to chronic glaucoma, which it thought to predispose a person to retinal vein occlusion (see Glaucoma).

SYMPTOMS

• Sudden loss of vision in one eye. Vision loss may be complete or partial.
• Sudden blurred vision in one eye.

• Other conditions, such as high blood pressure, diabetes mellitus, and polycythemia vera, are also associated with retinal vessel occlusion.

PREVENTION

• While there is no definitive way to prevent retinal vessel blockage, regular eye examinations may aid in early detection of potential disorders.

DIAGNOSIS

• Eye examination by an ophthalmologist is required.
• Complete patient history and physical examination may be needed to diagnose the underlying cause.

HOW TO TREAT IT

Arterial occlusions:
• A doctor may apply firm, intermittent pressure to the eye with the heel of the hand (pressing on the eye for a few seconds, suddenly releasing the pressure, then repeating the procedure), in an attempt to dislodge the blockage.
• Medications can be used or a small amount of fluid may be withdrawn from the front of the eye to suddenly lower eye pressure in hopes of propelling the blockage downstream to smaller vessels.
• Anticoagulant drugs, such as aspirin, heparin, or warfarin, may be administered to prevent further clot formation in some cases.
Venous occlusions:
• Ophthalmologists may use laser surgery to reverse vision loss from chronic swelling of the retina or to promote the regression of abnormal blood vessels that may arise as a complication of the disorder.
• Antihypertensive drugs may be prescribed to treat associated high blood pressure.
• Glaucoma medications may be necessary to treat associated glaucoma.

WHEN TO CALL A DOCTOR

• **EMERGENCY** Call an ambulance or see an ophthalmologist immediately if you experience sudden vision loss. 🏥

Reye's Syndrome

WHAT IS IT?

Reye's syndrome is a rare, life-threatening disorder that almost exclusively affects children under age 16, typically between ages six and eight. Although rare, cases have been reported in adults. Now widely recognized since it was first identified as a distinct disease in 1963, Reye's syndrome is characterized by swelling and inflammation of the brain and liver. The cause is unknown; however, aspirin may act as a trigger of the disease in children, especially when taken for viral infections such as influenza, chicken pox, or the common cold. Symptoms of Reye's syndrome generally appear during the recovery phase of the viral infection, and the disease may progress rapidly, resulting in a coma. The outcome is dependent upon the severity of the symptoms, especially the length of the coma. Reye's syndrome has been fatal in up to 50 percent of cases, but this percentage has been decreasing in recent years with advances in treatment. Patients who survive generally recover fully, with the exception of those few who suffer permanent brain damage. Early detection and treatment may limit damage from the disease and increase the likelihood of survival.

WHAT CAUSES IT?

• The cause of Reye's syndrome is unknown.
• Aspirin may trigger Reye's syndrome in children, especially when given for viral infections such as the flu or chicken pox.
• The primary damage is to the liver; brain injury results from the metabolic disturbances created by the acute liver abnormalities.

PREVENTION

• Do not give aspirin to children under 16 years of age. Acetaminophen or ibuprofen should be used instead to relieve pain and fever.

DIAGNOSIS

• Patient history and physical examination.
• Blood tests.
• Lumbar puncture (spinal tap).
• Liver biopsy may be done, but it is generally not needed. After local anesthesia is administered to the patient, the doctor inserts a needle under the ribs into the liver to extract a small sample of tissue for microscopic examination.

HOW TO TREAT IT

• Hospitalization in an intensive care unit is usually necessary.
• Intravenous fluids are given to restore blood electrolytes to normal and maintain blood glucose levels.
• Dexamethasone, a corticosteroid medication, may be given to reduce inflammation of brain tissue.
• Mannitol, a diuretic drug, may be administered to reduce pressure on the brain.
• Temporary dialysis may be necessary. Dialysis performs the functions of the kidneys by removing waste products and excess fluid from the blood when the kidneys cannot (see Renal Failure, Acute, for more information).
• A mechanical respirator may be necessary in the event the patient stops breathing.
• In some cases surgery may be performed to reduce swelling and pressure on the brain.

WHEN TO CALL A DOCTOR

• **EMERGENCY** Call an ambulance immediately if a child starts to vomit and becomes excessively drowsy in the aftermath of a viral infection. ▲

SYMPTOMS
• Severe nausea and vomiting.
• Drowsiness; lethargy.
• Mental confusion, hyperexcitability, disorientation, irritability, or memory loss.
• Severe symptoms: seizures, loss of consciousness, cessation of breathing.

Rheumatic Fever

WHAT IS IT?

Rheumatic fever is an inflammatory disease that occasionally occurs as a delayed complication of a streptococcal infection of the upper respiratory tract (usually strep throat). The disease is characterized by inflammation of one or more organ sites throughout the body, including the joints (hence the name "rheumatic," or joint-related, fever), the heart, the skin, and the central nervous system. Symptoms typically appear within one to five weeks after infection with group A streptococcal bacteria and include fever, painful and swollen joints, and a skin rash. Untreated attacks usually subside in about three months. With prompt diagnosis and treatment, the disease is usually short-lived, although symptoms may continue for as long as six months with severe heart involvement.

The most serious manifestations of rheumatic fever involve the heart muscle and valves. Congestive heart failure can develop and may be fatal. The only long-term complication of rheumatic fever is valvular heart disease, a thickening or distortion in the heart valves that prevents them from closing properly or opening fully. Such damage may not be detected for many years. About 15 percent of patients with rheumatic fever develop Sydenham's chorea (also known as St. Vitus' dance), which is characterized by emotional instability and involuntary jerking movements of the limbs or facial muscles. Rheumatic fever may occur in isolated instances or as part of an epidemic outbreak affecting numerous people, although in the United States, antibiotics and improved public health conditions have kept the incidence in check. Like strep infections in general, rheumatic fever is most common among children between the ages of five and 15.

WHAT CAUSES IT?

• Rheumatic fever is believed to result from an immune response by the body to specific strains of streptococcal bacteria. This immune reaction, and not the infection per se, produces the inflammatory lesions in the various tissues throughout the body.

PREVENTION

• Get prompt treatment for a sore throat that lasts longer than 48 hours, especially if accompanied by a fever. Timely administration of antibiotics may prevent the development of rheumatic fever.

DIAGNOSIS

• Patient history and physical examination. A characteristic heart murmur may be detected with a stethoscope if the disease has affected a heart valve.
• Blood tests for the presence of antibodies against streptococcal proteins.
• Throat culture, to detect a streptococcal infection.
• An electrocardiogram (ECG), a measurement of the heart's electrical activity, may be done to detect carditis or other heart abnormalities.

HOW TO TREAT IT

• Antibiotics, usually penicillin or erythromycin, are given to eliminate streptococcal bacteria even though they are usually absent by the time rheumatic fever occurs.
• Aspirin or another anti-inflammatory drug is usually given to control joint pain and swelling.
• For more severe inflammation, corticosteroids may be needed.
• For mild to moderate rheumatic fever, two to 12 weeks of bed rest are necessary.

SYMPTOMS

• Sore throat precedes the illness by some weeks.
• Swollen, painful joints, especially the knees, ankles, wrists, and elbows. Arthritis symptoms often move sequentially from one joint to another.
• Fever.
• Excessive fatigue.
• Evanescent raised, red patches on the skin, in a curved latticelike pattern.
• Small, painless, pea-size lumps or nodules beneath the skin, commonly appearing on the hands, elbows, knees, scalp, shoulder blades, and spine.
• Acute abdominal pain.
• Involuntary, jerky movements and extreme emotional instability (Sydenham's chorea).

Rheumatic Fever   *continued*

• Penicillin, taken daily by mouth or, less often, given by monthly injection, is continued for years to prevent reinfection.

• Preventive doses of penicillin or amoxicillin may be required prior to dental or surgical procedures throughout the patient's life.

• Sedatives and tranquilizers (such as diazepam or chlorpromazine) may be prescribed to treat Sydenham's chorea, the unusual complication of rheumatic fever that causes jerky, uncontrolled movements and mood swings.

WHEN TO CALL A DOCTOR

• If you have a sore throat that persists for more than 48 hours, especially if it is accompanied by a fever, consult your doctor. ▲

Rheumatoid Arthritis

WHAT IS IT?

Rheumatoid arthritis is a common, persistent systemic disorder that can cause inflammation of joints throughout the body. Joints contain a number of structures that allow for ease of movement. The ends of the bones in a joint are protected from rubbing together by an elastic cushioning material, known as cartilage. The entire joint is surrounded by a capsule, known as the synovial sac. A thin layer of tissue (synovial membrane) lines the sac and secretes synovial fluid, which provides lubrication to ease movement.

In the early stage of rheumatoid arthritis, the synovial membrane becomes inflamed and thickened, causing pain and limiting joint movement. As the disease progresses, the cartilage and the ends of the bones erode. The result is severe joint damage and deformity. Joint pain is often preceded by general, nonspecific symptoms, such as fever, fatigue, and loss of appetite. It may also be prefaced by stiffness in the joints, particularly in the morning.

The hallmark of the disorder is involvement of the small joints of the hands and wrists with painful, warm, swollen, tender, and reddish joints. The process can also involve the elbows, shoulders, knees, hips, ankles, feet, and neck. Symptoms tend to occur symmetrically; that is, joints on both sides of the body are usually affected at the same time. In some cases other organ systems of the body—including the eyes, heart, and lung—may become inflamed too.

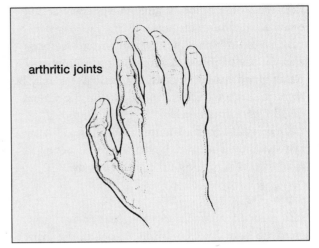

arthritic joints

As rheumatoid arthritis attacks and inflames joint tissues, joints may lose their shape and alignment, possibly resulting in severe deformity.

Symptoms occur in lengthy episodes that may be separated by remission periods of reduced or total absence of pain and stiffness. Between 50 and 75 percent of patients experience a remission within one to two years after the first episode.

Current research suggests that rheumatoid arthritis is an autoimmune disorder caused by an attack of the immune system on some of the body's own cells. The disease usually develops between the ages of 20 and 50, and its prevalence increases with age. Women are affected approximately three times more frequently than men. Treatment is aimed at relieving pain and inflammation, preventing joint deformity, and preserving function.

WHAT CAUSES IT?

- The cause of rheumatoid arthritis is unknown.
- Genetic factors play a role.
- Some theories suggest that a virus may be associated with the development of rheumatoid arthritis.
- Flare-ups of rheumatoid arthritis may be triggered by emotional stress or other concurrent illness.

PREVENTION

- There is no known way to prevent rheumatoid arthritis.

DIAGNOSIS

- Patient history and physical examination. There is no specific diagnostic test for rheumatoid arthritis;

SYMPTOMS

- Early symptoms, preceding obvious joint involvement: fatigue and weakness; low-grade fever; general feeling of poor health; loss of appetite and weight loss.
- Red, swollen, painful joints that may be warm to the touch. With long-term rheumatoid arthritis, joints may become bent and gnarled.
- Stiffness (often the second manifestation), especially after awakening in the morning.
- Red, painless skin lumps, known as rheumatoid nodules, on the elbows, knees, or toes.
- Chest pain and breathing difficulty.
- Dry mouth and dry, painful eyes.

Rheumatoid Arthritis   *continued*

long-term observation of joint changes may be necessary for definitive diagnosis.

• Blood tests for autoimmune rheumatoid factors; anemia may be found in almost half of patients. The white blood cell count is usually normal, but may be high (in active inflammation) or low (in the variant called Felty's syndrome).

• X-rays of the affected joints.

• Synovial fluid analysis. Under local anesthetic, synovial fluid is drawn from the affected joint.

HOW TO TREAT IT

• To reduce fever and treat pain, your doctor may prescribe large doses of aspirin, or one of the many other nonsteroidal anti-inflammatory drugs (NSAIDs), such as ibuprofen, naproxen, nabumetone, or salsalate.

• New medicines, dubbed COX-2 inhibitors, are becoming available that have pain-relieving and anti-inflammatory effects with a low risk of bleeding or stomach ulcers (common side effects of NSAIDs). Celecoxib (Celebrex) is the first of this new class to gain Food and Drug Administration approval.

• The current trend is to move patients more rapidly to other, more potent antirheumatic drugs if initial anti-inflammatories fail to control symptoms. Because of potential side effects, patients receiving such therapy must be closely monitored.

• Hydroxychloroquine, a drug used to treat malaria, may also be prescribed to relieve symptoms of rheumatoid arthritis. The drug's effects may not be felt for three to six months.

• A solution containing gold salts may be taken orally or injected to reduce inflammation and pain.

• Methotrexate, an antimetabolite drug, may be prescribed to subdue the immune system. If symptoms persist, immunosuppressants such as azathioprine or cyclophosphamide may be tried.

• Penicillamine, a penicillin derivative, may be prescribed to relieve symptoms if other drugs are ineffective (though its use is limited by a large number of side effects).

• Sulfasalazine appears to work by suppressing the immune response that is active in rheumatoid arthritis, and also as an anti-inflammatory agent.

• Minocycline is an antibiotic that acts more as an anti-inflammatory; it has modest benefit in some patients with early disease.

• Oral corticosteroids, such as prednisone, offer quick relief from symptoms of rheumatoid arthritis. Because prednisone has serious side effects when used for extended periods, it is often reserved for severe flare-ups of the disease or when other treatments are ineffective. Injection of corticosteroids into an affected joint may also be helpful.

• Researchers are developing drugs that target the mechanisms in the disease process and have the potential to prevent joint damage. In addition, innovative strategies such as combination therapy are being applied with encouraging results. Recent drug treatment advances include: Leflunomide, an immunomodulator that has antiproliferative activity as well as an anti-inflammatory effect, and etanercept, which inhibits the action of tumor necrosis factor (TNF), a naturally occurring substance that is overproduced in people with rheumatoid arthritis.

• Hot or cold compresses may provide pain relief.

• Get plenty of rest. People with rheumatoid arthritis often need over 10 hours of sleep a night, or eight hours a night and a two-hour nap during the day, and may need more during severe episodes.

• Creams or lotions containing capsaicin may be applied to relieve minor joint pain. Those containing camphor, menthol, or turpentine oil may mask pain and provide some relief from minor symptoms.

• Contrary to popular belief, there is no evidence that bee venom relieves or cures rheumatoid arthritis.

• Splints may be prescribed to relieve pain by immobilizing the joints during severe episodes.

• Your doctor may prescribe an exercise program or may advise you to see a physical therapist. While exercise that is too vigorous may worsen symptoms, some regular activity is necessary to maintain full range of motion of the joints and to prevent muscle deterioration (atrophy). Such programs outline gentle exercises that can be done to increase the range of motion of the joints.

• Some exercises are easier to perform in a pool or hot tub, because water helps support the body; these techniques should be discussed with your doctor or physical therapist.

• Surgery to remove the diseased synovial membrane

Rheumatoid Arthritis *continued*

from affected joints (synovectomy) may be performed in advanced cases.

• Surgery to remove the damaged joint and replace it with a mechanical joint (arthroplasty, or total joint replacement) may be performed in advanced cases. Almost 90 percent of the 150,000 joint replacements each year are of the hip or knee, but the shoulders, elbows, and joints in the hands and feet may be replaced as well. Discussion of the types of activities the patient would like to continue after joint replacement aids the surgeon in selecting the appropriate type of prosthesis and implantation technique, while making the patient more aware of the risks and limitations of surgery.

WHEN TO CALL A DOCTOR

• Make an appointment with a doctor if painful joints interfere with normal activities. ▲

Rheumatoid Arthritis, Juvenile

WHAT IS IT?

Juvenile rheumatoid arthritis is an uncommon childhood condition characterized by persistent or recurrent joint inflammation. Joints contain a number of structures and fluids that allow for ease of movement. The ends of the bones in a joint are protected from rubbing together by an elastic cushioning material (cartilage). The entire joint is surrounded by a capsule (synovial sac). A thin layer of tissue (synovial membrane) lines the sac and secretes synovial fluid, which provides lubrication to ease movement. But inflammation may thicken, erode, or otherwise damage these structures, causing pain and limiting movement. Current thinking is that juvenile rheumatoid arthritis is an autoimmune disorder, an attack by the immune system on some of the body's own cells. Most cases of juvenile rheumatoid arthritis have clinical features significantly different from those of the type of rheumatoid arthritis seen in adults (see Rheumatoid Arthritis for specific information about that disorder).

There are three main types of juvenile arthritis: pauciarticular and polyarticular juvenile rheumatoid arthritis, and Still's disease (also known as systemic juvenile arthritis). Pauciarticular juvenile rheumatoid arthritis, which accounts for approximately 40 percent of cases, causes pain, swelling, and stiffness in four or fewer joints. Polyarticular juvenile rheumatoid arthritis, a more severe form of the disease that accounts for another 40 percent of cases, causes pain, swelling, and stiffness in a number of joints throughout the skeleton. In Still's disease, which accounts for the remaining 20 percent of cases, the child may exhibit symptoms of general illness, including fever, rash, and abdominal pain that last for several weeks and precede symptoms of joint pain and stiffness by several months. Still's disease may cause inflammation of the eyes and lining of the lungs (pleura) or heart (pericardium). Unlike other forms of juvenile arthritis, Still's disease may also occasionally affect adults.

Joint symptoms of juvenile rheumatoid arthritis tend to occur in episodes of several weeks, separated by remission periods when symptoms subside. With frequent or severe episodes, bone growth may be uneven or abnormal. Permanent joint deformity and functional limitation occurs in over 30 percent of affected children after 10 years of follow-up.

Early-onset pauciarticular patients are typically very young girls (one to five years of age). They have the greatest risk for developing chronic eye inflammation, and have the best overall joint outcome. Late-onset pauciarticular patients (ages nine to 12) are more often boys; they often have tendinitis as well as arthritis affecting large joints (shoulders, hips, and knees) or the spine. Polyarticular juvenile rheumatoid arthritis may develop at any age, and girls are affected three times more often than boys. Still's disease may develop at any age, but the peak age of onset is one to six years of age. Boys and girls are equally affected. In many cases of Still's disease, symptoms disappear around the age of puberty. Patients with pauciarticular or polyarticular disease (approximately 40 percent) may have persistent joint symptoms. Treatment is aimed at relieving symptoms, preventing deformity, and maintaining optimal joint function throughout the duration of the disease.

WHAT CAUSES IT?

• The cause of juvenile rheumatoid arthritis is unknown, but genetic factors play a role.

SYMPTOMS

- Red, swollen, painful joints that may be warm to the touch.
- Stiffness, especially after awakening in the morning.
- Fatigue and muscle weakness.
- Fever that may spike as the day progresses. The child's temperature is often normal in the morning but may reach 103°F by the end of each day.
- Red or pink skin rash.
- General feeling of poor health.
- Abdominal pain.
- Loss of appetite and weight loss.
- Red, painful eyes from inflammation of the iris (pauciarticular).
- Chest pain; breathing difficulty (Still's disease).
- Anemia (all, but especially in Still's disease).
- Enlarged lymph nodes (Still's disease).

Rheumatoid Arthritis, Juvenile *continued*

PREVENTION

• There is no known way to prevent juvenile rheumatoid arthritis.

DIAGNOSIS

• Patient history and physical examination are needed. There is no specific diagnostic test for juvenile rheumatoid arthritis, and long-term observation may be necessary for definitive diagnosis.
• Blood tests will be taken.
• X-rays of the affected joints may be ordered.
• Synovial fluid analysis may be performed. In this procedure a local anesthetic is administered to desensitize the affected joint, and synovial fluid is then withdrawn from the joint capsule with a needle.

HOW TO TREAT IT

• To reduce fever and treat minor pain, your doctor may prescribe large doses of aspirin or one of the many other nonsteroidal anti-inflammatory drugs (NSAIDs), such as tolmetin or naproxen.
• Hot or cold compresses applied to the joints may offer some pain relief.
• Creams or lotions containing capsaicin may be applied to relieve minor joint pain. Preparations containing camphor, menthol, or turpentine oil may mask pain and provide some relief from minor symptoms.
• In severe cases, stronger medications may be prescribed to relieve pain and inflammation. The immunosuppressive drug methotrexate has been well tolerated and is effective, and is now the preferred second-line agent among most practitioners. Uncontrolled studies of sulfasalazine in children have been encouraging, but the drug has yet to be studied under double-blind, controlled conditions. Although injectable gold salt preparations have been useful, their role in treating patients has declined dramatically over the past 10 years (as the use of methotrexate has increased). Agents such as the antimalarial hydroxychloroquine, penicillamine, and oral gold salts are of little benefit.
• Corticosteroids, such as prednisone, offer quick relief from symptoms of juvenile rheumatoid arthritis but have serious side effects; they are used only in the smallest possible doses and only when other treatments prove ineffective. Oral prednisone has an important place, however, in the treatment of many patients with Still's disease, especially those with inflammation of the lining around the heart (pericarditis) and persistent fever. Intra-articular corticosteroids may be helpful for patients with limited joint involvement.
• Plenty of rest is required. Children with juvenile rheumatoid arthritis often need to sleep longer than average at night and may need to take naps during the day.
• Your child's doctor may prescribe an exercise program or may advise that your child see a physical therapist. While exercise that is too vigorous may worsen symptoms, some regular activity is necessary to prevent limitation of joint movements and to prevent muscle weakness and atrophy. Gentle exercises are taught to increase the range of motion in affected joints. Some movements are easier to perform in a pool or hot tub, since water helps support the body.
• Splints may be prescribed to relieve pain by immobilizing affected joints during severe episodes.
• Contact a local chapter of the Arthritis Foundation for information about support groups in your area.

WHEN TO CALL A DOCTOR

• Make an appointment with a doctor if your child develops painful or stiff joints. ⚠

Ringworm Dermatophytosis

WHAT IS IT?

Ringworm is a skin infection caused not by a worm but by several different species of fungus collectively referred to as tinea. The fungus causes scaly, round, itchy patches to develop on various parts of the body, including the scalp, groin, nails, feet, and the skin under the beard. Most people in the United States have had at least one form of ringworm, which is moderately infectious. Prompt treatment with topical antifungal agents usually clears up most cases within a few weeks.

WHAT CAUSES IT?

• Infection by one or more of the different tinea fungi causes ringworm. Exposure to animals (especially cats and dogs) with a fungal infection is one mode of transmission.

PREVENTION

• Do not share towels or shoes.
• Thoroughly dry the feet after taking a bath or shower, and after swimming.
• Avoid lengthy stays in an overheated, humid environment, like the areas around indoor swimming pools. Warmth, moisture, and darkness encourage the growth of fungi.

SYMPTOMS

• On the scalp: bald patches and scales.
• On the skin: round, red patches that grow to about one inch across. As the patch radiates outward, the central area heals, leaving a red ring where the infection remains active (hence the name "ringworm").
• Under a beard: an itchy, scaling rash.
• On the feet: dry scaling and fissuring of the skin between the toes and on the arch (athlete's foot).
• People with athlete's foot may develop a dermatitis (skin inflammation), possibly allergic, at other sites on the feet or hands. It clears when the fungal infection is fully treated.
• On the nails: red, swollen, and painful fingernails or toenails.

• Avoid contact with infected pets as much as possible. Seek prompt veterinary treatment for any skin conditions your pet exhibits.

DIAGNOSIS

• Ringworm is suspected by observation of the characteristic red-bordered rash.
• Culture and microscopic examination of skin, pus, or hair shafts may be needed to confirm the diagnosis.

HOW TO TREAT IT

• Ringworm can often be cured with over-the-counter antifungal creams or solutions, especially those containing clotrimazole, miconazole, or ketoconazole. Generally, these are applied once or twice daily; the infection should begin to fade within a week. Continuing treatment for the recommended amount of time will help ensure eradication of the fungus.
• If over-the-counter treatments fail, a more powerful oral agent (griseofulvin) or topical antifungal medication may be prescribed. Topical or low-potency corticosteroids may be prescribed as well to ease itching and speed healing.
• Keep affected areas as clean and dry as possible; talcum or medicated powder may be used.
• If a fungal infection begins to blister or ooze, apply damp compresses to help clear out the affected areas. Do not break blisters; this can spread the infection.
• Oral medication is recommended for ringworm of the scalp.
• If you have ringworm of the groin area (jock itch), wear cotton underwear and change it more than once a day. If your feet are affected (athlete's foot), change socks frequently to keep your feet dry.
• Sterilize any clothing, towels, or bedding that have touched the lesions.

WHEN TO CALL A DOCTOR

• Call your doctor if symptoms do not improve or if infection continues to spread after several weeks of over-the-counter treatment.
• Call a doctor if you develop new, unexplained symptoms, which may be side effects from the medications used to treat ringworm.
• Call your doctor if you suspect scalp ringworm.

Rocky Mountain Spotted Fever

WHAT IS IT?

Rocky Mountain spotted fever is an illness caused by a microorganism that infects humans through the bite of a tick. A severe headache, fever, and rash typically appear within one week of infection. The disease gets its name from the Rocky Mountain area where it was first reported, but its occurrence is widespread in the United States; cases are most common in the southern Atlantic states.

The wood tick and dog tick are the primary carriers, and either can be found in both city and woodland locales. More than 90 percent of cases occur between April 1 and September 30, the time of year when ticks are most prevalent. Children and adolescents account for nearly half of cases, primarily because of increased tick exposure through outdoor activity. Untreated, especially in older patients, Rocky Mountain spotted fever may result in heart failure, pneumonia, or coma, and is fatal in 20 to 30 percent of cases.

WHAT CAUSES IT?

• A bite from a tick infected with the microorganism *Rickettsia rickettsii.*
• The organism invades and multiplies in cells lining the arteries and veins throughout the body, causing vasculitis.

SYMPTOMS

• Severe headache.
• Chills and a high fever that reaches 103°F to 104°F within the first two days.
• A rash appears between the second and sixth day of illness. It begins at the wrists and ankles and within 24 hours spreads to the rest of the body and face. In about 10 percent of patients, the rash does not occur or is barely noticeable, particularly in males and persons with dark skin.
• Nausea and vomiting.
• Diarrhea and abdominal pain.
• A dry cough.
• Muscle aches.
• Heightened sensitivity to light.

PREVENTION

• Minimize contact with ticks and tick-infested areas.
• Wear protective clothing and use insect repellent on exposed skin and clothes.
• Inspect your body several times a day for ticks when visiting a tick-infested area.
• Check dogs for ticks; ticks may infect the animal and establish a host for further transmission.
• Remove an attached tick with tweezers: grasp it as close to the skin as possible, being careful not to squeeze the body of the tick, which may spew infectious microorganisms into the bloodstream. Pull the tick steadily upward without twisting. Do not handle it after removal. Transmission is unlikely unless the tick has been attached for a number of hours.
• Wash the bite area with soap and water or antiseptic to destroy any contaminants.

DIAGNOSIS

• A patient history should include any recent outdoor activities or travel in tick-infested areas.
• Microscopic examination of a biopsy of skin or rash is the only way to make a conclusive diagnosis early in the disease.

HOW TO TREAT IT

• Antibiotic drug therapy (usually doxycycline, tetracycline, or chloramphenicol) should be administered as early as possible in the course of illness. If treatment is delayed until the rash is widespread, therapy is less effective.
• If untreated, the illness often abates after two weeks and convalescence is usually rapid.

WHEN TO CALL A DOCTOR

• Call a doctor when there are symptoms of rash, fever, headache, and weakness, regardless of whether or not a tick bite is evident. Conclusive diagnosis and appropriate treatment are only available through a physician.

Rosacea

WHAT IS IT?

Rosacea is a chronic skin disorder frequently mistaken for the common form of acne typically seen in adolescence (acne vulgaris). Like acne, rosacea may be mild, moderate, or severe and may vary over time. It is characterized by variable degrees of redness, flushing, swelling, and blemishes around the nose, cheeks, and forehead.

Affecting one in 20 American adults (typically over age 30), rosacea is seen most often in women. In chronic or severe cases, rosacea may lead to rhinophyma (an overgrowth of tissues in the nose), resulting in a permanent red, swollen, or bulbous nose. Rosacea also commonly affects the eyes, leading to mild blepharitis or conjunctivitis (see Blepharitis and Conjunctivitis). Rarely, rosacea of the eyes is severe and may threaten sight; such severity requires immediate therapy by an ophthalmologist. Although there is no cure for rosacea, proper treatment can control symptoms, improve appearance, and prevent the condition from becoming worse.

WHAT CAUSES IT?

• In rosacea, the tiny blood vessels of the face become inflamed and dilated. The cause is unknown.
• People are more prone to develop rosacea and experience flare-ups if they have a family history of the condition, are fair-skinned (such as those of Celtic descent), or flush or blush easily. Flushing often occurs after ingesting alcohol, spicy foods, or hot drinks, after exposure to heat, or as an emotional response.
• Topical corticosteroid use may also lead to or aggravate rosacea.

PREVENTION

There is no known way to prevent rosacea. However, there are ways to prevent or minimize flare-ups:
• Avoid foods or drinks that cause flushing.
• If you are being treated by a doctor, do not stop therapy without consulting him or her. This may trigger a flare-up.
• Use only mild, water-soluble cleansers and moisturizers with no fragrance or astringents.
• Wash with tepid water rather than water that's too cold or too hot; dry the face by patting it gently with a towel.
• Topical products designed for acne vulgaris actually worsen rosacea and should not be used.
• Do not use steroids on the face.

DIAGNOSIS

• Patient history and physical examination are needed.

HOW TO TREAT IT

• Your doctor may prescribe topical or oral antibiotics to reduce redness and blemishes. Topical metronidazole or oral tetracycline (at the lowest dose to suppress the disorder) may be needed throughout life because rosacea tends to recur when therapy is discontinued. When used for rosacea, antibiotics are believed to have an anti-inflammatory effect rather than an antibacterial effect.
• Rosacea can be camouflaged with green-hued undercover or liquid makeup (green masks the redness). Once redness and blemishes disappear following treatment, laser surgery to remove dilated blood vessels is an option.
• Rhinophyma may be easily and quite effectively treated with laser or standard surgery by a dermatologist or plastic surgeon.

WHEN TO CALL A DOCTOR

• Contact your doctor if you notice facial flushing that lasts longer than usual, or if you develop pimples or swelling around the central area of the face. ▲

SYMPTOMS

Stages or degrees of severity of rosacea:
• Stage 1: Frequent, persistent facial flushing; fine visible blood vessels (telangiectasia); occasional stinging, burning, and a feeling that the skin is pulled tight across the face.
• Stage 2: More widespread facial redness accompanied by bumps, more prominent blemishes, and swelling of the nose and cheeks.
• Stage 3: Inflammation spreading across a wider area; swelling or enlargement of the nose (rhinophyma).

Roseola

WHAT IS IT?

Roseola is a common childhood viral infection. After a symptom-free incubation period of five to 12 days, a sudden high fever develops. The fever may persist for three to five days. During this time the child may become irritable and, in a few cases, experience febrile (fever-induced) seizures. On the fourth or fifth day of the illness, the fever subsides abruptly, and a rash appears on the torso.

The rash, consisting of small, red, flat areas, each about two millimeters in diameter, may quickly spread outward to the neck and face, as well as to the arms and legs. The rash often subsides after one or two days; in fact, in some cases it may only persist for a few hours. By the time the rash appears, the child typically feels better, has no fever, and is no longer contagious.

Roseola occurs exclusively in children, especially between the ages of six months and two years, and is more prevalent during the spring and fall than the other seasons. The disease is not a serious health risk, and no further complications arise after the infection subsides. Treatment is aimed at relieving symptoms while they last.

WHAT CAUSES IT?

• The human herpes virus 6 causes roseola.
• Exposure to an infected child may spread the virus to other children.

PREVENTION

• Follow proper sanitary measures, such as washing hands after using the bathroom and before handling food, to help prevent the spread of infectious disease.

• If possible, avoid exposing your child to another child with roseola.

DIAGNOSIS

• There is no specific test for roseola. Diagnosis is based on patient history and physical examination.
• Throat or blood cultures may be performed to rule out the possibility of other illnesses.

HOW TO TREAT IT

• Acetaminophen or ibuprofen may be given to reduce fever. Do not give aspirin, which may increase the risk of Reye's syndrome, a rare but life-threatening inflammation of the brain and liver in children (see Reye's Syndrome for more information).
• Anticonvulsant medications may be prescribed if seizures occur.
• Follow prevention tips, such as hand washing, to halt the spread of infection.
• Strenuous physical activity should be avoided during periods of high fever.

WHEN TO CALL A DOCTOR

• Call a doctor if a young child develops a high fever, with or without swollen glands. High fever can indicate a number of potentially serious disorders that may require professional treatment.
• **EMERGENCY** See your doctor immediately or go to an emergency room if your child experiences seizures. 🔺

SYMPTOMS

• Sudden onset of fever (possibly as high as 105°F).
• Irritability.
• Skin rash on the torso that usually spreads to the neck, face, arms, or legs.
• Sore throat.
• Swollen glands in the neck.
• Possible seizures.

Rotator Cuff Injury

WHAT IS IT?

Rotator cuff injury is an inflammation or tear in the tendons of the rotator cuff, the group of muscles and tendons that forms, in part, the covering around the shoulder joint. The muscles of the rotator cuff make it possible to lift and rotate the arm, and when the tendons are repeatedly stressed or torn, shoulder pain occurs and mobility of the arm becomes limited. In rotator cuff tendinitis, the humerus, or long bone of the upper arm, rubs against a tendon causing microscopic tears and inflammation. In rotator cuff tear, a more serious injury, a rupture of a tendon from the bone causes severe pain and may severely limit arm movement. Recovery from a rotator cuff injury depends on whether a tendon is inflamed (see Tendinitis for more information) or whether it is actually torn from the bone.

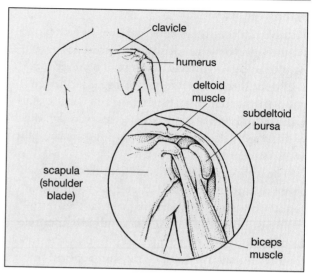

The structures of the rotator cuff lie just beneath the deltoid muscle, providing stability to the humerus where it enters the shoulder socket.

WHAT CAUSES IT?

• Repeated stress to the shoulder from activities such as sports or heavy labor.
• Trauma to the shoulder, such as falling on an outstretched arm or lifting heavy objects.
• Wearing out the shoulder by years of continual use, usually occurring between the ages of 60 and 75.

PREVENTION

• Exercises that increase strength and flexibility of the rotator cuff muscles will reduce the risk of injury.
• Avoid activities that cause shoulder soreness.

DIAGNOSIS

• Physical examination may include range of motion tests to determine the extent of injury. A mild tear is most painful when the arm is raised between 70 and 120 degrees; a complete tear often renders the arm incapable of being raised above the head.
• Arthrography (an x-ray technique using dye injection), MRI (magnetic resonance imaging), or ultrasound may be used to examine joint tissues.

HOW TO TREAT IT

• Ice the shoulder daily or after exercise.
• Take over-the-counter pain relievers such as aspirin, acetaminophen, ibuprofen, or naproxen.
• Partial immobilization with a sling may be recommended for a few days. Range of motion exercises are recommended as soon as possible after an injury to prevent a frozen or stiff shoulder. Physical therapy to show you specific exercises to strengthen the rotator cuff muscles may be helpful.
• If the above measures fail, a cortisone injection into the area of the tendon may reduce pain and inflammation.
• Surgery may be necessary for a torn tendon and for cases that do not respond to other treatments.

WHEN TO CALL A DOCTOR

• Call a doctor if routine motions such as lifting your arm to comb your hair become difficult and painful, or if you experience severe pain after trauma to the shoulder.

SYMPTOMS

• Tenderness in the shoulder region, often worse at night.
• Pain aggravated by rotating or lifting the arm, especially to an angle of 90 degrees or higher.
• Sudden, sharp pain in the shoulder that radiates toward the elbow.
• Pain and weakness in the shoulder that lasts several months or longer despite treatment.

Rubella

WHAT IS IT?

Rubella, also known as German measles, is a contagious viral infection. It is neither as severe nor as contagious as measles, another rash-producing viral infection. The most characteristic symptom of rubella is a nonitchy skin rash that lasts for a few days before fading. Symptoms vary widely between children and adults: Children may have few if any symptoms except the rash; adolescents and adults may develop more pronounced symptoms such as arthritis, encephalitis (infection of the brain), and thrombocytopenia (low amount of platelets in the blood). In any case, rubella is usually a mild infection that goes away on its own without complications. However, if contracted by a women in the first four months of pregnancy, the virus may cause miscarriage, stillbirth, or serious birth defects in the developing fetus, a condition known as congenital rubella syndrome. All women not immunized as children are therefore advised to receive the rubella vaccine.

WHAT CAUSES IT?

• A viral infection causes rubella.
• The virus may be spread by infected saliva expelled during coughing or sneezing, or by sustained, close contact (for example, within a household or school).

PREVENTION

• Children should be vaccinated with the MMR vaccine (a combination vaccine for measles, mumps, and rubella) at 12 to 15 months of age and again at four to six years. Children not reimmunized when they start school should receive a second dose of vaccine by 12 years of age.
• All women not immunized as children or who do not have evidence of immunity on blood tests should receive the rubella vaccine. Effective birth control should be used for three months after the vaccine, to prevent congenital rubella syndrome in a developing fetus. For this reason, pregnant women should not receive the rubella vaccine.

DIAGNOSIS

• Diagnosis is strongly suggested upon patient history and physical examination, although rubella can be easily mistaken for other viral illnesses. Cultures from the nose, throat, urine, or blood may confirm the presence of the virus.
• Blood tests that reveal antibodies to the virus can confirm diagnosis.

HOW TO TREAT IT

• Acetaminophen or ibuprofen may be given to a child to reduce fever and relieve headache. Do not give aspirin, which may increase the risk of Reye's syndrome, a rare but life-threatening inflammation of the brain and liver in children (see Reye's Syndrome for more information).

WHEN TO CALL A DOCTOR

• Call a doctor if you develop a stiff neck, severe headache, visual disturbances, or other symptoms of meningitis during or after a rubella infection (see Meningitis for more information).
• Call a doctor if you are pregnant, or suspect that you might be, and you believe you may have been exposed to rubella.
• See your doctor if you become pregnant and have not been immunized. ⚠

SYMPTOMS

• Rubella may have no symptoms.
• A mild skin rash that lasts for about three days, spreading from the face to the torso, arms, and legs before fading.
• Mild fever (102°F or lower).
• General feeling of poor health.
• Nasal discharge.
• Sore throat.
• Joint pain.
• Enlarged lymph glands.

Salivary Gland Disorders

WHAT IS IT?

The three sets of salivary glands, located at the sides of the mouth below the ears (parotid glands), below the jaw (submandibular glands), and in the floor of the mouth (sublingual glands), secrete saliva into the mouth through tiny ducts. Saliva aids in swallowing, prevents infection, and helps keep the mouth and teeth clean. The salivary glands can malfunction in a number of ways: too much or too little saliva may be produced; the glands may become infected; the ducts may be blocked by a plug, known as a stone; rarely, tumors (either cancerous or benign) may develop within the glands. Treatment depends upon the underlying problem. If one salivary gland needs to be removed (say, in the case of a malignant tumor), the remaining glands compensate and produce adequate amounts of saliva.

WHAT CAUSES IT?

• Bacteria and viruses may cause salivary gland infections (see Mumps or AIDS for more information).
• Chemicals in the saliva may solidify into a salivary duct stone.
• The cause of salivary gland tumors is unknown.
• Swelling of the salivary glands or a decrease in salivation may be caused by a number of factors, including: other disorders, such as diabetes mellitus, cirrhosis, Sjögren's syndrome, depression, and dehy-

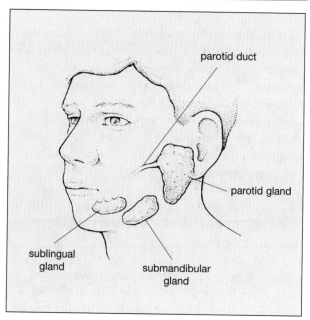

The salivary glands are each comprised of thousands of sacs that produce saliva, which is secreted into the mouth through ducts.

dration; treatments such as radiation therapy to the head and neck; and medications including antihistamines, antidepressants, and some combinations of antihypertensive drugs.
• Excessive salivation may be caused by certain salivary gland infections.

PREVENTION

• There is no known way to prevent salivary gland disorders.

DIAGNOSIS

• Patient history and physical examination, either by a physician or dentist.
• Dental x-rays.
• CT (computed tomography) scans.
• Biopsy of affected salivary glands.

HOW TO TREAT IT

• Antibiotics are prescribed to treat bacterial infections of the salivary glands.
• Antifungal agents may be needed to treat yeast infections of the mouth occurring in those with decreased saliva.
• Over-the-counter analgesics can be taken for pain

SYMPTOMS

• Decreased or increased salivation.
• Swelling around the mouth or in front of the ears. Painful swelling is associated with salivary gland infections and salivary duct stones; painless swelling that develops gradually may be due to salivary gland tumors or the conditions described above in "What Causes It?"
• Mouth pain, especially at mealtimes.
• Bad taste in the mouth (in salivary gland infection).
• Fever (in salivary gland infection).
• Increase in dental cavities and difficulty swallowing owing to decreased salivation (see Sjögren's Syndrome for more information).

Salivary Gland Disorders   *continued*

relief. Aspirin should never be given to children under the age of 16 (see Reye's Syndrome for more information).

• Sugarless gum or sour candies can help stimulate salivation. Increased fluid intake is also recommended for dry mouth.

• Saliva substitutes (solutions containing 2 percent methylcellulose) may be prescribed, especially to be used at night. In severe cases the drug pilocarpine may be prescribed to increase saliva production (see Sjögren's Syndrome for more information).

• Rinsing the mouth several times daily with a solution of salt or baking soda in warm water is advised to wash away pus from an infected salivary duct.

• Surgery may be performed to remove a stone blocking the salivary duct, to remove a tumor, or to widen the opening of the duct.

• Surgical removal of the entire salivary gland may be required for malignant tumors and may be advised in cases of recurrent infection.

• Radiation therapy may be needed to destroy cancerous cells. Prognosis for salivary tumors is quite favorable if they are detected early.

WHEN TO CALL A DOCTOR

• See your doctor if you develop pain or swelling in or around the mouth or if you experience an increase or decrease in saliva production. ▲

Sarcoidosis

WHAT IS IT?

Sarcoidosis is a relatively common disease character-ized by an accumulation of inflammatory cells that may occur in tissues throughout the body, most often in the lungs, lymph nodes, eyes, and skin. Although the cause is unknown, sarcoidosis is thought to be an autoimmune disorder—an attack of the immune system on certain of the body's own cells. Symptoms depend on which organs are affected; in many cases no symptoms appear at all.

Most cases of sarcoidosis subside spontaneously within two or three years; long-term or chronic sar-coidosis accounts for only 10 percent of cases. The most serious manifestations of sarcoidosis result from damage to the heart, eyes, and lungs. Symptoms may be relieved with corticosteroid drugs; however, since the disease may be mild and most cases subside even without treatment, the decision to prescribe cortico-steroids is based upon the likelihood of complica-tions developing in the lungs, eyes, or other organs. Sarcoidosis is more common between the ages of 20 and 40, although it may strike anyone at any age. In the United States, African Americans are affected more frequently and have more serious complica-tions than Caucasians.

WHAT CAUSES IT?

• The cause of sarcoidosis is unknown.

SYMPTOMS

• Sarcoidosis may cause no symptoms.
• Fatigue, aching muscles, general feeling of poor health.
• Fever.
• Breathing difficulty, dry cough, hoarseness, wheezing.
• Swollen lymph nodes.
• Blurred vision; painful, red, dry eyes; aversion to light (photophobia).
• Painful joints.
• Loss of appetite leading to weight loss.
• Reddish or brownish skin spots on the fore-arms, face, or legs; swollen bluish purple areas on the face.

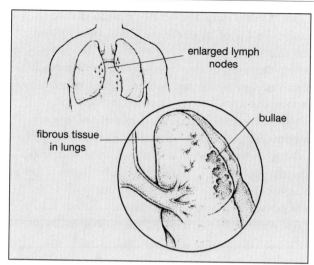

In sarcoidosis, the accumulation of inflammatory cells in various tis-sues may produce scarlike fibrous tissue or thin-walled blisters (bullae) in the lungs, and enlargement of the lymph nodes.

PREVENTION

• There is no known way to prevent sarcoidosis.

DIAGNOSIS

• Diagnosis is suspected from patient history, physical examination, and chest x-ray.
• Confirmation of the diagnosis requires a biopsy, often of lung tissue obtained by bronchoscopy (the passage of a thin, flexible viewing tube through the mouth and throat into the lungs).
• Skin lesions or other sites may be biopsied.
• Lung function tests may be performed.

HOW TO TREAT IT

• Corticosteroid drugs such as prednisone are pre-scribed to reduce inflammation and relieve symp-toms. When the lungs are involved, such therapy may be sustained for a year or more, then withdrawn to see if spontaneous remission has occurred. Relapses may require indefinite steroid therapy.
• Chloroquine (a drug usually used to treat malaria) is often useful in the treatment of skin lesions.

WHEN TO CALL A DOCTOR

• Call a doctor if you develop persistent shortness of breath, fever, unexplained weight loss, or other symptoms of sarcoidosis. 🩻

Scabies

WHAT IS IT?

Scabies is a disorder caused by a skin infestation of a burrowing mite. The tiny mite digs under the uppermost layer of the skin and lays several eggs. The skin becomes sensitized to the mite over a period of several weeks to several months, until finally a skin eruption of small blisters occurs, causing intense itching. Scratching may collect the mites and eggs under the fingernails and help transmit them to other parts of the body. The warm folds of the skin, such as those of the wrists, the underarms, the genitals and the webs between the fingers, are most commonly affected. In infants and small children, the blisters may be more generally distributed, appearing on the face and neck, palms, and soles. With treatment, itching usually subsides quickly, and all traces of the disease generally disappear within two to four weeks.

WHAT CAUSES IT?

• The female mite burrows into the upper layer of skin and lays two or three eggs daily for up to 60 days if undetected or untreated. Within three weeks newly hatched larvae mature and begin a continuing cycle of infestation. Itching is due to a reaction to the mite and its products.

• Physical contact with an infested person or with contaminated clothing or bedding may spread scabies. (Casual transmission, as between schoolmates, is uncommon.) Family members and bed mates are at the highest risk. Children under 15 are usually the first members of the family to get scabies.

• Crowded, institutional, or unsanitary living conditions also increase the risk.

PREVENTION

• Practice good personal hygiene; wash clothes and bedding often.

• Avoid physical contact with persons, clothing, or bedding that may be infested with scabies.

DIAGNOSIS

• Diagnosis is suspected upon visual inspection of burrows or lesions.

• Confirmation of the diagnosis requires observation of the mite upon microscopic examination of a skin scraping.

HOW TO TREAT IT

• Permethrin cream is the medication of choice for safety and effectiveness and should be applied after the skin has cooled following bathing. The medication is left on overnight and thoroughly washed off in the morning.

• Oral antihistamines (like diphenhydramine) may help ease itching, as may topical emollients.

• Antibiotics may be required to treat secondary bacterial infections.

• Bed linen and clothes used for two to three days prior to treatment should be thoroughly washed in hot water. The mite cannot live more than three days without a host.

• Family members, even without symptoms, may also be treated.

WHEN TO CALL A DOCTOR

• Call a doctor if you experience intense itching and over-the-counter remedies fail to relieve it. ▲

SYMPTOMS

• Small, red, itchy blisters, which break easily when scratched. Open blisters are prone to secondary infection.

• Severe itching, typically concentrated in the wrists, armpits, genitals, the folds of the breasts, buttocks, or elbows, and between the fingers. Itching is often worse at night or after a hot bath.

• Visible trailing burrows on the skin, especially between the fingers, which characteristically appear as dotted lines or wavy gray ridges resembling pencil marks.

• Small blisters without trailing burrows (indicating canine scabies, also highly contagious, acquired from a dog with mange).

• Severe scaling and crusting of the skin (in a rarer form known as Norwegian or crusted scabies, seen in persons with weakened immune systems and characterized by mild itching but extreme mite infestation).

Schizophrenia

WHAT IS IT?

Schizophrenia is a serious chronic mental disorder characterized by psychotic symptoms (such as hallucinations and delusions), rambling speech, impaired thinking, flat affect, and poor social functioning. The word "schizophrenia" means "split mind" and refers to the loss of reality that sometimes occurs. The onset of schizophrenia can be sudden (days, weeks, or months), but it usually develops slowly over the course of several years. Typically affecting about 1 percent of the general population, the peak onset in males is between the ages of 15 and 25; in females, between ages 25 and 35. Schizophrenia can be divided into five subtypes: catatonic, disorganized (also known as hebephrenic), paranoid, undifferentiated, and residual. Each type has its own set of characteristics, in addition to the general symptoms of schizophrenia.

About 25 percent of people with schizophrenia have a poor prognosis. They are unable to hold a job or live independently. Suicide attempts and episodes of depression are common during the course of the illness. Proper treatment and support enables 50 to 75 percent of people to be productive.

SYMPTOMS

- General symptoms: delusions (such as believing that a newscaster is speaking directly to them through the television); hallucinations (such as hearing voices in one's head of people who are not there); rambling or nonsensical speech; extremely disorganized behavior; inappropriate emotional responses or emotional detachment; minimal speech; and lack of willful movement.
- Catatonic type: minimal or stiff movement or stupor; excessive and erratic movements; negativity (refusal to go places or resistance when being physically moved); muteness; unusual movements, mannerisms, facial expressions, or postures; and senseless and uncontrollable repetition of a person's speech (words or phrases) or movements.
- Disorganized type: nonsensical speech that may be accompanied by silliness and laughter; lack of organization in the performance of basic daily activities such as showering, cooking food, and brushing of the teeth.
- Paranoid type: preoccupation with frequent hallucinations or one or more delusions of persecution.
- Undifferentiated type: general schizophrenia symptoms, but none of the catatonic, disorganized, or paranoid type symptoms.
- Residual type: continued evidence of the disorder, but no prominent or acute symptoms.

WHAT CAUSES IT?

The cause of schizophrenia is unknown. However, many experts believe it is linked to genetic as well as environmental factors, including:
- Complications before, during, and after birth (such as blood type incompatibilities, nutritional deficiency, and the flu).
- Certain types of brain damage (such as tumors or epilepsy).
- Drugs such as alcohol and cocaine occasionally induce schizophrenia-like episodes.

PREVENTION

- There is no known way to prevent schizophrenia, but relapses can be prevented through the use of neuroleptic and antipsychotic medications.

DIAGNOSIS

- Physical examination and patient history by a mental health professional are necessary.
- Depression and bipolar disorder should be ruled out (see Depression and Bipolar Disorder for more information).
- Laboratory tests may be done to rule out some underlying cause of symptoms, such as an adverse drug reaction or another medical condition (such as seizures, a brain tumor, Huntington's disease, or Alzheimer's disease).

HOW TO TREAT IT

- Antipsychotic drugs, such as haloperidol, risperidone, and olanzapine are typically prescribed. These drugs, while effective, can have serious side effects,

Schizophrenia *continued*

such as tardive dyskinesia (involuntary movements of the jaw, lips, tongue, and body). If conventional antipsychotic medications prove ineffective, your doctor may prescribe clozapine. This drug requires frequent monitoring by a doctor as it may lead to seizures and low white blood cell counts. Your doctor will administer weekly blood tests to measure white cell levels.

• Psychotherapy is an important part of the treatment of this and any mental illness.

• Community and familial support, in addition to medication, may help the individual to be productive in society and increase the time between relapses.

• Hospitalization may be necessary for severe episodes.

WHEN TO CALL A DOCTOR

Call a doctor if you or someone you know shows significant signs of schizophrenia. ▲

Scleritis and Episcleritis

WHAT IS IT?

Scleritis and episcleritis are inflammations of the protective outer layers of tissue that form the eyeball's shell. The deepest layer is the sclera, known commonly as the white of the eye. The transparent tissue covering the sclera is the episclera, which in turn is covered by a fine membrane called the conjunctiva. Inflammation of the episclera—or episcleritis—often resembles a localized form of conjunctivitis, but episcleritis is not accompanied by the watery or pus-filled discharge typical of conjunctivitis (see Conjunctivitis for more information). Episcleritis is usually a minor disorder that does not permanently damage the eye and generally resolves on its own within a week or two. Its presence occasionally indicates an underlying disease such as rheumatoid arthritis. Scleritis, a less common but more serious disease, most often occurs in association with an underlying systemic or autoimmune disorder, usually in people between the ages of 30 and 60.

SYMPTOMS

- A red or violet, slightly raised patch on the white of the eye, usually only a fraction of an inch in diameter.
- Sharp, severe eye pain that intensifies when the eye is moved.
- Dull, aching pain in one or both eyes, often worse at night. In some cases pain is severe.
- Aversion or increased sensitivity to light.
- Blurred vision.

WHAT CAUSES IT?

- The cause of episcleritis and scleritis is unknown.
- Both episcleritis and scleritis may be associated with a systemic disorder; that is, one affecting other organ systems in the body. Such disorders include autoimmune rheumatoid diseases (rheumatoid arthritis, scleroderma, systemic lupus erythematosus), inflammatory bowel disease, and tuberculosis.
- Herpes zoster involving the eye can lead to scleritis.

PREVENTION

- There is no way to prevent episcleritis or scleritis.

DIAGNOSIS

- Patient history and an eye examination by an ophthalmologist are required.
- An ultrasound of the eyeball may be conducted.
- A general physical examination by a medical doctor may be required to identify an associated underlying disease.

HOW TO TREAT IT

- In episcleritis, steroids in eyedrop or ointment form may be prescribed to reduce inflammation.
- The course of scleritis often parallels the activity and treatment of the associated systemic disorder. Corticosteroids, in tablet or eyedrop form, may reduce inflammation in some patients. Cycloplegic drugs may be administered to dilate the pupil, which may prevent scarring and alleviate pain somewhat. Immunosuppressive drugs may be prescribed in more severe cases.
- Surgery may be required for scleritis if the sclera has perforated.

WHEN TO CALL A DOCTOR

- If you suspect you have either scleritis or episcleritis, consult an ophthalmologist immediately.

Scleroderma Systemic Sclerosis

WHAT IS IT?

Scleroderma is an uncommon chronic multisystem disease characterized by a proliferative, destructive abnormality of small- and medium-size blood vessels, excessive collagen deposits in tissues, and an over-stimulated immune system. The disease, which means hardening (sclero) of the skin (derma), was initially thought to affect only the skin. It was later recognized that vital organs may be affected as well.

There appears to be an early inflammatory component. This may lead to fibroblasts and other cells that manufacture the protein collagen (a major component of connective tissue) to overproduce dense, inelastic, scarlike connective tissue. Circulation may be affected as the buildup of dense tissue chokes off blood flow through the tiny capillary blood vessels and small arterioles. When an internal organ (typically the esophagus, lungs, kidneys, or heart) is involved, fibrous tissue slowly infiltrates organ tissues. This may lead to life-threatening conditions such as severe lung disease or kidney failure. Scleroderma usually evolves gradually over a number of years; outcome depends on the organ system involved.

WHAT CAUSES IT?

• The cause of scleroderma is unknown, although it appears to be an autoimmune disorder (an attack by the body's defenses on healthy tissue). Exposure to silica dust, vinyl chloride, epoxy resins, and hydrocarbons can cause tight, thickened skin over the fingers (sclerodactyly), which differs from scleroderma.

PREVENTION

• There is no known way to prevent scleroderma.

DIAGNOSIS

• Frequently, the diagnosis may be determined upon patient history and physical examination alone.
• Blood tests and skin biopsy may be taken to rule out other connective tissue disorders.

HOW TO TREAT IT

• Treatment is aimed at minimizing symptoms and complications. Occasionally, the disease spontaneously improves.
• Immunosuppressive drugs such as azathioprine or penicillamine may help in some patients, but there is no solid proof that they improve the outcome.
• Skin lotions and bath oils may be used to soften the skin. Regular exercise and massage may help to maintain skin pliability as well.
• Antacids, frequent small meals, and elevation of the head of the bed are recommended for patients with heartburn. Medications such as histamine (H2) blockers or omeprazole may be helpful for esophagitis (inflammation or irritation of the esophagus).
• Drugs may be prescribed to aid circulation and so reduce the symptoms of Raynaud's phenomenon.
• Patients with scleroderma may have an associated polymyositis (muscle inflammation, sometimes involving the heart; see also Dermatomyositis). This should be detected early and treated aggressively with corticosteroids.
• Dialysis may be needed for impaired kidney function; high blood pressure (which occurs when the kidneys are affected) is treated with drug therapy.
• Patients with heart failure require treatment with digitalis and diuretics.

WHEN TO CALL A DOCTOR

• Call a doctor if patches of skin become tight, shiny, and inelastic or if you experience poor circulation, swallowing difficulty, or shortness of breath.

SYMPTOMS

• Distinctive, often painful change in skin color from white to blue as blood vessels constrict from cold, then to red as circulation returns during rewarming (Raynaud's phenomenon).
• Numbness or coldness in the fingers or toes.
• Shiny, waxy, or bluish appearance of skin.
• Puffiness, thickening, and tightening of the skin, especially on the face, arms, and hands.
• Changes in pigmentation.
• Joint pain and stiffness.
• Heartburn; tightness in the throat; swallowing difficulty.
• Shortness of breath after minimal exertion; fatigue; weakness; persistent slight fever.
• High blood pressure; signs of renal failure.

Scoliosis

WHAT IS IT?

Scoliosis is a sideways, or lateral, curvature of the spine. A curve to one side, most often in the thoracic (chest) portion of the spine, leads to compensatory bends in the lumbar (lower back) and cervical (neck) portions of the backbone. The resulting S-shape of the spine causes the chest cavity to be enlarged on the wide part of the curve and compressed on the narrow side. In severe cases with large curves, lung capacity can be seriously reduced resulting in heart and respiratory problems. The disorder is often accompanied by a forward or backward curvature, known respectively as kyphosis (humplike) and lordosis (swaylike).

Scoliosis usually begins in the years of rapid skeletal growth, between the ages of four and nine, or in the early teens. Adolescent girls are four times more likely to be affected than their male counterparts. Progression usually slows by early adulthood. When detected early, minor deformities may be halted by spine-strengthening exercises and by wearing a brace. More severe cases may require surgery. Scoliosis may worsen with age as a result of osteoporosis or loss of muscle strength.

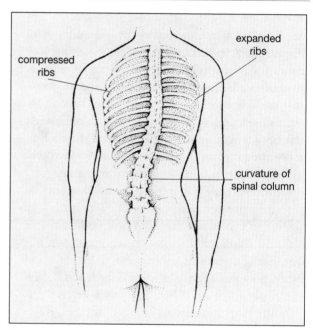

compressed ribs

expanded ribs

curvature of spinal column

Scoliosis compresses the rib cage on one side and expands it on the other. This may diminish lung capacity on the compressed side.

SYMPTOMS

- A visible S-shaped curve in the spine or noticeable deformity of the spine.
- Conspicuous hump of the upper back.
- Discernible flatness of the lower back with the loss of the normal curve.

WHAT CAUSES IT?

- In 80 percent of cases, the cause is unknown.
- In the remaining 20 percent of cases, scoliosis can be attributed to abnormalities such as weakness of the spinal muscles from neuromuscular disease, as in poliomyelitis; spinal injury, such as a fracture; or acquired or inherited defects in the vertebrae.

PREVENTION

- There is no known way to prevent scoliosis, but its progression may be arrested after it is diagnosed.

DIAGNOSIS

- Patient history and physical examination.
- Spinal x-rays.

HOW TO TREAT IT

- When the deformity is slight or associated with muscular weakness, exercises may be recommended. Bracing can be effective in children or adolescents with smaller curves.
- Frequent physician monitoring is necessary during the rapid growth years to detect significant changes in the curve.
- A hinged plaster jacket or adjustable metal brace, fitted by an orthopedic surgeon, may be used to immobilize the spine and to arrest the progression of the curvature.
- Progressing curvatures and curvatures greater than 45 degrees usually require surgery. Bone grafting with metal rods is done to straighten the spine and fuse it in this corrected position.

WHEN TO CALL A DOCTOR

- Call a doctor if you suspect scoliosis in yourself or your child. Early treatment can halt its progression.

Seizures

WHAT IS IT?

Seizures are alterations in neurologic function resulting from bursts of abnormal electrical activity in the brain. In normal brain function, electrical charges flow from one neuron to the other along pathways that establish orderly patterns of thought and behavior. Seizures are initiated by the sudden onset of repetitive, synchronized discharges from many neurons that can cause radical changes in consciousness, sensation, and muscle control. The many different types of seizures can be grouped into two broad categories: generalized and partial (or focal). In generalized seizures, abnormal electrical activity may occur anywhere in the brain, while in partial seizures, abnormal activity is isolated to one area of the brain.

Perhaps the best-known type of generalized seizure is the grand mal seizure: sudden loss of consciousness followed by violent full-body convulsions lasting several minutes. The patient has no memory of the event and is usually confused and drowsy for some time afterward. The petit mal seizure—another type of generalized seizure—is characterized by a blank look, staring, and loss of awareness, but not muscle convulsions. Like the grand mal, there is typically no memory of the event afterward. An untreated person may experience hundreds of petit mal seizures daily, each one lasting only a few seconds. However, these are only two of many different types of seizures.

Partial (or focal) seizures may trigger isolated, localized movements—such as chewing, lip smacking, or swallowing—or merely produce odd sensations, such as transient prickling or numbness. Disorders producing recurrent seizures are known as the epilepsies; seizures may also occur as one-time events, such as those triggered by high fevers in children. Epilepsy occurs in approximately 1 to 2 percent of the population. Generally, seizures last a few seconds to a few minutes at a time. Prolonged grand mal seizures (status epilepticus), or those that recur in rapid succession, require emergency medical treatment.

Although there is generally no cure, epilepsy can usually be controlled with a variety of anticonvulsant medications. Children with petit mal epilepsy often outgrow it as they reach late adolescence and young adulthood. For other types of seizures, anticonvulsant medication can often be discontinued after a patient has been seizure-free for two to five years. Finally, brain surgery is an option if seizures are severe or resistant to medication. After surgery, seizures may subside completely or almost completely, and mental functioning is often improved.

WHAT CAUSES IT?

- Sudden, explosive, highly synchronized firing of neurons in the brain—the cause of which is unidentifiable in about half of all cases.

SYMPTOMS

- Warning symptoms (known as an aura) prior to a seizure: sensations of strange odors, sounds, sights, or feelings; feeling of déjà vu; nausea. Each person generally has a consistent aura, although aura sensations vary widely from person to person.
- Petit mal or absence seizure: loss of awareness and lack of responsiveness; staring; twitching of the arm or head.
- Grand mal seizure: loss of consciousness; muscle rigidity followed by twitching or jerking; loss of bladder and bowel control. Most grand mal seizures are not preceded by an aura. After the seizure: no memory of the event; confusion; sleepiness; headache.
- Focal seizure: uncontrollable twitching of one part of the body, such as the hand, which may spread to nearby muscles or the entire body. The patient may remain conscious during a focal seizure.
- Temporal lobe seizure: loss of awareness; sudden, bizarre behavior, such as laughing or becoming angry for no apparent reason; repetitive lip smacking, chewing motions, or picking at clothes. Temporal lobe seizures may be preceded by an aura lasting a few seconds.
- Febrile seizure: rapid rise or fall in body temperature; loss of consciousness; muscle convulsions characteristic of a grand mal seizure. A febrile seizure is usually an isolated event that does not recur.

Seizures *continued*

- Brain damage due to prior head trauma, such as an automobile accident, sports injury, or a fall.
- Withdrawal from alcohol, illicit drugs, or anticonvulsant medication.
- Brain tumor or stroke.
- Infection of the brain or its surrounding tissues (see Meningitis and Encephalitis).
- High fevers, which commonly cause seizures in children under age five (febrile seizure).
- Congenital brain damage due to illness, injury, or infection during pregnancy that affects the development of the fetal nervous system.
- Chemical imbalances such as low blood sugar, calcium, or sodium levels, or severe vitamin deficiency.
- Conditions that affect the central nervous system, such as cerebral palsy and multiple sclerosis.
- Sleep deprivation or physical stress.

PREVENTION
- There is no known way to prevent epilepsy, but medications can control seizures in most cases.

DIAGNOSIS
- Patient history and physical examination.
- Electroencephalogram (EEG). In this procedure, electrodes are attached to the patient's head to measure electrical activity in the brain. A series of EEGs may be taken over a period of time to obtain a complete picture of brain activity.
- Skull x-ray; CT (computed tomography), PET (positron-emission tomography), or SPECT (single-photon emission computed tomography) scans of the brain; or MRI (magnetic resonance imaging) may be ordered.

- Proper diagnosis of the type of seizure is important for selecting the most appropriate drug treatment.

HOW TO TREAT IT
- Do not try to restrain someone having a seizure. If the person falls, try to ease the descent to the ground. Move objects out of the way to prevent accidental injury, then stand aside. Do not try to insert your fingers into the mouth of someone having a seizure; contrary to popular belief, people do not swallow their tongues during seizures, and attempting to force their mouth open may cause injury to them or you. After muscle convulsions have ceased, roll the person to one side to prevent choking on fluids or vomit. When the person regains consciousness, offer reassurance. The person may need to sleep for a while after a seizure.
- Treatment is unnecessary for seizures caused by high fevers in children.
- Anticonvulsant medications, such as carbamazepine, phenytoin, phenobarbital, valproate, gabapentin, tiagabine, topiramate, lamotrigine, ethosuximide, clonazepam, and primidone, may be prescribed.
- Brain surgery may be advised in severe cases to remove tumors, scar tissue, or vascular malformations, or to interrupt paths of abnormal electrical activity.

WHEN TO CALL A DOCTOR
- Call a doctor if you or your child suffers a seizure for the first time.
- **EMERGENCY** Call an ambulance if a seizure lasts for more than five minutes, or if the person has another seizure before regaining consciousness. 🔺

Septic Shock

WHAT IS IT?

Septic shock, a life-threatening medical emergency, is the result of an invasion of the bloodstream by infectious agents (septicemia), usually bacteria. In an inflammatory response to the infectious organisms or their toxic products, substances are released that cause blood vessels to dilate, cardiac output to decline, and fluids to leak from small blood vessels into the tissues. Blood pressure then drops precipitously (septic shock), starving the body's cells of oxygen-carrying blood. Cells begin to die.

Cell damage can rapidly lead to multiple organ-system failure of the liver, lungs, brain, kidneys, and heart. Failure of any of the vital organs can be fatal. Septic shock occurs most commonly among hospitalized patients, especially those with severe infections. Early recognition of the signs leading up to shock and immediate treatment are imperative. Full-blown septic shock is fatal in over two-thirds of cases despite modern therapeutic measures.

WHAT CAUSES IT?

• A bacterial infection is the most common cause of septic shock. Puncture wounds, deep cuts, burns, surgical procedures, or the use of a urinary catheter can introduce bacteria into the bloodstream.
• Rarely, viral or fungal infections cause septic shock.
• Risk factors for developing septic shock and for suffering more severe consequences include other disorders, such as diabetes mellitus, advanced cancer, and cirrhosis of the liver; severe injury or burns;

major surgeries; and a weakened immune system due to AIDS or treatment for cancer, for example. Newborns and the elderly are also at higher risk.

PREVENTION

• Obtain prompt treatment for bacterial infections, wounds, or burns.

DIAGNOSIS

• Diagnosis may be presumed immediately upon physical examination, patient history, and observation of characteristic symptoms. Because septic shock is an emergency, treatment is initiated prior to laboratory confirmation of diagnosis.
• Blood cultures provide a definitive diagnosis.

HOW TO TREAT IT

• Hospitalization in an intensive care unit is necessary.
• Intravenous antibiotics are administered to treat a bacterial infection.
• Intravenous fluids and blood transfusions are given to restore adequate fluid volume in the circulatory system and to counteract severe anemia, if present.
• If administration of fluids fails to restore blood pressure to acceptable levels, a vasopressor (blood vessel constricting) drug such as epinephrine or dopamine may be given to increase blood pressure.
• Mechanical respiration through a mask or nasal tubes may be required to supply adequate oxygen.
• Surgery to drain or remove infected tissue or to cleanse a wound of foreign material is performed as needed.

WHEN TO CALL A DOCTOR

• **EMERGENCY** Call an ambulance immediately if someone begins to hyperventilate and is confused and disoriented, with or without fever or nausea. ▲

SYMPTOMS

• Rapid, shallow breathing (hyperventilation).
• Changes in consciousness or mental state, such as confusion, agitation, disorientation, or coma.
• Sudden high fever and chills.
• Severe fatigue and weakness.
• Nausea and vomiting.
• Diarrhea.
• Decreased urine output.
• Prostration.
• Rapid heartbeat.

Shin Splints

WHAT IS IT?

Shin splints refer to pain in and around the large bone of the lower leg (tibia) due to exercise. While the exact cause is not known, shin splints appear to develop from excess stress or shock to the tibia and its surrounding tissues, such as occurs during running. The pain typically occurs on the inside portion of the leg. In severe cases, the tibia may gradually crack, forming a stress fracture.

These injuries are common among joggers, dancers, or anyone whose exercise routine or occupation involves pounding of the feet on hard surfaces. In most cases a few weeks of rest followed by a regimen of proper conditioning will allow a safe return to a full complement of normal activities.

WHAT CAUSES IT?

• Increased amount or intensity of exercise in legs not conditioned to the stress.
• Inadequate training or improper technique.
• Improper or worn-out footwear that no longer absorbs impact sufficiently.

PREVENTION

• Be sure to stretch your calf muscles thoroughly in your regular warm-up before exercise.
• Use proper athletic footwear with good cushion.
• Run on grass or dirt paths instead of on concrete.
• Avoid sudden increases in the intensity of your workout.

DIAGNOSIS

• Patient history and presentation of symptoms.
• Examination of the foot and lower leg helps to establish any anatomical predisposition.
• An x-ray or bone scan may be used to diagnose a hairline stress fracture when symptoms are prolonged or recurrent.

SYMPTOMS

• Pain of gradual or abrupt onset, which usually occurs during or just after exercise.
• Persistent aching pain in the front or side of the lower leg.

HOW TO TREAT IT

• Rest, usually for two or three weeks, is the most common recommendation and may be combined with physical therapy to strengthen any affected muscles.
• A temporary switch to low-impact activities such as bicycling or swimming is advised if high-impact exercise (like aerobic dancing or running) appears to have caused shin splints.
• Wear shoes that are well cushioned and provide good support.
• For pain, take over-the-counter anti-inflammatory drugs such as aspirin or ibuprofen.
• Ice packs may be recommended for swelling and inflammation.
• Heat, in the form of whirlpool or hot soaks, may reduce discomfort.
• Stretching exercises, particularly of the calf, and self-massage may ease pain.
• A podiatrist or orthopedist may recommend an orthotic device (a specially fitted insert) to place in your shoes. Orthotics may help to correct structural anomalies that promote repeated episodes of shin splints.

WHEN TO CALL A DOCTOR

• If shin pain persists for more than three weeks despite self-treatment, consult your doctor. You may be referred to a podiatrist or orthopedist for further evaluation and treatment.

Sinusitis

WHAT IS IT?

Sinusitis is an inflammation of one or more of the four sets of facial sinus cavities, usually due to infection. When irritated, the mucous membrane lining the sinus may swell and block the small drainage channels that permit mucus to flow into the nose. The buildup in pressure often results in headache, nasal congestion, and facial pain. Acute sinusitis is a common disorder that often follows a cold or flu; chronic sinusitis refers to persistent or recurrent episodes that are generally milder than acute cases. Sinusitis often subsides on its own and responds well to home treatment. In rare cases, however, infection may spread to the eyes or the brain, possibly leading to vision loss, meningitis, or brain abscess.

WHAT CAUSES IT?

• A viral or bacterial infection that spreads to the sinuses from the nose.
• Anatomical irregularities, such as a deviated septum.
• Nasal allergy resulting in swelling and polyps.
• Swimming in contaminated water.
• Infection spread from abscesses in the upper teeth.
• Chronic sinusitis may be caused by irritation from dust, air pollutants, or excessive exposure to tobacco smoke, or result from an untreated acute condition.

PREVENTION

• If you have allergies, limiting exposure to allergens and using antihistamines and/or nasal steroid sprays can help control sinusitis symptoms.

SYMPTOMS

• Headache pain and pressure concentrated over one or both eyes (frontal sinusitis).
• Pain in the cheek bones (maxillary sinusitis).
• Swelling of upper eyelids (ethmoid sinusitis).
• Tenderness over the affected sinus.
• Pain behind the eyes (sphenoid sinusitis).
• A yellowish green nasal discharge.
• Persistent nasal blockage and forced breathing through the mouth following a cold or flu.
• Fever and chills.
• Dental pain, usually in the upper jaw.

• When you have a cold, use a cool-mist humidifier and decongestants to promote drainage.
• Chronic sinusitis sufferers should avoid tobacco smoke and alcohol (its diuretic effect thickens mucus) and should drink plenty of liquids to loosen nasal secretions.

DIAGNOSIS

• Patient history and physical examination are needed.
• Removal of fluid from the maxillary sinus using a needle or endoscope-directed suction may be necessary to determine the type of bacterial infection.
• X-rays may be used to locate areas of blockage.

HOW TO TREAT IT

• Steam inhaled from a basin of hot water can thin the mucus and ease symptoms.
• Over-the-counter oral or nasal decongestants may reduce swelling. Nasal decongestants should not be used for more than three days. People with high blood pressure, heart disease, arrhythmias, or glaucoma should ask their doctor about decongestants.
• Nonprescription pain relievers, ice packs, or warm compresses may soothe sinus pain. In severe cases codeine may be prescribed.
• Antihistamines are used to treat allergic sinusitis.
• Steroid nasal sprays may be prescribed to reduce inflammation.
• Antibiotics are prescribed for bacterial infections. It may be necessary to use antibiotics for two to six weeks in difficult cases.
• Endoscopy (use of a lighted instrument) may be used to survey the sinuses and clear blockage.
• Surgery may be needed to drain sinuses in very rare cases. Early surgical drainage is often recommended for frontal sinusitis.
• Hospitalization and intravenous antibiotics are required for severe bacterial sinusitis.

WHEN TO CALL A DOCTOR

• Call a doctor if symptoms persist longer than two weeks or are accompanied by bloody nasal discharge.
• **EMERGENCY** See a doctor right away if you develop redness, pain, or bulging of an eye, paralysis of eye movements, or nausea and vomiting in association with other symptoms of sinusitis.

Sjögren's Syndrome

WHAT IS IT?
Sjögren's syndrome is a type of autoimmune disorder in which, for reasons unknown, the body's defenses against infection mistakenly attack cells in the salivary and lacrimal (tear) glands. The result is extreme dryness in the mucous membranes of the mouth and eyes, which may lead to dental cavities and corneal infections. Other glands may be affected too, such as those that produce vaginal lubrication. Vaginal dryness is thus a symptom in women, who develop Sjögren's syndrome nine times more often than men.

Nearly 60 percent of patients may develop other, nonglandular symptoms (such as fatigue and joint and muscle pain) over the course of the disease. The lungs, kidneys, blood vessels, and nervous system may also be affected, but less often. Lymph glands often become enlarged, and Sjögren's patients have a higher incidence of lymphoma (see Lymphoma, Non-Hodgkin's). The disorder may occur on its own or in conjunction with other autoimmune disorders; in fact, as many as 30 percent of those with rheumatoid arthritis also develop Sjögren's syndrome.

Sjögren's syndrome can begin at any time in life, including childhood, but typically starts after age 40. In uncomplicated cases symptoms can be eased with treatment, and the outlook is generally favorable.

SYMPTOMS
- Dry, red, painful eyes.
- Dry, painful mouth; swallowing difficulty; frequent dental cavities.
- Reduced ability to distinguish taste and smells.
- Hoarseness and dry cough that worsens in cold weather.
- Dry skin.
- Swelling of the salivary glands just in front of the ears (parotid glands).
- Vaginal dryness.
- Joint pain.
- Fatigue.
- Distinctive change of skin color from white to blue as blood vessels constrict in response to cold, and then to red as circulation returns during rewarming (Raynaud's phenomenon).

WHAT CAUSES IT?
- The cause of Sjögren's is unknown, although a hereditary predisposition appears to be involved.
- Other autoimmune disorders are linked to a higher risk of Sjögren's syndrome (see Rheumatoid Arthritis, Systemic Lupus Erythematosus, or Scleroderma).

PREVENTION
- There is no way to prevent Sjögren's syndrome.

DIAGNOSIS
- Patient history and physical examination.
- Blood tests for indicators of autoimmune activity.
- Biopsy and microscopic examination of a tissue sample from the salivary glands or lip.

HOW TO TREAT IT
- There is no cure for Sjögren's syndrome; treatment is aimed at relieving symptoms.
- Artificial tear solutions containing methylcellulose or saline eyedrops are used to treat dry eyes.
- Sugarless gum or sour candies may increase saliva.
- Increased fluid intake is important, but alcohol and caffeine can exacerbate dryness.
- Saliva-substitute solutions, which also contain methylcellulose, may be recommended. In severe cases the drug pilocarpine may be prescribed to increase saliva production.
- Vigilant dental hygiene is essential for the prevention of cavities.
- Antibiotics may be prescribed to treat associated bacterial infections in the eyes or eyelids.
- Over-the-counter water-based lubricants can be used to counteract vaginal dryness. Your doctor may recommend using a gel containing propionic acid.
- For dry skin, moisturizing creams should be applied right after bathing, while skin is still moist.
- In very severe cases corticosteroids such as prednisone or short-term courses of immunosuppressive drugs may be administered to treat life-threatening vital organ involvement, but this is uncommon.

WHEN TO CALL A DOCTOR
- Make an appointment with a doctor if you develop persistent dryness in the mucous membranes of the eyes, mouth, nasal passages, or vagina. ◪

Sleep Apnea

WHAT IS IT?

Sleep apnea is a disorder characterized by repeated cessation of breathing for brief periods during sleep. Most common among obese, middle-aged men, sleep apnea can usually be attributed to excessive relaxation during sleep of the muscles at the back of the throat—a consequence of getting older or gaining extra weight. The sagging folds of muscle and soft tissue may block the upper airway (obstructive sleep apnea) a dozen to hundreds of times a night. After 10 to 100 seconds, the demand for oxygen grows critical, and the sleeper gasps or snores abruptly in characteristically loud, staccato bursts in the struggle to regain normal breathing.

In a rare form of the disorder known as central sleep apnea, the airways remain open but the chest muscles and diaphragm are not stimulated to expand the lungs for repeated short periods. A third form, mixed sleep apnea, combines airway obstruction with central sleep apnea.

The sleeper rarely awakens fully during these gasping episodes but tends to arise tired and unrefreshed the next morning, because apnea prevents the sufferer from reaching deeper stages of sleep. Severe, persistent cases of sleep apnea may promote serious cardiovascular problems such as high blood pressure, abnormal heart rhythms, and heart failure. Treatment depends on the cause and severity of symptoms.

WHAT CAUSES IT?

• Excess body weight combined with loss of muscle tone at the base of the throat.
• Alcohol and sedatives promote apnea.
• Hormonal changes due to menopause may produce sleep apnea in some women.

SYMPTOMS

• Breathing cessation interrupted by loud, abrupt bursts of snoring or snorting.
• Excessive daytime sleepiness.
• Morning headache.
• Difficulty concentrating; memory loss; personality changes.

• Incidence increases with age.
• The cause of central sleep apnea is unknown.

PREVENTION

• Maintain a healthy weight.
• Avoid sleeping pills and do not consume alcoholic beverages within two or three hours of bedtime.

DIAGNOSIS

• Patient history and physical examination are necessary. History may include reports from roommates or bed mates. A tape recording of nighttime snoring may also be useful in making a diagnosis.
• Further evaluation at a sleep center may be recommended to pinpoint the underlying causes of sleep apnea and to devise a suitable treatment strategy.
• Laboratory tests may include chest x-rays, electroencephalogram, electrocardiogram, and tests of blood-oxygen levels, chest wall movement, and air movement through the nose and mouth during sleep.

HOW TO TREAT IT

• Weight loss is a key part of management for those who are overweight.
• A tennis ball may be sewn to the back of pajamas to prevent sleeping on one's back, a position that encourages episodes of sleep apnea.
• Medications such as the antidepressant protriptyline or the hormonal supplement medroxyprogesterone may relieve symptoms in some cases.
• A device known as continuous positive airway pressure (CPAP) may be prescribed. With CPAP, a mask is worn over the nose; air is forced through the mask throughout the night to keep the throat open.
• Surgery may be performed in some cases to improve breathing. Anatomical obstruction in the back of the throat may be corrected, or in life-threatening cases a small opening in the throat (tracheostomy) may be created to bypass the blocked airway.

WHEN TO CALL A DOCTOR

• Make an appointment with a doctor if you develop extremely loud snoring with periods of silence, or if excessive daytime sleepiness interferes with normal activities. 🛆

Spinal Cord Trauma

WHAT IS IT?

Injury to the spinal cord is a medical emergency that may result in severe and permanent disability. The spinal cord—which along with the brain comprises the central nervous system—is a bundle of nerve cells that travels almost the entire length of the spine, connecting the brain to the nerves in the rest of the body. The vertebrae, the small bones that make up the spine, form a bony tunnel that surrounds the cord and protects it from injury. However, if a blow is severe enough, or if the bones are weakened by disease, the spinal cord is vulnerable to damage.

Destroyed nerve cells cannot regenerate; injury to the spinal cord may thus result in permanent paralysis of the legs (paraplegia) or, in the case of a neck injury, the arms, torso, and legs (quadriplegia). About half of the cases of spinal cord injury involve the neck. However, partial or complete recovery may be expected in cases when neurons in the spinal cord have been traumatized but not completely destroyed. Outcome thus depends upon both the severity and the specific location of the injury. Damage to the spinal cord will affect nerves at the level of the injury and below.

WHAT CAUSES IT?

• Injury, from motor vehicle or sports accidents, falls, or gun shot wounds, is the most common cause of spinal cord trauma.
• Displaced or broken vertebrae can damage the spinal cord directly.

SYMPTOMS

• Intense localized back or neck pain.
• Swelling at the site of injury.
• Weakness, numbness, tingling, and impaired sensation in the limbs and torso below the injured area of the spinal cord.
• Paralysis of the legs (paraplegia) or of both the arms and legs (quadriplegia).
• Loss of bowel and bladder control.
• Erectile dysfunction (impotence).
• Breathing difficulty.
• Shock.

• Swelling of nearby tissues, or a blood clot, may compress the spinal cord.
• Trauma may damage the cord by interrupting its blood supply.
• People with bones weakened by osteoporosis, rheumatoid arthritis, or bone cancer are at greater risk for spinal cord damage.

PREVENTION

• Wear shoulder and lap belts when traveling in a car.
• Be sure water is sufficiently deep before diving.
• Wear protective gear when playing sports.
• Get enough calcium to reduce the risk of osteoporosis. Hormone replacement therapy may be recommended to postmenopausal women to prevent osteoporosis.

DIAGNOSIS

• Patient history and physical examination.
• X-rays of the spine.
• CT (computed tomography) scans or MRI (magnetic resonance imaging).
• X-rays may be taken after injection of a contrast medium (myelography) to outline the spinal cord.

HOW TO TREAT IT

• Call an ambulance immediately. Do not attempt to move someone who may have a spinal cord injury because any movement may cause further damage to the spinal cord.
• Careful immobilization of the head and back by means of traction, splints, and braces is necessary to prevent further damage.
• Oxygen may be supplied through a small tube inserted into the nose if breathing is impaired owing to paralysis of respiratory muscles.
• Intravenous methylprednisolone, a corticosteroid medication, may be administered within the first eight hours of injury to minimize the extent of nerve damage.
• Surgical decompression of the spinal cord may restore some function if cord damage is incomplete.
• Long-term use of a urinary catheter may be necessary if bladder control is lost.
• Special prescription support hose and anticoagulant drugs such as heparin help prevent the formation of

Spinal Cord Trauma *continued*

blood clots in immobilized limbs and the resultant pulmonary emboli.

• Tube feedings may be needed to provide ample nutrition.

• Wheelchairs may be needed for those with permanent paralysis.

• Frequent repositioning helps avoid skin breakdown (bed sores) over pressure points.

• Extensive physical therapy can prevent immobilization of joints and contractures of muscle.

• Occupational and emotional therapy help patients and their families cope with major lifestyle changes.

WHEN TO CALL A DOCTOR

• **EMERGENCY** Call an ambulance immediately if you suspect someone has sustained a back or neck injury. Do not attempt to move the person, and do not allow him or her to sit up. ▲

Spinal Stenosis

WHAT IS IT?

Spinal stenosis is a narrowing of the spinal canal, the cavity within the vertebral column through which the spinal cord passes. Nerves leaving and entering the spinal cord are called nerve roots; they pass through the vertebral column via small canals. Arthritic changes that cause overgrowth of vertebral bones may compress the spinal cord or the nerve roots, impairing sensation and muscle strength in the affected portion of the body. Most common among people in their 50s and 60s, spinal stenosis affects the lumbar (lower back) portion of the spine more than the cervical (neck) region. Symptoms include pain, numbness, and weakness in the lower back and legs. Aching in the buttocks, thighs, or calves during activity is a common feature of low back spinal stenosis.

WHAT CAUSES IT?

• Disorders that involve arthritic degeneration and abnormal overgrowth of bone tissue, such as osteoarthritis or Paget's disease (see these specific disorders), may cause spinal stenosis.

PREVENTION

• There is no way to prevent spinal stenosis.

DIAGNOSIS

• Patient history and physical examination. Reflexes in the legs are tested to assess nerve involvement.
• X-rays, sometimes with injected dyes (myelography).
• CT (computed tomography) scans or MRI (magnetic resonance imaging).

HOW TO TREAT IT

• Losing weight and toning the abdominal muscles with exercise may reduce pressure on the spine.

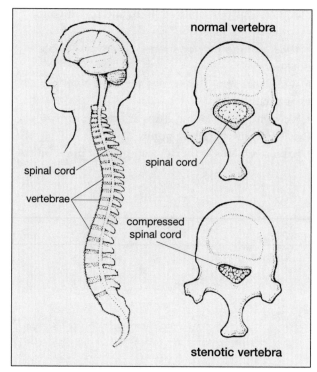

Overgrowth of the vertebrae narrows the spinal canal. This may compress the spinal cord or spinal nerves, causing pain and numbness.

Check with your doctor before beginning any weight-loss program or new exercise regimen.
• A lumbosacral support (a corset available at some pharmacies and medical-supply stores) may discourage motion that causes pain and help ease walking and exercise. It should not be worn all day, however.
• Anti-inflammatory drugs may relieve pain.
• If pain prevents normal activities despite self-care and medication, surgery to relieve pressure on the nerves (decompression surgery) may be warranted. The surgeon opens the spinal column where narrowing has occurred and removes the constricting bone or fibrous tissue. The opening through which nerve roots pass may be widened; if an excessive amount of bone is removed, the affected vertebrae may be fused together to increase spinal stability. Physical therapy may aid rehabilitation.

WHEN TO CALL A DOCTOR

• Call a doctor if you have persistent pain, numbness, or weakness in the back, legs, or neck, or if back pain accompanies changes in bowel or bladder function. ▲

SYMPTOMS

• Back pain that may radiate to the buttocks and legs. Pain worsens with activity.
• Numbness in the buttocks and legs.
• Weakness in the legs.
• Back pain with loss of or changes in bowel or bladder function.

Spinal Tumor

WHAT IS IT?

A spinal tumor is an abnormal growth of cells located either within the spinal cord itself or, much more often, in its surrounding membranes and tissues. The spinal cord, which along with the brain comprises the central nervous system, is a bundle of nerve cells encased in a protective membrane that travels almost the entire length of the spine, connecting the brain to the nerves in the rest of the body. Tumors affecting the spinal cord are uncommon; they may be either benign or malignant.

However, even benign tumors can compress the spinal cord, leading to irreversible paralysis (see Spinal Cord Trauma). They can also impinge upon nerves as they leave the spinal cord. Malignant tumors rarely originate in the spinal cord itself; most often, cancer compressing the spinal cord has spread from elsewhere in the body to the bones of the spine (vertebrae) or has originated in the vertebrae. Benign tumors usually grow slowly, but malignant tumors may increase in size in a matter of days; symptoms may be limited to back pain or may include numbness, loss of sensation, and weakness, generally beginning in the legs. Both benign and malignant tumors can damage the spinal cord by interrupting its blood supply. After diagnosis of a malignant tumor, rapid treatment is necessary to limit damage and to prevent irreversible paraplegia.

WHAT CAUSES IT?

• The cause of spinal tumors is unknown.
• Cancer that originates elsewhere in the body, such as the breast, lung, or prostate, may spread to the vertebrae.

PREVENTION

• There is no known way to prevent spinal tumors.
• Regular examinations of the breasts in women and the prostate in men aid in early detection and treatment of tumors in those areas (see Breast Cancer and Prostate Cancer for more information).

DIAGNOSIS

• Patient history and physical examination.
• X-rays of the spine.
• MRI (magnetic resonance imaging).
• CT (computed tomography) scans, with injection of a contrast material (myelography), in some cases.
• Lumbar puncture (spinal tap), to analyze a sample of cerebrospinal fluid.
• Biopsy of the tumor may be required to confirm the diagnosis.

HOW TO TREAT IT

• Surgery may be performed promptly to reduce compression of the spinal cord by removing part or all of the tumor.
• Large doses of corticosteroid drugs, such as dexamethasone, may be administered to reduce swelling.
• Radiation therapy may be required in addition to or instead of surgery to treat malignant tumors.
• Chemotherapy may be advised in some cases to treat malignant tumors.
• Physical, occupational, and emotional therapy may be recommended to patients and their families to help them cope with major lifestyle changes.

WHEN TO CALL A DOCTOR

• Call a doctor if you develop severe, persistent back pain, with or without numbness, tingling, or muscle weakness. △

SYMPTOMS

• Constant back pain that may spread in a horizontal band around the chest or abdomen. Pain may be described as a burning sensation and may worsen upon exertion, lying down, and coughing or sneezing.
• Numbness, tingling, and muscle weakness usually beginning in the legs.
• Loss of pain and temperature sensation below the site of the tumor.
• Loss of bladder and bowel control.

Spondylosis, Cervical

WHAT IS IT?

Cervical spondylosis is a general term for degeneration of the structures in the cervical (neck) region of the spine. The seven cervical vertebrae constitute the top portion of the spine—the long, flexible column of bones that supports the skeleton and protects the spinal cord. Flat, circular pads of cartilage known as intervertebral disks serve as cushions between the vertebrae and allow for smooth movement.

In spondylosis, rupture of a disk, or overgrowth of the vertebrae or the ligaments that support the spine, or a combination of these may compress the spinal cord or the nerves entering or exiting the spinal cord, causing pain and other symptoms (see Spinal Stenosis or Intervertebral Disk, Herniated, for more information). Spondylosis is common among those of middle age and older; many cases are mild and respond well to self-treatment.

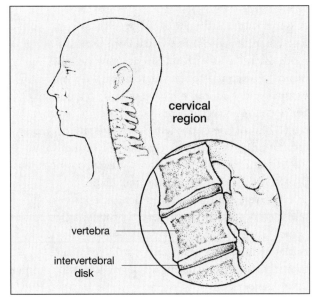

The cervical region of the spine is comprised of the seven uppermost vertebrae in the spinal column and their supporting structures.

WHAT CAUSES IT?

- The cause of spondylosis is unknown.
- Risk increases with age.
- Prior neck injuries may increase the risk of developing spondylosis.

PREVENTION

- There is no way to prevent cervical spondylosis.

DIAGNOSIS

- Patient history and physical examination are needed.
- Spinal x-ray, CT (computed tomography) scan, or MRI (magnetic resonance imaging) usually confirms the diagnosis.

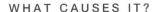

SYMPTOMS

- Pain and stiffness in the neck and shoulders. Pain may radiate to the arms and may worsen upon coughing or sneezing.
- Tingling or numbness in the hands and feet.
- Weakness in the arms and legs.
- Gait irregularities or walking difficulty in advanced cases.
- Impaired bladder or bowel control in very advanced cases.

- Myelography (injection of a contrast material into the space around the spinal cord to highlight spinal abnormalities during x-rays) is sometimes performed.

HOW TO TREAT IT

- Mild cases of cervical spondylosis may resolve on their own. Rest and immobilization of the neck with a brace may aid in recovery.
- Over-the-counter analgesics may be used for minor pain. For more severe cases prescription painkillers, muscle relaxants, or tranquilizers may be warranted.
- Traction therapy may be required if pain is persistent. This is usually done on an outpatient basis and, if effective, can be continued at home with a home traction unit.
- In advanced cases surgery may be performed to relieve pressure on the spinal nerves. Surgery may involve removing bony overgrowth in the vertebrae, fusing affected vertebrae together to prevent harmful joint movement, or both.
- Regular exercise or physical therapy may be recommended.

WHEN TO CALL A DOCTOR

- Call a doctor if persistent neck pain does not respond to self-treatment.

Sprains and Strains

WHAT IS IT?

A sprain refers to an injury to a ligament—one of the tough, fibrous cords that act as tethers to hold the bones together at the joint. Sprains occur at the joints when the adjacent bones are twisted or pushed too far. The ligaments can stretch and even tear, causing pain and loss of function. The most common joints to experience sprains are the knee, ankle, shoulder, and those in the fingers.

A strain refers to a muscle injury. As such, strains usually occur away from the joint, in the muscle tissue. The most commonly injured muscles are the hamstring at the back of the thigh and the gastrocnemius, or calf muscle. Athletes commonly suffer both sprains and strains.

WHAT CAUSES IT?

• Sprains occur as a result of an injury, when the joint is subjected to more physical force than it can withstand.
• Strains occur when a muscle is overstretched or overexerted, often from running or lifting a weight.
• Previous sprains may weaken the ligaments; recurrence is possible with only minor pressure.
• Strains increase with obesity and poor muscular conditioning.

PREVENTION

• Perform warm-up exercises before undertaking any strenuous physical activity.
• Engage in regular, moderate exercise to keep muscles and joints strong and flexible.

DIAGNOSIS

• Patient history and physical examination are needed.

SYMPTOMS

• Mild to severe pain in the affected joint that worsens with movement or the application of pressure.
• Swelling, redness, or bruising around the affected joint.
• In severe cases, loss of mobility in the affected joint.

• X-rays of the affected joint to rule out a bone fracture or other underlying problem.

HOW TO TREAT IT

First-aid measures for a sprain or strain can be easily remembered with the acronym RICE, short for rest, ice, compression, and elevation:
• *Rest* the injured area. Try not to move or put pressure on the affected joint. A sling or splint may be recommended to immobilize the joint and allow damaged ligaments or muscles to heal.
• *Ice* the affected area to reduce swelling. Apply ice daily (but for no longer than 20 minutes at one time) until the pain and swelling have resolved, and full motion and function have returned.
• *Compress* the joint by wrapping it in an elasticized bandage to help reduce swelling and pain.
• *Elevate* the joint to reduce swelling.
• In addition, take over-the-counter pain relievers to treat minor pain. Your doctor may prescribe stronger analgesics for more severe pain.
• Surgery may be required in severe cases to repair torn ligaments.
• After the pain has subsided, gently exercise the joint to regain strength and mobility. A physician or physical therapist may help devise an exercise program to aid in rehabilitation.

WHEN TO CALL A DOCTOR

• Call a doctor if symptoms do not respond to self-care treatments.
• Contact a doctor if you feel a joint shift, especially if it is accompanied by extreme pain, swelling, or loss of motion, or if the area turns black and blue.

Stomach Cancer

WHAT IS IT?

Stomach cancer results from the growth of malignant cells in the lining of the stomach. More than 90 percent of gastric cancers are adenocarcinomas, arising from cells lining the stomach wall; lymphomas account for 3 to 7 percent of stomach cancers (see Lymphoma, Non-Hodgkin's). For unknown reasons, the incidence of stomach cancer has decreased dramatically in the United States in the last 50 years; dietary factors and the refrigeration of foods (which has decreased the need for chemical preservatives) are thought to play roles in the decline. Adenocarcinomas often cause symptoms only after growing too large to be completely removed surgically; hence, early detection greatly increases the chances that treatment may be initiated in time.

WHAT CAUSES IT?

• Although the cause of stomach tumors is unknown, environmental factors appear to play a role. Geographic areas where colorectal cancer is common (such as the United States) often have a low incidence of stomach cancer.

• Consumption of foods containing nitrates or nitrites (chemicals commonly used in processed foods as preservatives) may increase stomach cancer risk. Salty, pickled, barbecued, or smoked foods are believed to pose the highest risk. Low consumption of vegetables and fruits may also raise risk.

• Surgical removal of a portion of the stomach (gas-trectomy), chronic inflammation of the stomach lining (gastritis), and pernicious anemia increase the odds of developing stomach cancer.

• Hereditary factors may be implicated: For reasons that are unknown, there is a higher incidence of stomach cancers among people with type-A blood.

• A type of lymphoma called MALT is linked to infection with the bacterium *Helicobacter pylori*.

PREVENTION

• Limit your intake of salty, pickled, and smoked foods (such as bacon, smoked or salted fish, and pickled vegetables) and increase your consumption of fruits and vegetables.

• Have regular checkups, especially a test for blood in the stool, to aid in early detection and treatment.

DIAGNOSIS

• Patient history and physical examination.

• Stool samples. Microscopic traces of blood in the stool may indicate digestive tract tumors.

• Tumors can be detected with x-rays done after the patient swallows barium to highlight the stomach.

• Gastroscopy must be performed, in which a thin, flexible, viewing tube (gastroscope) is passed into the stomach via the throat.

• Biopsy of the stomach lining may be taken with the gastroscope to confirm diagnosis.

HOW TO TREAT IT

• Surgery to remove as much of the tumor as possible is the primary treatment. Part or all of the stomach, nearby lymph nodes, the pancreas, and the spleen may also be removed if it is suspected that cancer may have spread to these sites.

• Radiation therapy may be administered instead of or in addition to surgery to relieve pain and bleeding.

• Survival rates for lymphomas of the stomach are improved with a combination of surgery and chemotherapy. In MALT, treatment with certain antibiotics and stomach acid inhibitors (such as omeprazole) can result in complete tumor regression.

WHEN TO CALL A DOCTOR

• Make an appointment with a doctor if you develop any symptoms of stomach cancer. ▲

SYMPTOMS

• No symptoms in most cases of small, surgically curable stomach cancers.
• Stomach discomfort or pain after meals that is not relieved by soothing foods or antacids.
• Loss of appetite and weight.
• Nausea and vomiting.
• Gas, heartburn, regurgitation, and belching.
• Abdominal fullness or bloating.
• Difficulty in swallowing.
• Weakness and fatigue.
• Anemia due to gastrointestinal bleeding.
• Black, tarry stools (due to bleeding).

Strabismus

WHAT IS IT?

Strabismus—a common disorder often referred to as crossed eyes—is a misalignment of the eyes. Normally, the six tiny muscles attached to each eye assure that the eyes work in parallel; coordinated eye movement allows for three-dimensional vision and proper depth perception. Impairment of the eye muscles or the nerves that control them may prevent the eyes from focusing together, resulting in double vision. In young children—in whom strabismus is most prevalent—the brain reacts to the double image by ignoring signals from the eye that deviates more often. If left untreated, this may result in permanent vision loss in the ignored eye (suppression amblyopia or lazy eye); a child will not simply outgrow strabismus. However, if amblyopia and strabismus are treated before the age of five or six, normal vision may be preserved. The earlier treatment is initiated, the greater the likelihood of a favorable outcome. When strabismus occurs in adults, it is often a sign of some underlying disorder.

WHAT CAUSES IT?

• Impaired development of the nerves to the ocular muscles or impaired development of the muscles themselves may cause strabismus in children.
• Hereditary factors may play a role.
• Increased risk is associated with farsightedness (hyperopia).
• In adults, strabismus may occur as a complication of an underlying disorder, such as diabetes mellitus, multiple sclerosis, cancer, or stroke.
• Fatigue, stress, or illness can sometimes cause temporary strabismus.

PREVENTION

• There is no known way to prevent strabismus.

SYMPTOMS

• Appears as if the two eyes are looking in two different directions.
• Impaired vision in the deviated eye.
• Double vision.
• Faulty depth perception.

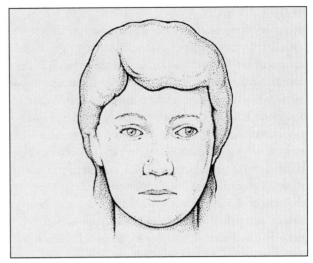

In divergent strabismus (shown here), the deviating eye turns outward; in convergent strabismus, the eye turns toward the bridge of the nose.

DIAGNOSIS

• Eye examination by an ophthalmologist can identify strabismus.
• Patient history and physical examination may be necessary, especially in adults, to diagnose an underlying disorder.

HOW TO TREAT IT

• Initial therapy involves attempts to force the brain to utilize the deviating eye. An eye patch or eyedrops that temporarily blur the vision may be used in the unaffected eye to encourage increased use of the amblyopic eye.
• Eyeglasses may be prescribed to correct farsightedness and other refractive (vision) conditions.
• Surgical repositioning of the muscles that control eye movement may be necessary to bring about realignment; more than one operation may be required.

WHEN TO CALL A DOCTOR

• Call a doctor or ophthalmologist if your child's eyes seem misaligned (although occasional crossed eyes in infants less than three months old is normal and nothing to worry about).
• Call a doctor or ophthalmologist if you develop double vision. ▲

Streptococcal Infections

WHAT IS IT?

Streptococcal infections are among the most common bacterial infections. There are many different strains of the bacteria; a number of them inhabit the mouth, intestine, and vagina without ill effect. However, these bacteria may cause infections elsewhere in the body, such as the skin or urinary tract (see Bladder Infection for more information), or produce symptoms if the immune system fails to prevent the bacteria from proliferating. The most common site of streptococcal infection is the throat. Strep may also infect the skin, ears, tonsils, urinary tract, heart valves, and other areas of the body. Most cases of strep respond well to antibiotics, although occasionally strep may lead to rheumatic fever or acute glomerulonephritis (see these disorders for more information).

WHAT CAUSES IT?

• Streptococcal bacteria may be spread through the air by the sneeze or cough of an infected person or by physical contact. Strep spreads easily in homes, schools, and other areas where people are in close and continued contact with one another.

• Infants, the elderly, and people with weakened immune systems, such as those infected with the human immunodeficiency virus (HIV) or undergoing chemotherapy for cancer, are at greater risk for the more serious complications of strep infections.

SYMPTOMS

• Symptoms depend on the location and nature of the specific infection, but may include the following:

• Fever.

• Headache.

• Swollen lymph glands.

• General feeling of poor health.

• Fatigue.

• Loss of appetite.

• Sudden, severe sore throat that is aggravated by swallowing.

• Nasal discharge.

• Red skin rash.

PREVENTION

• Wash hands frequently with soap and warm water, especially after visiting public places.

• Don't share towels or drinking glasses.

• Try to limit exposure to people who are coughing or sneezing.

DIAGNOSIS

• Patient history and physical examination.

• Throat culture (if strep throat is suspected).

• Culture of any lesion or discharge.

HOW TO TREAT IT

• Treatment varies depending on the location and nature of the infection. In general, antibiotics—usually penicillin or erythromycin—are prescribed to treat strep infections and must be taken for the full term prescribed (often 10 days or more). Stopping the medication early can result in an even more virulent recurrence of the infection (rebound infection). In severe cases antibiotics may be administered by injection.

• Over-the-counter pain relievers may be used to reduce pain and fever.

• Abscesses may need to be surgically drained.

WHEN TO CALL A DOCTOR

• Call a doctor if you develop sudden sore throat and fever.

• Call a doctor if a skin wound becomes infected, or if you or your child develops a red, crusting rash anywhere on the body. ▲

Stroke

WHAT IS IT?

A stroke is a medical emergency caused either by obstruction of an artery carrying blood to the brain or by rupture of one of the cerebral arteries. Because brain cells cannot regenerate, lack of oxygen from blockage of the blood supply may quickly lead to cell death and permanent brain damage.

Strokes are more likely to occur when arteries have been substantially narrowed by atherosclerosis (a buildup of plaques in the walls of the arteries). Blood flow through narrow arteries is reduced, and blood clots are more likely to form along the uneven surface of the plaque. A clot formed in a carotid artery in the neck or a cerebral (brain) artery can block the artery at the site. Clots may also form elsewhere, become detached, and ultimately block a cerebral artery, causing a stroke. About 80 percent of strokes are due to blockage in either an artery in the brain or in one of the carotid arteries in the neck. The remaining 20 percent result from a rupture of a brain artery (see Brain Hemorrhage for more information). This type of stroke is generally the most life-threatening, primarily because of the excessive pressure the hemorrhage exerts on brain tissue.

Although incidence is highest among those over age 65, a stroke may afflict anyone at any age. Symp-

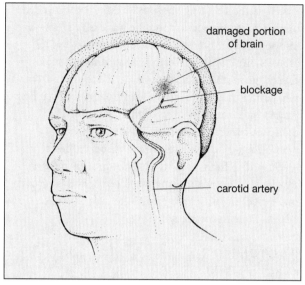

The carotid arteries are the main blood vessels from the heart to the brain. In the most common type of stroke, blockage in a cerebral or carotid artery cuts off the blood supply to a portion of brain tissue.

toms vary depending on the portion of the brain affected, but they often come on suddenly. Some patients will have temporary strokelike episodes (see Transient Ischemic Attack) prior to a stroke, which may resolve in minutes to a few hours. Strokes are the third leading cause of death in the United States, but the leading cause of disability. Prevention is key.

WHAT CAUSES IT?

• Blood clots that obstruct a carotid or cerebral artery are the most common cause of stroke.
• An embolus (a fragment of plaque, tissue, or blood clot) may develop in the heart and travel to the brain to cause a stroke. Emboli are most likely to develop in association with cardiac arrhythmias (especially atrial fibrillation), valvular heart disease, myocardial infarction, or cardiomyopathy (see these disorders for more information).
• An aneurysm (a balloonlike weak spot in an arterial wall) in a cerebral artery may burst or leak, resulting in a stroke.
• Hypertension is the greatest risk factor for stroke.
• Severely narrowed arteries due to atherosclerosis increase the risk of stroke.
• Use of cocaine or amphetamines may boost blood pressure dangerously high and cause a stroke.

SYMPTOMS

• Sudden, severe headache. (Stroke symptoms usually come on suddenly.)
• Weakness or paralysis on one or both sides of the face or body.
• Numbness and tingling in one or both arms or legs.
• Speech difficulty or loss; slurred speech.
• Nausea and vomiting.
• Total blindness or partial loss of vision, double vision, dilated pupils, or crossed eyes due to partial inability to move the eye.
• Dizziness, mental confusion, or sudden loss of consciousness.
• Memory loss.
• Inability to walk or coordinate limbs.
• Coma.

Stroke *continued*

• Risk is high among those who have experienced one or more transient ischemic attacks (TIAs)—a temporary blockage in an artery that lasts for less than 24 hours (usually only a few minutes) and causes no brain damage.
• A family history of stroke, early or premature heart attacks, atherosclerosis, or high blood pressure increases the risk of stroke.
• Smoking, alcohol abuse, high blood cholesterol levels, a diet high in fat (especially animal fat), obesity, lack of exercise, diabetes mellitus, and oral contraceptive use all may increase the risk of stroke.
• Risk increases with age.

PREVENTION

• Don't smoke.
• Eat a diet low in fat, cholesterol, and salt.
• Engage in moderate, regular exercise. Check with a doctor before beginning an exercise program.
• Lose weight if you are more than 20 percent overweight.
• Have no more than two alcoholic drinks a day.
• Low daily doses of aspirin or other antiplatelet drugs (such as ticlopidine, clopidogrel, and dipyridamole) may be prescribed to reduce the chances of blood clot formation in those who have had a TIA or are otherwise at high risk for stroke.
• Hypertension must be treated aggressively.
• The anticoagulant warfarin may be prescribed for those with atrial fibrillation and some other conditions to prevent blood clot formation.
• Patients who show evidence of substantial atherosclerotic narrowing in the carotid arteries (the two main blood vessels in the neck supplying the brain) may be good candidates for carotid endarterectomy, a surgical procedure to clear away plaque deposits in these arteries.

DIAGNOSIS

• Diagnosis is often made immediately upon examination by a doctor or emergency rescue technician.
• Blood tests are taken.
• CT (computed tomography) scans or MRI (magnetic resonance imaging) may be used to locate an abnormal blood vessel or an area of brain damage.

• Ultrasound scans of carotid arteries reveal narrowing due to atherosclerotic plaque.
• Angiography may be performed to locate the arterial blockage or aneurysm. In this procedure a tiny catheter is inserted into an artery in the groin (femoral artery) and threaded up to the carotid artery in the neck. A contrast material is injected to produce a clear x-ray image of the carotid and cerebral arteries.
• An electrocardiogram (ECG) is performed to detect a cardiac arrhythmia or heart damage from a myocardial infarction (heart attack).
• A cardiac ultrasound (echocardiography) may locate a source of blood clots in the heart.

HOW TO TREAT IT

• Emergency treatment and immediate hospitalization is necessary in the event of a stroke. Life support measures may be required.
• If a stroke is caused by arterial blockage due to a blood clot, thrombolytic (clot-dissolving) drugs, such as intravenous tPA, or anticoagulants, such as heparin or warfarin, should be initiated within three hours of the onset of symptoms.
• If the stroke is the result of a cerebral hemorrhage, physicians will immediately take measures to reduce blood pressure of hypertensive patients in order to minimize flow of blood from the ruptured artery.
• Long-term therapy following a stroke may include antiplatelet medications, such as aspirin, or blood thinners, such as warfarin, to prevent future clots.
• Special railings, braces, canes, wheelchairs, or other devices may be necessary to help increase mobility for those with partial paralysis.
• Physical, speech, occupational, and emotional therapy helps patients and their families cope with major lifestyle changes.
• Those with extensive disabilities may need a period of in-hospital rehabilitation or professional in-home medical care.

WHEN TO CALL A DOCTOR

• **EMERGENCY** Call an ambulance immediately if you or someone in your presence exhibits stroke symptoms. ▲

Styes

WHAT IS IT?

A stye is a common problem resulting from a bacterial infection that blocks an eyelash follicle. The infection causes a small, red, painful bump to form at the base of the eyelash. Generally, the stye enlarges over several days as the infected follicle fills with pus. It usually subsides within three to seven days, or it may rupture. The bump should not be squeezed; doing so may spread the infection and cause other styes to develop. In addition, the bacteria that produce styes are contagious, so care should be taken to avoid touching the eyes or sharing towels, washcloths, and cosmetics.

Styes are not a serious health risk, and they do not affect vision. Although styes often recur, they usually respond well to self-treatment. In some cases, however, an untreated stye may lead to cellulitis (a more widespread infection of the skin) of the eyelid.

WHAT CAUSES IT?

• Styes generally occur when an eyelash follicle becomes infected with staphylococcal bacteria.

PREVENTION

• Avoid touching the eyes.
• Wash hands frequently with soap and warm water.
• Do not share towels or washcloths.
• Change your towel and pillowcase often.
• Do not share eye makeup; replace cosmetics every four to six months.

DIAGNOSIS

• Diagnosis can usually be made upon visual inspection and does not normally require a visit to the doctor.
• If an abscess occurs, a culture of the pus is taken to identify the infectious agent.

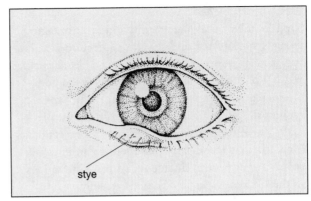

stye

When the follicle of an eyelash becomes infected, it produces a stye—a swollen, pus-filled bump on the eyelid.

HOW TO TREAT IT

• Hold a warm compress (a soft, clean towel or cloth that has been soaked in warm water and wrung out) against the affected eye for 10 to 15 minutes. Repeat the procedure two to four times a day until the stye drains (usually three to seven days). Use a new compress each time so as not to perpetuate the infection.
• Do not squeeze the stye; let it drain on its own.
• Antibiotic eye drops or ointment may be prescribed. Use as directed and be careful not to allow the tip of the bottle or tube to touch the eyes.
• A doctor may lance and drain a stye if it persists or enlarges despite treatment.

WHEN TO CALL A DOCTOR

• Call a doctor if a stye does not respond to self-treatment within a week or two, or if it enlarges despite treatment. ▲

> **SYMPTOMS**
> • A small, red, painful bump at the base of an eyelash.
> • A gritty sensation or a feeling that there is something in the eye.
> • Excessive watering of the affected eye.

Syphilis

WHAT IS IT?

Syphilis, a bacterial infection, is a highly contagious sexually transmitted disease. Once infection occurs, the bacteria travel quickly through the bloodstream and lymphatic system of the infected person and produce a wide variety of symptoms. If not treated, syphilis progresses through three main stages: primary (three to four weeks after infection), secondary (four to eight weeks later), and tertiary (one to 30 years after infection). Incidence of primary syphilis in the United States has declined steadily.

The skin lesions of both primary and secondary syphilis heal spontaneously over a period of several weeks to months. The secondary and tertiary stages are separated by a latent period during which the patient displays no symptoms and appears healthy. Latency usually lasts for years—often for a lifetime. A person infected with syphilis is extremely contagious during the primary and secondary stages, but not during the latent and tertiary phases. Adequate treatment with antibiotics during the primary or secondary stages cures the infection. Untreated syphilis that progresses to the tertiary stage may damage tissue in the heart, brain, spinal cord, eyes, and other organs, and can be fatal. Although tertiary symptoms appear in only about 30 percent of untreated patients, by the time these symptoms develop, tissue destruction is widespread, and antibiotic treatment is no longer effective. Therefore, early detection and treatment of syphilis are crucial.

WHAT CAUSES IT?

• Infection by the *Treponema pallidum* bacterium causes syphilis.
• Syphilis is spread by vaginal or anal intercourse. Those with multiple sexual partners are at higher risk.
• Syphilis has been strongly associated with drug use, especially crack cocaine.
• Infected pregnant women may transfer syphilis to the fetus.
• Persons with syphilis are at substantially increased risk for HIV infection.

PREVENTION

• Use latex condoms during sexual intercourse to reduce the risk of transmission. A mutually monogamous relationship is safest.

DIAGNOSIS

• Patient history and physical examination.
• Blood tests for antibodies against the bacteria.
• Microscopic examination of fluid from lesions.
• Lumbar puncture (spinal tap) can diagnose late central nervous system involvement (neurosyphilis).

HOW TO TREAT IT

• Intramuscular injections of penicillin can cure primary or secondary syphilis. Other antibiotics are used in people allergic to penicillin. Sexual partners should be treated as well.
• To prevent the spread of the syphilis, avoid sexual intercourse during treatment and until at least two follow-up examinations show no evidence of infection.

WHEN TO CALL A DOCTOR

• Call a doctor if you or your sexual partner develops a painless sore on the mouth or genital area.
• Call a doctor if you have had sexual contact with someone you suspect may have syphilis. ▲

SYMPTOMS

• Primary syphilis (three to four weeks after infection): a painless ulcer (chancre) on the penis, vagina, cervix, rectal area, or mouth; enlarged lymph nodes in the ulcer region.
• Secondary syphilis (four to eight weeks later): low fever; headache; sore throat; general feeling of poor health; hair loss; skin rash, especially on the palms of the hands and the soles of the feet; gray plaques in the mouth; painless, enlarged lymph nodes in the neck, armpit, or groin.
• Tertiary syphilis (five to 30 years after infection): loss of balance; loss of bladder control; sudden severe pains; loss of sensation in the legs, paralysis; erectile dysfunction (impotence); personality changes; dementia or insanity; blindness; symptoms of congestive heart failure due to damage to the aortic valve.

Systemic Lupus Erythematosus

WHAT IS IT?

Systemic lupus erythematosus, also known as lupus or SLE, is a persistent inflammation that may affect many organs throughout the body, including the skin and musculoskeletal, cardiovascular, renal, and neurological systems. Women are affected eight to 10 times more frequently than men. The precise cause of SLE is unknown. However, it is known that lupus is an autoimmune disorder: antibodies formed by the immune system attack some of the body's own cells. Inflammation typically occurs in the joints (arthritis), and inflammation of the skin may cause a characteristic butterfly rash on the face, as well as an increased sensitivity to the sun. Symptoms vary widely depending upon which organ systems are involved, and occur in a series of flare-ups or episodes separated by periods of normal or near-normal health. In severe cases SLE may lead to kidney or heart failure and can be fatal. However, SLE is often mild; many people never experience the most severe symptoms of the disease and, with treatment, are able to pursue a wide range of normal activities. An increased incidence of SLE is found among those of Asian or African descent and members of some Native American tribes. SLE usually develops between the ages of 15 and 35, although it may occur at any age. Currently, treatment is aimed at relieving the severity of episodes and limiting the progression of the disease.

SYMPTOMS

- Fever.
- Fatigue.
- General feeling of poor health.
- Loss of appetite and weight loss.
- Abdominal pain, nausea, and vomiting.
- Headache.
- Joint pain and swelling (see Rheumatoid Arthritis for more information).
- Red rash (butterfly rash) over both cheeks and the bridge of the nose, and rashes elsewhere on the body.
- Increased skin sensitivity to sun exposure.
- Small, painless ulcers in the mucous membranes of the nose and mouth.
- Blurred or worsening vision.
- Unusual bruising or bleeding; jaundice; dark urine; palpitations or irregular heartbeat (see Anemia, Hemolytic).
- Enlarged glands (lymph nodes).
- Swelling of the abdomen, the tissues around the eyes, and the ankles; weight gain; shortness of breath; decreased amount of urine (see Nephrotic Syndrome).
- Cough and chest pain (see Pleurisy).
- A tingling sensation or pain in the muscles, stiffness, spasms, seizures, numbness, or temporary paralysis.
- Emotional depression, anxiety, mental confusion, personality changes, or psychosis.

WHAT CAUSES IT?

- SLE is an autoimmune disorder, the exact underlying mechanisms of which remain unclear.
- Hereditary factors and sex hormones appear to play a role.
- Episodes may be triggered by ultraviolet radiation (as in sun exposure), infection, childbirth, abortion, or stress.
- Many drugs, including hydralazine (an antihypertensive), procainamide (a drug used to treat heart rhythm disturbances), and chlorpromazine (a tranquilizer), and certain foods, such as alfalfa sprouts, may cause a temporary lupuslike illness in some people; the illness disappears when the medication or food is discontinued.
- Some theories suggest that a virus may be responsible for the development of SLE.

PREVENTION

- There is no known way to prevent SLE.

DIAGNOSIS

- Patient history and physical examination. Long-term observation may be necessary for definitive diagnosis, which requires the presence of at least four of the symptoms of SLE.
- Blood tests for autoimmune antibodies, anemia, and decreased numbers of white blood cells and platelets.
- Urine tests for excessive protein and red blood cells.

Systemic Lupus Erythematosus   *continued*

• A kidney biopsy may be done. The doctor inserts a needle into the kidney through the back (under local anesthesia) to extract a small sample of tissue for microscopic examination.

• Lumbar puncture (spinal tap).

• CT (computed tomography) scans or MRI (magnetic resonance imaging).

HOW TO TREAT IT

• Treatment may be unnecessary for mild symptoms.

• Take aspirin or other over-the-counter pain relievers to reduce fever and treat minor pain.

• Apply warm compresses to relieve joint pain.

• Get plenty of rest. People with SLE often need over 10 hours of sleep a night and may need more during episodes of active disease.

• Oral corticosteroids such as prednisone may be prescribed to treat many of the major manifestations of lupus.

• Immunosuppressive drugs, including high doses of corticosteroids as well as chemotherapeutic medications, may also be prescribed to control disease activity.

• Hydroxychloroquine, an antimalarial drug, may be prescribed to relieve skin rash and the pain and swelling of arthritis.

• Warfarin, an anticoagulant, may be prescribed to prevent blood clots and reduce the possibility of heart attack and stroke.

• Your doctor may change your prescriptions for certain medications if they are suspected of causing drug-induced SLE.

• Apply a sunscreen lotion containing PABA (para-aminobenzoic acid) with a sun protection factor (SPF) of 15 or higher. Avoid exposure to direct sunlight between 10 a.m. and 2 p.m. whenever possible.

• Your doctor may recommend a low-salt diet. Calcium and vitamin D supplements may be advised for some patients.

• Dialysis may be needed to treat kidney failure. This procedure filters the blood artificially, removing waste products and excess fluid when the kidneys cannot (see Renal Failure, Chronic, for more information).

• A kidney transplant is an alternative to dialysis in cases of kidney failure.

WHEN TO CALL A DOCTOR

• Make an appointment with a doctor if you develop symptoms of SLE.

• Make an appointment with a doctor if, after being diagnosed with SLE, symptoms worsen or new symptoms develop. ▲

Tapeworm Infestation

WHAT IS IT?

Three common types of tapeworms (flat, segmented worms) can inhabit the digestive tract of humans: *Diphyllobothrium latum* (fish tapeworm), *Taenia saginatum* (beef tapeworm), and *T. solium* (pork tapeworm). Once inside the intestine, a tapeworm attaches itself to the intestinal wall with the suction cups and hooks on its head, and absorbs food through the entire surface of its body. Tapeworms vary in length from less than an inch to more than 30 feet, and some may survive for over 25 years in the body. Tapeworm larvae are most often ingested while eating raw or undercooked fish, beef, or pork; poor sanitary practices increase the risk of infestation. In humans, the adult worm remains in the intestine; however, the larvae of some tapeworms such as *T. solium* may form cysts in organs throughout the body (known as cysticercosis). While tapeworm infestation generally causes few if any symptoms, the cysts formed by the larvae may produce serious and widespread symptoms. Tapeworm infestation, although unpleasant, is easily treated.

WHAT CAUSES IT?

• Ingestion of raw or undercooked freshwater fish, beef, or pork that contains tapeworm cysts causes tapeworm infestation.

SYMPTOMS

• Hunger, fatigue, loss of appetite, and unintentional weight loss.
• Abdominal pain or discomfort.
• Diarrhea and excess gas.
• Nausea and vomiting.
• Anal itching or inflammation.
• White, mobile, ribbonlike worm segments in stool, clothing, or bedclothes.
• Fever, headache, muscle pain, seizures, bone fractures, eye pain, vision loss, memory loss, and personality changes (in advanced cases of cysticercosis).
• Symptoms of pernicious anemia (see this disorder for more information) due to the uptake of vitamin B_{12} by the fish tapeworm.

• Fish from lakes polluted with raw sewage are more likely to be infested.
• Poor sanitary conditions may promote infestation by tapeworm eggs.

PREVENTION

• Thoroughly cook fish, beef, and pork before eating.
• Avoid dishes made with raw meat or fish, such as steak tartare, sushi, ceviche, or inadequately cooked gefilte fish.
• Wash hands vigorously with soap and warm water after using the toilet and before handling food.

DIAGNOSIS

• Patient history and physical examination.
• Stool samples to detect eggs or worm segments.
• Abdominal x-rays. X-rays may be taken of other areas if cysticercosis is suspected.
• CT (computed tomography) scans or MRI (magnetic resonance imaging) may be done to detect cysts in the brain.

HOW TO TREAT IT

• Worm-killing medications, such as praziquantel, are prescribed. Duration of treatment and strength of dosage depend upon the type of tapeworm.
• Albendazole is recommended for cysticercosis.
• Injections of vitamin B_{12} may be administered to treat pernicious anemia associated with fish tapeworm infestation.
• Surgery is sometimes performed to excise cysts.
• Corticosteroid drugs may be prescribed to treat inflammation caused by a cyst.
• Anticonvulsant drugs may be prescribed to control seizures if brain infection is present.

WHEN TO CALL A DOCTOR

• Call a doctor if you notice worm segments or eggs in your stool or clothing, or if you develop unexplained hunger, fatigue, nausea, or abdominal pain.

Temporomandibular Joint Syndrome

WHAT IS IT?
Temporomandibular joint syndrome is characterized by pain and inflammation in the temporomandibular joints (TMJs), where both sides of the lower jaw (mandible) are attached to the skull. Normally, the muscles and ligaments in the TMJ stabilize, cushion, and guide the mandible's movements during eating, speaking, and other activities. TMJ syndrome occurs when these muscles and ligaments do not work together in a coordinated manner. For unknown reasons, 90 percent of TMJ sufferers are women, and most are young (20 to 40 years old).

WHAT CAUSES IT?
• Clenching and grinding the teeth (bruxism) is a common cause of TMJ syndrome. Bruxism often occurs during sleep, although the sleeper may be unaware of it.
• Emotional stress may lead to bruxism.
• Improper alignment of the teeth (malocclusion) is a common cause of TMJ syndrome.
• Bad posture (for example, thrusting the chin forward), a blow to the jaw, whiplash, or eating chewy foods can promote TMJ pain.
• Arthritis is an uncommon cause of TMJ syndrome.

PREVENTION
• Try not to grind the teeth or clench the jaw as a reaction to stress.
• See your dentist regularly.
• Practice correct posture to avoid muscle strain in the head and neck.

DIAGNOSIS
• Patient history and exam by a dentist or doctor.

• X-rays, CT (computed tomography) scans, or MRI (magnetic resonance imaging) of the TMJ may be done (although they usually show no abnormality).

HOW TO TREAT IT
• Follow prevention tips above.
• Take a nonprescription pain reliever.
• A hot or cold pack may offer temporary pain relief.
• At times when symptoms are particularly troublesome, eat soft foods and avoid chewing gum.
• Tranquilizers or muscle relaxants may be prescribed, and to reduce severe inflammation, corticosteroids may be injected into the TMJ.
• Your dentist may grind tooth surfaces to correct malocclusion, prescribe a removable plastic or rubber mold that fits over the teeth at night to prevent bruxism, or prepare a type of splint to be worn in the mouth during the day.
• Biofeedback (a technique for gaining voluntary control over certain of the body's reactions to stress and other stimuli) may be recommended. Relaxation training or physical therapy to lessen muscle tension may also be advised.
• In severe cases surgery may be recommended to repair damaged joint tissue and to correct bone defects. Surgery should only be considered as a last resort, however, because of the risk of severe complications. Always get a second opinion.

WHEN TO CALL A DOCTOR
• Call a doctor if symptoms of TMJ syndrome interfere with normal activities.

SYMPTOMS
• Headaches; earaches; or muscle aches in the neck, shoulders, or upper back.
• Pain and swelling in the jaw or at the TMJ.
• Clicking, popping, or scraping noises upon opening or closing the jaw.
• The jaw may temporarily lock in position.
• Tenderness of the muscles used for chewing.

Tendinitis

WHAT IS IT?

Tendinitis is inflammation of a tendon, one of the fibrous cords that join a muscle to a bone. Injury or repetitive overuse can cause microscopic tears and painful swelling in a tendon. Sites most commonly affected include the shoulder, the elbow (tennis or golfer's elbow), the wrist (de Quervain's tenosynovitis), the fingers (trigger finger), and the ankle (Achilles tendinitis). When the muscles in the affected area are used regularly despite pain, the injured tendon may be slow to heal. While many cases of tendinitis last no more than two weeks and are usually alleviated by rest and proper conditioning, repeated use of the injured tendon may lead to chronic tendinitis, characterized by scarring of the involved tissues and limited flexibility. Those over age 40 are most prone to the chronic form of tendinitis.

WHAT CAUSES IT?

• Overuse due to prolonged, repetitive movements as required by tennis, golf, bowling, and certain occupations, like carpentry and painting.
• Physical trauma, such as falling on an arm, twisting an ankle, or lifting heavy objects.
• Inadequate conditioning or insufficient warm-up prior to exercise.
• Degenerative changes owing to aging and years of continual use.
• Calcium deposits in a tendon (calcific tendinitis).

PREVENTION

• Avoid highly repetitive movements, or interrupt them with activities requiring other muscle groups.
• Engage in regular, moderate exercise to maintain strength and flexibility.

SYMPTOMS
• Pain in the affected area (often worse at night, disturbing sleep).
• Limited joint movement.
• Muscle spasms concurrent with pain.
• Sudden pain, often accompanied by a snapping sound, with the rupture of an Achilles tendon.

• Be sure to stretch and warm up adequately before engaging in exercise or other demanding physical activity.

DIAGNOSIS

• Patient history including recent physical activity.
• Physical examination may include palpation (physically touching and manipulating the area) and range of motion tests to determine the area and extent of the injury.
• Arthrography (injection of a contrast material into a joint to create a clear x-ray image of soft tissues) may be used to identify tendon damage.
• Ultrasound scans or MRI (magnetic resonance imaging) may be used to identify minor tears.

HOW TO TREAT IT

• Rest is essential, although gentle exercise may be advised to prevent stiffness. Slings or splints may be used for a few days to immobilize the injured area.
• Take over-the-counter anti-inflammatory drugs like aspirin, ibuprofen, or naproxen.
• Ice packs should be used immediately after an injury to reduce swelling. Do not apply ice to one area for more than 20 minutes at one time. After 72 hours, hot compresses may soothe discomfort and increase blood flow to speed healing.
• Corticosteroids may be injected directly into the affected area to relieve pain and inflammation (not routinely recommended for Achilles tendinitis, where injections may weaken or rupture the tendon).
• Surgery to repair the tendon may be required if the tendon is torn.
• Temporarily switch to low-impact exercise, like bicycling or swimming, if you suspect high-impact exercise is responsible.

WHEN TO CALL A DOCTOR

• Call a doctor if muscle or joint pain persists for more than two weeks and interferes with activities despite treatment with rest and pain relievers. 🛠

Testicular Cancer

WHAT IS IT?

Testicular cancer is the growth of malignant cells in the testicles. In almost all cases only one testicle is involved. While relatively rare, testicular cancer is the most common cancer among young men; incidence is highest between the ages of 15 and 34, and quite rare beyond age 40. The disease disproportionately affects white men. Prognosis is often good, though it depends heavily on whether the cancer has spread to other organs. The cure rate is very high when testicular cancer is detected and treated early.

WHAT CAUSES IT?

• The cause is unknown, but the incidence is significantly higher among men in whom one or both testicles failed to descend from the abdominal cavity into the scrotum before birth (cryptorchidism).
• Other predisposing factors include a history of inguinal hernia in childhood (see Inguinal Hernia) and testicular inflammation that occurs in conjunction with mumps (see Orchitis and Mumps).

PREVENTION

• There is no way to prevent testicular cancer, but vigilant monthly self-examination can aid in early detection, which promises a very favorable prognosis. The best time to perform self-examination is after a warm shower, when the scrotum is soft and pliable.

DIAGNOSIS

• Patient history and physical examination are needed. A special bright light can be shined through

---

SYMPTOMS

• A firm, painless lump or nodule in one of the testicles.
• A feeling of heaviness or hardness in a testicle.
• Rarely, testicular pain or hydrocele (fluid around the testes; see Hydrocele).
• Breast growth or nipple tenderness.
• In advanced cases: swollen lymph glands; abdominal or back pain; urinary difficulty; fatigue; weight loss; cough or breathing difficulty (due to spread of cancer to the lungs).

---

the scrotum to aid in diagnosis; tumors will appear opaque, while most other abnormalities (such as a hydrocele or a spermatocele) will appear translucent.
• Blood tests for specific biochemical markers of testicular cancer can be used to track the response to treatment and detect the recurrence of cancer.
• An ultrasound scan can confirm the presence of a solid mass.
• Chest x-rays and CT (computed tomography) scans of the abdomen and pelvis are used to evaluate the stage of any tumors and to determine whether cancer has spread beyond the testicle. Treatment strategy depends heavily upon results of these tests and the type of cell causing the cancer, determined by microscopic examination of testicular tissue.

HOW TO TREAT IT

• Once a tumor is detected by diagnostic procedures, the affected testicle must be removed. (A biopsy to confirm diagnosis is not done since it may promote the spread of the cancer.)
• The course of further treatment depends on the cell type of the tumor. Seminomas are treated with radiation to pelvic and abdominal lymph nodes. Other types of cancer (nonseminomas) require surgical removal of these lymph nodes or chemotherapy.
• Chemotherapy is used if either type of cancer has spread to other sites in the body. These treatments may result in infertility.
• Men who discover they have testicular cancer and wish to have children in the future may consider preserving sperm in a sperm bank prior to treatment. The approximate two-week delay in therapy appears to have little effect on outcome.
• The removed testicle may be replaced with a prosthesis; fertility is maintained if the other testicle is unaffected. If need be, regular hormone injections can be given to preserve normal sexual functioning.

WHEN TO CALL A DOCTOR

• Make an appointment with your doctor right away if you discover a lump on one of your testicles. While any testicular abnormality is cause for concern, an actual lump is frequently a sign of cancer, and the sooner treatment is sought, the greater the likelihood of a complete cure. ◢

Testicular Torsion

WHAT IS IT?

Each testicle is suspended within the scrotum from one of the two spermatic cords. These cords, in addition to providing a conduit for sperm manufactured in the testis, contain blood vessels that supply the testicle. Testicular torsion involves an abnormal twisting of a testicle and its spermatic cord, so that testicular blood supply is cut off (strangulation). The condition is extremely painful, and if prompt treatment is not obtained, permanent damage may occur within hours, rendering the affected testicle unable to produce sperm. In 90 percent of cases, torsion involves only one testicle; sperm production still occurs in the unaffected testicle, and fertility persists despite a diminished sperm count.

In rare cases the testicle somehow becomes untwisted by itself, resulting in immediate relief. Subsequent evaluation by a physician is essential nonetheless, so that recurrence can be prevented and more serious disorders, including testicular cancer, may be ruled out. Testicular torsion is most common between the ages of 12 and 18, although it can happen at any age, including infancy.

WHAT CAUSES IT?

• Testicular torsion usually occurs spontaneously for no apparent reason; indeed, it may even occur during sleep.
• The patient may be predisposed to the condition because of a congenital abnormality or weakness in the structures within the scrotum.
• Torsion sometimes occurs following very strenuous activity.

SYMPTOMS

• Excruciating pain and tenderness in the affected testicle. Pain may radiate into the lower abdomen.
• Swelling, unusual firmness, and redness of the scrotum.
• Affected testicle may appear to be positioned higher than normal.
• Nausea and vomiting.
• Faintness or fainting.

PREVENTION

• Testicular torsion is difficult to anticipate and thus difficult to prevent; in any case, use an athletic supporter when engaged in strenuous physical activities.

DIAGNOSIS

• Patient history and physical examination suggest the diagnosis. Because testicular torsion is an emergency, treatment is generally initiated at once, without any special tests.
• An ultrasound scan may be done to rule out other disorders (such as epididymitis or strangulated hernia) that produce similar symptoms.
• Diagnosis is confirmed by visual inspection of the twisted spermatic cord during the minor surgical procedure used to correct testicular torsion.

HOW TO TREAT IT

• Immediate medical treatment is imperative. The doctor will first attempt to properly reposition the testicle by gentle manipulation.
• If manipulation fails, a small incision is made in the scrotum and the testicle is rotated to untwist the spermatic cord.
• In most cases—whether torsion is corrected by manipulation or surgery—the testicle is surgically anchored to the side of the scrotum (orchiopexy) to prevent recurrences. As a precaution, the unaffected testicle may be anchored in place too.
• If treatment is not received soon enough (within a few hours), the testicle begins to atrophy and may have to be removed (orchiectomy).

WHEN TO CALL A DOCTOR

• **EMERGENCY** Get immediate medical attention for any severe testicular pain or injury. Even if the pain eases on its own, the likelihood of recurrence or complications warrants examination by a doctor.

Tetanus

WHAT IS IT?

Tetanus is a life-threatening disease. It is caused by a toxin produced by bacteria that typically enter the body as a dormant form (spore) through a deep cut or puncture wound. The spores require an environment with a low oxygen content for about seven to 10 days to be activated to the growing form of the bacteria that produces the toxin. The toxin travels along nerves to the spinal cord, where it produces muscle rigidity and spasms. Tetanus is sometimes called lockjaw, because difficulty opening the mouth is often the first symptom; rigidity may become so severe the jaw is frozen shut.

The bacterial spores of Clostridium tetani are found worldwide in soil, dust, animal feces, and, occasionally, human feces. Incidence is highest in rural areas with warm climates or in any population that is not immunized or is only partially immunized. People over the age of 50 are most commonly affected, usually because they have not gotten booster vaccinations.

Severity ranges from mild muscle stiffness to convulsive spasms that can choke or suffocate the victim by blocking the respiratory airway. The illness usually lasts from four to six weeks. Infection rarely occurs when a person is properly immunized. Aggressive treatment has reduced the overall mortality rate to less than 25 percent in the United States, and incidence is now rare in this country.

SYMPTOMS

- Muscle rigidity and pain, typically in the jaw, neck, back, and abdomen.
- Muscle spasms, often first felt in the jaw and neck, which may progress to painful spasms throughout the body.
- Pain and tingling at the wound site.
- Swallowing or breathing difficulty.
- Grimacing due to involuntary constriction of facial muscles.
- Irritability.
- Drooling.
- In severe cases: high fever, profuse sweating, rapid heartbeat, or heart rhythm disturbances.

WHAT CAUSES IT?

- Tetanus is caused by bacterial infection from C. tetani, which usually enters the body through a wound. Less often, tetanus follows a burn, surgery, or injection of illicit drugs into the skin.

PREVENTION

- Immunization should be initiated in early infancy. The DTP vaccine (diphtheria, tetanus, and pertussis) is most often used.
- Get a booster shot every five to 10 years or after sustaining a deep wound.
- Clean wounds with soap and water and apply an antiseptic, such as hydrogen peroxide.

DIAGNOSIS

- Patient history should include any prior tetanus immunization, allergic reactions to immunizations or penicillin, and recent wounds.
- Diagnosis is generally based on characteristic clinical findings.
- Wound cultures may be taken, although not all patients with tetanus produce a positive test result.

HOW TO TREAT IT

- Deep, often surgical cleansing of the wound is commonly performed to eliminate invading bacteria.
- Antitoxin should be administered immediately to neutralize the bacterial toxin.
- Antibiotics (usually penicillin, doxycycline, or metronidazole) are administered intravenously.
- Muscle relaxants, such as diazepam (Valium), may be used to relieve muscle stiffness.
- Neuromuscular blockers (drugs that block nerve-to-muscle signals) may be administered to control violent spasms, especially if they threaten breathing.
- For patients with severe breathing difficulty, tracheostomy (the implantation of a breathing tube through a surgical opening in the throat) may be needed, along with mechanical ventilation.
- Tetanus vaccine may be administered.

WHEN TO CALL A DOCTOR

- **EMERGENCY** Get immediate medical attention whether or not a wound is present if you begin to suffer from unusual muscle spasms and stiffness.

Thrombophlebitis

WHAT IS IT?

Thrombophlebitis is inflammation of a vein (usually in an extremity, especially one of the legs) that occurs in response to a blood clot in the vessel. When it occurs in a vein near the surface of the skin, it is known as superficial thrombophlebitis, a minor disorder commonly identified by a red, tender vein. Deep-vein thrombophlebitis (affecting the larger veins farther below the skin's surface) is more serious. It may produce less-pronounced symptoms at first—indeed, half of all cases are asymptomatic—but carries the risks of pulmonary embolism (when the clot detaches from its place of origin and travels to the lung) and chronic venous insufficiency (impaired outflow of blood through the veins), resulting in dermatitis, increased skin pigmentation, and swelling. Thrombophlebitis is common; incidence is higher among women and older people.

WHAT CAUSES IT?

• Stagnation of blood flow due to immobility. This is common among bedridden patients (such as heart patients and those who have undergone any type of major or orthopedic surgery, especially of the hip or knee) and healthy persons who sit or lie still for an extended period—for example, on a long trip.
• Blood vessel injury, caused by trauma, intravenous catheters or needles, chemotherapeutic agents, or infectious organisms.
• Conditions that increase the tendency for blood to coagulate, such as a familial deficiency in anticlotting factors or disorders like systemic lupus erythematosus.
• Pregnancy and varicose veins are associated with a higher risk of superficial thrombophlebitis.

SYMPTOMS
• Superficial thrombophlebitis: a red, engorged, cordlike vein, associated with localized swelling, pain, or tenderness.
• Deep-vein thrombophlebitis: generalized swelling, warmth, and redness in the affected limb; distention of superficial veins; bluish skin color in the limb or toes (cyanosis); rarely, fever and chills.

• Deep-vein thrombophlebitis is associated with a number of different cancers.

PREVENTION

• Stand up and walk around often on long trips.
• Following a heart attack or major surgery, low doses of an anticoagulant such as heparin or warfarin may be recommended. Getting up and walking around again as soon as possible is also advised.

DIAGNOSIS

• Superficial thrombophlebitis can usually be diagnosed from patient history and physical examination alone. Deep-vein thrombophlebitis is more elusive and often requires further tests.
• Venography (x-rays following the injection of a contrast material into the affected vein) is a highly accurate means of identifying an obstructing clot.
• Ultrasound may be used to identify altered blood flow caused by an obstructing clot.

HOW TO TREAT IT

• Superficial thrombophlebitis may be treated with warm compresses and anti-inflammatory drugs to relieve discomfort, and elevation of the affected limb to reduce swelling. A few days of rest are advised.
• Hospitalization may be required for deep-vein thrombophlebitis. Bed rest and elevation of the affected limb are essential. An anticoagulant, usually heparin, is administered intravenously for seven to 10 days to inhibit further clotting. Oral anticoagulants such as warfarin are then given for three to 12 months depending on the thrombophlebitis site.
• Thrombolytic (clot-dissolving) agents such as streptokinase or urokinase may be administered in some cases to completely resolve the condition.
• Special elastic support stockings may be prescribed to aid circulation in the lower limbs.
• Surgery may be advised to tie off the affected vein to prevent the clot from migrating to the lungs (pulmonary embolism).

WHEN TO CALL A DOCTOR

• Call a doctor if you have a painful, swollen vein that does not disappear in a few days, or if you have unexplained swelling in an arm or leg. 🔺

Thyroid Cancer

WHAT IS IT?

Thyroid cancer is the growth of malignant cells in the thyroid, a gland comprising two large lobes flanking the windpipe (trachea) at the base of the neck. There are four basic types of thyroid cancer: papillary, follicular, medullary, and anaplastic.

Papillary carcinoma accounts for over 80 percent of thyroid cancers. Such tumors tend to grow very slowly and often take years to spread to other sites. Follicular carcinoma, the second most common type, is also slow growing, but like papillary carcinoma, it can spread to the lungs and to bone tissue. Medullary carcinomas are considerably more rare; they are aggressive but highly curable if detected and treated while still confined exclusively to the thyroid. Anaplastic carcinomas are more common in the elderly, and are highly malignant—death usually occurs within six months of diagnosis. Fortunately, they are the least common form of thyroid cancer.

The majority of cases of thyroid cancer occur between ages 25 and 65, and women are more commonly affected than men. While the prognosis depends heavily upon the type of malignancy involved and the age of the patient, the outlook is generally quite good, and the mortality rate is low.

WHAT CAUSES IT?

• The cause of thyroid cancer is unknown, but previous radiation therapy to the thyroid area (for acne, enlarged thymus gland, tonsils, or adenoids) is a significant risk factor, especially if it was administered during infancy or early childhood. Malignancies may appear as early as five years or as late as 30 years after radiation.

• Exposure to radioactive fallout is associated with an increased incidence of thyroid cancer.

• Medullary carcinoma frequently occurs as a genetic disorder in members of the same family. Familial medullary carcinoma is often associated with a type of adrenal tumor (see Pheochromocytoma) and overgrowth of the parathyroid glands (see Hyperparathyroidism).

• Papillary and follicular carcinoma (the two most common types) also appear to be linked to hereditary factors.

PREVENTION

• Avoid x-rays to the neck or upper chest areas as much as possible.

• Frequent screening for elevated calcitonin levels is recommended (see Diagnosis below) in family members of patients with medullary cancer.

DIAGNOSIS

• Patient history should include any childhood radiation treatments, as well as any family history of thyroid cancer.

• Physical examination of the nodule to identify whether it is solitary or part of a cluster, common in benign goiters (see Goiter and Thyroid Nodules).

• A fine-needle biopsy (use of a small-gauge needle and syringe to take a tissue sample for examination under a microscope) may identify malignant cells.

• When medullary carcinoma is suspected, blood levels of calcitonin, a thyroid hormone, are measured. (High calcitonin levels may indicate medullary carcinoma.) Genetic testing is now available to determine susceptibility in family members of patients with medullary carcinoma.

• Radioiodine thyroid scanning may be used to determine if the nodule is "cold," or nonfunctioning; 10 percent of cold nodules are malignant.

• Ultrasound may determine the consistency of the tumor or mass.

• Suppressive doses of thyroid hormone may be given to see whether the nodule shrinks or disappears, indicating a benign tumor.

SYMPTOMS

• A firm or hard, usually painless lump in the front of the neck.

• Swelling in the neck (goiter).

• Swallowing difficulty.

• Hoarseness or changes in the voice.

• Cough, possibly bloody.

• Breathing difficulty.

• Unexplained bone fractures (occurs with follicular carcinoma).

• Severe flushing or diarrhea (occurs with medullary carcinoma).

Thyroid Cancer *continued*

HOW TO TREAT IT

• Near-total surgical removal of the thyroid (thyroidectomy) is done in almost all cases. Removal of surrounding lymph nodes and other tissues may also be warranted.

• The absence of thyroid tissue following thyroidectomy requires lifetime supplementation with thyroid hormone (thyroxine), which also reduces the risk of cancer recurrence.

• Radioactive iodine therapy may be used to destroy thyroid tissue left behind after thyroidectomy or to treat thyroid cancer that has spread to the lungs or the bones.

• Treatment for rare anaplastic carcinoma primarily involves supportive therapy to make the patient as comfortable as possible.

WHEN TO CALL A DOCTOR

• Call a doctor as soon as you detect an unusual lump in your neck, especially if it rapidly increases in size. Although thyroid cancer is rare, all such growths warrant examination. ▲

Thyroid Nodules

WHAT IS IT?

Thyroid nodules are solid lumps arising in the thyroid gland. The thyroid, consisting of two large lobes on either side of the windpipe at the base of the neck, produces thyroid hormone, which regulates body growth and metabolism. Nodules usually grow slowly over many years. They appear singularly or in clusters (benign nodular goiter) and usually are not detectable until they have grown to at least one centimeter in size. The greatest concern of a solitary nodule is the possibility of cancer, although this is uncommon. The vast majority of solitary nodules are cysts or benign tumors (adenomas), which affect about 4 percent of the adult population. Nodules are classified according to their production of thyroid hormone. "Warm" nodules mimic normal thyroid cells in this regard. "Hot" nodules overproduce thyroid hormone and are virtually always benign (see Hyperthyroidism for more information). "Cold" nodules underproduce thyroid hormone.

WHAT CAUSES IT?

• The cause of thyroid nodules is unknown, but incidence is higher among people who received x-ray treatment to the thyroid area in infancy or childhood. Women are affected more often than men.

PREVENTION

• There is no known way to prevent thyroid nodules.

DIAGNOSIS

• A thyroid scan with radioactive iodine or technetium to identify if the nodule is hot, warm, or cold.
• Patient history including any radiation treatments in infancy or childhood.
• Physical examination to determine whether the lump is solitary or in a cluster.
• Thyroid function tests to measure thyroid hormone levels.
• Ultrasound scans to identify cysts.
• If the nodule is cold, fine-needle biopsy (use of a small-gauge needle and syringe to take a tissue sample for examination under a microscope) is used to rule out cancer.

HOW TO TREAT IT

• If a needle biopsy shows no evidence of cancer and thyroid function tests are normal, regular follow-up with thyroid function tests is all that is required.
• If the nodule is a fluid-filled cyst, needle drainage may be done.
• Hot nodules associated with hyperthyroidism are treated with radioactive iodine or surgery.
• Near-total thyroidectomy is recommended if cancerous cells are detected in a needle biopsy.
• Treatment for hypothyroidism may subsequently be needed if excess thyroid tissue is removed or destroyed by radioactive iodine therapy (see Hypothyroidism for more information).
• If the findings are equivocal on fine-needle biopsy, thyroid hormone may be administered to observe whether the nodule shrinks over the ensuing six to 12 months.

WHEN TO CALL A DOCTOR

• Call a doctor as soon as possible if you detect an unusual lump in your neck. A complete evaluation is imperative. ▲

SYMPTOMS

• A solid, usually painless lump in the front of the neck, near the windpipe or Adam's apple.
• Possibly, in the case of "hot" nodules, symptoms of hyperthyroidism (see Hyperthyroidism for more information).
• Substantial swelling in the neck in cases of benign nodular goiter.
• Rarely, breathing or swallowing difficulty, if nodules grow large enough to become obstructions.

Thyroiditis

WHAT IS IT?

Thyroiditis is inflammation of the thyroid, the gland at the base of the neck that produces thyroid hormone (thyroxine), crucial in the regulation of body growth and metabolism. There are three types of thyroiditis: acute, subacute, and chronic. Although inflammation of the thyroid gland is common to all three, they differ significantly in terms of symptoms, cause, and outcome. Acute thyroiditis is extremely rare. Subacute thyroiditis is self-limited, meaning it resolves spontaneously without treatment, usually in a matter of months. Chronic thyroiditis, the most serious of the three, may lead to tissue destruction and scarring of the thyroid; indeed, it is the leading cause of insufficient thyroid hormone production in adults (see Hypothyroidism).

WHAT CAUSES IT?

• Acute thyroiditis is rare, resulting from direct infection of the thyroid following a penetrating neck wound or, more rarely still, a bacterial infection elsewhere in the body that spreads to the thyroid via the bloodstream.

• The cause of subacute thyroiditis is unknown, although it is often preceded by a viral infection of the upper respiratory tract, suggesting some association with the body's response to infection.

• The cause of chronic thyroiditis is also uncertain, but evidence is strong that it involves autoimmune activity (an attack by the body's defenses on its own healthy tissue). Hereditary factors may play a role.

• A painless and typically temporary form of thyroiditis affects about one in 20 women after they give birth (postpartum thyroiditis). Either hyper- or hypothyroidism may occur transiently.

PREVENTION

• There is no known way to prevent thyroiditis.

DIAGNOSIS

• Patient history and physical exam are necessary.

• Blood levels of thyroid hormone, thyroid-stimulating hormone, and antibodies to the thyroid gland are measured.

• A scan of the thyroid may be taken after administration of radioactive iodine to evaluate thyroid function.

• A fine-needle biopsy, extracting tissue directly from the thyroid, may be done to rule out thyroid cancer in patients with chronic thyroiditis.

HOW TO TREAT IT

• Antibiotics are used to treat the infection associated with acute thyroiditis.

• Because subacute thyroiditis resolves on its own, treatment is aimed at relieving symptoms only. Aspirin or other pain relievers may ease inflammation and tenderness. Beta-blocker medications are helpful at treating the symptoms of hyperthyroidism. Corticosteroids such as prednisone may sometimes be used.

• Some patients with subacute thyroiditis may develop transient hyper- or hypothyroidism, which may require brief periods of treatment with, respectively, either beta-blockers or thyroid hormone.

• Treatment for chronic thyroiditis primarily consists of thyroid hormone (thyroxine) replacement to correct hypothyroidism (see Hypothyroidism).

WHEN TO CALL A DOCTOR

• Call a doctor if you suffer from pain or swelling in the neck; pain in the ears, lower jaw, or back of the head; fatigue, unexplained weight gain, or other symptoms of hypothyroidism. ▲

SYMPTOMS

• Acute thyroiditis: fever; swelling, pain, or tenderness in the front of the neck.

• Subacute thyroiditis: pain and tenderness in the front of the neck, especially upon swallowing or the application of pressure; fever; local swelling; pain in one or both ears. Symptoms may develop gradually or come on suddenly.

• Chronic thyroiditis: painless swelling in the neck (see Goiter); symptoms of hypothyroidism (see Hypothyroidism), including fatigue, unexplained weight gain, constipation, dry skin, and intolerance to cold.

Tics

WHAT IS IT?

Tics are abrupt, involuntary, repeated movements (motor tics) or vocalized sounds (vocal or phonic tics). They usually develop during childhood and may gradually disappear with time or persist into adulthood. Their nature, severity, and frequency vary from case to case. With effort, tics can usually be suppressed for short periods of time. They tend to become more pronounced during periods of stress or excitement and disappear when the person is distracted or deeply absorbed.

The most common and severe condition that causes tics is called Gilles de la Tourette's syndrome. More common among boys than girls, Tourette's syndrome is usually a lifelong illness that normally begins before the age of 21. It is characterized by frequent, multiple motor and vocal tics that may wax and wane throughout the course of the illness. Tourette's syndrome may also be accompanied by behavioral disturbances such as obsessive-compulsive disorder, attention and learning difficulties, or sleep disorders. Treatment of tics varies considerably depending on the nature and severity of the individ-

ual case. Mild cases require no treatment or can be treated with behavioral therapy. Tics that cause discomfort or embarrassment, or that otherwise interfere with daily life, may be treated with one of several drugs. Tourette's syndrome usually requires lifetime drug treatment.

WHAT CAUSES IT?

• The cause of simple tics is unknown. They may develop as a means of relieving psychological tension.
• Tourette's syndrome is usually genetically inherited.

PREVENTION

• There is no known way to prevent tics or Tourette's syndrome.

DIAGNOSIS

• Medical history and physical examination are needed.

HOW TO TREAT IT

• In people with simple, transient tics, symptoms usually disappear without treatment within one to several years.
• Mild cases may be treated with behavioral therapy, during which the patient learns to control the tic.
• Drug therapy is indicated in more severe, persistent cases (such as Tourette's syndrome) when tics cause physical or social discomfort. Several types of medications can be effective, including anticonvulsants, antipsychotics, tranquilizers, antidepressants, and the antihypertensive drug clonidine. These are all powerful drugs that may produce bothersome side effects.

WHEN TO CALL A DOCTOR

• If you or your child develops a simple tic or multiple tics, make an appointment with a doctor. You may be referred to a behavioral therapist or other specialist for further examination or treatment. ▲

SYMPTOMS

• Repetitive movements or sounds, usually first appearing during childhood. Motor tics usually involve one or more muscle groups in the face, shoulders, or arms, but other parts of the body may be affected. They may be simple (blinking, raising the eyebrows, nose or mouth twitching, head turning, shoulder shrugging, or a specific facial grimace) or complex (leg kicking, jumping). Vocal or phonic tics also vary in complexity from sniffing or throat clearing to echolalia (compulsive repeating of words or phrases uttered by other people) or coprolalia (compulsive swearing and repeating vulgar phrases).
• Symptoms of Tourette's syndrome: multiple, complex motor tics; grunting, barking, or coprolalia; obsessive-compulsive behavior, poor attention span, learning difficulties, and sleep disorders.

Tinnitus

WHAT IS IT?
Tinnitus is the perception of sound in the absence of an external source. The perceived sound is variously described as ringing, buzzing, hissing, or even roaring, whistling, or pounding. Almost everyone experiences intermittent tinnitus once in a while (especially in a quiet room), and it is nothing to worry about. Persistent tinnitus, however, can be extremely distressing psychologically, may interfere with sleep, and is sometimes a sign of a more serious underlying disorder. Treatment depends upon identifying the underlying problem.

WHAT CAUSES IT?
• Tinnitus can be associated with all types of hearing loss and may be a symptom of almost any ear disorder, including labyrinthitis, Ménière's disease, otitis media, otosclerosis, acoustic neuroma, and presbycusis (see these disorders for more information).
• Certain conditions can produce an actual sound near the ear that an examiner can hear with a stethoscope. This phenomenon is known as objective tinnitus and can be caused by increased intracranial pressure, an aneurysm, temporomandibular jaw disorders, normal blood flow through an artery or vein, or a tumor pressing on a blood vessel or nerve.
• Drugs such as caffeine, aminoglycosides, aspirin, propranolol, levodopa, and quinidine can cause tinnitus.
• In some cases no cause can be established.

PREVENTION
• Prompt antibiotic therapy can avert the disorder in cases of otitis media or other ear infections.
• Noise-induced tinnitus can be prevented by avoiding loud sounds or using ear plugs or muffs.

SYMPTOMS
• Persistent or intermittent noises in one or both ears (often described as ringing, buzzing, hissing, humming, whistling, roaring, or pounding).
• Hearing loss.
• Sleep disturbances.
• Emotional distress.

• Drug-induced tinnitus can be prevented by avoiding the drugs mentioned above.

DIAGNOSIS
• A patient interview and physical examination, including a detailed description of the sounds and when they occur, are conducted.
• Audiometry (hearing tests) may be used to measure any hearing loss.
• X-rays or ultrasound scans may be used to detect a tumor or other abnormality.

HOW TO TREAT IT
• Background sound or static (white noise) from a radio or television may successfully mask tinnitus and help sufferers to fall asleep.
• Sedatives may be prescribed to alleviate chronic sleep disturbance, although this is not recommended as a long-term solution.
• Hearing aids can amplify ambient sound and drown out tinnitus.
• In more severe cases tinnitus masking may be prescribed by an otolaryngologist (ear, nose, and throat specialist). Masking utilizes white noise or a more pleasant sound that often successfully inhibits tinnitus for several hours after use.
• Tinnitus and depression may co-exist. Consult your doctor if you develop any symptoms of depression (see Depression for more information).
• Tinnitus clinics and support groups are available in most major cities. They offer programs that improve coping skills.
• Surgery may be used to correct an underlying disorder, such as a tumor, but may be ineffective in eliminating the tinnitus.

WHEN TO CALL A DOCTOR
• Call a doctor if ringing, buzzing, or other sounds disrupt daily activities or sleeping habits. Your physician may refer you to an otolaryngologist for further evaluation and treatment. ▲

Tongue Disorders

WHAT IS IT?

Tongue disorders are characterized by changes in the texture and appearance of the tongue's surface. They may result from poor oral hygiene or indicate a medical problem. Glossitis is inflammation of the tongue, in which the whole tongue becomes extremely smooth, swollen, red, and painful. Geographic tongue also involves inflammation, but in sometimes sensitive migrating patches. Macroglossia is an abnormally enlarged tongue. Hairy tongue and discolored tongue are more unsightly than painful, and both can usually be remedied by good oral hygiene. Tongue cancer, the most serious disorder, primarily affects people over 40. A small ulcer or a raised white patch (leukoplakia) may be the earliest sign of cancer, although most leukoplakias do not become malignant. Tongue cancer may spread rapidly to surrounding tissues in the gums, lower jaw, or lymph nodes in the neck; detection before cancer spreads is essential for a favorable prognosis.

WHAT CAUSES IT?

• Hairy tongue and discolored tongue (in which papillae, the small projections on the tongue, become elongated or darkened) may be caused by tobacco, foods, or medications such as antibiotics. Poor oral hygiene is a contributing factor.

• Tongue disorders may be a sign of an underlying ailment, such as systemic lupus erythematosus, candidiasis, psoriasis, or syphilis. Disorders associated with glossitis include a deficiency of vitamin B_{12} (pernicious anemia) or other B vitamins, scarlet fever, toxic shock syndrome, and infection (particularly herpes simplex, which may also cause cold sores on the tongue). Down syndrome, intrauterine hypothyroidism (cretinism), and overproduction of growth hormone by a pituitary tumor (see Acromegaly) can cause macroglossia.

• Chronic irritation due to smoking, alcohol, jagged teeth, or dentures can cause leukoplakia or glossitis.

• Tongue cancer is often associated with smoking and alcohol use (especially in combination).

• Hairy leukoplakia may be a complication of HIV infection.

PREVENTION

• Brush or scrape the tongue when you brush your teeth to promote good oral hygiene.

• See a dentist at least once a year.

• Avoid tobacco (smokers have a high incidence of tongue cancer) and excessive use of alcohol.

DIAGNOSIS

• Examination and patient history are often sufficient.

• Tongue biopsy (removal of a small tissue sample for analysis) may be performed when cancer is suspected.

HOW TO TREAT IT

• Treatment is directed at the underlying cause. For example, if a tongue disorder is caused by a vitamin deficiency, dietary guidelines or vitamin supplements may be recommended. Ill-fitting dentures or jagged teeth should be remedied by a dentist.

• A mild salt solution, antiseptic mouthwash, or topical ointment may soothe discomfort or kill germs.

• Antibiotics may be used when the disorder includes minor bacterial infections (as in glossitis).

• Tongue cancer may require surgical excision of all affected tissue, followed by radiation therapy. Tumors that have spread may also require chemotherapy.

WHEN TO CALL A DOCTOR

• Call a doctor if your tongue is sore, swollen, or stiff, or if symptoms persist for more than three days.

SYMPTOMS

• A painful, red, swollen tongue that glistens and is extremely smooth (glossitis).

• Painless red patches that heal then reappear on other parts of the tongue (geographic tongue).

• Elongated papillae that make the tongue look hairy (hairy tongue).

• A painless, raised white patch that may become firm or rough (leukoplakia).

• Discoloration of the tongue ranging from yellowish white to brown-black (hairy tongue).

• Bad breath.

• Excessive salivation.

• Difficulty swallowing.

• Stiffness of the tongue.

Tonsillitis

WHAT IS IT?

Tonsillitis is inflammation, from infection, of the tonsils (the infection-fighting lymph tissue located on either side of the back of the mouth). It is most common in children between the ages of five and 15—although it can occur at any age—and is characterized by a severe sore throat. Once considered a nuisance and frequently removed surgically, the tonsils are now known to serve an immune system role. They are also the respiratory system's first line of defense, trapping and neutralizing infectious agents before they can penetrate the bronchial passages. Children's tonsils are normally large; they reach their maximum size at around age six or seven and then start to shrink. Because of their continuous exposure to infectious agents, the tonsils sometimes become overwhelmed by infection, resulting in tonsillitis.

Although tonsillitis usually goes away on its own within a week, it still warrants a physician's attention to identify the infectious agent. Bacterial infections, particularly strep throat, require prescription medication, because an immunologic reaction to products formed by group A streptococci causes glomerulonephritis or rheumatic fever (see these disorders for more information). A serious infection can also lead to peritonsillar abscess, an accumulation of pus in the tissues around the tonsils. Chronic, recurrent tonsillitis may require surgery (tonsillectomy).

WHAT CAUSES IT?

• Viruses are the most common cause; bacteria account for some 40 percent of cases. Germs that cause tonsillitis are usually spread via hand-to-hand and hand-to-mouth contact.

SYMPTOMS

• Sore, red, raw throat; swallowing difficulty.
• Gray or white patches on the tonsils or the soft palate.
• Fever.
• Headache.
• Swollen lymph nodes in the jaw and neck.
• Nausea, vomiting, and abdominal pain (common in children).

PREVENTION

• Normal infection-fighting measures can help reduce the incidence of tonsillitis. Chief among these is frequent hand washing, especially in winter when germs are spread more easily owing to close indoor contact. Young children should be taught to cover their mouths when they sneeze or cough.
• Prompt treatment will limit transmission to others.

DIAGNOSIS

• Patient history and physical examination are necessary. Streptococcal tonsillitis cannot be distinguished from viral causes by its clinical features.
• Throat swabs are cultured to identify the underlying infectious agent and so determine the proper treatment.
• More rapid tests are available to quickly identify group A streptococci.

HOW TO TREAT IT

• Antibiotics are prescribed for streptococcal or other bacterial infections and must usually be taken for at least 10 days.
• Acetaminophen or other nonprescription pain-relieving and fever-reducing medications are recommended to relieve discomfort. Do not give aspirin to those under 16 years of age, however, as it may trigger a potentially life-threatening disorder (see Reye's Syndrome for more information).
• Gargling with a salt-water solution several times a day may relieve sore throat.
• Surgical drainage may be required if an abscess develops.
• If tonsillitis becomes chronic, or tonsil size interferes with breathing or swallowing, surgical removal of the tonsils (tonsillectomy) may be recommended. This procedure is often done on an outpatient basis.

WHEN TO CALL A DOCTOR

• Call a doctor if a sore throat does not go away within 48 hours, especially if accompanied by fever.
• Call a doctor if a sore throat worsens, especially on one side, despite antibiotic therapy.

Tooth Abscess

WHAT IS IT?

A tooth abscess is a pus-filled sac that forms in the tissues surrounding a tooth's root. It usually occurs when bacteria penetrate the hard outer layers of a tooth and spread to the pulp (the blood vessels and nerves that make up the soft core of each tooth), causing the pulp to die. The body's white blood cells' response to bacteria and dead pulp tissue results in pus, which may spread to the surrounding tissue and cause a painful abscess. Left untreated, the abscess may erode a channel through the jawbone to the gum or the skin of the face or neck, forming a boil. The boil may eventually burst, relieving pain. If the infection does not drain, it will spread to other parts of the body. The abscess may also cause swelling in the side of the face or lymph nodes in the neck, severe pain, and difficulty opening the mouth.

WHAT CAUSES IT?

• The most common cause is tooth decay. It erodes the tooth's outer layers; bacteria then enter the pulp.
• An abscess may result when gingivitis or periodontitis goes unchecked, as bacteria proliferate in gaps between the teeth and gums.
• An abscess may develop after injury to a tooth.
• Occasionally, tooth pulp dies spontaneously for no apparent reason; resulting pus may form an abscess.

PREVENTION

• Practice careful oral hygiene (see Gingivitis). See a dentist at least once a year.

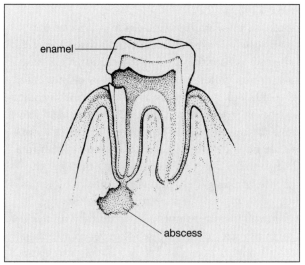

An abscess may result when plaque eats through the tooth's outer protective enamel, allowing bacteria to invade the soft inner tissues.

• Have decay treated promptly (see Tooth Decay).
• Undergo root canal treatment or extraction of the infected tooth before an abscess can form.

DIAGNOSIS

• Dental examination and x-rays.

HOW TO TREAT IT

• Rinse with warm salt water to ease pain until you can see a dentist.
• Aspirin or another pain reliever can help reduce discomfort. Stronger analgesics may be prescribed.
• The dentist may drill a small hole through the crown of the infected tooth into the pulp, to release the pus. The pulp cavity and root canals are cleaned out and disinfected (root canal procedure). After the infection has subsided, the cavity is filled and the tooth is fitted with a crown. (Severe infection must be drained surgically to prevent the spread of infection to other parts of the body.)
• If the tooth cannot be saved, it will be extracted.
• Antibiotics may be given to fight infection.

WHEN TO CALL A DOCTOR

• The pain of a tooth abscess usually prompts a visit to the dentist as soon as possible. But if pain eases as an abscessed boil bursts, or if swelling has spread to the face or neck, see a dentist immediately.

SYMPTOMS

• Persistent aching or throbbing in the affected tooth. Severe pain when biting or chewing.
• Difficulty opening the mouth or swallowing.
• Sensitivity to hot or cold foods and drinks.
• Tenderness, redness, or swelling in the gum around the affected tooth.
• A foul taste in the mouth if the abscess forms a boil and bursts.
• Swelling and tenderness of the lymph nodes in the side of the face.
• Fever and general malaise.

Tooth Decay

WHAT IS IT?

Tooth decay is caused by bacteria that normally dwell inside the mouth. These bacteria combine with food particles and mucus to form dental plaque, a sticky, colorless film that builds up on the teeth. The bacteria in plaque breaks down sugars to produce acids. Without proper oral hygiene, these acids may gradually erode the tooth's hard protective layer of enamel, forming cavities. Once the acids have penetrated the enamel, they can then attack the softer layers of tissue inside the tooth (the dentin and the pulp, which contain nerves and blood vessels), resulting in a toothache. Eventually, bacteria may invade the dentin and pulp, causing an infection that leaves the tooth vulnerable to a potentially dangerous abscess, characterized by severe pain and infection of the jaw. For this reason, tooth decay should be treated promptly.

WHAT CAUSES IT?

• Poor dental hygiene causes tooth decay.
• Sugary or starchy foods and drinks may promote tooth decay.

PREVENTION

• Brush your teeth at least twice a day, using a soft bristle toothbrush and a fluoride toothpaste. Scrub with a gentle circular motion, then brush vertically, away from the gums. Brush your tongue too; it collects the same bacteria that stick to the teeth.
• Floss daily. Ease the floss between the teeth, forming a crescent against one side of a tooth. Gingerly scrape up and down, from just under the gum line to the top of the teeth.
• Fluoride mouth rinses offer additional protection.

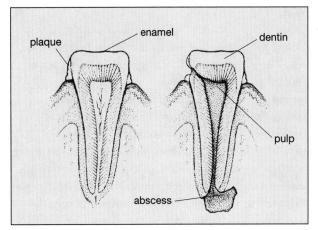

Dental plaque may erode the tooth's outer protective enamel so that bacteria can invade the soft dentin and pulp, leading to an abscess.

• Ask your dentist about the benefits of irrigation devices such as Waterpik or plaque removal devices such as Interplak.
• Schedule a dental checkup at least once a year.
• Limit your consumption of sugary drinks and sweet, starchy, or sticky foods.

DIAGNOSIS

• A dental examination is performed.
• Dental x-rays may be taken.

HOW TO TREAT IT

• For a toothache, use ice packs, aspirin, or acetaminophen until you receive professional help. (Schedule an appointment with a dentist immediately.)
• The decayed section of tooth will be drilled, abraded, or lasered and then filled with a metal alloy or plastic resin.
• If a tooth is severely decayed and in danger of being lost, a root canal may be needed. The nerve and pulp of the tooth are removed leaving only the hollow tooth and roots. The cavity is then sterilized and filled with cement, and the tooth is fitted over with a metal or porcelain crown.
• In the case of extensive decay or an abscess, extraction may be required if the tooth cannot be restored.

WHEN TO CALL A DOCTOR

• See a dentist regularly. Make an appointment promptly if you develop a toothache. ▲

SYMPTOMS

• Early decay has no symptoms.
• Increased tooth sensitivity to heat and cold.
• Toothache, especially after eating sweet or sour foods. Pain may grow more intense and persistent as decay worsens.
• Bad breath and an unpleasant taste in the mouth.

Toxic Shock Syndrome

WHAT IS IT?

Toxic shock syndrome (TSS)—most commonly linked to tampon use—is a reaction to bacterial toxins. The number of TSS cases in the United States peaked in the late 1970s and early 1980s among young women using certain brands of superabsorbent tampons, and it has dropped dramatically since these tampons were taken off the market. TSS may be triggered by other causes and can affect older women, men, and children as well. It is a potentially serious condition that requires prompt medical attention. If left untreated, TSS can produce complications such as a severe drop in blood pressure (shock), or liver or kidney failure. Most patients recover fully with treatment in one to two weeks, but TSS can recur (for example, with subsequent menstrual periods), and in rare cases, it can be fatal. Overall incidence of TSS is now low, and in general, judicious tampon use is safe. However, women who use tampons during menstruation should be aware of the typical symptoms of TSS and should seek immediate medical attention if any of these symptoms appears.

WHAT CAUSES IT?

• Toxic shock syndrome is usually caused by *Staphylococcus aureus* bacteria, which produce toxins that are absorbed into the bloodstream. In the case of tampon-associated infection, the precise relationship between tampons and TSS is still in question; it is believed that tampon insertion may cause tiny breaks in the skin, which become infected, or that superabsorbent tampons that are left in place too long may trap the bacteria in the vagina and provide a favorable environment for bacterial growth.

• TSS may result from other *Staph. aureus* and streptococcal infections, occurring in conjunction with infected scrapes or burns, abscesses, osteomyelitis, or postsurgical infections. Over the past 10 years, increasing numbers of TSS cases have been caused by streptococcal organisms—typically associated with an infected wound.

PREVENTION

• Change tampons several times a day, or alternate tampons with sanitary napkins. Never use a tampon overnight or between menstrual periods.
• Use lower-absorbency tampons.
• If you have experienced TSS in the past, avoid using tampons altogether.
• Clean and disinfect surface cuts and scrapes, and cover them with an antibiotic cream.
• Change wound dressings often, or as directed by your doctor.

DIAGNOSIS

• Patient history (including tampon usage) and physical examination are necessary.
• Blood tests help to rule out other disorders that can cause similar symptoms.
• Vaginal tissue or discharge may be cultured to confirm the diagnosis.

HOW TO TREAT IT

• If using a tampon, remove it immediately.
• In most cases hospitalization and intravenous administration of antibiotics are required.
• Intravenous fluid replacement is necessary for patients who have gone into shock.
• Further treatment may be needed for the complications of TSS, such as renal failure.

WHEN TO CALL A DOCTOR

• **EMERGENCY** Seek medical help immediately if you experience the symptoms of TSS. 🔺

SYMPTOMS
• Sudden, high fever (above 102°F).
• Vomiting and diarrhea.
• A deep red rash, most often on the palms of the hands or soles of the feet. After one to two weeks, the skin begins to peel.
• Aching or severe muscle pain.
• Headache.
• Bloodshot eyes.
• Sore throat.
• Vaginal bleeding or discharge.
• Dizziness, weakness, disorientation, or fainting.

Transient Ischemic Attack

WHAT IS IT?

A transient ischemic attack (TIA) occurs when blood flow to part of the brain is interrupted by a temporary blockage in an artery supplying the brain. The pathological mechanism of a TIA is identical to that of certain kinds of stroke (see Stroke), except that normal circulation is restored within 24 hours and no permanent brain damage occurs. Most TIAs resolve within a few minutes to an hour. Symptoms appear suddenly and vary considerably depending on the part of the brain affected. Although TIA symptoms disappear completely without treatment, they often recur. Prompt medical attention is important: TIAs are a warning sign of an impending stroke.

WHAT CAUSES IT?

• The majority of TIAs are associated with atherosclerosis, a buildup of plaques in the walls of the arteries. A TIA may develop when a plaque becomes substantial enough to reduce blood supply locally in an artery supplying the brain. More commonly, however, a TIA occurs when a small fragment of a plaque that has broken off from a blood vessel, or a blood clot (embolus), usually from the heart, travels to an artery supplying the brain and lodges in a site already narrowed by atherosclerosis.

• Major risk factors for TIAs include high blood pressure, heart disease, diabetes, smoking, and aging.

PREVENTION

• Seek treatment for any predisposing condition, such as hypertension, diabetes, or heart disease.

• Don't smoke.

• Lose weight if you are overweight.

SYMPTOMS

• Sudden weakness, tingling, or numbness, usually affecting only one side of the body.

• Double vision or temporary blindness in one eye.

• Speech difficulty.

• Dizziness and loss of balance or coordination.

• Lightheadedness, confusion, or amnesia.

• Headache or eye pain.

DIAGNOSIS

• Patient history and physical examination are needed to rule out other disorders such as epileptic seizures and migraines.

• Blood tests are taken to rule out disorders like hypoglycemia.

• Imaging studies may be done, such as magnetic resonance imaging (MRI) of the brain or ultrasound scans of the carotid arteries.

• Cerebral arteriography (injection of a contrast material into the blood vessels supplying the brain to highlight them during x-ray imaging) may be performed in some cases.

HOW TO TREAT IT

• Drugs that inhibit blood clot formation may be prescribed. Aspirin—the most commonly used antiplatelet agent—is usually tried first. More powerful anticoagulants such as warfarin and heparin may be warranted in some cases.

• Measures to control hypertension and blood cholesterol levels (including drug therapy) are undertaken if needed.

• Patients who have experienced one or more TIAs, who are healthy enough to have surgery, and who show evidence of substantial atherosclerotic narrowing in the carotid arteries (the two main blood vessels in the neck supplying the brain) may be good candidates for carotid endarterectomy—a surgical procedure to clear away plaque deposits in the arteries. This technique is not appropriate for all patients, but in those who do qualify, it has been shown to reduce the risk of having a stroke in the future.

WHEN TO CALL A DOCTOR

• If you experience the symptoms of a TIA, visit a doctor immediately. Do not ignore symptoms just because they go away by themselves. ◼

Trench Mouth

WHAT IS IT?

Trench mouth is a painful gum infection that was widespread among soldiers in the trenches during World War I, hence its name. Also known as necrotizing ulcerative gingivitis or Vincent's disease, trench mouth is a noncontagious, relatively rare condition that usually affects young adults, ages 15 to 35, though it can occur at any age. Symptoms generally appear suddenly over the course of one to two days, and they can be mild or severe. The infection destroys gum tissue, usually the gum tips between the teeth (papillae). Craterlike ulcers that bleed spontaneously may form where the papillae have been damaged, and gums may become so painful that eating is difficult. A grayish film of decayed gum tissue develops over the damaged areas. Fever, malaise, and swollen lymph nodes are common. Severe or recurrent trench mouth can damage the underlying supporting bone and tissue in the mouth and lead to eventual tooth loss. In most cases prompt treatment results in marked improvement within five days. However, if follow-up dental care is not maintained after an acute episode of trench mouth, recurrence and eventual tooth loss is possible.

WHAT CAUSES IT?

• Trench mouth is caused by infection from bacteria that normally inhabit the mouth in harmless numbers. It may occur when gingivitis or periodontitis is left untreated, allowing bacteria to proliferate.
• Smoking, lack of sleep, inadequate nutrition, poor dental hygiene, and emotional stress increase the risk of getting trench mouth.
• Trench mouth may occur when the immune system is weakened by a more serious disease, such as leukemia or AIDS.

PREVENTION

• Practice careful oral hygiene (see Gingivitis for more information) and see a dentist at least once a year for a routine cleaning and checkup.
• Do not smoke.
• Eat a balanced, nutritious diet.
• Get adequate amounts of rest.

DIAGNOSIS

• Examination of the teeth and gums by a dentist is necessary.

HOW TO TREAT IT

• A topical anesthetic is applied, and the gums are cleaned thoroughly; bacteria and dead tissue are removed from the gum surface. The mouth is then flushed with warm water or saline.
• At a later visit, the dentist will remove surface plaque and calculus—a buildup of minerals and bacterial products—from the teeth (dental scaling).
• Antibiotics may be prescribed to fight bacteria.
• Frequent rinsing with a dilute hydrogen peroxide mouthwash is recommended.
• Take aspirin or another pain medication to help ease pain.
• During recovery, avoid hot, spicy foods, alcohol, and tobacco; get plenty of rest; eat a well-balanced diet; and brush teeth gently and cautiously.
• A series of follow-up dental visits may be required.
• In severe cases when infection has spread to other parts of the body, hospitalization and intravenous antibiotics may be required.

WHEN TO CALL A DOCTOR

• If you suspect you have trench mouth, especially if your symptoms are accompanied by a fever, see a dentist immediately. 🛗

> ### SYMPTOMS
> • Red, swollen, painful gums.
> • Highly sensitive gums that may bleed profusely with even slight pressure.
> • A grayish film over the gums.
> • Bleeding ulcers on the gums.
> • Bad breath and a foul taste in the mouth.
> • Fever and general malaise.
> • Swelling in the lymph nodes under the jaw.

Trichinosis

WHAT IS IT?

Trichinosis is a parasitic disease often spread through raw or undercooked meat, especially pork. Most cases are mild and cause few if any symptoms. Trichinosis is transmitted to humans who ingest the larvae of a parasitic roundworm found in the muscles of infected animals. These larvae mature into adult worms in the lining of the intestine. The fertilized female can produce thousands of larvae that may migrate throughout the body and form cysts in the muscles of the host. These cysts can persist indefinitely. If symptoms do occur, those resulting from infestation of the intestine generally begin within one to two days after eating the infected meat. Symptoms due to muscle involvement typically begin a week later and subside gradually after a few weeks, but they sometimes last for several months. Severity depends on the number of larvae consumed and the condition of the host's immune system.

In many people, trichinosis resolves on its own; however, treatment is necessary if larval cysts in the muscles of the host produce significant muscle inflammation. Rarely, the infection may cause serious, even fatal complications involving the heart, lungs, or central nervous system. The incidence of trichinosis in the United States has dropped greatly over the past few decades thanks to public health regulations, but it is still important to cook all meat thoroughly, particularly pork and pork products, as well as wild game (such as bear, wolf, coyote, fox, horse, boar, and walrus).

SYMPTOMS

- Early symptoms (within a few days of ingestion): nausea and vomiting; diarrhea and abdominal pain or cramps; fever; sometimes prostration.
- Later symptoms (one to three weeks after ingestion): swelling around the eyes; red eyes; muscle pain and tenderness; severe weakness; fever; itching or burning skin.
- Possible more serious symptoms: coughing up bloody phlegm, paralysis, delirium, coma, heart failure.

WHAT CAUSES IT?

- Trichinosis is caused by the roundworm *Trichinella spiralis,* which lives in the intestines and muscles of many species of animals. The disease is transmitted to humans by ingestion of undercooked meat from such animals. Larvae from intestinal worms enter the bloodstream and muscles where they form cysts that can induce an inflammatory response and lead to damage to the heart, lungs, and brain.

PREVENTION

- Cook pork and other meat thoroughly. Pork should be cooked until all pink portions turn white or gray.
- As an alternative precaution, store meat for at least 20 days in a deep freezer before cooking it.

DIAGNOSIS

- Patient history (including recent food consumption history) is taken. Physical examination may reveal characteristic signs of trichinosis infection.
- Blood tests will reveal an elevated eosinophil count and antibodies against *T. spiralis.*
- Stool analysis may detect worms and larvae.
- The most definitive test is a muscle biopsy to detect the presence of the *T. spiralis* larvae.
- If possible, a portion of the suspect meat is analyzed.

HOW TO TREAT IT

- In mild cases treatment may not be necessary.
- Mebendazole may be prescribed to kill the worms and so relieve symptoms. Mebendazole kills larvae as well as adult worms, but it should not be used in children or pregnant women.
- Acetaminophen or aspirin may be used to reduce fever and ease discomfort.
- When the heart is affected, bed rest is necessary until symptoms subside.
- Corticosteroid drugs may be prescribed to reduce inflammation in severe cases, or for patients who have an allergic response to the parasite.

WHEN TO CALL A DOCTOR

- If you experience the symptoms of trichinosis, especially if you have eaten pork within the past several weeks, see a doctor as soon as possible.

Tuberculosis

WHAT IS IT?

Tuberculosis, also known as TB, is a chronic infection with a specific type of bacterium (*Mycobacterium tuberculosis*) that usually affects the lungs. Although contagious, TB is not as easy to catch as other respiratory infections, since repeated and prolonged exposure to airborne particles from coughing or sneezing is usually necessary to permit sufficient numbers of the bacteria into the lungs. Overcrowded, impoverished living conditions and frequent contact with others who are sick with TB are significant risk factors. In the United States a large proportion of people with TB were born in countries with high rates of the disease.

The infection has two distinct stages. First, bacteria are inhaled into the lungs, where most are destroyed by the immune system. Bacteria that are not destroyed are trapped by the immune system inside hard, walled capsules, known as tubercles, which are composed of a number of different types of cells. TB bacteria cannot cause damage or symptoms while encased in the tubercles, and in many people the disease never progresses beyond this point. Only a small fraction of those infected will develop active disease, the second stage of TB.

Active disease appears if the bacteria escape control of the tubercles and infect other sites in the lungs. Bacteria may also invade the bloodstream and the lymphatic system and spread throughout the body. A few people develop active disease within weeks of the initial infection, but in most cases the second stage does not appear until years or decades later. Factors such as aging, a weakened immune system, and poor nutrition increase the risk that the

bacteria will break through the tubercle walls. Most commonly, active TB destroys lung tissue and severely impairs breathing, but it may also affect other parts of the body, including the brain, lymph nodes, kidneys, and gastrointestinal tract. Untreated TB may be fatal.

Sometimes known as the white plague for the ashen complexion of its victims, TB is a leading killer worldwide despite the development of effective drug treatment. In addition, the disease experienced a resurgence in the United States between 1985 and 1992. With strengthened public health measures, however, the rate of TB has fallen substantially in recent years.

A significant factor that contributed to the resurgence of TB, including drug-resistant TB, was nonadherence to treatment by people with the disease. A combination of drugs must be taken for six to nine months to cure the illness. These drugs kill the weakest bacteria first; stronger, more resistant bacteria survive the initial assault and must be attacked steadily over time. However, because symptoms fade after a few weeks, many people do not complete the entire course of treatment. This practice may lead to a relapse with an even more deadly form of the disease. Taking the medication for only a few weeks or months favors survival and growth of the strongest bacteria, creating an infection resistant to some or all drug therapy. To fight TB effectively, and to prevent the growth of drug-resistant strains of the bacteria, it is important that proper courses of treatment are strictly followed. In the United States it is generally recommended that all treatment for TB be directly supervised by a nurse or other health worker to assure compliance. Directly observed therapy (DOT) has been shown to result in high cure rates and low levels of drug resistance.

Another major contributor to the resurgence of TB was the AIDS epidemic. The weakened immune defenses of AIDS patients result in the rapid spread of bacteria after an infection.

WHAT CAUSES IT?
• Bacterial infection causes tuberculosis.
• TB is spread through the air by the sneeze or cough of an infected person.

SYMPTOMS
• Persistent cough, possibly producing bloody sputum.
• Chest pain.
• Shortness of breath.
• Fever.
• Fatigue.
• Night sweats.
• Loss of appetite; weight loss.

Tuberculosis *continued*

• Those who live in crowded or unsanitary areas, including the poor, migrant farm workers, and the homeless, are at higher risk for TB.

• People from nations with high rates of TB, such as countries in Latin America, Asia, or Africa, may harbor the TB bacteria and be at risk for becoming sick.

• People with weakened immune systems, such as those infected with the human immunodeficiency virus (HIV) or undergoing treatment for cancer, are at greater risk for TB.

• Others at high risk for TB include infants, the elderly, people with diabetes, intravenous drug users, the malnourished, health-care workers, prison guards, and family members of those with TB.

• TB spreads more easily in confined, poorly ventilated spaces, including jails, nursing homes, tenements, homeless shelters, and even hospitals.

PREVENTION

• A vaccine against TB, called BCG, is widely used around the world—but its use is discouraged in the United States. BCG helps reduce the risk of serious TB in children. However, it may provide adults with little or no protection against the disease.

• Antibiotics may be administered to people who test positive for TB but have no evidence of active disease. These drugs prevent development of second-stage TB by destroying the bacteria trapped within the tubercles. The most commonly used medicine is isoniazid, which should be taken for nine months. A newer treatment employs the drugs rifampin and pyrazinamide, which must be taken for two months.

DIAGNOSIS

• Patient history and physical examination.

• Chest x-rays.

• Tuberculin skin test. A small amount of protein derived from mycobacteria is injected into the skin on the arm, and the area is examined after a day or two. A slightly raised, hard, red patch of skin at the site indicates the presence of TB (although not necessarily active disease). However, a positive TB skin test may also result from prior immunization with BCG.

• Sputum smears and culture. Examining sputum for TB bacteria is essential. The smear shows if TB-like organisms are present; smears are negative, however, in many patients who have TB, and some positive smears may be caused by organisms other than TB. The results of the culture may take three to six weeks to develop. A positive culture confirms diagnosis.

• Bone marrow biopsy. A sample of bone marrow is usually taken from the hip bone.

• Bronchoscopy (the use of a thin, hollow, flexible tube passed through the mouth into the windpipe to view the main bronchial passages).

HOW TO TREAT IT

• A combination of three or four antibiotics—isoniazid, rifampin, pyrazinamide, and ethambutol, the most effective drugs against TB—is prescribed for six to nine months. After two months the treatment is usually reduced to only isoniazid and rifampin. The antibiotics must be taken for the full term prescribed, both to cure the infection and to prevent the development of drug-resistant TB strains. Supervised treatment is recommended.

• Resistant strains of bacteria may require treatment with a combination of additional drugs.

• Patients should get plenty of rest until symptoms subside.

• TB sufferers should sneeze or cough into disposable tissues to prevent the spread of infection.

• Hospitalization in an isolation room with adequate ventilation may be necessary to prevent the spread of TB until the infection has been brought under control.

• Surgery to remove damaged lung tissue may be performed in advanced cases of drug-resistant TB.

WHEN TO CALL A DOCTOR

• Call a doctor if you develop a persistent cough, chest pain, night sweats, and shortness of breath.

• If you have been exposed to someone sick with TB, your doctor or local health department can perform a TB skin test.

Typhoid Fever

WHAT IS IT?

Typhoid fever is a contagious bacterial infection that involves the intestine and lymphatic system. Rare in the United States, typhoid fever is common in developing countries, especially in areas with poor sanitation. Symptoms develop gradually over three weeks; fever, chills, and headache occur first. Left untreated, typhoid fever may result in life-threatening intestinal perforation and bleeding.

Some people become symptom-free carriers of the disease when the typhoid bacteria lodge in the bile or in gallstones. The bacteria may then periodically migrate to the bowel and be excreted in the feces, thereby contaminating ground water or vegetation fertilized with human waste. Typhoid fever responds well to antibiotics. Severe symptoms are unlikely with early treatment, although about one in five patients relapses.

WHAT CAUSES IT?

• Typhoid is caused by *Salmonella typhi,* a bacterium that invades the wall of the small intestine.
• Typhoid fever is spread by water and food contaminated with the fecal matter of an infected person.
• Nearly 5 percent of former patients become chronic carriers—people who carry the bacteria and spread the disease but have no symptoms themselves.

SYMPTOMS
• Persistent fever and chills. Fever is higher in the morning.
• Headache.
• Abdominal pain.
• General feeling of poor health.
• Muscle aches.
• Nausea and vomiting.
• Constipation or diarrhea.
• Loss of appetite and weight.
• Pale, reddish skin rash ("rose spots") on the shoulders, chest, and back, lasting for three to four days.
• Nosebleeds.
• Personality changes and delirium; coma; seizures in children.

• Flies may spread the bacteria and cause epidemics; this is more common in areas with poor sanitation.

PREVENTION
• Wash hands with soap and warm water often, especially after using the toilet or before handling food. (Infected people should use a separate toilet and wash hands or don gloves before handling others' food.)
• Get a typhoid vaccine (though it's only partially effective) before traveling to high-risk areas.
• When traveling abroad or in areas with poor sanitation, drink only bottled water or other bottled beverages, and eat only well-cooked foods and fruit you can peel yourself. Do not use ice.

DIAGNOSIS
• Laboratory tests are required for diagnosis.

HOW TO TREAT IT
• Do not take aspirin or other over-the-counter pain relievers for typhoid fever unless prescribed by your doctor. These medications may lower blood pressure; aspirin may also promote gastrointestinal bleeding.
• The antibiotic chloramphenicol is most often prescribed to treat typhoid fever in developing countries. Other antibiotics, such as ciprofloxacin or trimethoprim-sulfamethoxazole, can also be effective.
• Intravenous fluids and electrolytes (mineral salts) may be administered to treat dehydration.
• Antidiarrheal drugs or narcotics may be warranted to relieve diarrhea and cramps.
• Blood transfusions may be necessary in the event of intestinal bleeding.
• Dexamethasone, a corticosteroid drug, may be used in severe cases involving the central nervous system to treat delirium, seizures, or shock.
• Emergency surgery may be necessary to repair intestinal perforation.
• Several months of antibiotic treatment may eliminate bacteria from chronic carriers; surgical removal of the gallbladder (cholecystectomy) is occasionally necessary.

WHEN TO CALL A DOCTOR
• Call a doctor if you develop persistent fever and chills along with other symptoms of typhoid fever. ⚠

Urethritis

WHAT IS IT?

Urethritis is an inflammation of the urethra, the thin tube that carries urine out of the body from the bladder. Often caused by a bacterial infection, urethritis may produce distinctly different symptoms in men and women. Infectious agents (including chlamydia, gonorrhea, and herpesvirus) transmitted during sexual activity may cause urethritis in both men and women, but women may not exhibit any symptoms. In symptomatic women, urethritis may be difficult to distinguish from a bladder infection; however, treatment is similar in either case (see Bladder Infection for more information). Urethritis may also be caused by nonsexually transmitted infections; such infections are most common among women.

WHAT CAUSES IT?

• In women, urethritis often results from an infection caused by bacteria that normally inhabit the anal area with no ill effect. If these bacteria enter the urinary tract, urethritis may ensue.
• Urethritis may result from sexual transmission of the herpesvirus or the bacteria that cause chlamydia or gonorrhea.
• Prolonged use of a urinary catheter increases the risk of urethritis.
• Sexual activity may bruise the urethra in women and promote inflammation.
• Some soaps, bath oils, and vaginal douches may irritate the urethra.

PREVENTION

• Use condoms during sexual intercourse to help decrease the risk of infection.

• Good hygiene is recommended, especially prior to sexual activity. Use mild, unscented soap. Showers are less likely to promote urethritis than baths.
• To flush bacteria from the vaginal tract, women should drink some water prior to sexual intercourse and urinate within 15 minutes afterward; if necessary, they should use a water-soluble lubricant (not petroleum jelly) to decrease the risk of bruising during intercourse.
• After using the bathroom, women should wipe from front to back to avoid spreading fecal bacteria to the urethra.
• Women should not douche unless otherwise instructed by a doctor.
• People who have recurrent episodes of urethritis should drink at least eight glasses of liquid a day and should avoid caffeine and alcohol, which may irritate the bladder.

DIAGNOSIS

• Patient history and physical examination.
• Microscopic examination and culture of urethral discharge and urine.

HOW TO TREAT IT

• Antibiotics, prescribed to treat bacterial infections, should be taken for the full term as directed; stopping the medication too early may result in a more serious and more difficult-to-treat rebound infection. For sexually transmitted diseases, only one partner may exhibit symptoms, but it is likely that the symptomless partner is also infected. Therefore, both partners need to be treated to prevent a self-perpetuating cycle of reinfection.
• Analgesics may be administered to relieve pain.
• Cranberry juice can increase the acidity of urine and enhance the effectiveness of some medications for urinary tract infections.

WHEN TO CALL A DOCTOR

• Call a doctor if you or your partner experiences painful, frequent urination, or if you notice an abnormal discharge from the vagina or penis. ▲

SYMPTOMS
• Burning on urination.
• Frequent urination with only small amounts of urine passed on each occasion.
• Urgent need to urinate.
• Blood in the urine.
• Yellowish discharge from the urethra.
• Lower abdominal pain.
• Painful sexual intercourse in women.

Urinary Incontinence

WHAT IS IT?

Urinary incontinence, the partial or complete inability to control the urge to urinate, is a very common problem in older people (and twice as common in women). Incontinence is not, however, an inevitable consequence of aging; it is caused by some underlying disorder. There are different types of incontinence: stress and urge incontinence are two of the most common.

Stress incontinence occurs when some activity (coughing, laughing, or lifting, for example) temporarily increases the pressure on the bladder, causing a small amount of urine to be released. Urge incontinence occurs when a sudden need to urinate is accompanied by an inability to control the bladder, sometimes releasing large amounts of urine. Incontinence causes embarrassment, depression, and social isolation, and is often the final reason why people are placed in nursing homes.

Specific treatment and the degree of success achieved with them depend on the underlying cause. But in most instances, incontinence can at least be controlled if not eliminated.

WHAT CAUSES IT?

• Abnormalities of the detrusor muscle, which contracts to force urine out of the bladder.
• Weakness, due to childbirth, of the muscles of the pelvic floor that support the bladder and control urine flow.
• Age-related changes in the urinary tract, such as bladder shrinkage.
• Atrophy of the urethra due to decreased estrogen production in postmenopausal women.
• Medications, including diuretics, sleeping pills, and tranquilizers.

SYMPTOMS
• Urine leakage when coughing or during lifting or other activities that increase pressure on the bladder.
• Partial or complete inability to control the bladder.
• Involuntary, unpredictable urination.

• Poorly controlled diabetes mellitus (sugar in the urine creates large amounts of urine to be voided).
• Urinary tract infections.
• Damage to the nerves that control bladder function, causing either excessive bladder contraction or loss of sensation governing the urge to urinate.
• Surgery or radiation therapy of the pelvic area.
• Obstruction of the flow of urine, for example, due to an enlarged prostate or urethral stricture.
• Psychological disorders including depression.

PREVENTION
• Hormone replacement therapy may be prescribed for postmenopausal women.

DIAGNOSIS
• Patient history and physical examination.
• An "incontinence chart" or voiding record of the time, amount, and circumstances of urination.
• Catheterization of the bladder to measure amount of urine remaining in the bladder after urination.
• Observation of the effects of filling the bladder using a catheter.
• Microscopic examination and culture of urine.

HOW TO TREAT IT
• Education is important. Sometimes mere interpretation of the incontinence chart will lead to complete or greatly improved bladder control.
• In many cases bladder control can be regained with techniques known as bladder training (for urge incontinence) and Kegel exercises (for stress incontinence). Bladder training begins by scheduling a bathroom visit every two hours, whether the patient needs to go or not. The interval is gradually increased by a half hour at a time, toward a goal of four-hour intervals. In many cases the body adapts to this schedule, eliminating incontinence. Kegel exercises involve repetitive contractions of the pelvic-floor muscles to strengthen them and prevent stress incontinence.
• Biofeedback—a technique using electronic equipment that provides visual and auditory feedback to increase patient awareness and control of the bladder muscles—may improve or even cure incontinence in certain patients.

Urinary Incontinence   *continued*

• Anticholinergic drugs (which block the neuro-transmitter acetylcholine), imipramine, and estrogen are sometimes helpful in treating incontinence.

• Antibiotics may be prescribed to treat an associated bacterial infection.

• Your doctor should be consulted if you think that any medications may be contributing to incontinence.

• Adult diapers and pads may actually promote complications, so they are not recommended for anything but very short-term use unless otherwise advised by a doctor.

• A bedside toilet may help with nighttime urgency. Avoid drinking excess fluids for two to three hours prior to going to bed.

• Surgery may be used to relieve pressure on bladder nerves, reduce blockage of the urethra, or repair damaged muscles or other structures.

• In rare, severe cases an indwelling catheter may be indicated.

WHEN TO CALL A DOCTOR

• Call a doctor if you experience any bladder control problems. ▨

Uterine Cancer

WHAT IS IT?

Uterine cancer is the growth of malignant cells in the uterus. The term uterine cancer is often used interchangeably with endometrial cancer, because uterine malignancy most often develops in the endometrium, or uterine lining. Malignant tumors may also develop in the muscular wall of the uterus (uterine sarcoma), although this is relatively rare.

Endometrial cancer is the most common pelvic gynecological cancer; it almost always affects postmenopausal women between the ages of 50 and 70. Endometrial cancer tends to grow and spread slowly, and so with early detection and treatment, it is highly curable.

WHAT CAUSES IT?

• The cause of uterine cancer is unknown.
• Obesity, high blood pressure, diabetes mellitus, endometrial hyperplasia, endometrial polyps, polycystic ovary disease, and a late menopause with heavy bleeding are all associated with an increased risk of uterine cancer. (See these specific disorders for more information.)
• Long-term use of unopposed estrogen replacement therapy (without progesterone) in postmenopausal women is associated with a higher incidence of endometrial cancer.
• Tamoxifen, a drug used in the treatment of breast cancer, may increase the risk of uterine cancer.
• Endometrial cancer is more common in women who have had few or no children; it is less frequent in those who have used oral contraceptives.

PREVENTION

• In high-risk (non-ovulating) women, uterine cancer may be prevented with cyclical use of progestational drugs. Regular pelvic examinations during and after menopause are advised to aid in early detection and treatment of any abnormalities.
• Postmenopausal estrogen replacement should be accompanied by a progestational agent or frequent endometrial biopsies.

DIAGNOSIS

• Patient history and gynecological examination are necessary.
• Diagnosis of endometrial cancer requires an endometrial biopsy or dilatation and curettage (D&C). In these procedures the cervical canal is dilated so that an instrument can be passed into the uterine cavity to biopsy the endometrium.
• Pelvic ultrasound scans may be done to detect tumors (whether benign or malignant).
• A Pap smear (performed during a pelvic examination) may reveal the presence of malignant cells in the cervix (see Cervical Cancer), but it is not a reliable way to detect endometrial cancer.

HOW TO TREAT IT

• The primary treatment for uterine cancer is a total hysterectomy (surgical removal of the uterus), in addition to removal of the cervix, fallopian tubes, both ovaries, a portion of the upper vagina, and neighboring lymph nodes.
• Cancers in their earliest stage (noninvasive and with normal-appearing cells) may be treated by hysterectomy alone, without further measures.
• If cancer is believed to have advanced beyond the earliest stage, radiation therapy is initiated in addition to surgery. Both external and internal radiation may be used; in internal radiation, small radioactive pellets are implanted in or near the tumor site for 48 to 72 hours at a time.
• Progestational agents are used in the treatment of endometrial cancer; chemotherapy has not proved to be effective in most cases.

WHEN TO CALL A DOCTOR

• Call a gynecologist if you develop heavy vaginal bleeding or if you experience vaginal bleeding between periods or after menopause. ⚠

SYMPTOMS

• Vaginal bleeding after menopause.
• Heavy, persistent, or unusual (sometimes watery or blood-streaked) vaginal discharge.
• Lower abdominal pain and weight loss in advanced stages.

Uterine Prolapse

WHAT IS IT?

Uterine prolapse is a protrusion of the uterus into the vagina. It occurs when the pelvic muscles and supporting ligaments, which normally hold the uterus in place, become injured or weakened. In mild prolapse a portion of the uterus descends into the top of the vagina. In more severe cases the uterus may protrude through the vaginal opening. Uterine prolapse is often accompanied by a bulging of the bladder (cystocele) or the urethra (urethrocele) into the front wall of the vagina, or a bulging of the rectum into the back wall of the vagina. Mild cases of uterine prolapse may not require treatment. If symptoms become more pronounced, treatment options include special exercises, a device that physically supports the uterus (a pessary), and surgery.

WHAT CAUSES IT?

• Injury or weakness of the pelvic muscles, usually from multiple or unattended childbirths, is the most common cause of uterine prolapse.
• Obesity, diabetes mellitus, chronic bronchitis, asthma, certain generalized defects in supporting tissues, and a retroverted uterus (uterus is tipped toward the back of the body) increase the risk.
• Heavy lifting or straining may contribute to uterine prolapse if pelvic muscles are already weakened.
• Rarely, uterine prolapse may appear in infants.

PREVENTION

• Kegel exercises to strengthen the muscles supporting the uterus may be recommended after childbirth.

SYMPTOMS

• In many women, no symptoms.
• Discomfort, pain, or a sensation of heaviness or fullness in the lower abdomen and vagina.
• Abnormal vaginal discharge or bleeding.
• Uncomfortable sexual intercourse.
• Pain in the lower back.
• Anal pain or a sensation of "sitting on a ball."
• Urinary urgency or frequency; constipation.
• Visible protrusion of the uterus through the vaginal opening (in severe cases).

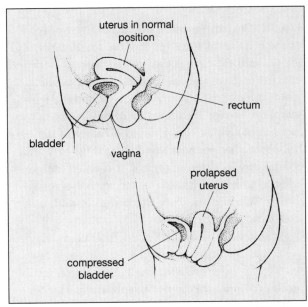

A slackening or stretching of the pelvic muscles may cause the uterus to prolapse and slide into the vaginal canal, compressing the bladder.

• If necessary, weight reduction may be advised.
• Estrogen replacement may be recommended for postmenopausal women.

DIAGNOSIS

• Gynecological examination.

HOW TO TREAT IT

• Avoid tight pants, belts, or girdles.
• Minimize straining during urination and bowel movements.
• A small plastic, rubber, or silicone ring known as a pessary may be used to provide support for a mildly prolapsed uterus or when surgery is warranted but the patient has serious medical problems and cannot endure it. The pessary is inserted into the vagina and positioned against the cervix. The pessary should be removed, cleaned, and reinserted every few months.
• Surgery (hysterectomy) may be performed to remove a severely prolapsed uterus, but the supporting tissues must be sutured to avoid prolapse of the vagina after uterine removal.

WHEN TO CALL A DOCTOR

• Call a doctor if you develop pelvic pain or discomfort or unusual pelvic protrusion.

Uveitis and Iritis

WHAT IS IT?

Uveitis is an inflammation of the uvea, the portion of the eye that includes the iris, the ciliary body, and the choroid. The iris is the colored portion of the eye that controls the opening and closing of the pupil; the ciliary body is a muscle behind the iris that helps change the curvature of the lens so as to focus light rays; and the choroid is a layer of the eyeball containing essential blood vessels. When uveitis is primarily localized in the iris, it is called iritis or, when it affects the iris and the ciliary body, anterior uveitis. When it primarily affects the choroid, it is known as posterior uveitis.

Attacks of anterior uveitis, the most common variety, usually subside within a few days to a few weeks with no permanent damage; however, recurrence is common. Posterior uveitis may persist for months or years even with treatment and cause irreversible scarring of delicate structures within the eye, including the retina (the layer of nerve cells that converts light rays into nerve impulses). If left untreated, uveitis of either type may lead to permanent vision loss and complications, including glaucoma, cataracts, and retinal detachment. A rare form of uveitis occurs when an injured eye that is severely inflamed for several weeks triggers inflammation of the uvea in the uninvolved eye. This condition, known as sympathetic ophthalmia, can result in severe vision loss in both eyes and requires prompt medical attention. Uveitis is a relatively rare disorder and most often affects young adults.

WHAT CAUSES IT?

- In most cases the cause of uveitis is unknown.
- An autoimmune reaction (in which the body's natural defenses inappropriately attack healthy tissue) may be responsible.
- Bacterial, viral, and fungal infections are potential causes.
- Systemic disorders (those affecting entire organ systems of the body) such as rheumatoid arthritis, ankylosing spondylitis, toxoplasmosis, Crohn's disease, ulcerative colitis, and sarcoidosis may cause uveitis.

PREVENTION

- There is no known way to prevent uveitis.

DIAGNOSIS

- A thorough examination by an ophthalmologist is necessary.

HOW TO TREAT IT

- A cycloplegic (iris-paralyzing) drug such as atropine sulfate may be administered. Immobilizing the inflamed iris and ciliary body may prevent scarring and alleviate pain somewhat. When such drugs are used, the pupil remains constantly dilated in one position, making the eye extremely sensitive to light; dark glasses are therefore recommended during the treatment period, even while indoors.
- Topical anti-inflammatory corticosteroid eye drops are usually prescribed. For more severe cases, oral or injected steroids may be required.
- Long-term steroid use increases the risks of cataracts and glaucoma, so frequent monitoring by an ophthalmologist is essential.
- Some causes of uveitis require cytotoxic drugs to treat the underlying disorder.
- Aspirin may help reduce inflammation and eye pain.

WHEN TO CALL A DOCTOR

- Any persistent or serious eye pain and even the slightest loss of vision warrant a prompt examination by an ophthalmologist.

SYMPTOMS
- Moderate to severe eye pain.
- Aversion to light.
- Blurred vision.
- Spots in the field of vision.
- Redness in the eye.
- Pupil contraction.
- Excessive tearing.

Vaginal Cancer

WHAT IS IT?

Vaginal cancer—the growth of malignant cells in the vagina—is rare, representing less than 2 percent of all gynecologic cancers. Most cases of vaginal cancer occur in women over the age of 50. However, some types may affect young women during adolescence or early adulthood, and one very rare type appears in children under five. Vaginal cancers are highly treatable and often curable; outlook is optimistic with early detection and treatment.

WHAT CAUSES IT?

• The cause of vaginal cancer is unknown.
• Women whose mothers took the synthetic hormone DES (diethylstilbestrol) during pregnancy are at greater risk for vaginal cancer.
• Previous radiation therapy to the pelvic region carries a higher risk of the disease.
• Women who have had cervical dysplasia or cervical cancer have an increased risk.
• A history of untreated genital warts is associated with vaginal cancer.

PREVENTION

• There is no way to prevent vaginal cancer, but regular pelvic examinations and Pap smears are advised to aid in the early detection and treatment of any abnormalities.
• Women whose mothers took the drug DES during pregnancy should have periodic pelvic examinations and Pap smears of the vagina as well as the cervix at least once a year.

DIAGNOSIS

• Patient history and gynecologic examination are necessary.
• A Pap smear (involving the scraping of a small sample of cells from the cervix and vagina for microscopic inspection) may reveal the presence of malignant cells.
• Colposcopy (use of a special magnifying scope designed to examine the female reproductive system) may be used to view the vagina in detail. A biopsy may be taken at the time of the colposcopy.

HOW TO TREAT IT

• In the very earliest stage of vaginal cancer, a cream containing the chemotherapeutic medication fluorouracil may be applied intravaginally for five to 10 days.
• Laser surgery may be performed to eliminate a single tumor that has not spread.
• Radiation therapy may be used in addition to or instead of surgery to destroy cancerous cells. Both external and internal radiation may be administered; in internal radiation, small radioactive pellets are implanted in the body near the tumor site for 48 to 72 hours at a time.
• Conventional surgery may be performed to remove the cancerous region of the vagina and some neighboring tissue. If a large portion of vaginal tissue is to be removed, a skin graft and plastic surgery can be performed to reconstruct a functional vagina. In more severe cases a hysterectomy (removal of the cervix and uterus) or a radical hysterectomy (removal of the cervix and uterus as well as the upper vagina, fallopian tubes, neighboring lymph nodes, and possibly the ovaries) may be advised.

WHEN TO CALL A DOCTOR

• Call a gynecologist if you develop abnormal vaginal itching, bleeding, or pain. ⚠

SYMPTOMS

• Vaginal bleeding between menstrual periods or after menopause.
• Firm, raised ulcer or bump in the vagina.
• Vaginal pain or itching. Pain may be worse upon urination and during sexual intercourse.

Vaginitis

WHAT IS IT?

Vaginitis is a common inflammation of the vaginal lining and the vulva, the folds of skin surrounding the vaginal opening. It is often a result of infection by one of various microorganisms, but vaginitis may also be caused by irritation from soaps or medications, an allergic reaction, or hormonal changes. The three most common types of vaginitis are candidiasis (yeast infection), trichomoniasis (infection by a tiny, one-celled organism called a protozoan), and bacterial vaginosis (or nonspecific vaginitis). Although irritating, vaginitis is not a serious health risk, and it typically subsides quickly with treatment. Recurrent or persistent cases may be associated with an underlying medical condition.

WHAT CAUSES IT?

• Bacterial, fungal, or protozoal infections.
• An allergic reaction to or irritation by substances in spermicides, douches, soaps, or bath oils may produce vaginitis.
• Trichomoniasis may be spread through sexual intercourse.
• Oral corticosteroids, antibiotics, and oral contraceptives may make vaginitis more likely.
• Certain conditions including pregnancy, malnutrition, poor health, and diabetes mellitus carry a greater risk of vaginitis.
• A decrease in estrogen levels in postmenopausal women may thin the vaginal lining and cause atrophic vaginitis.

SYMPTOMS

• Profuse vaginal discharge. Discharge may be heavy, white, thick, and odorless (candidiasis); greenish yellow, frothy, and foul-smelling (trichomoniasis); white or gray, and fishy-smelling (bacterial vaginosis); thin, white or blood-streaked, and foul-smelling (atrophic vaginitis).
• Vaginal and vulvar pain or itching. Pain may be worse upon urination and during sexual intercourse.
• Bright reddish color to the vulva.

PREVENTION

• Shower daily, using a mild, unscented soap in the vaginal area.
• Use condoms during sexual intercourse to help decrease the risk of infection.
• Wear cotton undergarments and pantyhose with a cotton crotch. Avoid nylon undergarments, which do not breathe. Do not share underwear, towels, or swimsuits.
• After a bowel movement, wipe from front to back to prevent the bacteria that normally inhabit the anal area from contacting the vagina.
• Do not use vaginal douches unless advised to do so by your doctor.

DIAGNOSIS

• Pelvic examination.
• Microscopic examination or a culture of vaginal discharge.

HOW TO TREAT IT

• An antifungal medication such as miconazole or clotrimazole is prescribed in the form of vaginal suppositories or cream to treat candidiasis (yeast infection). These medications are now available over the counter. Oral antifungal medication such as ketoconazole may be prescribed in severe cases that do not respond to topical therapy.
• Metronidazole, an antimicrobial drug, is administered to both sexual partners for trichomoniasis and should be taken for the full term prescribed. Only one partner may exhibit symptoms, but both need to be treated to prevent a perpetual cycle of reinfection.
• Metronidazole or various antibiotics may be prescribed to treat bacterial vaginosis.
• Topical or oral estrogens may be prescribed for atrophic vaginitis.
• If a medication is suspected as the cause of vaginitis, a change in prescription may be warranted.
• Abstinence from sexual intercourse may be advised until treatment is completed.

WHEN TO CALL A DOCTOR

• Call your gynecologist if you experience vaginal itching, burning, or pain, or if you notice any abnormal vaginal discharge.

Valvular Heart Disease

WHAT IS IT?

Valvular heart disease is characterized by damage to or a defect in one of the four heart valves: the mitral, aortic, tricuspid, or pulmonary. The mitral and tricuspid valves control the flow of blood between the atria and the ventricles (the upper and lower chambers of the heart). The pulmonary valve controls the flow of blood from the heart to the lungs, and the aortic valve governs blood flow between the heart and the aorta, and thereby the blood vessels to the rest of the body. The mitral and aortic valves are the ones most frequently affected by valvular heart disease.

Normally functioning valves ensure that blood flows with proper force in the proper direction at the proper time. In valvular heart disease, the valves become too narrow and hardened (stenotic) to open fully, or are unable to close completely (incompetent). A stenotic valve forces blood to back up in the adjacent heart chamber, while an incompetent valve allows blood to leak back into the chamber it previously exited. To compensate for poor pumping action, the heart muscle enlarges and thickens, thereby losing elasticity and efficiency. In addition, in some cases blood pooling in the chambers of the heart has a greater tendency to clot, increasing the risk of stroke or pulmonary embolism (see Stroke and Pulmonary Embolism for more information).

The severity of valvular heart disease varies. In mild cases there may be no symptoms, while in advanced cases, valvular heart disease may lead to congestive heart failure (see Congestive Heart Failure) and other complications. Treatment depends upon the extent of the disease.

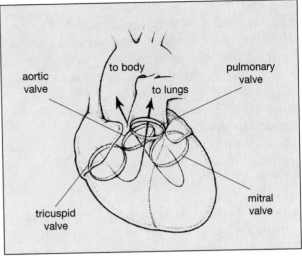

When the heart's ventricles contract, the aortic and pulmonary valves open to allow blood to be pumped out to the body and lungs, respectively. As the ventricles relax between beats, the aortic and pulmonary valves close, while the mitral and tricuspid valves open, allowing the ventricles to fill with blood again before the next contraction.

WHAT CAUSES IT?

• Rheumatic fever may cause valvular heart disease.
• Bacterial endocarditis, an infection of the inner lining of the heart muscle and heart valves (endocardium), is a cause of valvular heart disease.
• High blood pressure and atherosclerosis may damage the aortic valve.
• A heart attack may damage the muscles that control the heart valves.
• Congenital abnormalities of the heart valves may be present.
• Heart valve tissue may degenerate with age.
• Other disorders such as carcinoid tumors, rheumatoid arthritis, systemic lupus erythematosus, or syphilis may damage one or more heart valves (see these specific disorders for more information).
• Methysergide, a medication used to treat migraine headaches, and some diet drugs may promote valvular heart disease.
• Radiation therapy (used to treat cancer) may be associated with valvular heart disease.

PREVENTION

• A heart-healthy lifestyle is advised to reduce the risks of high blood pressure, atherosclerosis, and heart attack.

SYMPTOMS

• Symptoms of congestive heart failure: shortness of breath and wheezing after limited physical exertion; swelling of feet, ankles, hands, or abdomen (edema).
• Palpitations; chest pain (may be mild).
• Fatigue.
• Dizziness or fainting (with aortic stenosis).
• Fever (with bacterial endocarditis).

Valvular Heart Disease *continued*

DIAGNOSIS

• Patient history and physical examination. The doctor listens for distinctive heart sounds, known as heart murmurs, that indicate valvular heart disease.

• An electrocardiogram (ECG), to measure the electrical activity of the heart, regularity of heartbeats, thickening of heart muscle (hypertrophy), and heart-muscle damage from coronary artery disease.

• Stress testing (measurement of blood pressure, heart rate, ECG changes, and breathing rates while the patient walks on a treadmill).

• Chest x-rays.

• Echocardiogram (use of ultrasound waves to create a moving image of the valves as the heart beats).

• Cardiac catheterization: the threading of a catheter into the heart chambers to measure pressure irregularities across the valves (to detect stenosis) or to observe backflow of an injected dye on an x-ray (to detect incompetence).

HOW TO TREAT IT

• Don't smoke; follow prevention tips for a heart-healthy lifestyle. Avoid excessive alcohol consumption, excessive salt intake, and diet pills—all of which may raise blood pressure.

• Your doctor may adopt a "watch and wait" policy for mild or asymptomatic cases.

• A course of antibiotics is prescribed prior to surgery or dental work for those with valvular heart disease, to prevent bacterial endocarditis.

• Long-term antibiotic therapy is recommended to prevent a recurrence of streptococcal infection in those who have had rheumatic fever.

• Antithrombotic (clot-preventing) medications such as aspirin or ticlopidine may be prescribed for those with valvular heart disease who have experienced unexplained transient ischemic attacks, also known as TIAs (see this disorder for more information).

• More potent anticoagulants such as warfarin may be prescribed for those who have atrial fibrillation (a common complication of mitral valve disease) or who continue to experience TIAs despite initial treatment. Long-term administration of anticoagulants may be necessary following valve replacement surgery, because prosthetic valves are associated with a higher risk of blood clots.

• Balloon dilatation (a surgical technique involving insertion into a blood vessel of a small balloon that is led via catheter to the narrowed site and then inflated) may be done to widen a stenotic valve.

• Surgery to repair or replace a damaged valve may be necessary. Replacement valves may be artificial (prosthetic valves) or made from animal tissue (bio-prosthetic valves). The type of replacement valve selected depends on the patient's age, condition, and the specific valve affected.

WHEN TO CALL A DOCTOR

• **EMERGENCY** Call an ambulance if you experience severe chest pain.

• Call a doctor if you develop persistent shortness of breath, palpitations, or dizziness. ▲

Varicocele

WHAT IS IT?

A varicocele is an enlarged, knotty, swollen (varicose) vein in the scrotum. Veins are the vessels that return blood to the heart after oxygen has been delivered to the body's tissues. All along the walls of the veins are valves that permit blood to flow in only one direction. Varicose veins occur when these valves become weak or defective, allowing blood to flow backward or stagnate within the vein. Varicoceles are simply varicose veins in the scrotum; they are not a serious health risk and in many cases do not require treatment. However, varicoceles may lead to infertility in some men. It is thought that the pooled blood in the engorged vein may increase testicular temperature and impair blood flow; both can inhibit sperm cell production. In such cases fertility may improve when the varicocele is surgically treated. Varicoceles are quite common, affecting about 10 percent of all men.

WHAT CAUSES IT?

• Weak or defective valves in the veins leading from the testicles may produce a varicocele.
• Infrequently, an obstruction of the vein due to a tumor or blood clot may lead to a varicocele.

PREVENTION

• There is no known way to prevent varicocele.
• Regular testicular examination aids in early diagnosis and treatment of any abnormalities (see Testicular Cancer for more on testicular examination).

DIAGNOSIS

• Testicular examination, involving gentle palpation

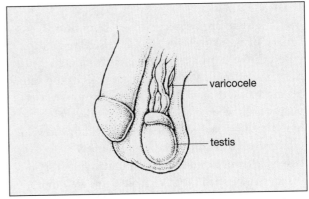

Each testis is suspended from a spermatic cord. Varicose veins along the spermatic cord produce a knotty, swollen varicocele.

of the testicles and scrotum, is performed by the doctor to determine the size and consistency of any lumps.
• A special bright light can be shined through the scrotum to aid in diagnosis; varicoceles are opaque and do not allow the light to shine through, while other abnormalities (such as a hydrocele or a spermatocele) appear translucent.
• An ultrasound examination may be performed to confirm the diagnosis.
• Seminal fluid is analyzed in infertile men.

HOW TO TREAT IT

• In many cases treatment is unnecessary.
• Wear an athletic supporter or snugly fitting briefs to provide extra support for the scrotum and to relieve pain.
• Surgery to remove the enlarged veins through a small incision in the scrotum may be performed to improve fertility. Other remaining veins compensate for the absent ones.
• An x-ray approach (angiography) can be used to block blood flow to the enlarged vein, thus sealing off the varicocele.

WHEN TO CALL A DOCTOR

• Call a doctor if you feel an unusual lump in the scrotum. While a varicocele is not a serious health risk, all such lumps should be examined by a doctor to rule out cancer.
• Call a doctor if you are concerned that a varicocele may be impairing fertility. ▲

SYMPTOMS

• Painless swelling on one side of the scrotum (almost always the left) that may disappear when lying down. The swollen area may feel like a mass of soft tubes or worms when pressed gently.
• Pain or sensation of heaviness in the scrotum during hot weather or after strenuous physical activity.

Varicose Veins

WHAT IS IT?

Varicose veins are twisted, swollen veins near the surface of the skin. Veins are the vessels that return blood to the heart after oxygen has been delivered to the body's tissues. Valves along the walls of the veins permit blood to flow in only one direction. Varicose veins occur when weak or defective valves allow blood to flow backward or stagnate within the vein. Chronic obstruction of the veins can also cause varicose veins, but in most cases no underlying abnormality can be identified. Varicose veins are quite common, though women are affected twice as often as men. Usually appearing in the legs, varicose veins may also occur in the anus, where they are known as hemorrhoids (see Hemorrhoids for more information). While not a serious health risk, varicose veins can be eliminated for cosmetic reasons or if they cause discomfort.

WHAT CAUSES IT?

• The cause of most cases is unknown.
• Chronic venous (vein) obstruction may play a role.
• Hereditary factors appear to have an effect. People of Irish or German descent are at highest risk.
• Other risk factors include pregnancy, prolonged standing or sitting, obesity, lack of exercise, and increased age.

PREVENTION

• Maintain a healthy weight and engage in regular, moderate exercise.
• Avoid standing or sitting for long periods.
• Elevate the legs above hip level periodically throughout the day. Do not cross your legs.
• Avoid tight shoes, belts, or other restrictive clothing.

SYMPTOMS

• Enlarged, swollen, knotted clusters of purple veins.
• Edema (swelling in the legs).
• Aching or a sensation of heaviness in the legs.
• Itching skin above the affected veins.
• Skin discoloration and ulcers on the inner aspect of the ankles (in advanced cases).

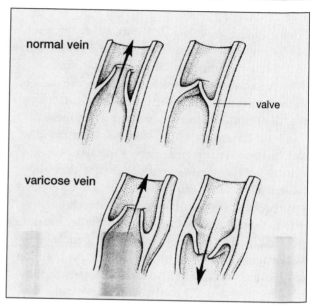

In a normal vein, valves permit blood to flow in only one direction. In a varicose vein, defective valves never fully close, allowing backflow.

DIAGNOSIS

• Diagnosis may be made by observation of veins and does not require a doctor.
• In some cases x-rays may be taken after a contrast medium is injected into the veins (venography) to highlight them.

HOW TO TREAT IT

• Follow prevention tips.
• Raise the foot of your bed from two to four inches with blocks to aid circulation at night.
• Avoid scratching itchy skin above varicose veins; this may cause ulceration or profuse bleeding.
• Special elastic support stockings that prevent blood from pooling in the veins may be recommended.
• For superficial varicose veins, sclerotherapy (injection of chemicals that harden and shrink the vein) is an option. Blood is rerouted through other veins.
• Surgical ligation (tying off) and removal (stripping) of the varicose vein is the definitive therapy in severe cases. Other veins compensate for the absent one(s).

WHEN TO CALL A DOCTOR

• Call a doctor if symptoms of varicose veins interfere with normal activities, or if you develop skin ulcers over the veins. ▲

Vitiligo

WHAT IS IT?

Vitiligo is the patchy depigmentation of skin due to loss of melanocytes in the skin. Melanocytes, located in the epidermis (the surface layer of the skin) and eyes, are cells that produce melanin, a dark pigment that gives skin its color and protects against ultraviolet radiation. People with darker skin produce more melanin than those with pale skin. In vitiligo, melanocytes are lost and white spots develop at these locations. Some people may exhibit just a few small white or depigmented patches, while others may have widespread depigmentation. The cause of vitiligo is unknown; however, it may be an autoimmune disorder, in which the body's defenses mistakenly destroy some of its own cells—in this case, melanocytes. People of any skin color may be affected, but the condition is more apparent in those with darker skin. Vitiligo is a relatively common condition that does not pose a health risk, but it may be quite psychologically distressing.

SYMPTOMS
- Irregular patches of depigmented, white skin. Patches are commonly located on the hands, face, groin, and folds of skin, and may be symmetrically distributed on the body. Patches may slowly spread to cover large areas of the body.
- White hairs within depigmented patches.

WHAT CAUSES IT?

- Vitiligo may be an autoimmune disorder. The underlying cause is unknown, but hereditary factors play a role.
- Vitiligo may be associated with other disorders such as autoimmune thyroid disease, diabetes mellitus, adrenal insufficiency, and pernicious anemia.
- Skin injury, burns, and inflammatory skin disorders may trigger the local loss of pigment in people with vitiligo.

PREVENTION

- There is no known way to prevent vitiligo.

DIAGNOSIS

- Patient history should include any exposure to caustic chemicals or solvents. (These can cause chemical leukoderma or chemical pigment destruction, which are different from vitiligo.)
- Diagnosis can usually be made solely by observation of characteristic skin changes.
- A special light (Wood's lamp) may be shined on the skin in a dark room to identify vitiliginous patches in fair-skinned patients.

HOW TO TREAT IT

- To keep skin as evenly pigmented as possible, try to avoid exposure to direct sunlight between the hours of 10 a.m. and 2 p.m. Block the sun's rays by wearing protective clothing, such as hats and long sleeves, whenever possible. Apply a sunscreen lotion that has a sun protection factor (SPF) of 30 or higher. Reapply often, especially after swimming or perspiring heavily.
- Over-the-counter cosmetic creams and dyes are available to cover depigmented areas with a color that matches your skin tone.
- Photochemotherapy (PUVA) may be used to try to stimulate skin repigmentation. PUVA is controlled exposure to ultraviolet A (UVA) light, in combination with psoralen (P), a drug that increases the skin's sensitivity to UVA wavelengths. A minimum of two sessions each week is necessary, and many sessions may be required before any improvement is seen, if it occurs at all.
- Creams containing fluorinated steroids may be prescribed to stimulate repigmentation of the skin.
- In cases of widespread vitiligo, bleaching the unaffected skin with hydroquinone to match depigmented areas may be considered.

WHEN TO CALL A DOCTOR

- Make an appointment with a doctor if you find mere cosmetic coverage of vitiliginous patches of skin to be unsatisfactory.

Von Willebrand's Disease

WHAT IS IT?

Von Willebrand's disease is the most common inherited blood coagulation disorder, caused by a deficiency in a blood clotting factor known as von Willebrand's factor. Von Willebrand's factor promotes clotting in two ways: first, it is an essential component in the mechanism that causes platelets to gather and adhere to one another at the site of an injury; second, it acts as a carrier for Factor VIII (also known as antihemophilic factor), a crucial protein in the process of clot formation. A deficiency in von Willebrand's factor thus results in uncontrolled bleeding due to inadequate platelet activity and decreased levels of active Factor VIII.

Von Willebrand's disease affects both men and women alike (unlike hemophilia, which only leads to bleeding in men; see Hemophilia for more information). The severity of symptoms varies widely—most cases are mild, with episodes of excessive bleeding presenting a risk only after surgery. Unlike hemophilia, most people with von Willebrand's disease need not limit their level of physical activity. Treatment of bleeding episodes consists of transfusions of essential clotting factors from donated blood, or administration of a medication that stimulates the release of von Willebrand's factor into the blood.

SYMPTOMS
- Easy bruising.
- Frequent nosebleeds.
- Heavy bleeding from cuts, during menstrual periods, and after surgery or tooth extraction.
- Blood in the urine or stool.
- Swollen, painful joints (uncommon compared to hemophilia).

WHAT CAUSES IT?
- A genetic deficiency of von Willebrand's factor, a clotting factor in the blood, causes von Willebrand's disease. This condition is a genetically dominant trait, meaning it can be inherited by offspring if even only one parent carries the affected gene.

PREVENTION
- There is no way to prevent von Willebrand's disease, although those with a family history of it may benefit from genetic counseling when considering having a child.

DIAGNOSIS
- Patient history (including family history) and physical examination.
- Blood tests to measure bleeding time and blood levels of von Willebrand's factor and Factor VIII.

HOW TO TREAT IT
- Do not use medications such as aspirin that promote bleeding.
- Infusions of cryoprecipitate, a product containing concentrated clotting factors rich in von Willebrand's factor and derived from donated blood, may be administered.
- Infusions of desmopressin (DDAVP), a medication that stimulates the release of von Willebrand's factor and Factor VIII from blood vessel endothelia, may be administered to stop bleeding.
- For women with a severe form of von Willebrand's disease, oral contraceptives may be prescribed to suppress unusually heavy menstrual bleeding.
- Patients may be advised to wear a medical bracelet identifying them as having a blood clotting disorder.
- Surgeons or dentists should be informed of the condition prior to surgery or tooth extraction, so that DDAVP or cryoprecipitate can be given and other precautions taken to prevent uncontrolled bleeding during and after the procedure.

WHEN TO CALL A DOCTOR
- **EMERGENCY** Call an ambulance for any episode of prolonged, uncontrolled bleeding.
- All blood relatives of someone with von Willebrand's disease may want to be tested for the disorder.

Warts

WHAT IS IT?

Warts are common, benign skin growths caused by a viral infection. Usually appearing on the hands, elbows, face, and soles of the feet, warts may also be located on the genitals (see Genital Warts for more information). Nongenital warts are harmless and only mildly contagious. There are a number of different types of warts, named for their location on the body and their appearance: common warts (verrucae vulgaris) are most often seen on the hands and fingers; plantar warts are located on the soles of the feet (see Plantar Warts); periungual warts are located around the nails of fingers and toes; digitate warts are small fingerlike projections that appear on the scalp; filiform warts are thin, threadlike projections commonly found around the face and neck; flat warts occur in groups of up to several hundred at a time. Many warts disappear spontaneously within one or two years, or they may be removed by a variety of treatments. Because the virus may be present in neighboring tissues, recurrence is common. As people grow older, however, most develop an immunity to warts.

WHAT CAUSES IT?

• Warts are caused by the human papillomavirus (HPV), of which there are more than 60 types. The virus enters the skin through tiny breaks and can be transmitted by direct physical contact with another person or, for example, through contact via a shower room floor with skin shed from a wart. For the most part, warts are only mildly contagious (with the exception of genital warts).
• People with weakened immune systems—such as those infected with the human immunodeficiency virus (HIV) or undergoing treatment with immuno-suppressant drugs following organ transplant—have a higher risk for widespread, persistent warts.
• Contrary to popular belief, you cannot get warts from handling frogs or toads. The wartlike bumps on these amphibians contain poison to protect against enemies, but are unrelated to actual warts, which are caused by a virus found only in humans.

PREVENTION

• You can use an electric razor or depilatory in lieu of a conventional razor to prevent nicks that may promote the spread of warts on the face.
• Do not scratch existing warts.

DIAGNOSIS

• Diagnosis can be made by observation of the characteristic appearance and does not require a doctor.

HOW TO TREAT IT

• In healthy people most warts (including genital warts) will heal without treatment in six months to three years, when the body develops an immune response.
• Wart removal preparations containing salicylic or lactic acid are available over the counter. Do not use these wart removal preparations to remove facial or genital warts; such preparations are too harsh for sensitive facial and genital skin.
• Warts may be removed by freezing them off with liquid nitrogen (cryosurgery), by laser surgery, or by electrocautery (burning warts off with an electric current). These treatments can be painful, may leave scars, and are not recommended for young children.
• Topical tretinoin (Retin-A), a vitamin A derivative, may be prescribed to treat flat warts.
• Your doctor may apply caustic chemical solutions such as cantharidin or trichloroacetic acid to destroy the warts.

WHEN TO CALL A DOCTOR

• Make an appointment with a doctor or dermatologist if you want warts removed; if you are over age 45 and develop warts (new or unusual skin growths should be evaluated to rule out skin cancer); or if you or your sexual partner develops genital warts. ◮

SYMPTOMS

• Bumps or lesions on the skin. Warts may be pale or dark, rough or smooth, raised or flat; appearance depends on the location of the wart and the human papillomavirus type.
• Clusters of multiple warts.
• Thin hornlike projections.
• Bleeding or itching (in some cases).

Whooping Cough Pertussis

WHAT IS IT?

Whooping cough, also known as pertussis, is a highly contagious, potentially serious, bacterial infection of the respiratory tract. Symptoms occur in three distinct stages, each lasting several weeks. The disease may affect anyone, but it is most dangerous when severe coughing interferes with breathing in children and infants; pneumonia, seizures, and encephalopathy can be serious complications in young infants. Pertussis in older children and adults results in mild symptoms such as nasal congestion and cough. Fortunately, the incidence of whooping cough has declined sharply in the United States since the introduction of the pertussis vaccine in the 1940s. The vaccine does not provide indefinite immunity, but it protects children during the ages when they are most at risk.

WHAT CAUSES IT?

• An infection with the bacterium *Bordetella pertussis* causes whooping cough.
• Whooping cough is spread through the air by the sneeze or cough of an infected person. The infection may spread easily in families, schools, and day-care centers; those living in overcrowded or unsanitary conditions are at heightened risk. Infants younger than six months and those born prematurely are also at increased risk for the disease.

SYMPTOMS

• First or catarrhal stage (resembling an ordinary cold and lasting 10 days to two weeks): nasal discharge; sneezing; mild cough; general feeling of poor health.
• Second or paroxysmal stage (lasting four to six weeks): episodes of severe coughing, sometimes followed by a characteristic "whoop" as air is inhaled sharply at the end of a coughing spasm; bulging eyes and neck veins; blue tinge to the skin during a coughing spasm due to lack of oxygen; vomiting induced by efforts to expel thick sputum; seizures (rare).
• Third or convalescent stage: coughing spasms that become milder and less frequent.

PREVENTION

• A combination vaccine that protects against diphtheria, tetanus, and pertussis, known as DTP, provides immunity from pertussis for a number of years. A new derivation of the vaccine, DTaP (acellular pertussis vaccine), is currently recommended and has fewer side effects of fever and redness at the injection site. Children should receive the DTaP vaccine at two, four, six, and 18 months of age. A DTaP booster shot is given between the ages of four and six years, just before the child starts school.
• A 14-day course of preventive antibiotics may be administered to household members or schoolmates if a child develops whooping cough. Children under seven years of age who are unimmunized or have received fewer than four doses of DTP or DTaP vaccine may be given a booster shot; younger children should be continued on their regular vaccination schedule.

DIAGNOSIS

• Patient history and physical examination during the paroxysmal stage usually establishes the diagnosis.
• Throat culture.
• Chest x-ray if pneumonia is suspected.

HOW TO TREAT IT

• Treatment with antibiotics during the first stage may limit or prevent more severe symptoms. Antibiotics administered during the second stage do not alter the course of the infection but can reduce the degree of contagion. Fourteen days of antibiotic therapy is recommended.
• Supportive care is aimed at making the patient as comfortable as possible. Plenty of fluids and frequent small meals are recommended.
• Hospitalization in an isolation room may be necessary for infants, especially those younger than six months of age. Oxygen and intravenous fluids and nutrients may be administered.

WHEN TO CALL A DOCTOR

• Call a doctor if a child's cold persists or worsens.
• **EMERGENCY** Call an ambulance if a child turns blue or stops breathing. ⚠

Wilson's Disease

WHAT IS IT?

Wilson's disease is a rare inherited disorder marked by a defect in the body's ability to excrete copper. Consequently, excess copper accumulates in body tissues—primarily the liver and brain—causing organ damage and a myriad of possible symptoms and complications. The disorder is present from birth, but symptoms are rare before age six. Half of those affected remain asymptomatic through adolescence, and in rare cases the disease will not be apparent until adulthood.

Treatment is essential whether or not symptoms are present. Untreated Wilson's disease can lead to hepatitis, cirrhosis, and brain damage, often before age 20, and is ultimately fatal. Early detection and treatment of Wilson's disease can prevent symptoms and complications entirely. Children whose siblings or parents have the disease should be tested at birth. With lifelong treatment, prognosis is excellent.

SYMPTOMS

- Fatigue, weakness, loss of appetite, and jaundice, resembling viral hepatitis.
- Muscle rigidity, spasms, and tremors.
- Walking difficulty.
- Swallowing difficulty; drooling.
- Progressive intellectual impairment; speech difficulties; psychological deterioration; personality changes; bizarre behavior.
- In advanced stages, symptoms due to chronic active hepatitis or cirrhosis, including swelling and fluid accumulation in the abdomen and vomiting of blood (see Hepatitis, Acute, and Cirrhosis for more information).
- Lightheadedness; paleness (pallor); heart palpitations, chest pain, or shortness of breath on exertion (due to associated anemia).
- Cessation of menstruation (amenorrhea).

WHAT CAUSES IT?

- A recently discovered genetic defect prevents the normal excretion of copper in the bile and leads to excess storage of copper.

PREVENTION

- There is no way to prevent Wilson's disease, but a family history of the disorder warrants diagnostic testing so that symptoms and complications may be prevented by early detection and treatment.

DIAGNOSIS

- Patient and family history; physical examination.
- Blood tests show low levels of the copper-carrying protein ceruloplasmin, as well as anemia.
- Urine tests may show increased levels of copper.
- Diagnosis is confirmed by a liver biopsy (removal of a small sample of liver tissue) showing excessive levels of copper.
- Detection of a Kayser-Fleischer ring—a green or golden deposit of copper in the cornea—may require a special examination by an ophthalmologist.

HOW TO TREAT IT

- Treatment with penicillamine, a medication that binds copper, removes copper from the body by increasing its excretion in the urine. In about 10 percent of patients, allergy to penicillamine develops, occasionally requiring the administration of prednisone. In some cases trientine or zinc acetate may be prescribed instead of penicillamine.
- Because penicillamine counteracts vitamin B_6 (pyridoxine), supplements of pyridoxine are given to avoid damage to the nervous system.
- Intake of foods high in dietary copper—including mushrooms, nuts, dried fruit, liver, shellfish, and chocolate—may be restricted.
- Regular lifelong checkups are necessary to detect for side effects of the medication and to monitor the effectiveness of therapy by measuring copper levels in the urine.
- In advanced cases where cirrhosis of the liver is extensive, a liver transplant may be advised.

WHEN TO CALL A DOCTOR

- Call a doctor if you or your child develops tremors, psychological changes, fatigue, or jaundice, especially if there is a family history of Wilson's disease.

Index

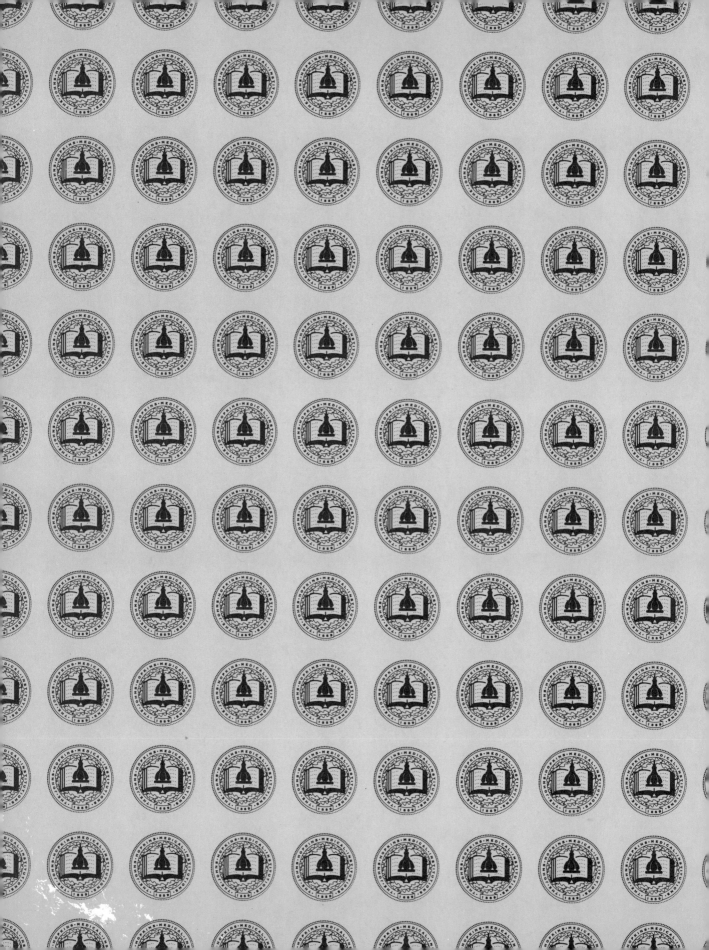